Axonal Regeneration in the Central Nervous System

NEUROLOGICAL DISEASE AND THERAPY

Advisory Board

1. Handbook of Parkinson's Disease, *edited by William C. Koller*
2. Medical Therapy of Acute Stroke, *edited by Mark Fisher*
3. Familial Alzheimer's Disease: Molecular Genetics and Clinical Perspectives, *edited by Gary D. Miner, Ralph W. Richter, John P. Blass, Jimmie L. Valentine, and Linda A. Winters-Miner*
4. Alzheimer's Disease: Treatment and Long-Term Management, *edited by Jeffrey L. Cummings and Bruce L. Miller*
5. Therapy of Parkinson's Disease, *edited by William C. Koller and George Paulson*
6. Handbook of Sleep Disorders, *edited by Michael J. Thorpy*
7. Epilepsy and Sudden Death, *edited by Claire M. Lathers and Paul L. Schraeder*
8. Handbook of Multiple Sclerosis, *edited by Stuart D. Cook*
9. Memory Disorders: Research and Clinical Practice, *edited by Takehiko Yanagihara and Ronald C. Petersen*
10. The Medical Treatment of Epilepsy, *edited by Stanley R. Resor, Jr., and Henn Kutt*
11. Cognitive Disorders: Pathophysiology and Treatment, *edited by Leon J. Thal, Walter H. Moos, and Elkan R. Gamzu*

12. Handbook of Amyotrophic Lateral Sclerosis, *edited by Richard Alan Smith*
13. Handbook of Parkinson's Disease: Second Edition, Revised and Expanded, *edited by William C. Koller*
14. Handbook of Pediatric Epilepsy, *edited by Jerome V. Murphy and Fereydoun Dehkharghani*
15. Handbook of Tourette's Syndrome and Related Tic and Behavioral Disorders, *edited by Roger Kurlan*
16. Handbook of Cerebellar Diseases, *edited by Richard Lechtenberg*
17. Handbook of Cerebrovascular Diseases, *edited by Harold P. Adams, Jr.*
18. Parkinsonian Syndromes, *edited by Matthew B. Stern and William C. Koller*
19. Handbook of Head and Spine Trauma, *edited by Jonathan Greenberg*
20. Brain Tumors: A Comprehensive Text, *edited by Robert A. Morantz and John W. Walsh*
21. Monoamine Oxidase Inhibitors in Neurological Diseases, *edited by Abraham Lieberman, C. Warren Olanow, Moussa B. H. Youdim, and Keith Tipton*
22. Handbook of Dementing Illnesses, *edited by John C. Morris*
23. Handbook of Myasthenia Gravis and Myasthenic Syndromes, *edited by Robert P. Lisak*
24. Handbook of Neurorehabilitation, *edited by David C. Good and James R. Couch, Jr.*
25. Therapy with Botulinum Toxin, *edited by Joseph Jankovic and Mark Hallett*
26. Principles of Neurotoxicology, *edited by Louis W. Chang*
27. Handbook of Neurovirology, *edited by Robert R. McKendall and William G. Stroop*
28. Handbook of Neuro-Urology, *edited by David N. Rushton*
29. Handbook of Neuroepidemiology, *edited by Philip B. Gorelick and Milton Alter*
30. Handbook of Tremor Disorders, *edited by Leslie J. Findley and William C. Koller*
31. Neuro-Ophthalmological Disorders: Diagnostic Work-Up and Management, *edited by Ronald J. Tusa and Steven A. Newman*
32. Handbook of Olfaction and Gustation, *edited by Richard L. Doty*
33. Handbook of Neurological Speech and Language Disorders, *edited by Howard S. Kirshner*
34. Therapy of Parkinson's Disease: Second Edition, Revised and Expanded, *edited by William C. Koller and George Paulson*
35. Evaluation and Management of Gait Disorders, *edited by Barney S. Spivack*
36. Handbook of Neurotoxicology, *edited by Louis W. Chang and Robert S. Dyer*
37. Neurological Complications of Cancer, *edited by Ronald G. Wiley*
38. Handbook of Autonomic Nervous System Dysfunction, *edited by Amos D. Korczyn*

39. Handbook of Dystonia, *edited by Joseph King Ching Tsui and Donald B. Calne*
40. Etiology of Parkinson's Disease, *edited by Jonas H. Ellenberg, William C. Koller, and J. William Langston*
41. Practical Neurology of the Elderly, *edited by Jacob I. Sage and Margery H. Mark*
42. Handbook of Muscle Disease, *edited by Russell J. M. Lane*
43. Handbook of Multiple Sclerosis: Second Edition, Revised and Expanded, *edited by Stuart D. Cook*
44. Central Nervous System Infectious Diseases and Therapy, *edited by Karen L. Roos*
45. Subarachnoid Hemorrhage: Clinical Management, *edited by Takehiko Yanagihara, David G. Piepgras, and John L. D. Atkinson*
46. Neurology Practice Guidelines, *edited by Richard Lechtenberg and Henry S. Schutta*
47. Spinal Cord Diseases: Diagnosis and Treatment, *edited by Gordon L. Engler, Jonathan Cole, and W. Louis Merton*
48. Management of Acute Stroke, *edited by Ashfaq Shuaib and Larry B. Goldstein*
49. Sleep Disorders and Neurological Disease, *edited by Antonio Culebras*
50. Handbook of Ataxia Disorders, *edited by Thomas Klockgether*
51. The Autonomic Nervous System in Health and Disease, *David S. Goldstein*
52. Axonal Regeneration in the Central Nervous System, *edited by Nicholas A. Ingoglia and Marion Murray*

Additional Volumes in Preparation

Handbook of Multiple Sclerosis: Third Edition, *edited by Stuart D. Cook*

Axonal Regeneration in the Central Nervous System

edited by

Nicholas A. Ingoglia
New Jersey Medical School–UMDNJ
Newark, New Jersey

Marion Murray
Medical College of Pennsylvania/Hahnemann University
Philadelphia, Pennsylvania

MARCEL DEKKER, INC. NEW YORK • BASEL

ISBN: 0-8247-0410-X

This book is printed on acid-free paper.

Headquarters
Marcel Dekker, Inc.
270 Madison Avenue, New York, NY 10016
tel: 212-696-9000; fax: 212-685-4540

Eastern Hemisphere Distribution
Marcel Dekker AG
Hutgasse 4, Postfach 812, CH-4001 Basel, Switzerland
tel: 41-61-261-8482; fax: 41-61-261-8896

World Wide Web
http://www.dekker.com

The publisher offers discounts on this book when ordered in bulk quantities. For more information, write to Special Sales/Professional Marketing at the headquarters address above.

Current printing (last digit):
10 9 8 7 6 5 4 3 2 1

PRINTED IN THE UNITED STATES OF AMERICA

AUTHOR'S NOTE

The work described in these chapters summarizes the current state of research into regeneration of axons in the Central Nervous System of vertebrates. We need to remember that these advances are the result of basic scientific research carried out by dedicated scientists in all fields of biology, even those apparently distant from the issues of regeneration research. The remarkable developments in this research give hope that greatly improved treatments for brain and spinal cord injuries will soon be available. Indeed this work has also been stimulated by the appreciation that we have for those who suffer from the devastating consequences of brain and spinal injury and for their families. We would like to dedicate this volume to those individuals - to the famous, such as Christopher Reeve, whose unstinting efforts to raise awareness of the emotional, physical and monetary costs of spinal injury have been so important to the recent advancement of the research efforts, and to the less famous, such as Adam Shapiro, a boy struggling to recover and rebuild a life after his spinal injury, who has reminded us of the courage, the hope, and effort and ultimately the optimism that this requires and who recently sent us this note:

Hi. My name is Adam Shapiro and I am 15 years old. In September of 1996 I broke my neck (C3-C4) leaving me an incomplete quadriplegic. My mom and I check the Internet every day to see if there is any new information on spinal cord nerve regeneration. I have come a long way. I started off on a ventilator, and could not move anything. It took me three months to get off the ventilator, and that is when I started conditioning my body. At this time I am able to walk with a walker, but my arms are considerably weaker than my legs.. If you could please e-mail me back, I am very anxious to get involved in new treatments that you are conducting now on humans, I would greatly appreciate it, or if not please keep me in mind in the future. Thank you so much for your time…

Finally, on a more personal note, we would like to dedicate this volume to our friend, our teacher, our mentor and our colleague, Bernice Grafstein, who led us into this field and so changed our scientific lives.

PREFACE

One of the most fundamental questions in neuroscience is why certain neurons respond to axotomy by robustly regrowing a new axon while others do not. This basic difference between neurons in lower vertebrates and mammalian peripheral nerves on the one hand, and nerves found in the central nervous system (CNS) of mammals on the other, has been the launching pad for the experimental lives of countless former and current researchers and in many cases has led to lifelong commitments to try to understand this elemental fact of neural life. What is perhaps most vexing about our inability to understand the reasons why mammalian central neurons fail to regenerate following injury is the enormous impact this has on the human condition. Each year thousands of patients become victims of brain or spinal cord injuries resulting in varying degrees of cognitive loss or paralysis. Once these neurons have been severed they are not likely to recover. To these patients we can, at present, offer little in the way of treatment. But we offer much in the way of hope. The hope springs from the enormous progress that has been made in the past 30 or so years in understanding the molecular and cellular events occurring in systems that are successful in regenerating new axons and, more recently, in the analysis of mammalian central neurons where abortive regeneration and cell death are still the general consequences of axotomy but where there is now clear evidence for regrowth following certain experimental interventions.

Our view of the scientific problem, and thus our approach to solving it, has been shaped in large part by the studies of Santiago Ramon y Cajal (1928) who wrote in the early part of this century: *"My observations, made in the optic nerve and spinal cord...demonstrated also that the incapability of regeneration is not a fatally irresistible law, but is a secondary outcome of a physical or chemical environment unfavorable for the growth of the sprouts...."* These observations focused our thoughts and research strategies on the glial barriers ("scars") to nerve growth. But we know today that, while an impenetrable barrier (or inhibitory proteins on the membranes of cells in the region of the injury) is likely to play an important role in the failure of a neuron to grow a new axon, other factors such as cell survival, the genetic growth program of the damaged neuron, the response of neurons to growth and guidance factors and, perhaps, the failure of a cut axon to reseal may all play roles in the successful regrowth of a new axon. As was true for Cajal, modern researchers have generally favored the optic nerve and spinal cord as models to study the issue of axonal regeneration and recovery of function, and the contributions in this volume largely reflect those models. We believe, however, that the lessons learned from the optic nerve and spinal cord are generalizable to other parts of the CNS.

The goal of this book is to summarize some of the major research contributions in nerve regeneration reported over the past 30 years and then show how these discoveries have led to the current strategies to promote axonal regeneration in the mammalian CNS. Part I deals with reviews of studies primarily in the visual system of lower vertebrates where axotomy has been shown to result in nerve regeneration, functional recovery and remarkable fidelity in the re-establishment of synaptic connections. These studies were stimulated by the pioneering work of Roger Sperry and provide a backdrop against which to view efforts to stimulate regeneration in the CNS of mammals.

In Part II, the correlation between developmental age and the ability of nerves to regenerate is addressed. Cut axons can regenerate in early stages of embryonic development and regenerating axons can penetrate glial scars in embryos. But at some point, that ability is lost. What changes? What are the environmental developments that prevent nerve growth?

In Part III, the most extensive section of the book, the response of mammalian neurons to axotomy is examined at the cell body, at the site of injury, and in the distal nerve segment where new growth will occur. The questions of why some neurons die following injury, and specifically what induces apoptosis following axotomy, are addressed. Also, the genomic response to axotomy is reviewed, with a description of the genes transcribed in successfully regenerating neurons and a comparison with those transcribed in neurons incapable of regrowth. The consequences of that transcription, those proteins that are selectively or preferentially synthesized, are also presented. Perhaps one of the most neglected areas of research in this field is the response at the site of nerve injury. Here, early inflammatory cell and glial responses to injury as well as the resealing of cut axons, reactions that are critical in preventing neuronal cell death, are reviewed. The distal nerve segment (undergoing Wallerian degeneration in the initial period after axotomy and supporting axon elongation, if it occurs, in the latter stage) must form a permissive and supporting environment for growing axons if successful regeneration is to occur. Contributions in this section range from a description of the genes induced in glia/Schwann cells following axotomy and during regeneration and the way in which growing axons might induce the expression of those genes. The final topic in this section is a description of the factors (both positive and negative) that influence axonal elongation.

Theoretically, factors that stimulate axonal growth (and/or neutralize those molecules that block neurite extension) could be used to promote regeneration following axotomy in the CNS and experiments describing these approaches are presented in Part IV.

In these chapters, contributors report on their attempts to promote regeneration in the CNS by using one or a combination of techniques dictated primarily by the results of basic studies described in earlier chapters. Thus, protecting a cell from apoptosis following axotomy must be a prime objective of any therapeutic interventional strategy and is dealt with in the opening chapter. A hospitable terrain (such as the one made by Schwann cells in the PNS) must also be created, and several chapters are devoted to the use of peripheral nerve, olfactory ensheathing cells, and fetal cell transplants to create an environment that can support regeneration. Neurotrophic agents can protect cells from apoptosis following axotomy and may also stimulate axonal outgrowth; successes and failures using these agents are reviewed. The use of antibodies to myelin inhibitory proteins has led to successful regrowth of fibers in the spinal cord of rats, with some functional recovery. In one of the most recent approaches to effecting regeneration of cut axons, gene therapy is being used to deliver trophic and survival factors to injured neurons. In the penultimate chapter in this section, initial results from studies in which fetal CNS tissue has been applied to injured human spinal cord are described. Finally, a review of the obstacles to regeneration faced by an injured CNS neuron and a description of the experiments that have attempted to overcome them are presented, followed by therapeutic recommendations in what may be our best hope at encouraging significant regeneration following CNS damage.

In the last part, called "*Perspective,*" a senior researcher gives a personal view of the maturation of the field and discusses where best to focus future studies in our attempt to restore function following injury or diseases of the central nervous system.

This book will serve as an important resource for all basic neuroscientists, especially those interested in the growth and regeneration of neurons. In addition, this volume should be a critical reference for clinical neurologists, neurosurgeons, orthopedic surgeons, physiatrists and physical therapists, who will find the contents informative and useful in their understanding of the problem of nerve repair. Finally, it is hoped that this book will be read by molecular and cellular biologists who may know little about the nervous system, but who share our concern for the fundamental question being asked and for the human consequences of our inability to answer it. And perhaps upon reading a passage, one of these scientists will assemble some pieces of the puzzle and make a connection that has thus far eluded the rest of us, put the book down for a moment and say, "Wait! I have an idea… ."

Nicholas A. Ingoglia and Marion Murray

CONTENTS

PART V. PERSPECTIVE

CONTRIBUTORS

Anderson, Douglas K., Ph.D. Department of Neuroscience, University of Florida Brain Institute, Gainesville, Florida
email: anderson@ufbi.ufl.edu

Bähr, Mathias, Ph.D. Neurologische University of Tübingen, Germany
email: mathias.baehr@uni-tuebingen.de

Beazley, Lynda D., Ph.D. Department of Zoology, University of Western Australia, Nedlands, Australia
email: lynb@cyllene.uwa.edu.au

Benowitz, Larry I., Ph.D. Department of Neurosurgery, Children's Hospital, Harvard Medical School, Boston, Massachusetts
email: benowitz@a1.tch.harvard.edu

Bittner, George D., Ph.D. Department of Zoology, University of Texas, Austin,Texas
email:bittner@mail.utex

Bunge, Mary B., Ph.D. The Miami Project, University of Miami School of Medicine, Rm 1044, Miami, Florida
email: mbunge@miamiproj.med.miami.edu

Chaudhary, P., Ph.D. Department of Neurosurgery, Oregon Health Sciences University, Portland, Oregon
email: Priya_chaudary@yahoo.com

David, Samuel, Ph.D. Centre for Research in Neuroscience, The Montreal General Hospital Research Institute and McGill University, Montreal, Quebec, Canada
email: mcsl@musica.mcgill.ca

Fawcett, James W., Ph.D. Department of Physiology, Cambridge University-Physiology Laboratory Cambridge, England
email: JF108@CAM.AC.UK

Fernandes, Karl J. L., Ph.D. CORD (Collaboration On Repair Discoveries) University of British Columbia, Vancouver, Canada
email: fernande@cord.ubc.ca

Fessler, Richard G. M.D., Ph.D. Department of Neurosurgery, University of Florida, Gainesville, Florida

Fischer, Itzhak, Ph.D. Department of Neurobiology & Anatomy, MCP Hahnemann University, Philadelphia, Pennsylvania
email: Itzhak.Fischer@drexel.edu

Fishman, Harvey M. Ph.D. Department of Physiology & Biophysics, University of Texas Medical Branch, Galveston, Texas
email: hfishman@utmb.edu

Gillen, Clemens, Ph.D. Department of Molecular Pharmacology, Gruenenthal GmbH Aachen, Germany
email: clemens.gillen@popmail.oche.de

Grafstein, Bernice, Ph.D. Department of Physiology and Biophysics, Joan and Sanford I. Weill Medical College of Cornell University, New York, New York
email: bgraf@med.cornell.edu

Grumet, Martin, Ph.D. W. M. Keck Center for Collaborative Neuroscience, Department of Cell Biology and Neuroscience, Rutgers State University of New Jersey, Piscataway, New Jersey
email: mgrumet@rci.rutgers.edu

Himes, B. Timothy, Ph.D. Department of Neurobiology & Anatomy, MCP Hahnemann University, Philadelphia, Pennsylvania
email: bthimes@drexel.edu

Hirsch, S. Department of Neurology,University of Tübingen, Tübingen, Germany

Ingoglia, Nicholas A. Ph.D. Departments of Pharmacology/Physiology and Neuroscience, New Jersey Medical School–UMDNJ, Newark, New Jersey
email: ingoglia@umdnj.edu

Irwin, Nina A. Ph.D. Department of Neurosurgery, Children's Hospital Harvard Medical School, Boston, Massachusetts
email: irwin_c@a1.tch.harvard.edu

Jing, Y. M.D. Department of Neurology, Beijing Tong Ren Hospital, Capital University of Medical Sciences, Beijing, China

Kreutzberg, Georg W. M.D. Department of Neuromorphology, Max Planck Institute Psychiatry, Planegg-Martinsried, Germany

Leon, Steven M.D. Neurosurgery, Children's Hospital and Brigham and Women's Hospital Boston, Massachusetts

Leppert, C. Department of Biology Univ Konstanz, Konstanz, Germany

Liu, Y., Ph.D. Department of Neurobiology & Anatomy, MCP Hahnemann University, Philadelphia, Pennsylvania

Mannion, Richard, Anaesthesia - Neural Plasticity Research Group, Massachusetts General Hospital, Charlestown, Massachusetts
email: mannion@helix.mgh.harvard.edu

McKerracher, Lisa J., Ph.D. Department of Pathology, University of Montreal Faculty of Medicine, Montreal, Quebec, Canada
email: mckerral@ere.umontreal.ca

Murray, Marion, Ph.D. Department of Neurobiology & Anatomy, MCP Hahnemann University, Philadelphia, Pennsylvania
email: murray@drexel.edu

Nachman-Clewner, Michele, Ph.D. Department of Neuroscience, New Jersey Medical School –UMDNJ, Newark, New Jersey

Plant, Giles W. Ph.D. CTEC and Department of Anatomy and Human Biology Nedlands, Western Australia
email: gplant@anhb.uwa.edu.au

Raisman, Geoffrey, M.D., Ph.D. The Norman and Sadie Lee Research Centre, Division of Neurobiology, National Institute for Medical Research, The Ridgeway, London, UK
email: graisma@nimr.mrc.ac.uk

Raivich, Gennadij, Ph.D. Department of Neuromorphology, Max-Planck Institute Psychiatry, Planegg-Martinsried, Germany
email: raivich@neuro.mpg.de

Ramón-Cueto, Almudena, M.D. Ph.D. Ctr Molec Biol-Severo Ochoa, Fac De Ciencias, Univ. Autonoma De Madrid Canto Blanco, Madrid, Spain
email:aramon@cbm.uam.es

Reier, Paul J. Ph.D. Department of Neurological Surgery, University of Florida College of Medicine, JHM Health Center, Gainesville, Florida
email: reier@ufbi.ufl.edu

Schwab, Martin E, Ph.D. Department of Neuromorphology, University of Zurich & Swiss Federal Institute of Technology, Zurich, Brain Research Institute, Zurich, Switzerland
email: schwab@hifo.unizh.ch

Sharma, Sansar C. Ph.D. Department of Ophthalmology, New York Medical College, Valhalla, New York
email: Sharma@nymc.edu

So, Kwok-Fai, Ph.D. Department of Anatomy, Faculty of Medicine, University of Hong Kong, Hong Kong, China
email: hrmaskf@hkucc.hku.hk

Steeves, John D. Ph.D. CORD (Collaboration On Repair Discoveries) University of British Columbia, Vancouver, Canada
email: STEEVES@cord.ubc.ca

Stuermer, Claudia A. O. Ph.D. Department of Biology, University of Konstanz, Konstanz, Germany
email: claudia.stuermer@uni-konstanz.de

Tabibiazar, R. M.D. Department of Medicine, Stanford University School of Medicine, Palo Alto, California

Tessler, Alan R. M.D. Department of Neurobiology and Anatomy, MCP Hahnemann University, Philadelphia, Pennsylvania
email: atessler@drexel.edu

Tetzlaff, Wolfram G, M.D. Ph.D. CORD (Collaboration On Repair Discoveries) Departments of Zoology and Surgery, University of British Columbia, Vancouver, Canada
email: tetzlaff@cord.ubc.ca

Thoenen, Hans, M.D. Department of Neurobiochemistry, Max-Planck Institute of Neurobiology, Planegg-Martinsried, Germany
email: ashdown@neuro.mpg.de

Thompson, Floyd J. Ph.D. Department of Neuroscience, University of Florida College of Medicine, Health Science Center, Gainesville, Florida
email: thompson@ufbi.ufl.edu

Townes-Anderson, Ellen S. Ph.D. Department of Neuroscience, New Jersey Medical School–UMDNJ, Newark, New Jersey
email: andersel@umdnj.edu

Wirth, Edward D. III, M.D. Ph.D. Department of Neuroscience, University of Florida, Gainesville, Florida
email: wirth@ufbi.ufl.edu

Woolf, Clifford J. M.D., Ph.D. Anesthesia-Neural Plasticity Research Group, Massachusetts General Hospital, Charlestown, Massachusetts
email: woolf.clifford@mgh.harvard.edu

Yip, Henry, Ph.D. Department of Anatomy, Faculty of Medicine, University of Hong Kong, Hong Kong, China
Email: hkfyip@hkusua.hku.hk

Zhang, Nan, Ph.D. Department of Neuroscience, New Jersey Medical School–UMDNJ, Newark, New Jersey
email: zhangn@umdnj.edu

Foreword

HALF A CENTURY OF REGENERATION RESEARCH

Bernice Grafstein

Department of Physiology and Biophysics, Joan and Sanford I. Weill Medical College of Cornell University, New York, New York

"I feel convinced that the time is propitious for a professionally calculated risk in research on central nervous regeneration, for, though the path is beset with many insurmountably appearing difficulties, yet the stakes are high, and they are human."

(Pearce Bailey, 1955)

"From the controversial to the self-evident is a very small step."

(Paul A. Weiss, personal communication, ca. 1968)

I. INTRODUCTION

In medical science there is always a tension between following the search for knowledge, wherever it may lead, and the need to find the cure for a particular disease. This is especially true in the field of central nervous system regeneration: the wayward pursuit of the mysteries of growth and repair in the most complex organ of the body is balanced by the exigency of alleviating the suffering that is produced when it is injured.

Awareness of this suffering, particularly the suffering produced by spinal cord injury, has increased notably since World War II (Bailey, 1955). At that time, the introduction of antibiotics, together with advances in nursing care and rehabilitation (the outstanding names in this field are those of Sir Ludwig Guttmann in England and Howard Rusk in the U.S.A.), enormously increased the likelihood of survival from spinal cord injuries. This gave great impetus to a resurgence of interest in regeneration research, leading to a half century of remarkable progress and increasing optimism about our prospects of devising meaningful interventions in this area. Thus, in seeking a perspective on our accomplishments, it is valuable to focus on what has happened in this period, rather than, as is more usual, to look back to the prescient writings of our 19th century predecessors[1].

Contemplating the changes that have occurred in this half-century, we can identify the scientific contributions that have been made by a number of important figures, and how their ideas have led to alterations in our thinking about the nature of the neuronal response to injury, about what factors regulate regeneration, and about what interventions can be used to promote regeneration. Important as this may be, however, it is only part of the story. Conspicuous changes have also occurred in the ways that information is disseminated and exchanged among regeneration-research scientists. This may be one consequence of the increase in our numbers, which may be proportionately even greater than the staggering increase in the number of scientists that have entered the field of neuroscience overall. Another striking change has been the increase in the resources devoted to research on regeneration. Increased funding from Federal sources has been at least partly the result of efforts by scientists to raise the awareness of legislators about the economic and emotional costs of central nervous system trauma. It also reflects the concerted efforts of many members of the lay public, operating through voluntary health agencies, particularly those concerned with spinal cord injury, who have been effective not only on the Federal level, but also, to a remarkable degree recently, at the level of State government. These are the three principal themes of this chapter – how our thinking has evolved, how our scientific community has evolved, and how our relationship with the spinal cord injury community has evolved. In all of these, however, I can only give snapshots, based on my own experience in regeneration research and my acquaintance with some of the people involved.

II. HALF A CENTURY OF IDEAS ABOUT REGENERATION

A convenient point of departure for a "then-and-now" overview is the book "Central Nervous System Regeneration", edited by William F. Windle (1955)[2]. This volume contains papers by some of the scientists whom we now recognize as

[1] This may be my rationalization for limiting this overview to the period of my own experience. Reconstructing historical events is always a difficult task – the artifacts that remain for posterity to unearth represent only a small and haphazard sample of the temporal unfolding of events, and the record is further distorted by the self-interest, wishful thinking and faulty recollection of the record-keepers. Necessary information about the social and intellectual context of the time is usually deficient. This article undoubtedly suffers from some of the same limitations.

[2] The book was the product of a meeting in May, 1954, convened by the National Institute of Neurological Diseases and Blindness, at that time directed by Dr. Pearce Bailey, when Dr. Windle was Chief of the Laboratory of Neuroanatomical Sciences.

II. HALF A CENTURY OF COMMUNICATION AMONG REGENERATION SCIENTISTS

Windle's book of 1955 also presents an interesting starting point for considering the changes that have occurred during this half-century with respect to opportunities for essential exchanges of scientific information and for initiating collaborations among scientists with common interests. Small invitational meetings of the kind that this book was based on have been a very effective means of promoting these interactions, and in fact a significant part of Windle's scientific legacy was a series of conferences that he subsequently initiated that brought together outstanding workers in regeneration research. The first of these took place in Palm Beach, Florida in 1970 (Guth and Windle, 1970), and they continued at approximately 2-year intervals for more than a decade (see Veraa and Mendell, 1986). These conferences were effective not only because they were the venue for the presentation of new findings relevant to nervous system regeneration, but also because they focused attention of the participating scientists on the underlying concern for improving the well-being of patients with spinal cord injuries. Although only a fraction of the presentations dealt directly with central nervous system injury, the participants were exposed to many notable advances in related fields that emphasized functional and morphological plasticity, especially nervous system development on the cellular and molecular level[16].

The Florida conferences were each limited to the relatively small number of invited participants, but their influence is likely to have been much broader, since they were the model for an increasing number of meetings, in both the USA and abroad, featuring nervous system regeneration and development[17]. A notable development was the establishment by the U.S. Veterans Administration of the Office of Regeneration Research Programs, directed by Frederick Seil. This led to a series of conferences at the Asilomar Conference Center in California, beginning in 1985, which were open to all interested scientists and featured not only invited presentations but poster sessions for voluntary contributions, thus extending their reach to a many-fold larger number of investigators involved in regeneration research.

And there is no question that this number is continually expanding. In addition to specialized symposia in many international locales, an increasing number

---

[16] Important advances in research related to nervous system regeneration were also the subject of some of the symposia organized by the Neurosciences Research Program, which was founded by Francis O. Schmitt in the early 1960's and subsequently directed by Gerald Edelman. Although attendance at these symposia was by invitation only, summaries of the presentations were published in the Neurosciences Research Program Bulletin, which provided for rapid dissemination of important new findings in many cutting-edge areas of neuroscience.

[17] Evidence of this is the dedication to Windle of the proceedings of one such meeting (Haber et al., 1963)

of papers dealing with nervous system regeneration on every level are being given at the meetings of the Society for Neuroscience (the membership of which has now grown to about 30,000 from an initial 600-700 in 1971). A Neurotrauma Society and an International Society for Neurotrauma have been established, and are the sponsors of the Journal of Neurotrauma, which is an important site for publication of papers on regeneration research, although by no means the only one. Indeed, a major outlet for such work is the journal Experimental Neurology, which was founded by William Windle in 1959, and still retains its high impact in the field, yet another tribute to Windle's dedication and foresight.

III. HALF A CENTURY OF FOCUS ON THE CLINICAL IMPORTANCE OF REGENERATION RESEARCH

Here again we have to pay homage to William Windle's leadership. Although he had escaped getting a medical degree in his youth, he was always mindful of the clinical relevance of his research (Clemente, 1985). He was disappointed that the meeting he had so perspicaciously organized in 1954 had little effect in stimulating scientific interest and support (Windle, 1981). It was not until 15 years later that a new opportunity to recruit scientists to the cause of regeneration research presented itself. That was when Alan Reich, himself a paraplegic, who was then president of the National Paraplegia Foundation, induced Windle to organize a conference to reconsider what might be done towards a cure for spinal cord injury. That conference in Florida in 1970 was attended by a number of spinal cord injury victims and their family members as well as scientists and clinicians. The outcome was the declaration that the enigma of regeneration in the central nervous system was soluble, and that the path toward the solution was clear, based on exciting new findings in many areas of basic research, which redefined how the problem might be approached (Guth and Windle, 1970). As we know, it was to be the first in a series of such conferences, which were strongly supported by lay interest groups and individual donors concerned with the consequences of spinal cord injury[18].

What was especially remarkable about that conference in 1970 for many of the scientists attending it was that it was the first occasion for them to have direct contact with people with spinal cord injuries. This aroused a sense of urgency about the necessity of pushing progress in the field, independent of the scientific priorities. It also energized the efforts of the patients and concerned lay people. A number of such voluntary groups subsequently materialized, anxious to attract scientists to the problem of spinal cord injury, and determined to raise funds to facilitate their research. An important and lasting outcome of the efforts of some of the lay interest groups was their funding of research projects and fellowships

---

[18] This was in addition to core support from a number of government agencies, including, at various times, the NIH, the U.S. Veterans Administration, and the Social Rehabilitation Service of the Department of Health, Education and Welfare.

for young investigators, such as the programs that are currently sponsored by the Spinal Cord Research Foundation of the Paralyzed Veterans of America, by the Eastern Paralyzed Veterans Association, and by the Christopher Reeve Paralysis Foundation[19]. Support from a lay group made it possible to develop an important experimental tool – objective criteria for assessing recovery from spinal cord injury by behavioral methods (Goldberger et al., 1990). One major fund-raising effort resulted in the establishment of The Miami Project to Cure Paralysis, which is a separate institute at the University of Miami School of Medicine that brings together basic scientists and clinical specialists from various disciplines to conduct research and develop treatments for the sequelae of spinal cord injury. Another consequence of the conferences that Windle organized was the establishment of a prominent prize, the Wakeman Award for Research in the Neurosciences, which continues to be bestowed by Duke University.

Lay interest groups have played an especially important role in raising public awareness about the problem of spinal cord injury, including political lobbying for increased support for regeneration research[20]. At least partly in response to these efforts the U.S. Congress identified spinal cord injury as a special area of concern to which Federal funding should preferentially be directed [21]. An even more dramatic result has been the response of various State governments, including Florida, Kentucky and Virginia, and more recently New York and New Jersey (and California expected soon), in making appropriations available for regeneration research. For example, lobbying by lay people has been directly credited with eliciting an appropriation of several million dollars for the newly established New York State Spinal Cord Injury Research Board, with a mandate to "solicit, identify and support meritorious research targeting spinal cord injury and its devastating effects."

These advances in the understanding of research on spinal cord injury and the importance of support for such research have come at a time of increasing public awareness of the momentousness of nervous system disease and the efforts of scientists and clinicians to find means to deal with it. When Congress desig-

---

[19] I can name here only some of the major groups that have been involved in this effort. There are many others, not only in the U.S.A., but also in Canada and England, and other countries in Europe.

[20] The prominent actor Christopher Reeve, who suffered a spinal cord injury a few years ago, has been determinedly making great efforts to give visibility to the problems of living with this disability, and the urgency of bringing relief to its victims.

[21] An early landmark was the establishment by the National Institute of Neurological and Communicative Disorders and Stroke of an ad hoc Subcommittee on Growth and Regeneration in the Central Nervous System (Carter, 1975). The documents produced by the Subcommittee provided a stimulating review of the then current status of research in the field and a blueprint for further experimentation (Experimental Neurology, 48, no. 3: 1-251, 1975).

nated the 1990's as "The Decade of the Brain", this became an opportunity for special efforts to communicate with the public and educate them about recent accomplishments and current directions in neuroscience research. For example, programs of the Society for Neuroscience have included initiatives for communicating research advances to the press and to science teachers. Especially notable in the area of public communication have been the programs of the Charles A. Dana Foundation, which is engaged in promoting awareness of public and personal benefits of brain research. These programs have included recruiting neuroscientists into the Dana Alliance for Brain Initiatives, which sponsors many nervous system disease-related publications and information campaigns. Among these is an annual "Brain Awareness Week", with the Dana Alliance coordinating the activities of close to 200 organizations throughout the nation [22], which has been especially effective, for example, in bringing information about the nervous system to schoolchildren. Research on central nervous system regeneration has correspondingly benefited from this rising tide of interest in neuroscience.

In the present volume, we see that the approach to the problem of alleviating human suffering from central nervous system injury appears in many guises that may not immediately seem to be related to the central issue – regeneration in lower animals, developmental mechanisms, cell death, gene expression in peripheral nerves, treatment of degenerative diseases. This oblique approach has been used for half a century; can it be that we have made so little inroad into the problem? On the contrary, we now see a great many new paths to try. Some of the questions, great and small, that perplexed us in 1955 – do younger animals really regenerate better, does the response of the glial cells affect regeneration, what changes occur in a nerve cell when regeneration begins, how can a growing axon identify its appropriate path, do genes matter – no longer seem to be such conundrums. If we don't know the answers, at least we are closer to defining the questions in a way that should be answerable. And the words – "promote", "enhance", "transplantation", "therapy", "treatment" – these words now have a concrete meaning for us, very different from half a century ago.

> *I believe that this conference will be counted a success if we are able to ... bring out those doubts and complexities which trouble you, because obviously future thinking and investigative work to be productive must be based just upon this.*
>
> *(Louis B. Flexner, 1955)*

---

[22] And recently extended to Europe as well.

ACKNOWLEDGMENTS

I am indebted to my colleagues, Nicholas Ingoglia and Marion Murray, for the opportunity to write this article. I am proud to think that their training as Fellows in my laboratory influenced them toward their important contributions in the field of regeneration research. I am grateful to Dr. Sabine Brauckmann for making available to me some of her unpublished material on the scientific theories of Paul Weiss and Roger Sperry.

I dedicate this article to my friends in wheelchairs, whose courage has been a stimulus to my research and a personal inspiration. I would like to mention especially Alan A. Reich, Richard P. Veraa, Henry G. Stifel III, and the late Robert Moss.

REFERENCES

Bailey P (1955) Foreword. In: *Regeneration in the Central Nervous System* (Windle WF, ed), pp vi-ix. Springfield: Thomas CC.

BardeYA, Edgar D, Thoenen H (1983) New neurotrophic factors. Ann Rev Physiol 45: 601-612.

Bracken MB, Shephard MJ, Hellenbrand KG, et al. (1985) Methylprednisolone and neurological function 1 year after spinal cord injury. Results of the National Acute Spinal Cord Injury Study. J Neurosurg 63: 704-713.

Bracken MB, Shepard MJ, Collins WF, et al. (1992) Methylprednisolone or naloxone treatment after acute spinal cord injury; 1 year follow-up data. Results of the second National Acute Spinal Cord Injury Study. J Neurosurg 76: 23-31.

Carter S (1975) Preface. Exp Neurol. 48, no. 3: 1-2.

Clemente CD (1955) Structural regeneration in the mammalian central nervous system and the role of neuroglia and connective tissue. In: *Regeneration in the Central Nervous System* (Windle WF, ed), pp 147-161. Springfield: Thomas CC.

Clemente CD (1985) In memoriam William Frederick Windle (1898-1985). Exp Neurol 90: 1-20.

Cuénod M, Cowan WM (eds) (1975) *The Use of Axonal Transport for Studies of Neuronal Connectivity* . Amsterdam: Elsevier Press. 365 pp.

David S, Aguayo AJ (1981) Axonal elongation into peripheral nervous system "bridges" after central nervous system injury in adult rats. Science 214: 931-933.

Eisen JS (1999) Patterning motoneurons in the vertebrate nervous system. Trends Neurosci 22: 321-326.

Flexner LB (1955) Introduction of the conference. In: *Regeneration in the Central Nervous System* (Windle WF, ed), pp xiii-xiv. Springfield: Thomas CC.

Gardner, D (1993) Static determinants of synaptic strength. In: *The Neurobiology of Neural Networks* (Gardner D, ed), pp 21-70. Boston: MIT Press.

Glees P (1955) Studies of cortical regeneration with special reference to cerebral implants. In: *Regeneration in the Central Nervous System* (Windle WF, ed), pp 94-111. Springfield: Thomas CC.

Goldberger ME, Bregman BS, Vierck CJ Jr, Brown M (1990) Criteria for assessing recovery of function after spinal cord injury: behavioral methods. Exp Neurol 107: 113-117.

Grafstein B (1969) Axonal transport: communication between soma and synapse. In: *Advances in Biochemical Psychopharmacology, vol. 1* (Costa E, Greengard P, eds), pp 11-25. New York: Raven Press.

Grafstein B (1971) Transneuronal transfer of radioactivity in the central nervous system. Science 172: 177-179.

Grafstein B (1986) The retina as a regenerating organ. In: *The Retina: A Model for Cell Biology Studies, Part II* (Adler R, Farber DB, eds), pp 275-335. New York: Academic Press.

Grafstein B (1995) Axonal transport: function and mechanisms. In: *The Axon* (Waxman SG, Kocsis JD, Stys PK, eds), pp 185-199. New York: Oxford.

Grafstein B, Forman DS (1980) Intracellular transport in neurons. Physiol Rev 60: 1167-1283.

Grafstein B, Murray M (1969) Transport of protein in goldfish optic nerve during regeneration. Exp. Neurol. 25: 494-508.

Grimm LM (1971) An evaluation of myotypic respecification in axolotls. J Exp Zool 178: 479-496.

Guth L, Windle WF (1970) The enigma of central nervous regeneration. Exp Neurol, Suppl 5: 1-43.

Haber B, Perez-Polo JR, Hashim G, Giuffrida-Stella AM (1983) *Nervous System Regeneration.* New York: Liss. 560 pp.

Hall ED (1992) The neuroprotective pharmacology of methylprednisolone. J Neurosurg 76: 13-22.

Hamburger V (1955) Regeneration in the central nervous system of reptiles and of birds. In: *Regeneration in the Central Nervous System* (Windle WF, ed), pp 47-53. Springfield: Thomas CC.

Hamburger V, Levi-Montalcini R (1949) Proliferation, differentiation and degeneration in the spinal ganglia of the chick embryo under normal and experimental conditions. J Exp Zool 111: 457-502.

Hoffman H (1955) Axoplasm, its structure and regeneration. In: *Regeneration in the Central Nervous System* (Windle WF, ed), pp 112-126. Springfield: Thomas CC.

Holder N, Mills J, Tonge DA (1982) Selective reinnervation of skeletal muscle in the newt *Titurus cristatus*.. J Physiol 326: 371-384.

Holtzer H (1955) Comments on regeneration as opposed to neogenesis of amphibian neurons. In: *Regeneration in the Central Nervous System* (Windle WF, ed), pp 81-83. Springfield: Thomas CC.

Langley JN (1895) Note on regeneration of pre-ganglionic fibres of the sympathetic. J Physiol (Lond) 18: 280-284

Levi-Montalcini R (1955) Neuronal regeneration in vitro. In: *Regeneration in the Central Nervous System* (Windle WF, ed), pp 54-65. Springfield: Thomas CC.

Levi-Montalcini R (1966) The Nerve Growth Factor: its mode of action on sensory and sympathetic nerve cells. Harvey Lect 60: 217-259.

Levi-Montalcini R (1987) The Nerve Growth Factor 35 years later. Science 237: 1154-1162.

Littrell JL (1955) Apparent functional restitution in Piromen treated spinal cats. In: *Regeneration in the Central Nervous System* (Windle WF, ed), pp 219-228. Springfield: Thomas CC.

McDonald JW et al. (1999) Repairing the damaged spinal cord. Scient Amer 281 (no. 3): 65-73.

McEwen BS, Grafstein B (1968) Fast and slow components in axonal transport of protein. J. Cell. Biol. 38: 494-508.

McGrath PA, Bennett MR (1979) The development of synaptic connections between different segmental motoneurones and striated muscles in the axolotl limb. Dev Biol 69: 133-145.

Moskowitz PF, Oblinger MM (1995) Sensory neurons selectively upregulate synthesis and transport of the β_{III}-tubulin protein during axonal regeneration. J Neurosci 15: 1545-1555.

Politis MJ, Ederle K, Spencer PS (1982) Tropism in nerve regeneration in vivo. Attraction of regenerating axons by diffusible factors derived from cells in distal nerve stumps of transected peripheral nerves. Brain Res 253: 1-12.

Puchala E, Windle WF (1977) The possibility of structural and functional restitution after spinal cord injury. A review. Exp Neurol 55: 1-42.

Purves D, Lichtman JW (1985) *Principles of Neural Development.* Sunderland, MA: Sinauer. 433 pp.

Rosenblatt F, Farrow JT, Herblin WF (1966) Transfer of conditioned responses from trained rats to untrained rats by means of a brain extract. Nature 209: 46-48.

Scott D Jr (1955) Conduction over regenerated central nervous system neurons. In: *Regeneration in the Central Nervous System* (Windle WF, ed), pp 181-194. Springfield: Thomas CC.

Scott D Jr, Liu CN (1963) The effect of nerve growth factor on regeneration of spinal neurons in the cat. Exp Neurol 8: 279-289.

Sperry RW (1947) Nature of functional recovery following regeneration of the oculomotor nerve in amphibians. Anat Rec 97: 293-316.

Sperry RW (1950) Myotypic specificity in teleost motoneurons. J Comp Neurol 93: 277-288

Sperry RW (1955) Functional regeneration in the optic system. In: *Regeneration in the Central Nervous System* (Windle WF, ed), pp 66-76. Springfield: Thomas CC.

Sperry RW (1959) The growth of nerve circuits. Scient Amer 201 (no.5): 68-75.

Sperry RW (1963) Chemoaffinity in the orderly growth of nerve fiber patterns and connections. Proc Nat Acad Sci USA 50: 703-710.

Sperry RW (1965) Selective communication in nerve nets: Impulse specificity vs. connection specificity. In: *Specificity in the Neurosciences* (Weiss PA, ed), Neurosci Res Prog Bull 3: 37-43.

Sperry R (1982) Some effects of disconnecting the cerebral hemispheres. Science 217: 1223-1226.

Sperry RW and Arora HL (1965) Selectivity in regeneration of the oculomotor nerve in the cichlid fish, *Astronotus ocellatus*.. J embryol Exp Morphol 14: 307-317.

Stuart EG (1955) Tissue reactions and possible mechanisms of Piromen and desoxycorticosterone acetate in central nervous system regeneration. In: *Regeneration in the Central Nervous System* (Windle WF, ed), pp 162-170. Springfield: Thomas CC.

Su QN, Namikawa K, Toki H, Kiyama H (1997) Differential display reveals transcriptional up-regulation of the motor molecules for both anterograde and retrograde axonal transport during nerve regeneration. Eur J Neurosci 9: 1542-1547.

Tessier-Lavigne M, Goodman CS (1996) The molecular biology of axon guidance. Science 274: 423-433.

Thompson DW (1917) *On Growth and Form*. Cambridge: Cambridge University Press.

1

Molecular Determinants of Retinal Axon Pathfinding in Fish

Claudia A. O. Stuermer and Christian A. Leppert
University of Konstanz, Konstanz, Germany

I. INTRODUCTION

The fish visual pathway has received continuous attention from researchers whose interest was initially focused on the exploration of rules governing the establishment of the precisely organized retinotopic map of retinal ganglion cell (RGC) axons on the optic tectum (Sperry, 1963; Gaze, 1970; Jacobson, 1970). Here, the ability of the system to restore a retinotopic map and normal vision was advantageous and it was believed that regeneration recapitulates development which - as we know now - is only partially true. The continuous growth of the system brings with it specific problems for the preservation of the retinotopic order of axon terminal arbors in the tectum and for the guidance of growth cones. Older views on the internal organization of the pathway (Attardi and Sperry, 1963) had to be revised (Stuermer and Easter, 1984a; Easter and Stuermer, 1984). This brought with it the discovery that regenerating axons behave differently from embryonic axons in their growth toward tectum and in their progression to their retinotopic termination sites in the tectum (Stuermer and Easter, 1984b; Schmidt et al., 1988) which they nevertheless recognize and find. This, in turn, led to the conclusion that terminal arbor deployment by regenerating axons is apparently under the control of the same gradients of molecules as in embryos and in the continuously growing adult (Gierer, 1987; Walter et al., 1987a,b; Vielmetter and Stuermer, 1989).

That axon regeneration per se is a remarkable property of this system and requires a special response of the affected neurons after axotomy has been realized (Grafstein, 1986). But the importance of the environment of the cut axons and, in particular, the role of the glial cells has only become clear when axon growth inhibitors were identified (this volume, chapter by Schwab; Schwab et al., 1993).

More recently, the zebrafish has become a central object for studies of vertebrate early development and the generation of hundreds of mutants provides increasing information about the genes and gene regulation operating in embryogenesis. As a result some of the genes essential for brain and retinotectal development are now known (Development V. 123, the Zebrafish issue, 1996). In addition, using more conventional strategies, molecular components involved in axon growth and pathfinding have been identified in fish through antibodies, antibody perturbation experiments and cDNA cloning. With these different approaches we are gradually obtaining new information about molecular determinants of retinal axon pathfinding.

In this review, we briefly summarize rules of order in this pathway and discuss in greater detail the role of identified molecular components which either have been shown to contribute to pathfinding, or by their special spatiotemporal expression pattern, are very likely to be used by the system for growth and regeneration, guidance and the generation of order.

In the first section we will discuss molecular determinants of RGC axon pathfinding in the embryo and early larvae. The second section reviews pathfinding of young axons from newborn RGCs during the ongoing growth of retina and tectum in adults. Finally, we consider selected parameters for RGC axon regeneration following optic nerve transection.

II. RGC DIFFERENTIATION, PATHFINDING AND RETINOTOPIC MAPPING IN ZEBRAFISH EMBRYOS

A. The spatiotemporal pattern of RGC differentiation

The pattern of RGC differentiation in zebrafish is unusual compared to other vertebrates. Morphological analysis (Schmitt and Dowling, 1999), backfilling RGCs through their axons (Burrill and Easter, 1995) and use of markers for developing RGCs (Laessing and Stuermer, 1996) showed that the first RGCs that differentiate are localized in the ventronasal retina in the 28 hpf (hours postfertilization) embryo. These first RGCs and the next ones to follow express cell surface proteins of the immunoglobulin superfamily (IgSF), in particular neurolin, the homolog of chicken SC-1/DM-GRASP/BEN (Laessing et al., 1994, Kanki et al., 1994, Laessing and Stuermer, 1996).

RGC differentiation in the embryo, as evidenced by neurolin expression, progresses in a pattern that anticipates the annular growth of the retina (Fig. 1). This takes place by the addition of new neurons from roughly 3 days of embryogenesis onwards and continues into adulthood (Johns, 1977; Paschke et al., 1992, and see section 2). After the ventronasal group, RGCs in dorsal, ventral and

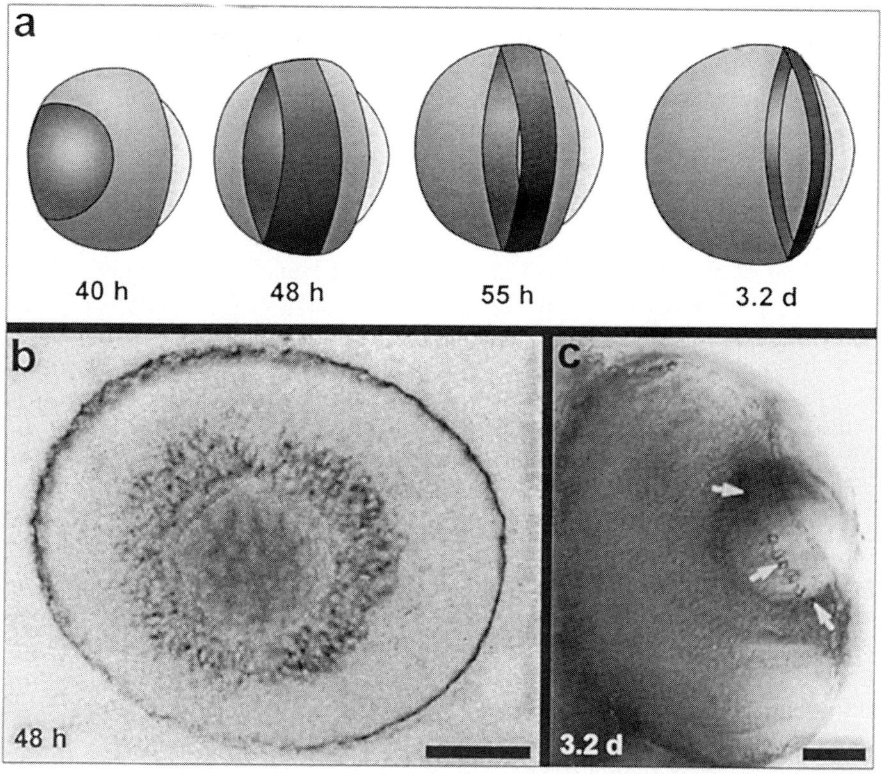

Figure 1 Pattern of RGC differentiation in the zebrafish embryo. a) Schematic representation of RGC differentiation which first encompasses the central retina, and then progresses in rings towards the retinal periphery where from 3.5 days onwards new RGCs are added at the retinal peripheral margin. The stage of the embryo in hours (h) is given below each retina. b) The annular arrangement of neurolin mRNA expressing RGCs is exemplified in the 48 h old fish. (c) The mRNA expressing cells added at the margin of the retina from 3.5 days onwards are marked by arrows. Scale bars, 100 µm.

finally temporal aspects of the eye acquire neurolin and upon closure of the choroid fissure, the differentiating RGCs are organized in rings centered on the optic disk (Laessing and Stuermer, 1996). By the time the more peripheral (younger) RGCs differentiate and synthesize neurolin (between 30-40 hpf), the older ones downregulate expression of this protein, indicating that neurolin functions in the early events of RGC differentiation and perhaps in growth cone guidance. The very first RGC axons from the ventronasal cluster are neurolin positive and so are the emerging axons from the next differentiating RGCs (Laessing and Stuermer, 1996). Neurolin`s function in RGC axon pathfinding was characterized in adult goldfish (section 2) (Ott et al., 1998; Leppert et al., 1999) and here, axonally expressed neurolin seems to represent a receptor for a guidance component at or around the optic disk. The spatiotemporal pattern of neurolin expression by RGCs and RGC axons in the zebrafish embryo indicates that this cell surface recognition protein may also contribute to RGC growth cone guidance for the first differentiating RGCs, and does play such a role in developing motor axons (Ott et al., 1999).

B. Cell surface proteins on RGC axons

In addition to neurolin, RGCs in the embryonic eye express Gap-43, E587 antigen (Giordano et al., 1997; Weiland et al., 1997), L1.1 and L1.2 (Tongiorgi et al., 1995), NCAM (Bernhardt et al., 1996), and a homolog of R-cadherin (Liu et al., 1998). The contribution of these proteins to aspects of axon growth and pathfinding was analyzed in other systems and species and some of them in the adult retina (see section 2). In zebrafish embryos, E587 antigen is involved in the formation of orderly tracts in many parts of the developing nervous systems (Weiland et al., 1997) and seems to also mediate axon fasciculation in the embryonic eye (H. Ott, M. Bastmeyer and C.A.O. Stuermer, unpublished observations).

Strikingly different from the above IgSF members which basically mark all differentiating RGCs is the expression pattern of TAG-1. TAG-1 mRNA and protein are localized in RGCs and RGC axons in the 48 hpf nasal retina and are absent from the temporal retinal half (Warren et al., 1999; Lang et al., 1999). TAG-1 antibodies selectively label nasal axons in the optic nerve and tract. This implies that TAG-1 in zebrafish embryos is involved in defining position dependent differences perhaps with consequences for RGC growth cone navigation and targeting in the tectum.

C. RGC axon pathfinding mistakes in zebrafish mutants

Domains and sites providing guidance cues to developing RGC axons and the mistakes the axons make were highlighted by the zebrafish mutants generated in the large-scale Tuebingen screen (see zebrafish issue of Development, 1996). Some of these mutants with defects in RGC navigation have been analyzed in more detail and will be briefly described below.

One of the first tasks of an emerging RGC growth cone is to advance towards the choroid fissure and through this structure into the prospective optic nerve. This path is made up of primitive glial cells (Macdonald et al., 1997). These cells express noi (no isthmus), a member of the zebrafish Pax family of transcription regulators (Lun and Brand, 1998), and line the choroid fissure and optic stalk/nerve up to its junction with the optic tract. In noi^{-} mutants, the fissure fails to close and glial cell differentiation is compromised resulting in RGC axon pathfinding errors. Fasciculation is affected, some axons grow ipsilaterally or towards the anterior commissure or in aberrant routes after crossing the midline (Macdonald et al., 1997).

In noi^{-} mutants, the expression of netrin-1 and -2, important guidance cues with chemoattractive and chemorepulsive function depending on the type of axon and system (Tessier-Lavigne and Goodman, 1996), is reduced in the choroid fissure/optic stalk. However, in contrast to results in netrin knock-out mice where RGC axons fail to exit the eye (Deiner et al., 1997), fish axons still find their way through the fissure into the nerve (Macdonald et al., 1997). This indicates the existence of additional guidance cues or that weak residual netrin expression levels suffice for RGC axon guidance into this structure.

Analysis of the noi^{-} mutant has thus elucidated a role of the primitive glia lining the primary path of the embryonic RGC axons. The molecules on or around these glial cells which are perceived by the RGC growth cones and the axonally expressed receptors mediating recognition and directed growth remain to be identified.

Several other mutants were obtained with RGC axon pathfinding defects. In some of these mutants, RGC axons fail to cross the midline (Karlstrom et al., 1996; Brand et al., 1996), indicating that this area provides important cues for RGC growth cones as is the case for a variety of CNS neuron types throughout the developing CNS (review: Mueller, 1999). Additional cues appear to reside in the optic tract as is indicated by mutants with aberrant behavior of RGC axons along this portion of the pathway (Karlstrom et al., 1996). Moreover, others show abnormal growth of RGC axons within the retina. All this is indicative of the existence of many guidance cues and axonal receptor systems governing each segment of the RGC growth cone`s long journey to its target.

Furthermore, mutants with striking retinotopic disorders in mapping of RGC axons were discovered (Trowe et al., 1996) with problems along the dorsoventral and anterior-posterior axis (Picker et al., 1999). Recent evidence from birds and mice has highlighted the importance of specific ephrins and Eph-receptors in anterior-posterior mapping (reviewed in Mueller, 1999; O'Leary et al., 1999). Molecular cloning of the zebrafish homologs (Brennan et al., 1997), analysis of their expression and use of the ace (acerebellar) mutant (Picker et al., 1999), allowed an assessment of their function for RGC mapping in the embryo.

D. The retinotopic order of RGC axons in the tectum

Labeling small groups of RGCs with red and green fluorescent dyes and tracing the path of the axons into the tectum has previously revealed that RGC axons in zebrafish embryos terminate directly at retinotopically appropriate sites (Stuermer, 1988a).

Temporal and nasal axons arrive at the anterior edge of the developing tectum at about the same time (between 46-48 hpf), invade the tectal neuropil and develop their terminal arbors with striking precision: temporal axons in the anterior tectum, nasal axons in the posterior half (Stuermer, 1988). The arbors of a small group of RGCs from opposite retinal positions are localized to small distinct areas of the tectum and do not overlap. That their intratectal path and their ability to recognize retinotopic target areas is likely to be under the control of tectal cues was suggested by the finding that nasal axons pass anterior regions and steer toward their destination in the posterior tectum in the absence of their partner axons from the temporal retina, and vice versa. Moreover, the formation of the map occurs in the absence of normal impulse activity (Stuermer et al., 1990; Kaethner and Stuermer, 1994).

Time-lapse videomicroscopic observations of individual dye-filled RGC axons from defined retinal positions allowed viewing of the direct progression of growth cones toward their destined tectal area (Kaethner and Stuermer, 1992). Here, the growth cones changed their behavior and divided to explore and branch extensively over a small area of the tectal neuropil. This behavior was entirely in accordance with the hypothesis that gradients of tectal guidance molecules are involved in retinotopic mapping (Gierer, 1987). Results from a series of ingenious tissue culture choice assays with chick RGC axons and membranes from opposite ends of the chick tectum strongly supported the view that membrane-bound molecules are expressed in a graded manner over the anterior-posterior extent of the tectum (Walter et al., 1987a,b) and that temporal and nasal axons possess differential sensitivity for these membrane bound guidance components. The tectal components were identified as members of the GPI-linked ephrins, ephrin A2 and A5 which interact with transmembrane Eph receptor tyrosine kinases on RGC axons (Drescher et al. 1995; for details see reviews: Mueller, 1999; O'Leary et al., 1999).

E. Mapping mistakes in the ace mutant

The ace mutant is deficient in FGF8 expression which is normally synthesized by cells at the midbrain-hindbrain boundary (Reifers et al., 1997). FGF8 is required for the induction of engrailed expression which in turn is required for the graded expression of ephrin A2 and ephrin A5 (Logan et al., 1996; O'Leary et al., 1999). Both of these ephrins are more strongly expressed in the caudal tectum. The gradient of ephrin A5 is steep and extends toward midtectal levels, whereas ephrin A2 declines more gradually from posterior high to anterior low levels (Picker et al., 1999). There is evidence in support of the notion that temporal axons express high levels of Eph-receptors to which ephrin A5 and A2 bind, and that this interaction impairs the advance of temporal axons (or causes their collapse). Temporal RGC axons are thus being “prevented” from elongating into the posterior tectum. A differential and perhaps graded sensitivity of temporal and nasal axons may assist them in terminating at the appropriate position along the anterior-posterior tectal extent (Drescher et al., 1997).

In the ace mutants, ephrin A5 and A2 gradients fail to be generated and as a consequence, temporal and nasal RGCs form overlapping terminal arbor fields (Picker et al., 1999). Unexpected was the finding that terminal arbor expansion also occurred to some extent in the dorsal-ventral dimension which would have been expected to be patterned by different members of the ephrin/Eph-receptor family (Holash et al., 1997).

Another observation of interest resulted from ace mutant analysis. The invading RGC axons displayed quite abnormal fascicles upon entering the tectum and failed to form a dorsomedial and ventrolateral brachium (Picker et al., 1999) which, in wildtype embryos, are selectively chosen by RGC axons of the ventral and dorsal retinal halves (Stuermer, 1988a). This gives reason to speculate that ephrin and Eph-receptors are involved in sorting RGC axons along their path to the tectum (Orioli and Klein, 1997). This aspect of RGC guidance remains to be specifically analyzed, and it will be interesting to see which role the unevenly expressed IgSF members, especially TAG-1, may play in axon sorting.

Since new RGC axons from the retinal margin in adult fish undergo sorting and resorting similar to that which takes place in embryos, we may predict that the same recognition molecules are operating for the establishment of ordered pathways during the continuous growth of the system, as well as during axonal regeneration (see below).

III. RULES OF ORDER, AXONAL RECOGNITION MOLECULES AND RGC AXON GUIDANCE IN THE ADULT RETINOTECTAL PATHWAY

A. RGC axons are ordered by age and retinal sectorial origin

A striking feature of the fish retinotectal system is its continuous growth, involving the addition of new neurons to retina and the optic tectum (Johns, 1977; Meyer, 1978; Raymond and Easter, 1983). The differentiating ganglion cells at the peripheral margin of the retina extend growth cones which fasciculate with one another and with their immediate forerunners on their path to the optic disk (Easter et al., 1984; Stuermer et al., 1992). During their progression into the optic nerve head they join to form a coherent bundle in the optic nerve and tract (Scholes, 1979; Easter et al., 1981; Bastmeyer et al., 1990). In addition to being ordered by age, RGC axons in the nerve are ordered by sectorial retinal origin. Axons from the dorsal retina are flanked on one side by temporal and temporoventral axons and on the other side by nasal and ventronasal axons (Easter et al., 1981). In the tectum, young axons follow a path according to their dorsal and ventral retinal origin and pass through the ventrolateral and dorsomedial brachia into the corresponding tectal halves (Attardi and Sperry, 1963; Stuermer and Easter, 1984a) where they sequentially leave their age-matched partner axons to elaborate terminal arbors in retinotopically appropriate regions (Easter and Stuermer, 1984; Stuermer, 1984). As far as has been analyzed, these new RGCs express the same growth-associated and surface recognition proteins (and more) as developing RGCs in the embryo (Stuermer et al., 1992). Older and more centrally located RGCs have downregulated the expression of these proteins. These growth cones may require the same and perhaps additional cues for their growth to their targets as those in the embryonic eye. However, the environment encountered by the new growth cones is more complex than that of its forerunners. Moreover, the distance they have to cover is much larger than in the embryo, several centimeters in adult goldfish as opposed to some hundred μm in the embryo. Furthermore, the newly added axons must elaborate their terminal arbors at tectal sites occupied by older axons. This requires a translocation of RGC terminal arbors in the tectum, a process known as "shifting" or "sliding" connections (Stuermer and Easter, 1984; Easter and Stuermer, 1984; Reh and Constantine-Paton, 1984). It serves to preserve a geometrically simple and well-organized retinotopic map. Guidance of added axons and synapse reformation of old arbors with retinotopically appropriate tectal neurons implies that tectal cues such as the relevant ephrins/Eph receptors and additional guidance components involved in targeting (review: Mueller, 1999), must be present in a pattern that allows old and new terminal arbors to adjust their position according to the continuously changing molecular tectal coordinates (Stuermer, 1984). How this is regulated is beyond the present state of knowledge.

We also lack insight into molecular determinants governing the various aspects of order and pathway decisions displayed by RGC axons in the adult nerve and tract, except for those discussed below.

B. Selective expression of cell surface recognition proteins by new RGCs and growing RGC axons

In this continuously growing system, we found specific cell surface recognition proteins expressed in a spatiotemporal pattern that directly reflects this growth pattern (Stuermer et al., 1992; Stuermer, 1998). These proteins selectively mark axons which are growing and hence are called growth-associated surface proteins, whereas older RGCs and axons downregulate their expression. Antibodies against these proteins therefore mark young growing axons in the retina in their peripherocentral growth and the bundle of new axons in the nerve and tract. Some stain these axons along their course through the tectum.

This growth-associated pattern is revealed by antibodies against NCAM 180/140 (Bastmeyer et al., 1990), against the L1-related E587 antigen (Vielmetter et al., 1991a), against neurolin (Paschke et al., 1992; Laessing et al., 1994), antibody M802 against a GPI-linked surface protein of unknown identity (Stuermer et al., 1992; Lang et al., 1998a), and partially with anti-TAG-1 antibodies (Lang et al., 1999). Antibodies against intracellular proteins, such as GAP-43 and reggie-1 and –2, show the same specificity for young RGCs and axons (Schulte et al., 1997; Lang et al., 1998b).

As most of the growth-associated surface proteins belong to cell adhesion molecules (CAMs) of the IgSF (Stuermer, 1998), they are expected to function in axon outgrowth, elongation and selective fasciculation, perhaps mediating the selective fasciculation of the young RGC axons and growth cone elongation along forerunners. However, this view turned out to be oversimplified, at least in the case of neurolin.

Consistent with its identity as an L1-related CAM (Vielmetter et al., 1991a; Giordano et al., 1997), E587 antigen is a growth supportive substrate for RGC axons (Bastmeyer et al., 1995). In vitro, antibodies interfere with RGC axon growth on E587 antigen as a substrate and cause axons to defasciculate (see also Fig. 7). Moreover, they lead to a reduction in growth velocity of growth cones elongating in association with other RGC axons (Bastmeyer et al., 1995).

Tissue culture experiments with DM-GRASP/SC-1/BEN in chick embryos (Burns et al., 1991; Tanaka et al., 1991) suggested a similar function of the homolog of this CAM in fish (i.e. neurolin). With neurolin and neurolin antibodies, however, none of the expected functions were observed (Leppert et al., 1999). Neurolin is not a substrate for axon growth, neurolin antibodies have a very weak effect on fasciculation and no influence on growth velocity. In light of results from *in vivo* experiments, presented below, the quasi-negative outcome of the *in vitro* tests appear plausible.

C. E587 antigen and neurolin functions *in vivo*

1. E587 antigen mediates selective fasciculation of age matched axons

The overall growth of goldfish and the growth of the goldfish retina can be markedly enhanced by special growth promoting maintenance (Bastmeyer et al., 1995). Over a period of three months, goldfish raised in this way exhibit a 100% increase in the diameter of their retina. This amounts to roughly 50,000 new RGCs and RGC axons. When these rapidly growing fish receive repeated injections of Fab fragments of polyclonal E587 antisera into the vitreous of one eye (with the other eye receiving control injections of non-immune Fabs or buffer) the order of RGC axon fascicles is notably disturbed. The fasciculation of new growth cones from newborn RGCs is delayed (Fig. 2a,b). The fascicles of newly added RGC axons are broader and crossing of fascicles is frequent (Fig. 2b, 3a,b). Thus, the presence of E587 antigen on young axons promotes their association into tight and orderly bundles thereby contributing to the age-related order of RGC axons in the fish retina (Bastmeyer et al., 1995; Ott et al., 1998).

As a consequence of the disturbed fasciculation in the retina, the fascicle order of young RGC axons in the optic nerve was also disrupted (Ott et al., 1998). Instead of forming one (or two) coherent bundle(s), the young axons were scattered over the nerve's cross sectional area, indicating that the young axons had lost their ability to recognize each other and to associate by retinal circumferential origin, i.e. age.

In addition to the loss of their age-related order, the order by their origin from dorsal, ventral, nasal and temporal retina (as described above) seems also to be lost in the nerves of E587 blocked fish (Ott et al., 1998). An additional interesting aspect was revealed by these results: the young growing axons are apparently capable of joining "old" axons in "old" fascicles. This would indicate that these alternative pathways are growth permissive (see section 3), although old axons are surrounded by fully differentiated glial cells and are myelinated by oligodendrocytes.

Thus, blockade of one cell adhesion/recognition protein on growing RGC axons causes significant pathfinding errors in the retina and in the optic nerve.

2. Neurolin is involved in RGC axon guidance to the optic disk

Perturbation experiments using polyclonal and monoclonal anti-neurolin antibodies, revealed that neurolin's contribution to axon fasciculation is minor, yet its role in axon guidance is significant. In the presence of neurolin Fabs, growing RGC axons fail to reach the optic disk (Ott et al., 1998). At around the last 50% of their growth toward the disk, RGC axons grow in loops and circles (Fig. 2c, 3c), indicating they have lost orientation. These pathfinding errors are significantly different from those elicited by E587 Fabs. Disturbing E587 antigen function reduced the fascicle order but did not prevent axon arrival at the optic disk (Fig. 2).

The finding that neurolin-blocked axons fail to reach the optic disk indicates that the disk is an intermediate target for growing RGC axons (Leppert et al., 1999). Therefore, one may expect the presence of guidance cues, for newly added RGC axons, at or around the disk. Under this premise, the highly aberrant routes of RGC axons suggest that neurolin is a receptor (or part of a receptor complex) for a retinal axon guidance component within the retina (Fig. 5), which assists growing axons in their disk-oriented growth.

Application of monoclonal anti-neurolin antibodies against Ig domain 1, 2 or 3, show that Ig domain 2 is essential to neurolin`s function in axon guidance (Leppert et al., 1999). Antibodies against Ig domain 1 and 3 affected fasciculation in that axons within one fascicle were separated instead of being tightly bound. But the antibody against Ig domain 2 caused axon growth in abnormal routes including loops and circles. The observation of live growth cones in isolated ex-vivo retina wholemounts supports the importance of Ig domain 2. Under the influence of anti-Ig domain 2 antibody, RGC growth cones turned away from the optic disk and erred through regions outside their normal fascicle tracks (Fig. 4). In these regions the velocity of the growth cones fell to a third of normal (Leppert et al., 1999), indicating that the fascicular pathway is superior to extrafascicular routes in its growth promoting properties.

Neurolin may therefore represent a multifunctional surface protein mediating close binding of neighboring axons and participating in growth cone guidance to the optic disk, in the presence of an axon guidance component whose identity and distribution is unknown at present. The observation that neurolin-blocked axons lose orientation at around 50% of their path from the margin to the disk suggests that this guidance component extends up to midretinal levels. Quite remarkable is

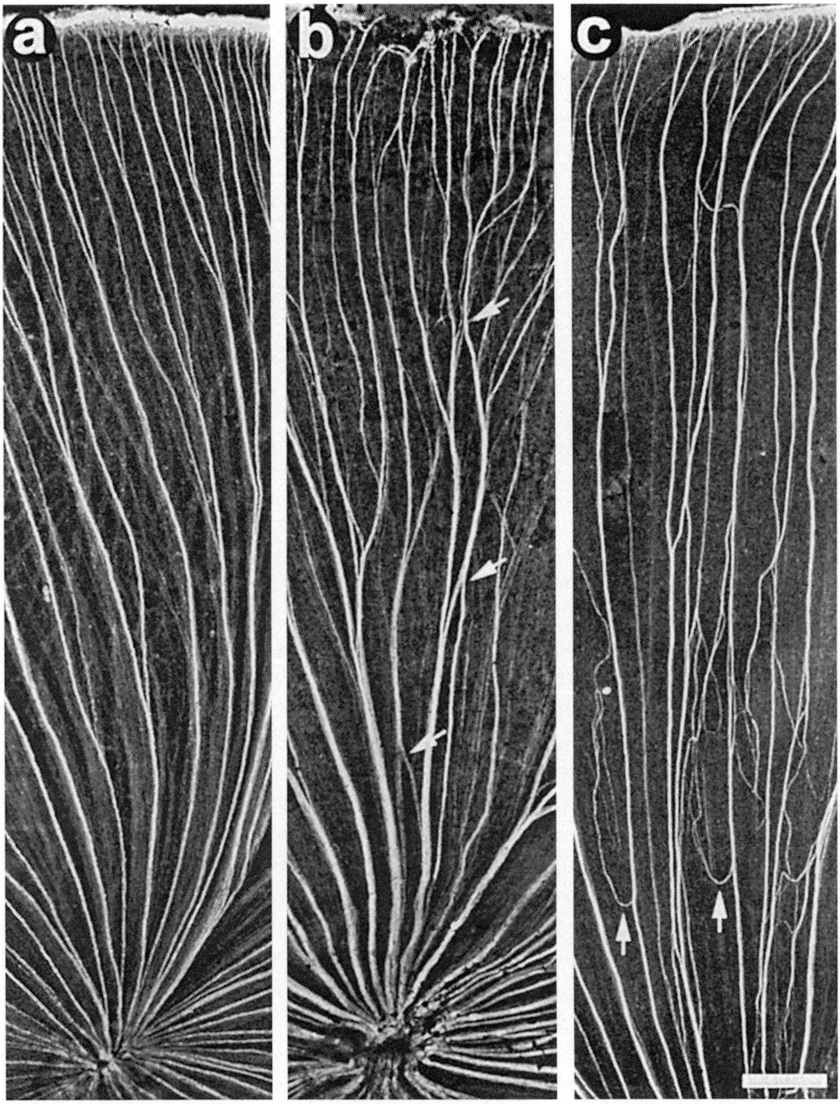

Figure 2 Segments of a goldfish retina showing RGC axons on their path from the retinal margin (top) to the optic disk (bottom). In (a), the normal order of young axons in fascicles is shown. The retina in (b), was exposed to E587 antibodies, the retina in c, to anti-neurolin. (b) When exposed to E587 antibodies the young axon fascicles have lost their normal order. Fascicles cross each other or split (arrows) and are broader than in controls. (c) When neurolin on the axons is blocked, many axons fail to reach the optic disk. Instead, they depart from their fascicle of origin, turn (arrows), grow in the opposite direction and fail to arrive at the disk. Scale bar, 200μm.

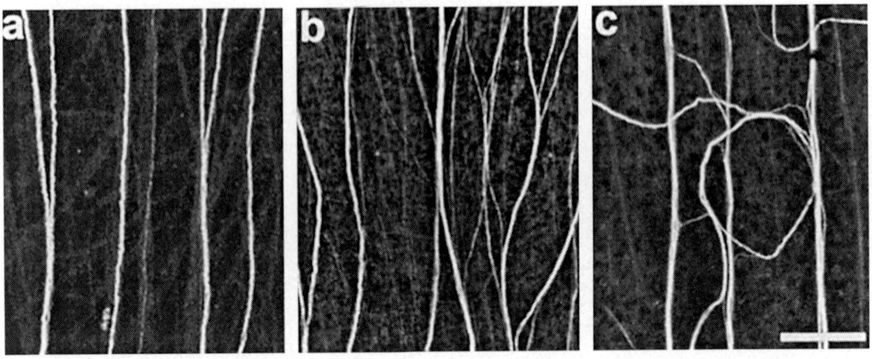

Figure 3 Comparison of the fascicle order in (a) the control retina, (b) after E587 blockage and (c) after blockage of neurolin. Antibodies against E587 antigen disrupt the fascicles, however, axons still grow towards the disk. Neurolin-blocked axons, in contrast, grow in highly aberrant routes, lose orientation and grow, as demonstrated here, in circles. Scale bar, 100μm.

the turning and growth in circles of the neurolin-blocked axons. This turning away from the disk-directed pathway may mean that the axons become responsive to a repulsive signal when neurolin is blocked. If neurolin operated in response to an attractive signal the axons might cease to advance but not necessarily grow off the track into the opposite direction and through a less favorable environment. A promising strategy employed to find the presumed ligand is the use of a tagged neurolin construct which is expected to bind the ligand-expressing cells and tissues and which can be used to isolate and identify the guidance component (Diekmann et al., 1999).

That members of the IgSF subserve a function as receptor for axon guidance components has been demonstrated, for instance, in the case of DCC which is required for the growth of axons toward a netrin source (Keino-Masu et al., 1996). Interestingly, in netrin knock-out mice, RGC axons do grow toward and arrive at the optic disk but fail to enter the optic nerve head (Deiner et al., 1997). As netrins and netrin receptors seem to be present not only in the embryonic fish visual pathway (Straehle et al., 1997) but even in the adult (Leppert and Stuermer, unpublished observations; Fig. 5), it appears that RGC growth cone guidance from the retina into the nerve depends on the netrins. However, growth towards and arrival at the disk seems to require neurolin and its interaction with the still unidentified neurolin ligand.

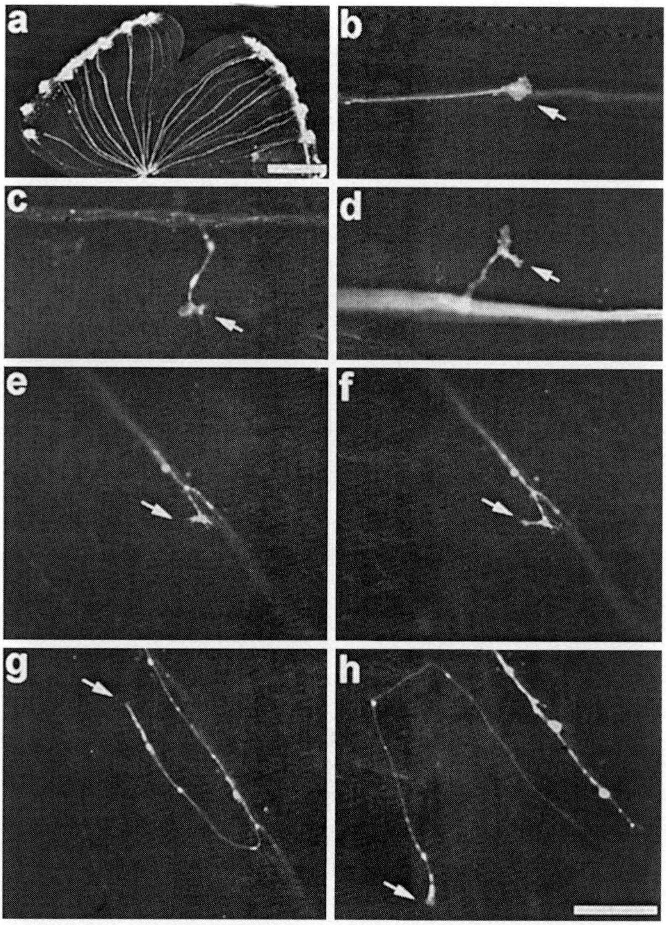

Figure 4 Antibody against Ig domain 2 of neurolin causes aberrant growth of RGC growth cones as observed in ex vivo time lapse videorecordings. Fluorescent dyes were applied to the margin of the isolated retina to stain young growing axons. The labeled growth cones in control retinae (b, arrow) follow the fascicle track toward the optic disk (to the right in b-d). Under the influence of antibodies against Ig domain 2 (c-h), growth cones exit at right angles from the fascicles (arrows in c,d) and take abnormal routes. (e-h) This growth cone was followed over 24 hours. After its exit from its fascicle (arrows in e,f), this growth cone turns into the opposite direction (arrow in g) and grows away from the optic disk (to the lower right hand corner). On its further path outside the fascicles it turns again at quasi right angles and errs through extrafascicular territories (arrow in h). Scale bar, 1mm (a); 50 μm (b-h).

D. Position dependent differences in intraretinal axon guidance

The situation is more complicated than described above insofar as defects in the orderly axon growth pattern provoked by the antibodies against E587 antigen or neurolin are restricted to dorsal RGC axons (Ott et al., 1998; Leppert et al., 1999), although ventral RGC axons express the proteins at seemingly similar levels and bind antibodies to an extent that does not seem to differ from that on dorsal RGC axons.

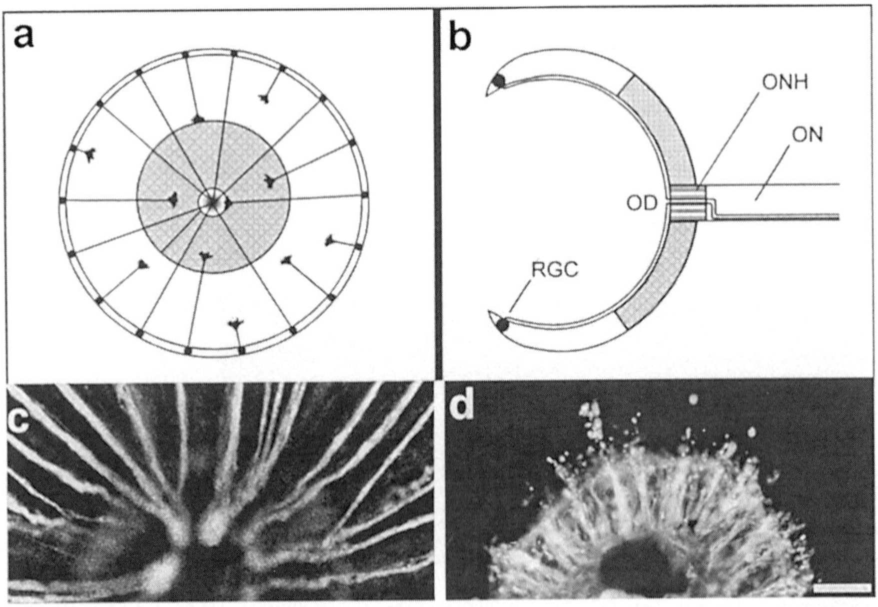

Figure 5 Guidance of RGC axons in their intraretinal path and into the optic nerve. Schematic representation of the growth cones` path from the retinal margin to the optic disk at the center of the retina (a). From experiments with anti-neurolin antibodies it appears that growth cones respond to a guidance component presumably localized around the optic disk (stippled region in a,b). b) Lateral view on the retina and optic nerve to illustrate the path of RGC growth cones to the optic disk, their passage into the optic nerve head (ONH) and optic nerve (ON). After axons have been guided to the optic disk they enter into the ONH. The patterned region (ONH) marks the zone at which axons turn to exit the retina and to enter into the optic nerve head and optic nerve. In this region, netrin seems to be expressed (d) and may be responsible for guidance of RGC axons into the ONH. As indicated in c, the RGC axons merge in this zone where elongated netrin-expressing glial cells reside (d). Scale bar, 50 μm.

While there is no direct explanation for this difference in RGC growth cone behavior, it is possible that proteins such as the ephrins and Eph-receptors with a position-dependent expression pattern may interact with the Ig family members (Zisch et al., 1997) or that other Ig family members and receptor/ligand systems are responsible for fasciculation and guidance of ventral RGC axons in fish.

Newly added RGCs seem to express most or all of the proteins which are synthesized by differentiating RGCs in the embryo. This also applies to TAG-1. TAG-1 is strongly expressed only by growing RGC axons of the nasal retina and is weakly expressed by RGCs in the temporal retinal half (Lang et al.,1999) As discussed in section 1, the functional consequence of this uneven expression is not known. But by its uneven expression TAG-1 is implicated to participate in the control of some position-dependent growth behavior of the axons, be it in selective fasciculation or target interaction or both.

From these findings it follows that the many Ig family members co-expressed on young growing axons may each fulfill a specific function in one or more parts of the RGC axonal path. Quite extensive work lies ahead of us to clarify their mutual interactions, interactions with ECM proteins and cooperation with members of other receptor/ligand systems.

Surface recognition proteins which guide axons along the path through the optic nerve, across the chiasm and into the tract and tectum have not been identified in the adult (yet growing) fish visual system. However, from the spatiotemporal expression patterns of some of the relevant growth-associated proteins follows the prediction that cues involved in guiding embryonic axons, mediating their mutual recognition and creating their order are quite likely to be present in the adult for growth and guidance of growing axons of newly added RGCs. Moreover, the molecular system involved in guiding RGC axons to their retinotopically appropriate regions must be continuously operating in fish, for homing in of new RGC axons and for the translocation of resident "older" RGC arbors to their actual appropriate sites.

IV. RETINAL AXON REGENERATION FOLLOWING OPTIC NERVE TRANSECTION

The fish visual pathway is a prime example of a selfrepairing CNS system. The lesioned RGC axons are able to regenerate and restore a retinotopically organized projection on the tectum. They also undergo timely interactions with glial cells which lead to remyelination of regenerated RGC axons soon after they begin to restore synaptic connections with the tectum (Wolburg, 1978; Ankerhold et al., 1995). This results in efficient spike propagation, synaptic transmission and recovery of normal vision (Northmore and Masino, 1984). Clearly, this requires the regulated expression of many genes in the affected neurons, in the glial cells and in the environment through which the axons pass as well as in the target tissue where the axons arborize.

The capability for complete functional repair in the fish visual pathway is outstanding and in striking contrast to the poor regenerative capacity of the lesioned mammalian visual system, where neurite growth inhibitors block axon regeneration (this volume, chapter by Schwab). Such inhibitors were not found in fish (Stuermer, 1995; Lang et al., 1996). The properties of glial cells, however, are considered in other chapters of this book. We will concentrate here on selective aspects; the reexpression of growth-associated proteins by axon-regenerating fish RGCs; the induction of one of these proteins in glial cells; the abnormal pathways and the restoration of a retinotopic map.

A. The reaction of the retinal ganglion cells

Among the many genes whose expression is induced in RGCs by axotomy are transcription factors (Herdegen et al., 1993), cytoskeletal elements (Jian et al., 1996; Asch et al., 1998; Bormann et al., 1998; Hieber et al., 1998), mediators of axon growth such as GAP-43 (Benowitz et al., 1981; Skene, 1989) and other intracellular signaling molecules (Ballestero et al., 1997; Schmidt, 1998) and cell surface recognition proteins which function in axon growth and guidance in the embryo and in newborn RGCs in the adult. In situ hybridization and immunostaining experiments have shown re-expression of NCAM (Bastmeyer et al., 1990; Bernhardt et al., 1996), the L1-like E587 antigen (Giordano et al., 1996), L1.1, L1.2 (Tongiorgi et al., 1995), neurolin (Paschke et al., 1992), TAG-1 (Lang et al., 1999), and reggie-1 and -2 (Schulte et al., 1997). With antibodies, the surface proteins NCAM, E587 antigen, neurolin, and M 802 antigen were shown to reappear on the RGC axons on their "old" portion within the retina (Fig. 6) and on the newly generated (i.e., regenerating) axon on its path into the optic tectum.

There are temporal differences in the onset of re-expression and downregulation of these proteins, as well as spatial expressional differences. In the case of TAG-1, the positional differences in expression observed in the embryo (section 1) and normal adult were retained insofar as only nasal RGCs strongly re-expressed this protein in the lesioned system (Lang et al.,1999).

The fact that they are re-expressed indicates that they are required or advantageous for the regenerative growth of the RGC axons, particularly since this controlled re-expression is not observed in mammals (Stuermer, 1998). However, the signals that control the upregulation and downregulation of these proteins are not known, nor are the functions of each of the many re-expressed proteins understood.

When regenerating axons cross the lesion site and pass through the nerve and tract, they lose their original order by both retinal cicumferential origin, i.e., age, and retinal sectorial origin (Stuermer and Easter, 1984b; Stuermer, 1988b,c; Bastmeyer et al., 1990; Vielmetter et al., 1991a). Since the age-related order of RGC axons in the nerve is dependent on the spatiotemporally restricted expression

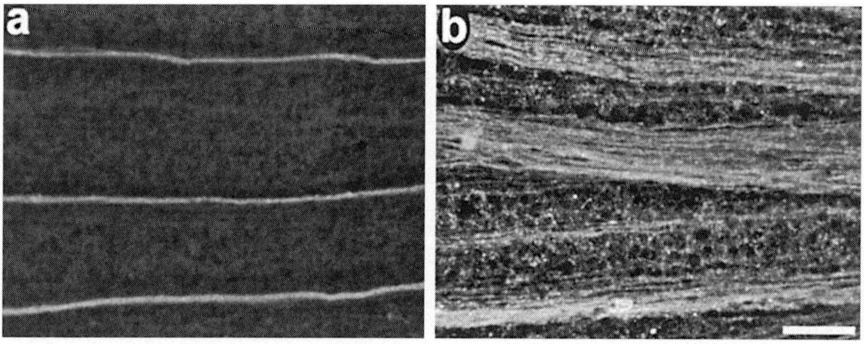

Figure 6 Re-expression of growth-associated surface proteins on retinal axons. In the normal retina, only the fascicles of young axons express the proteins on their surface (a) here exemplified for M802 antigen, whereas following optic nerve transection, all RGCs and RGC axons re-express this surface protein (b). The retinal peripheral margin is to the left, the optic disk on the right side. Scale bar, 100μm.

of growth-associated surface recognition proteins such as E587 antigen, a reasonable assumption is that this rule of order is broken because all regenerating axons reexpress E587 antigen and other IgSF members simultaneously (Stuermer et al., 1992). Since E587 antigen promotes axon growth, axons re-expressing E587 antigen may represent the preferred substrate for later emerging growth cones which (as occurs during normal development, section III) fasciculate with their forerunners during regeneration irrespective of their retinal regional origin.

B. The reaction of the optic nerve/tract glial cells

Following optic nerve transection, the regenerating RGC axons form growth cones at their proximal stumps (Lanners and Grafstein, 1980), grow across the site of lesion, assisted by fibroblast-like cells which bridge the gap created by the cut (Hirsch et al., 1995), and progress into the old fascicles where they encounter glial cells including oligodendrocytes and myelin debris.

Evidence available to date suggests that oligodendrocytes and CNS myelin do not inhibit growing RGC axons (Bastmeyer et al., 1991; Strobel and Stuermer, 1994; Wanner et al., 1995; review: Stuermer, 1995; Lang et al., 1996) nor do astrocytes form impenetrable glial scars (Hirsch et al., 1995). Instead, the glial cells and in particular oligodendrocytes appear to assist RGC axon regeneration, *in vitro* and *in vivo*.

In vitro, fish oligodendrocytes are highly growth supportive and promote growth not only of fish RGC axons but also of regenerating rat RGCs (Bastmeyer et al., 1993; Ankerhold et al., 1998). E587 antigen contributes significantly to axon growth along oligodendrocytes and also mediates adhesion between growth cones and the glial cells (Fig. 7). This was demonstrated by the fact that E587 antibodies disturb this interaction (Ankerhold et al., 1998).

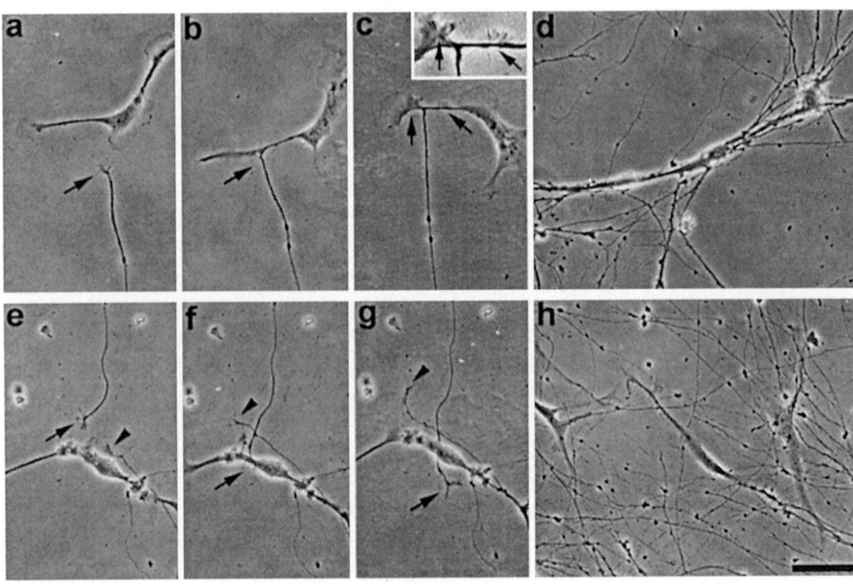

Figure 7 Interaction of regenerating growth cones with fish oligodendrocytes in vitro. (a-d) When the growth cone of an axon (arrow) makes contact with an oligodendrocyte (b), adhesion of the axon to the cell is so strong, that the axon is stretched when the cell moves (c). The insert in c shows the growth cones on the cell surface (arrows). (d) In cultures with many RGC axons, they grow preferentially along the long axis of the oligodendrocyte. (e-h) In presence of antibodies against E587 antigen, growth cones (arrow, arrowhead) cross the oligodendrocytes and continue to grow past them, or grow freely across the cells in denser cultures (h). Scale bar, 50μm.

E587 antigen may also participate in the interaction of regenerating axons with oligodendrocytes in the lesioned nerve much as in tissue culture assays, because regenerating fish RGC growth cones have also been found in direct contact with the surface of oligodendrocytes *in vivo* (Strobel and Stuermer, 1994). Moreover, recent findings revealed that oligodendrocytes *in vivo* are induced to express E587 antigen by optic nerve lesion (Ankerhold et al., 1998). The appearance of E587 antigen in oligodendrocytes in fact marks oligodendrocyte dedifferentiation. The interaction of regenerating axons with oligodendrocytes may stimulate growth cone elongation and/or the association of oligodendrocytes with regenerating axons for remyelination. When oligodendrocytes redifferentiate they synthesize myelin marker molecules such as 36K protein and MBP (Ankerhold and Stuermer, 1999) and reform a myelin sheath around regenerated axons. This coincides with the downregulation of E587 antigen. Thus, the expression of E587 antigen by RGC axons and in glial cells occurs in perfect temporal correlation.

Still, the timely expression of one protein hardly accounts for the success of RGC axon regeneration through the nerve. Among the many molecules with potential effects on regrowing axons which are synthesized in the lesioned visual pathway are laminin (Hopkins et al., 1985), chondroitin sulphateproteoglycans (Battisti et al., 1992) and other proteoglycans, HNK-1 (possibly on immunoglobulin family proteins) (Battisti et al., 1992), fibronectin (Hirsch et al., 1995) and tenascin (Bernhardt et al., 1996). Upregulation of L1.1, L1.2 and NCAM mRNAs has also been observed in optic nerve/tract glial cells (Bernhardt et al., 1996). These observations speak for the view that the lesioned fish visual pathway - in addition to lacking inhibitors - undergoes substantial changes allowing axonal regeneration to be successful.

C. Re-establishment of a retinotopic RGC axon terminal order in spite of aberrant pathways

The disorder among regenerating axons in the nerve distal to the site of lesion persists (Stuermer and Easter, 1984b; Stuermer, 1988b,c; review: Stuermer, 1988d): dorsal and ventral axons are mixed in the brachia and pass through both the dorsomedial and ventrolateral halves of the tectum in fascicles of abnormal internal order. In the layer below, axons form numerous side branches in all directions and it appears as if they widely explore the tectal territories before finally developing their terminal arbors at retinotopically appropriate sites (Schmidt et al., 1988; Stuermer et al., 1988b,c).

The fact that they do find their retinotopic target area suggests that the relevant recognition systems on axons and in the optic tectum are present. Although it has not been examined whether the ephrins, Eph-receptors and additional candidate guidance molecules are expressed by the regenerating axons and their target cells, results obtained over the years speak strongly for their continued presence in this system. In the famous Bonhoeffer stripe assay (Walter et al.,

1987a,b), where cell surface membranes of anterior and posterior tectum are laid down side by side in alternate lanes, the regenerating fish RGC axons do make the correct choices, i.e. temporal RGC axons grow preferentially on anterior tectal membranes and avoid the lanes containing membranes of the posterior tectum (Vielmetter and Stuermer, 1989). That regenerating axons are guided by molecular components related to those that provoke this behavior in birds and mammals was supported by several lines of evidence: regenerating fish RGC axons recognize the same difference between anterior and posterior tectal membranes when these were derived from the fish or embryonic chick tectum (Vielmetter et al., 1991b), and they lose the ability to respond when the tectal membranes of chick and fish were pretreated with the enzyme PIPLC (phosphoinositol-specific phospholipase C) which cleaves GPI-anchored proteins. The relevant ephrins (A2 and A5) as well as another guidance component (RGM) are GPI-anchored and are lost by this treatment (review: Mueller, 1999).

Because these assays (Vielmetter and Stuermer, 1989) were performed with membranes from normal adult goldfish tecta, the proper sorting of the axons suggests that the relevant ephrins and guidance components are expressed by the tectum throughout the fish`s life. This implies that the relevant and corresponding receptor systems on the axons (review: Mueller, 1999) are operating. In the normal adult, these may either be expressed by the young growing axons only and then become more widely re-expressed during regeneration or they are present in the retina continuously irrespective of age or lesion but in correspondence with retinal positional identity. As some of the relevant probes have recently become available, ephrin A2 and A5 expression in the tectum and the Eph-receptor distribution in the retina can be determined and will be compared to the above predictions.

V. SUMMARY AND FUTURE DIRECTIONS

In summary, events observed during regeneration in the fish retinotectal pathway indicate that a regulated expression of genes in fish correlates with axon regeneration and may thus be causally involved in this process and required for repair of this pathway

The present state of knowledge suggests that molecular components involved in axon growth and guidance are regulated in the fish visual pathway in a way that is perfectly adapted to its specific mode of development. Moreover, the system has the ability to re-activate genes for growth and guidance allowing regeneration and repair to occur. An important goal for future research is to identify the regulatory elements (factors) which control the regulation of gene expression in RGCs and in their environment.

ACKNOWLEDGMENTS

Work from our laboratory discussed in this article has been supported by grants of the DFG (Deutsche Forschungsgemeinschaft), an EC grant and by the FCI (Fond der Chemischen Industrie).

REFERENCES

Ankerhold R, Kaethner RJ, Stuermer CAO (1995) Morphology of oligodendrocytes in the goldfish optic tract and their fate after optic nerve transection. Soc Neurosci Abstr 21:42.

Ankerhold R, Leppert CA, Bastmeyer M, Stuermer CAO (1998) E587 antigen is upregulated by goldfish oligodendrocytes after optic nerve lesion and supports retinal axon regeneration. Glia 23:257-270.

Ankerhold R, Stuermer CAO (1999) The fate of oligodendrocytes during retinal axon degeneration and regeneration in the goldfish visual pathway. J Neurobiol 41:572-584.

Asch WS, Leake D, Canger AK, Passini MA, Argenton F, Schechter N (1998) Cloning of zebrafish neurofilament cDNAs for plasticin and gefiltin: increased mRNA expression in ganglion cells after optic nerve injury. J Neurochem 71:20-32.

Attardi DG, Sperry RW (1963) Preferential selection of central pathways by regenerating optic fibers. Exp Neurol 7:46-64.

Ballestero RP, Wilmot GR, Agranoff BW, Uhler MD (1997) gRICH68 and gRICH70 are 2',3'-cyclic-nucleotide 3'-phosphodiesterases induced during goldfish optic nerve regeneration. J Biol Chem 272:11479-11486.

Bastmeyer M, Schlosshauer B, Stuermer CAO (1990) The spatiotemporal distribution of N-CAM in the retinotectal pathway of adult goldfish detected by the monoclonal antibody D3. Development 108:299-311.

Bastmeyer M, Beckmann M, Schwab ME, Stuermer CAO (1991) Growth of regenerating goldfish axons is inhibited by rat oligodendrocytes and CNS myelin but not by goldfish optic nerve/tract oligodendrocytelike cells and fish CNS myelin. J Neurosci 11:626-40.

Bastmeyer M, Bähr M, Stuermer CAO (1993) Fish optic nerve oligodendrocytes support axonal regeneration of fish and mammalian retinal ganglion cells. Glia 8:1-12.

Bastmeyer M, Ott H, Leppert CA, Stuermer CAO (1995) Fish E587 glycoprotein, a member of the L1 family of cell adhesion molecules, participates in axonal fasciculation and the age-related order of ganglion cell axons in the goldfish retina. J Cell Biol 130:969-976.

Battisti WP, Shinar Y, Schwartz M, Levitt P, Murray M (1992) Temporal and spatial patterns of expression of laminin, chondroitin sulphate proteoglycan and HNK-1 immunoreactivity during regeneration in the goldfish optic nerve. J Neurocytol 21:557-573.

Benowitz LI, Shashoua VE, Yoon MG (1981) Specific changes in rapidly transported proteins during regeneration of the goldfish optic nerve. J Neurosci 1:300-307.

Bernhardt RR, Tongiorgi E, Anzini P, Schachner M (1996) Increased expression of specific recognition molecules by retinal ganglion cells and by optic pathway glia accompanies the successful regeneration of retinal axons in adult zebrafish. J Comp Neurol 376:253-264.

Bernhardt RR (1999) Cellular and molecular bases of axonal pathfinding during embryogenesis of the fish central nervous system. J Neurobiol 38:137-160.

Bormann P, Zumsteg VM, Roth LW, Reinhard E (1998) Target contact regulates GAP-43 and alpha-tubulin mRNA levels in regenerating retinal ganglion cells. J Neurosci Res 52:405-419.

Brand M, Heisenberg CP, Jiang YJ, Beuchle D, Lun K, Furutani-Seiki M, Granato M, Haffter P, Hammerschmidt M, Kane DA, Kelsh RN, Mullins MC, Odenthal J, Van Eeden FJM, Nüsslein-Volhard C (1996) Mutations in zebrafish genes affecting the formation of the boundary between midbrain and hindbrain. Development 123:179-190.

Brennan C, Monschau B, Lindberg R, Guthrie B, Drescher U, Bonhoeffer F, Holder N (1997) Two Eph receptor tyrosine kinase ligands control axon growth and may be involved in the creation of the retinotectal map in the zebrafish. Development 124:655-664.

Burns FR, Von Kannen S, Guy L, Raper JA, Kamholz J, Chang S (1991) DM-GRASP, a novel immunoglobulin superfamily axonal surface protein that supports neurite extension. Neuron 7:209-220.

Burrill JD, Easter SS, Jr. (1995) The first retinal axons and their microenvironment in zebrafish: Cryptic pioneers and the pretract. J Neurosci 15:2935-2947.

Diekmann H, Leppert CA, Bastmeyer M, Stuermer CAO (1999) The optic disk-directed growth of retinal axons is severely impaired by a monoclonal antibody against the second Ig-domain of goldfish neurolin. 1rst European Zebrafish Meeting, Tuebingen (abstract).

Deiner MS, Kennedy TE, Fazeli A, Serafini T, Tessier-Lavigne M, Sretavan DW (1997) Netrin-1 and DCC mediate axon guidance locally at the optic disc: Loss of function leads to optic nerve hypoplasia. Neuron 19:575-589.

Drescher U, Kremoser C, Handwerker C, Loeschinger J, Noda M, Bonhoeffer F (1995) In vitro guidance of retinal ganglion cell axons by RAGS, a 25 kDa tectal protein related to ligands for Eph receptor tyrosine kinases. Cell 82:359-370.

Drescher U, Bonhoeffer F, Müller BK (1997) The Eph family in retinal axon guidance. Curr Opin Neurobiol 7:75-80.

Easter SSJ, Rusoff AC, Kish PE (1981) The growth and organization of the optic nerve and tract in juvenile and adult goldfish. J Neurosci 1:793-811.

Easter SSJ, Bratton B, Scherer SS (1984) Growth-related order of the retinal fiber layer in goldfish. J Neurosci 4:2173-2190.

Easter SSJ, Stuermer CAO (1984) An evaluation of the hypothesis of shifting terminals in goldfish optic tectum. J Neurosci 4:1052-1063.

Gaze RM (1970) The Formation of Nerve Connections. London: Academic Press.

Gierer A (1987) Directional cues for growing axons forming the retinotectal projection. Development 101:479-489.

Giordano S, Laessing U, Ankerhold R, Lottspeich F, Stuermer CAO (1997) Molecular characterization of E587 antigen: An axonal recognition molecule expressed in the goldfish central nervous system. J Comp Neurol 377:286-297.

Grafstein B (1986) The retina as a regenerating organ. In: The retina: a model for cell biology studies, part III.

Herdegen T, Bastmeyer M, Bähr M, Stuermer CAO, Bravo R, Zimmermann M (1993) Expression of JUN, KROX, and CREB transcription factors in goldfish and rat retinal ganglion cells following optic nerve lesion is related to axonal sprouting. J Neurobiol 24:528-543.

Hieber V, Dai X, Foreman M, Goldman D (1998) Induction of alpha1-tubulin gene expression during development and regeneration of the fish central nervous system. J Neurobiol 37:429-440.

Hirsch S, Cahill MA, Stuermer CAO (1995) Fibroblasts at the transection site of the injured goldfish optic nerve and their potential role during retinal axonal regeneration. J Comp Neurol 360:599-611.

Holash JA, Soans C, Chong LD, Shao H, Dixit VM, Pasquale EB (1997) Reciprocal expression of the Eph receptor Cek5 and its ligand(s) in the early retina. Dev Biol 182:256-269.

Hopkins JM, Ford-Holevinski TS, McCoy JP, Agranoff BW (1985) Laminin and optic nerve regeneration in the goldfish. J Neurosci 5:3030-3038.

Jacobson M (1970) Developmental Neurobiology. New York: Holt Rinehart and Winston.

Jian X, Szaro BG, Schmidt JT (1996) Myosin light chain kinase: expression in neurons and upregulation during axon regeneration. J Neurobiol 31:379-391.

Johns PA (1977) Growth of the adult goldfish eye. III: Source of the new retinal cells. J Comp Neurol 176:343-357.

Kaethner RJ, Stuermer CAO (1992) Dynamics of terminal arbor formation and target approach of retinotectal axons in living zebrafish embryos: A time-lapse study of single axons. J Neurosci 12:3257-3271.

Kaethner RJ, Stuermer CAO (1994) Growth behavior of retinotectal axons in live zebrafish embryos under TTX-induced neural impulse blockade. J Neurobiol 25:781-796.

Kanki JP, Chang S, Kuwada JY (1994) The molecular cloning and characterization of potential chick DM-GRASP homologs in zebrafish and mouse. J Neurobiol 25:831-845.

Keino-Masu K, Masu M, Hinck L, Leonardo ED, Chan SS, Culotti JG, Tessier-Lavigne M (1996) Deleted in Colorectal Cancer (DCC) encodes a netrin receptor. Cell 87:175-185.

Karlstrom RO, Trowe T, Klostermann S, Baier H, Brand M, Crawford AD, Grunewald B, Haffter P, Hoffmann H, Meyer SU, Müller BK, Richter S, Van Eeden FJM, Nüsslein-Volhard C, Bonhoeffer F (1996) Zebrafish mutations affecting retinotectal axon pathfinding. Development 123:427-438.

Laessing U, Giordano S, Lottspeich F, Stuermer CAO (1994) Molecular characterization of fish neurolin: a growth associated cell surface protein and member of the immunoglobulin superfamily in the fish retinotectal system with similarities to chick protein DM-GRASP/SC-1/BEN. Differentiation 56:21-29.

Laessing U, Stuermer CAO (1996) Spatiotemporal pattern of retinal ganglion cell differentiation revealed by the expression of neurolin in embryonic zebrafish. J Neurobiol 29:65-74.

Lang DM, Ankerhold R, Stuermer CAO (1996) Axonal regeneration in the fish and amphibian CNS: myelin-associated neurite growth inhibitors and adaptive plasticity of glial cells. In: Cell Biology and Pathology of Myelin: Evolving Biological Concepts and Therapeutic Approaches. (Juurlink BHJ, Devon RM, Doucette JR, Schreyer DJ, Verge VM, K. eds), New York: Plenum Press.

Lang DM, Leppert CA, Wiechers M, Stuermer CAO (1998a) Mab M802 recognizes a 48 kDa GPI-anchored surface protein involved in axonal guidance. Europ J Neurosci 10 (Suppl):274.

Lang DM, Lommel S, Jung M, Ankerhold R, Petrausch B, Laessing U, Wiechers MF, Plattner H, Stuermer CAO (1998b) Identification of reggie-1 and reggie-2 as plasmamembrane-associated proteins which cocluster with activated GPI-anchored cell adhesion molecules in non-caveolar micropatches in neurons. J Neurobiol 37:502-523.

Lang DM, Klisa C, Warren JT, Stuermer CAO (1999) TAG-1 in the fish visual system: expression pattern and functional studies. 1rst European Zebrafish Meeting, Tuebingen (abstract).

Lanners HN, Grafstein B (1980) Early stages of axonal regeneration in the goldfish optic tract: an electron microscopic study. J Neurocytol 9:733-751.

Leppert CA, Diekmann H, Paul C, Laessing U, Marx M, Bastmeyer M, Stuermer CAO (1999) Neurolin Ig domain 2 participates in retinal axon guidance and Ig domains 1 and 3 in fasciculation. J Cell Biol 144:339-349.

Liu O, Sanborn J, Marrs A, Raymond PA (1998) Expression of R-cadherin in zebrafish suggests a role in guidance of retinal axons. Soc Neurosci Abstr 24:306.

Logan C, Wizenmann A, Drescher U, Monschau B, Bonhoeffer F, Lumsden A (1996) Rostral optic tectum acquires caudal characteristics following ectopic *Engrailed* expression. Curr Biol 6:1006-1014.

Lun K, Brand M (1998) A series of zebrafish *no isthmus* alleles of the *pax2.1* gene reveals multiple signaling events in development of the midbrain-hindbrain primordium. Development 125:3049-3062.

Macdonald R, Scholes J, Strähle U, Brennan C, Holder N, Brand M, Wilson SW (1997) The Pax protein Noi is required for commissural axon pathway formation in the rostral forebrain. Development 124:2397-2408.

Meyer RL (1978) Evidence from thymidine labeling for continuing growth of retina and tectum in juvenile goldfish. Exp Neurol 59:99-111.

Mueller BK (1999) Growth cone guidance: First steps towards a deeper understanding. Annu Rev Neurosci (in press).

Northmore DPM, Masino T (1984) Recovery of vision in fish after optic nerve crush: a behavioral and electrophysiological study. Exp Neurol 84:109-125.

O'Leary DDM, Yates PA, McLaughlin T (1999) Molecular development of sensory maps: representing sights and smells in the brain. Cell 96:255-269.

Orioli D, Klein R (1997) The Eph receptor family: axonal guidance by contact repulsion. Trends Genet 13:354-359.

Ott H, Bastmeyer M, Stuermer CAO (1998) Neurolin, the goldfish homolog of DM-GRASP, is involved in retinal axon pathfinding to the optic disk. J Neurosci 18:3363-3372.

Ott H, Bastmeyer M, Stuermer CAO (1999) Functions of neurolin (DM-GRASP/SC-1) in guidance of motoaxons in embryonic zebrafish. 1rst European Zebrafish Meeting, Tuebingen (Abstract)

Paschke KA, Lottspeich F, Stuermer CAO (1992) Neurolin, a cell surface glycoprotein on growing retinal axons in the goldfish visual system, is reexpressed during retinal axonal regeneration. J Cell Biol 117:863-875.

Picker A, Brennan C, Reifers F, Clarke J, Holder N, Brand M (1999) Requirement for the zebrafish mid-hindbrain boundary in midbrain polarisation, mapping and confinement of the retinotectal projection. Development (in press).

Raymond PA, Easter SS Jr (1983) Postembryonic growth of the optic tectum in goldfish. I. Location of germinal cells and numbers of neurons produced. J Neurosci 3:1077-1091.

Reh TA, Constantine-Paton M (1984) Retinal ganglion cell terminals change their projection sites during larval development of *Rana pipiens*. J Neurosci 4:442-457.

Reifers F, Böhli H, Walsh EC, Crossley PH, Stainier DYR, Brand M (1998) *Fgf8* is mutated in zebrafish *acerebellar* (*ace*) mutants and is required for maintenance of midbrain-hindbrain boundary development and somitogenesis. Development 125:2381-2395.

Schmidt JT, Turcotte JC, Buzzard M, Tieman DG (1988) Staining of regenerating optic arbors in goldfish tectum: progressive changes in immature arbors and a comparison of mature regenerated arbors with normal arbors. J Comp Neurol 269:565-591.

Schmidt JT (1998) Up-regulation of protein kinase C in regenerating optic nerve fibers of goldfish: immunohistochemistry and kinase activity assay. J Neurobiol 36:315-324.

Schmitt EA, Dowling JE (1999) Early retinal development in the zebrafish, *Danio rerio*: light and electron microscopic analyses. J Comp Neurol 404:515-536.

Scholes J (1979) Nerve fibre topography in the retinal projection to the tectum. Nature 278:620-624.

Schulte T, Paschke KA, Laessing U, Lottspeich F, Stuermer CAO (1997) Reggie-1 and reggie-2, two cell surface proteins expressed by retinal ganglion cells during axon regeneration. Development 124:577-587.

Schwab ME, Kapfhammer JP, Bandtlow CE (1993) Inhibitors of neurite growth. Ann Rev Neurosci 16:565-595.

Skene JHP (1989) Axonal growth-associated proteins. Annu Rev Neurosci 12:127-56.

Sperry R (1963) Chemoaffinity in the orderly growth of nerve fiber patterns and connections. Proc Natl Acad Sci USA 50:703-710.

Straehle U, Fischer N, Blader P (1997) Expression and regulation of a *netrin* homologue in the zebrafish embryo. Mech Dev 62:147-160.

Strobel G, Stuermer CAO (1994) Growth cones of regenerating retinal axons contact a variety of cellular profiles in the transected goldfish optic nerve. J Comp Neurol 346:435-448.

Stuermer CAO (1984) Rules for retinotectal terminal arborizations in the goldfish optic tectum: A whole-mount study. J Comp Neurol 229:214-232.

Stuermer CAO, Easter SSJ (1984a) Rules of order in the retinotectal fascicles of goldfish. J Neurosci 4:1045-1051.

Stuermer CAO, Easter SSJ (1984b) A comparison of the normal and regenerated retinotectal pathways of goldfish. J Comp Neurol 223:57-76.

Stuermer CAO (1988a) Retinotopic organization of the developing retinotectal projection in the zebrafish embryo. J Neurosci 8:4513-4530.

Stuermer CAO (1988b) Trajectories of regenerating retinal axons in the goldfish tectum: I. A comparison of normal and regenerated axons at late regeneration stages. J Comp Neurol 267:55-68.

Stuermer CAO (1988c) Trajectories of regenerating retinal axons in the goldfish tectum: II. Exploratory branches and growth cones on axons at early regeneration stages. J Comp Neurol 267:69-91.

Stuermer CAO (1988d) Navigation of normal and regenerating axons in the goldfish. In: The making of the nervous system. (Parnavelas, Stern and Stirling, eds.) Oxford University Press, Oxford.

Stuermer CAO, Rohrer B, Münz H (1990) Development of the retinotectal projection in zebrafish embryos under TTX-induced neural-impulse blockade. J Neurosci 10:3615-3626.

Stuermer CAO, Bastmeyer M, Bähr M, Strobel G, Paschke K (1992) Trying to understand axonal regeneration in the CNS of fish. J Neurobiol 23:537-550.

Stuermer CAO (1995) Glial cells and regeneration in lower vertebrates. In: Neuroglial cells (Kettenmann, Ransom eds), pp 905-915. London: Oxford University Press.

Stuermer CAO (1998) Ig superfamily molecules in neural regeneration in the CNS. In: Immunoglobulin Superfamily Molecules in the Nervous System (Sonderegger P ed), pp 235-269. Harwood Academic Publisher.

Tanaka H, Matsui T, Agata A, Tomura M, Kubota I, McFarland KC, Kohr B, Lee A, Phillips HS, Shelton DL (1991) Molecular cloning and expression of a novel adhesion molecule, SC1. Neuron 7:535-545.

Tessier-Lavigne M, Goodman CS (1996) The molecular biology of axon guidance. Science 274:1123-1133.

Tongiorgi E, Bernhardt RR, Schachner M (1995) Zebrafish neurons express two L1-related molecules during early axonogenesis. J Neurosci Res 42:547-561.

Trowe T, Klostermann S, Baier H, Granato M, Crawford AD, Grunewald B, Hoffmann H, Karlstrom RO, Meyer SU, Müller B, Richter S, Nüsslein-Volhard C, Bonhoeffer F (1996) Mutations disrupting the ordering and topographic mapping of axons in the retinotectal projection of the zebrafish, *Danio rerio*. Development 123:439-450.

Vielmetter J, Stuermer CAO (1989) Goldfish retinal axons respond to position-specific properties of tectal cell membranes in vitro. Neuron 2:1331-1339.

Vielmetter J, Lottspeich F, Stuermer CAO (1991a) The monoclonal antibody E587 recognizes growing (new and regenerating) retinal axons in the goldfish retinotectal pathway. J Neurosci 11:3581-3593.

Vielmetter J, Walter J, Stuermer CAO (1991b) Regenerating retinal axons of goldfish respond to a repellent guiding component on caudal tectal membranes of adult fish and embryonic chick. J Comp Neurol 311:321-329.

Walter J, Henke-Fahle S, Bonhoeffer F (1987a) Avoidance of posterior tectal membranes by temporal retinal axons. Development 101:909-913.

Walter J, Kern-Veits B, Huf J, Stolze B, Bonhoeffer F (1987b) Recognition of position-specific properties of tectal cell membranes by retinal axons in vitro. Development 101:685-696.

Wanner M, Lang DM, Bandtlow CE, Schwab ME, Bastmeyer M, Stuermer CAO (1995) Reevaluation of the growth-permissive substrate properties of goldfish optic nerve myelin and myelin proteins. J Neurosci 15:7500-7508.

Warren JT, Chandrasekhar A, Kanki JP, Rangarajan R, Furley AJ, Kuwada JY (1999) Molecular cloning and developmental expression of a zebrafish axonal glycoprotein similar to TAG-1. Mech Dev 80:197-201.

Weiland UM, Ott H, Bastmeyer M, Schaden H, Giordano S, Stuermer CAO (1997) Expression of an L1-related cell adhesion molecule on developing CNS fiber tracts in zebrafish and its functional contribution to axon fasciculation. Mol Cell Neurosci 9:77-89.

Wolburg H (1978) Growth and myelination of goldfish optic nerve fibers after retina regeneration and nerve crush. Z Naturforsch 33:988-996.

Zisch AH, Stallcup WB, Chong LD, Dahlin-Huppe K, Voshol J, Schachner M, Pasquale EB (1997) Tyrosine phosphorylation of L1 family adhesion molecules: Implication of the Eph kinase Cek5. J Neurosci Res 47:655-665.

2

Axonal Regeneration in the Primary Visual Pathway of Goldfish and Rats

Larry I. Benowitz, Steven Leon, Raymond Tabibiazar, Yun Jing and Nina Irwin

Laboratories for Neuroscience Research in Neurosurgery, Children's Hospital, Department of Surgery and Program in Neuroscience, Harvard Medical School, Boston, Massachusetts

I. INTRODUCTION

Our sensory world, like that of many other species, is dominated by vision. This, combined with the accessibility of the retina and its efferent projections to experimental manipulations, has made the primary visual pathway a gateway for understanding neural development, sensory processing, and the response of neurons to injury. Across vertebrate species, there has been a remarkable conservation in the cellular and molecular organization of the retina and its efferent projections. However, one striking difference between amniotic and anamniotic vertebrates is in their ability to regenerate axons of the optic nerve after injury.

In its glial make-up, the mammalian optic nerve is a typical central nervous system (CNS) pathway, rich in oligodendrocytes and white matter astrocytes (Ramon y Cajal, 1928). As in other pathways of the mammalian CNS, axons arising from retinal ganglion cells (RGCs) are unable to regenerate through the optic nerve if they are damaged in mature animals. The consequences of this are dire: injured axons rapidly undergo anterograde and retrograde degeneration, and within a few days, the ganglion cells begin to undergo apoptotic cell death, culminating in a near-complete loss of this cell population and a permanent loss of vision. This sequence of events is not inevitable, however. Under the right set of conditions, mature mammalian RGCs can survive axotomy and go on to regenerate their axons. In cell culture, RGCs from mature animals will regenerate their axons when grown with astrocytes, serum, or other growth factors (Wigley and Berry, 1988; Thanos et al., 1989; Schulz et al., 1990; Meyer et al., 1994; Meyer-Franke et al., 1995; Jo et al., 1999). Moreover, *in vivo*, RGCs can extend severed axons long distances through a peripheral nerve graft (So et al., 1985; Aguayo et al., 1991) and, if stimulated by appropriate trophic factors, even into the optic nerve itself (Berry, 1996). Thus, by identifying the factors that stimulate the survival and growth of axons from retinal ganglion cells, some degree of visual recovery may become a reality.

II. OPTIC NERVE REGENERATION IN LOWER VERTEBRATES: MOLECULAR CHANGES

The situation in lower vertebrates is very different from that in mammals. Almost all RGCs survive injury to the optic nerve, and go on to reestablish the correct pattern of connections with their central targets within a month or so (Sperry, 1963; Jacobson, 1991). Axon regeneration is characterized by a shift in the ganglion cells' program of gene expression (Grafstein and Murray, 1969). The most striking change is a 100-fold increase in the synthesis of GAP-43, a phosphoprotein that is localized on the cytoplasmic surface of growing axonal membranes and growth cones (Benowitz et al., 1981, 1983; Skene & Willard, 1981a,b; Heacock & Agranoff, 1982; Perry et al., 1986; LaBate & Skene, 1989). GAP-43 induction begins within 2 days of axotomy and remains high for 2-3 weeks, during the period of rapid axon growth and synaptogenesis. In the primary visual pathway of mammals, deletion of the GAP-43 gene by homologous recombination disrupts axon pathfinding at the optic chiasm and alters the distribution of retinal fibers in the diencephalon (Strittmatter et al., 1995; Kruger et al., 1998). In contrast, overexpression leads to exuberant synaptic growth (Aigner et al., 1995). In addition to its role in development, the persistent expression of GAP-43 in associative regions of the mature CNS is linked to activity-dependent synaptic plasticity (Benowitz & Routtenberg, 1997). At a molecular level, GAP-43 shows an association with the submembrane cytoskeleton (He et al., 1997) and the membrane fusion apparatus (Coopersmith et al., 1998; Haruta et al., 1997). Thus, during axonal regeneration, it is likely to play a role in membrane addition, growth cone motility, axon targeting, and/or synaptic tuning events.

The expression of several transmembrane adhesion proteins of the immunoglobulin superfamily also shifts during optic nerve regeneration. Increases in gene expression occur for neurolin, a homologue of mammalian DM-GRASP, which has been shown to participate in axon fasciculation within the retina and optic nerve (Paschke et al., 1992; Ott et al., 1998); L-1 (Vielmetter et al., 1991; Blaugrund et al., 1992; Bernhardt et al., 1996), which is also implicated in fasciculation and pathfinding (Ott et al., 1998); and N-CAM, which contributes to adhesive interactions and axon guidance through homophilic binding (Bastmeyer et al., 1990; Bernhardt et al., 1996), interactions with the FGF receptor (Doherty et al.,

1996), and regulation of GAP-43 phosphorylation (Meiri et al., 1998). An upregulation of two other cell surface proteins, reggie-1 and -2, occurs as well (Schulte et al., 1997).

Regeneration of the goldfish optic nerve is also accompanied by a significant upregulation of the intermediate filament proteins gefiltin (ON-1) and plasticin (Glasgow et al., 1992, 1994), along with the microtubule subunit α-1 tubulin (Bormann et al., 1998). These changes presumably contribute to rebuilding the axonal cytoskeleton and establishing the scaffold required to transport membranous organelles. Expression of one or more members of the jun family of transcription factors occurs (Herdegen et al., 1993), though the relationship of this to the observed changes in effector gene products is not yet known. Finally, there is a marked increase in soluble cyclic nucleotide phosphodiesterases (Ballestero et al., 1997), and several other proteins that remain to be characterized (Skene & Willard, 1981a; Benowitz & Lewis, 1983; Perry et al., 1987).

In experimental paradigms in which mammalian retinal ganglion cells are induced to regenerate their axons, there is a striking upregulation in the expression of GAP-43 (Doster et al., 1990; Meyer et al., 1994; Schaden et al., 1994; Berry et al., 1996), the cell adhesion molecule L1 (Jung et al., 1997), and a member of the jun family of transcription factors (Hull and Bähr, 1994). While many other changes are no doubt taking place, the patterns of gene expression underlying axon regeneration in goldfish and rat RGCs appear at first glance to be similar.

III. WHAT INDUCES GOLDFISH RETINAL GANGLION CELLS TO REGENERATE THEIR AXONS?

While the molecular changes that accompany optic nerve regeneration in lower vertebrates have been investigated in some detail, relatively little attention has been paid to the signals that trigger this process. Explant studies provided the first clue that the inductive signals arise from a source extrinsic to the retina. If goldfish RGCs are stimulated to begin regenerating their axons *in vivo* for 1-2 weeks ('priming'), they continue to extend axons when explanted into serum-containing media (Landreth and Agranoff, 1976, 1979). However, if regeneration is not initiated *in vivo*, 'naive' RGCs show little growth when explanted. These observations suggest that regeneration is triggered by something that is available to RGCs *in vivo*, but which is not intrinsic to the retina nor present in the culture media. We therefore carried out 'complementation' studies to identify factors which, when added to RGCs, enable them to regenerate their axons even without being 'primed' *in vivo*. These studies utilized dissociated cultures highly enriched in RGCs (Schwartz & Agranoff, 1982; Schwalb et al., 1995). When maintained in serum-free, defined media, dissociated RGCs remained viable for several weeks but failed to extend axons. The addition of factors secreted by optic nerve glia stimulated dramatic outgrowth (Schwalb et al, 1995, 1996: Fig. 1). Upon size fractionation, the principal axon-promoting factor proved to be a small molecule,

< 1 kilodalton in mass, which was tentatively named axogenesis factor-1 (AF-1). AF-1 induced the same level of outgrowth from RGCs regardless of whether cells had been primed to begin regenerating their axons *in vivo*; in the absence of AF-1, even primed retinal ganglion cells failed to show appreciable growth (Fig. 2). These findings support the hypothesis that AF-1 is a key determinant of regenerative growth *in vivo,* and suggest that, the priming phenomenon might be explained by the need for RGCs to remain exposed to optic nerve glia to trigger the regenerative program.

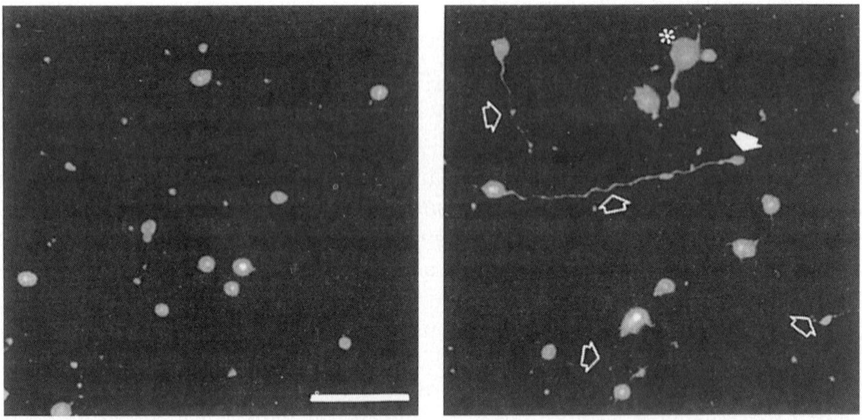

Figure 1 Factors secreted by the goldfish optic nerve glia induce RGCs to extend axons. Left: In defined media, goldfish retinal neurons remain viable (as demonstrated by metabolism of 5,6-carboxyfluorescein diacetate), but show little outgrowth. Right: The addition of media conditioned by optic nerve glia induces cells 10-17 μm in diameter to extend one or two processes of a uniform caliber (open arrows); these sometimes terminate in a prominent growth cone (closed arrow). Retrograde labeling shows that the responsive cells are RGCs (Schwalb et al., 1995). Bar = 100 μm.

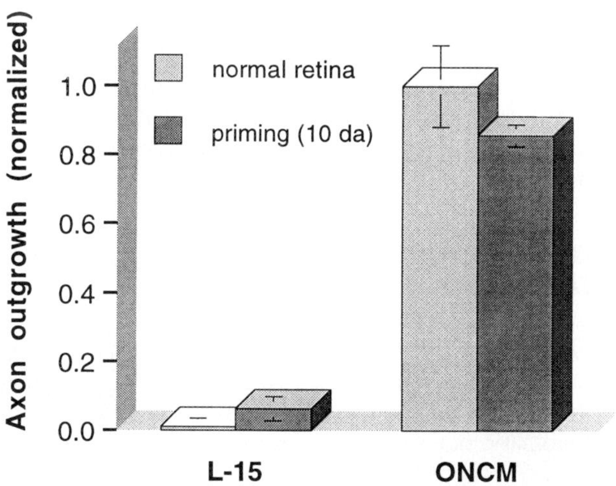

Figure 2 Factors secreted by optic nerve glia induce the same level of outgrowth from RGCs irrespective of "priming". RGCs were dissected either from previously unoperated animals (light bars) or from goldfish in which axon regeneration had proceeded *in vivo* for 10 days after an optic nerve crush (dark bars: "priming"). In the presence of factors secreted by optic nerve glia, 'naive' and primed RGCs showed the same level of outgrowth. In the absence of glial factors, both failed to extend axons. Thus, optic nerve-derived factors induce all of the outgrowth seen in primed RGCs, whereas in the absence of these factors, there is no effect of priming; these factors therefore, appear to be necessary and sufficient for outgrowth. Outgrowth was measured as the percent of phase-bright cells (10-17 μm diameter) extending one or two processes of uniform caliber more than 5 cell diameters in length. Results were normalized by subtracting the level of growth seen in negative controls, then dividing by the net growth in positive controls (partially purified AF-1). Data represent means from 4 wells per condition ± SEM. Counting was carried out blind to the identity of samples (Schwalb et al., 1996).

Optic nerve glia also secrete a larger axon-promoting factor, probably a polypeptide. In our earlier work, chromatography pointed to a peak of biological activity at 12 kDa and a second one at 70 kDa. With procedural refinements, however, the 12 kDa species appears to be a proteolytic fragment of AF-3, the larger protein (R. Tabibiazar and L. Benowitz, unpublished observations). Even at saturating concentrations, AF-3 promotes much less outgrowth than AF-1. A host of polypeptide growth factors were tested for their ability to mimic the effects of AF-3 (Schwalb et al., 1995). Of these, only recombinant rat ciliary neurotrophic factor (CNTF) was active (ED50 ~5 ng/ml: R. Tabibiazar, L. Benowitz, unpublished observations). Whether AF-3 is related to CNTF remains to be determined. A number of small differentiation factors (e.g., retinoic acid, taurine, small peptides) were investigated for their ability to mimic AF-1's actions. None showed any activity except for the purine nucleosides, which led to a surprising discovery about intracellular signaling mechanisms.

IV. STIMULATION OF GROWTH THROUGH A PURINE NUCLEOSIDE-SENSITIVE PATHWAY

We investigated whether purine nucleosides or nucleotides might induce growth, perhaps by acting upon one or more of the well-characterized purine receptors (Burnstock, 1990; Linden, 1998). Low micromolar concentrations of either adenosine or guanosine induced dramatic outgrowth, whereas pyrimidine nucleosides were inactive (Fig. 3a, lanes 1-5). The effects of adenosine and guanosine were not, however, mediated through extracellular purine receptors. P1 (adenosine) receptors were ruled out since a non-hydrolyzable agonist for all of the known extracellular adenosine receptors (2-chloroadenosine, 2-CA) was inactive; at the same time an antagonist of the A1 and A2 receptors (8-p-sulphophenylthioinosine, 8-PST) failed to block the effects of adenosine (Fig. 3b, lanes 1,2). P2 (purine nucleotide) receptors were likewise ruled out, since adenosine mono-, di- and triphosphate showed little or no activity. Moreover, the purine nucleosides were not serving as precursors to cyclic nucleotides that might act as intracellular second messengers, since non-hydrolyzable, membrane-permeable analogs of cAMP or cGMP failed to stimulate outgrowth (Fig. 3a, lanes 7,8). One remaining possibility, that adenosine acts by virtue of being converted to a metabolite, proved to be correct. When we prevented adenosine from being hydrolyzed to inosine (using the adenosine deaminase inhibitor deoxycoformycin, DCF), adenosine not only failed to stimulate growth, but actually proved to be cytotoxic (Fig. 3b, lane 3). As anticipated from this result, inosine stimulated extensive outgrowth, with an EC50 of 11 μM. Inosine and guanosine were both found to act upon an intracellular target, and failed to induce growth in the presence of a purine transport blocker (nitrobenzylthioinosine, NBTI: Fig. 3b, lanes 5,6).

Studies in pheochromocytoma PC12 cells provide a hint about the intracellular target of the purine nucleosides. In PC12 cells and some peripheral ganglionic neurons, nerve growth factor (NGF) stimulates cell survival as well as neurite outgrowth. The purine analog 6-thioguanine (6-TG) selectively blocks NGF-induced neuritogenesis, which correlates with the inhibition of a 47-49 kDa serine-threonine kinase (N-kinase: Volonte et al., 1989; Greene et al., 1990; Batistatou et al., 1992). In light of the structural similarities among 6-TG, inosine, and guanosine (Fig. 4a), we hypothesized that the two purine nucleotides might act as agonists at the same site at which 6-TG functions as an antagonist. One prediction from this hypothesis is that inhibiting the N-kinase should block axon outgrowth

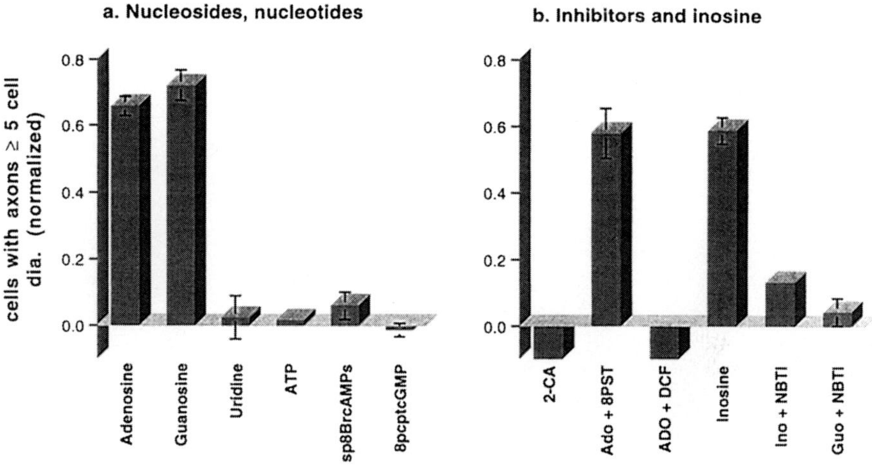

Figure 3 Purinergic effects on axon outgrowth. (a) Effects of purine nucleosides and nucleotides. Goldfish retinal ganglion cells were grown in defined media and treated with the indicated nucleosides, nucleotides, or analogs. Extensive outgrowth was obtained from the purine nucleosides adenosine and guanosine, but not from any of the pyrimidines (only uridine shown here). None of the purine nucleotides induced growth, including membrane-permeable, non-hydrolyzable analogs of cAMP (8-bromoadenosine-3',5' cyclic monophosphorothioate, sp8BrcAMPs) and of cGMP (8-(4-chlorophenylthio) guanosine-3',5'-cyclic monophosphate, 8pcptcGMP). All compounds were tested between 1-1000 μM; results shown here are at 100 μM, a concentration that yielded results in cases in which any response was seen. Data are normalized as described in the legend to Fig. 2. (b) Further studies on purinergic effects: inosine is the active metabolite of adenosine, and acts through an intracellular mechanism. lane 1: 2-CA, a non-hydrolyzable adenosine analog that acts as an agonist at all known adenosine receptors, fails to stimulate growth. lane 2: Further evidence that adenosine is not stimulating growth through adenosine receptors comes from the failure of 8-PST, an antagonist of A1 and A2 receptors, to stimulate growth. lane 3: Evidence that adenosine must be hydrolyzed to stimulate growth comes from the fact that DCF, an inhibitor of adenosine deamidation, blocks the activity of adenosine. lane 4: Inosine, the product of adenosine deamidation, stimulates outgrowth. lanes 5, 6: Evidence that inosine and guanosine act through an intracellular mechanism comes from the observation that NBTI, an inhibitor of purine transport across the membrane, blocks their activity.

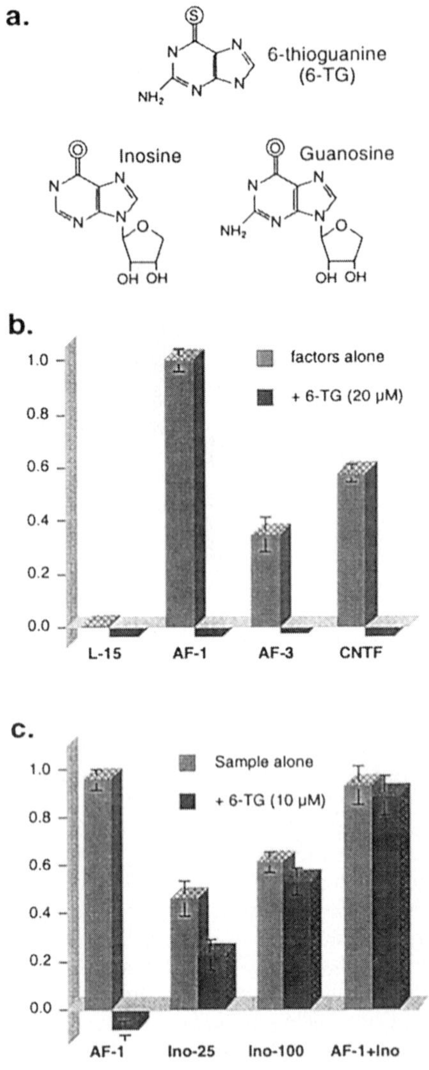

Figure 4 Evidence that purine nucleosides may act upon the intracellular target that is inhibited by 6-thioguanine. (a) Structural similarities among the purine analog 6TG, inosine, and guanosine. 6-TG, which blocks growth and inhibits N-kinase, differs from the growth-promoting nucleosides inosine and guanosine by the absence of the ribose group and the substitution of a sulfhydryl group for oxygen. (b) 6-TG inhibits the outgrowth induced by AF-1, AF-3 or CNTF to a level below baseline. Thus, the effects of all three factors on outgrowth may be mediated through a purine-sensitive mechanism. (c) Inosine and 6-TG act competitively. Outgrowth induced by 25 μM inosine is only partly affected by 10 μM 6-TG, while outgrowth induced by 100 μM is unaffected. At 100 μM, inosine restores the full level of growth induced by AF-1 to its original level in the presence of 6-TG.

from goldfish RGCs. This proved to be correct at 10 μM, 6-TG blocked outgrowth initiated by AF-1, AF-3, or CNTF but did not affect cell survival (Fig. 4b). A second prediction is that inosine would act competitively with 6-TG to restore growth. As shown in Fig. 3c, outgrowth stimulated by a near-saturating concentration of inosine was partially affected by 6-TG, but higher levels of inosine overcame this blockade. In addition, inosine restored the full level of growth induced by AF-1 in the presence of 6-TG (Fig. 4c). While these studies support the possibility that inosine acts by stimulating the N kinase, other possibilities cannot yet be ruled out, e.g., that inosine activates some pathways that are 6-TG insensitive.

As mentioned above, one hallmark of axon regeneration in the visual system is the dramatic upregulation of GAP-43 expression. As shown in Fig. 5, GAP-43 is induced by AF-1, inosine, and guanosine. Moreover, GAP-43 induction by growth factors is blocked by 6-TG but restored by inosine. Thus, at least this one facet of axon growth appears to be mediated through the purine-sensitive transduction step. It will be important to determine whether other gene products associated with regenerative growth *in vivo* are likewise regulated through this pathway.

V. INVOLVEMENT OF OTHER SIGNAL TRANSDUCTION PATHWAYS

In PC12 pheochromocytoma cells, stimulation by NGF leads to the phosphorylation of several key tyrosine residues on trkA, the high affinity NGF receptor, which allows for the docking of shc and other adapter proteins. This leads to the subsequent activation of several downstream signaling pathways (reviews: Greene and Kaplan, 1995; Segal and Greenberg, 1996), two of which have been implicated in neurite outgrowth: one involves the mitogen-activated protein kinase cascade (MAPK: Cowley et al., 1994), and the other, activation of phosphatidylinositol-3 kinase (PI3-K: Kimura et al., 1994; Kita et al., 1998). In goldfish retinal explant cultures, inhibition of PI 3-K signaling with wortmannin has been reported to partially inhibit neurite outgrowth (Lavie et al., 1997). In dissociated goldfish RGCs, two inhibitors of PI3-K signaling, wortmannin and LY294002, failed to block outgrowth stimulated by AF-1, but blocked c. 50% of the growth stimulated by inosine (Benowitz et al., 1998). Quantitatively similar results were obtained with PD098059, which inhibits MEK-1 and -2 activity and therefore blocks MAPK phosphorylation (Alessi et al., 1995). Like LY294002, PD098059 had little effect on AF-1-induced growth but blocked much of the growth stimulated by inosine. When combined, LY294002 and PD098059 blocked all outgrowth stimulated by inosine, but still left much of the activity of AF-1 unimpeded (Fig. 6a). From these studies, it appears that inosine-induced growth requires MEK and PI3-kinase to be active, whereas AF-1 may stimulate additional signaling pathways that lead to axon growth (Fig. 6b). More work is needed to clarify the relationship between the purine-sensitive mechanism and other signaling pathways.

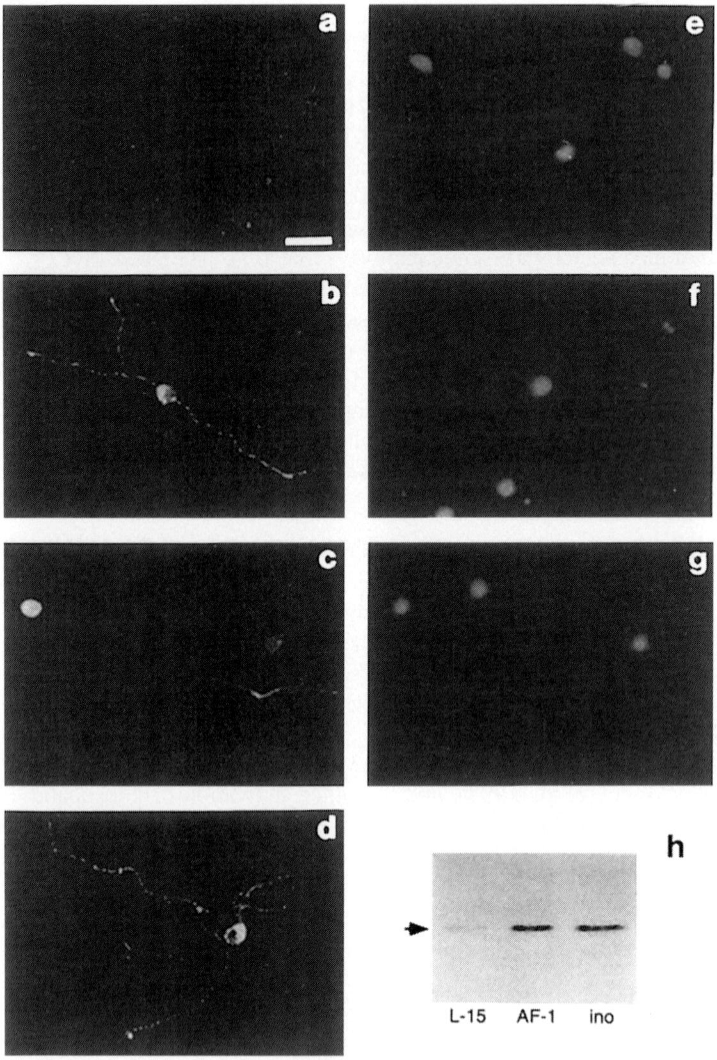

Figure 5 GAP-43 induction parallels axon outgrowth. (a,c,e,g). Goldfish RGCs were immunostained with a primary antibody to recombinant zebrafish GAP-43 (courtesy C. Stuermer, Univ. Konstanz) and a fluorescent secondary antibody (b,d,f): same field as a, c, e, stained with DAPI to visualize cell nuclei. (a,b) Negative controls maintained for 6 days in defined media show little GAP-43. (c,d) Cells treated with AF-1 extend axons and express GAP-43. (e,f) Cells grown with 100 μm inosone or 100 μm guanosine. (h) Western blot showing GAP-43 induction in RGCs grown in culture, scraped and prepared for protein separation by SDS-PAGE. Guanosine, not shown here, induces a similar level of GAP-43 expression as inosine.

VI. MAMMALIAN RETINAL GANGLION CELLS

In mature mammals, the rapid death of RGCs that occurs after intraorbital injury to the optic nerve can be attenuated with a variety of trophic factors or by directly manipulating elements of the cell death pathway (e.g., caspase inhibitors or over-expression of the bcl-2 gene: Kermer et al., 1998; Bonfanti et al., 1996). Trophic factors that enhance RGC survival *in vivo* include brain-derived growth factor (BDNF: Mansour-Robaey et al., 1994), CNTF (Mey and Thanos, 1993), acidic or basic fibroblast growth factor (FGF: Sievers et al., 1987), neurotrophin- 4/5 (NT-4/5: Cohen et al., 1994), and glial-derived neurotrophic factor (GDNF: Koeberle and Ball, 1998). Implanting Schwann cells intravitreally, or grafting a segment of peripheral nerve onto the distal end of a cut optic nerve, also enhances RGC survival, and this may involve factors that remain to be identified. In homogeneous RGC cultures, Meyer-Franke et al. (1995) found that BDNF, CNTF, insulin-like growth factor-1 (IGF-1), NT-4/5, leukemia inhibiting factor (LIF), basic FGF, transforming growth factor-β (TGF-β), and insulin each had a partial effect in enhancing cell survival. These partial effects could be increased several-fold by combining several polypeptide growth factors while at the same time increasing physiological activity or directly elevating intracellular cAMP levels. In the presence of forskolin, the combination of BDNF (or NT-4/5), insulin (or IGF-1), and CNTF (or LIF) allowed most retinal ganglion cells to survive for several weeks. Addition of an as yet unidentified factor derived from CNS oligodendrocytes had a further effect on survival (Meyer-Franke et al., 1995). Thus, unlike the situation in peripheral neurons, where a single target-derived factor may control cell survival, the survival of RGCs depends upon the level of physiological activity and the availability of growth factors from more than one tissue source (e.g., target cells, sheath cells).

Besides attenuating cell death, Schwann cells enable RGCs to regenerate their axons. This enhancement of regeneration has variously been ascribed to (a) the presence in Schwann cells of neurotrophic factors that are absent in CNS glia; (b) synthesis by Schwann cells of cell surface or basement membrane molecules favorable to growth, e.g., laminin; and/or (c) an absence in Schwann cells of factors that inhibit axonal growth, e.g., myelin associated glycoprotein (MAG: McKerracher et al., 1994; Mukhopadhyay et al., 1994), NI-250 or NI-35 (Nogo: Caroni and Schwab, 1988; Weibel et al., 1994). In support of the latter hypothesis, antibodies to NI-250 applied to the injured optic nerve have some effect in enhancing axon regeneration past the injury site (Weibel et al., 1994). However, even without altering the inhibitory influences of oligodendrocytes, the presence of appropriate trophic factors may enable RGCs to regenerate their axons into the optic nerve (Berry et al., 1996; Lucius et al., 1998). Following optic nerve injury in adult rats, implanting a sciatic nerve fragment or dissociated Schwann cells into the vitreous induces RGCs to extend local neurites (Cho and So, 1992), upregulate GAP-43 expression (Ng et al., 1995), and regenerate their axons past the injury site several millimeters into the distal optic nerve (Berry et al., 1996). Identificaa.

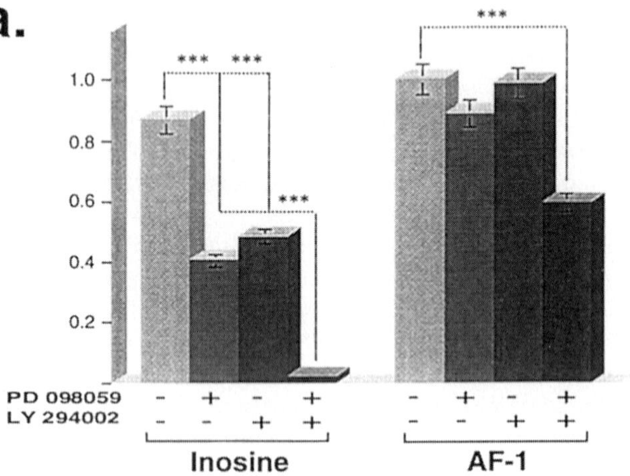
***
***
***
***
1.0
0.8
0.6
0.4
0.2
PD 098059
LY 294002
Inosine
AF-1

b.

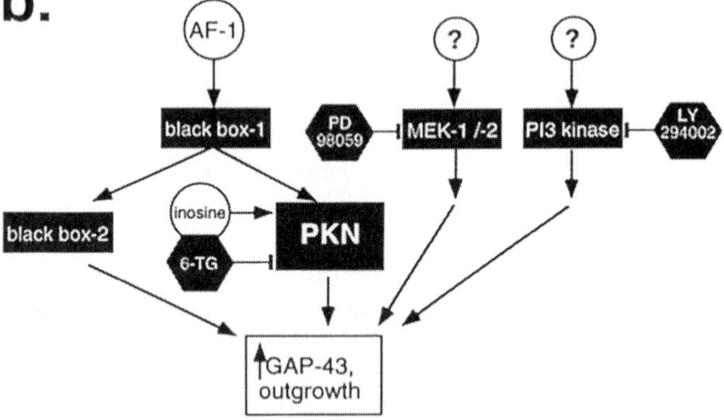
AF-1
?
?
black box-1
PD 98059
MEK-1 /-2
PI3 kinase
LY 294002
black box-2
inosine
PKN
6-TG
GAP-43, outgrowth

tion of the active factor(s) is an issue of paramount interest.

In dissociated RGCs cultured from juvenile rats, CNTF and LIF were found to stimulate lengthy axon regeneration and induce GAP-43 expression (Fig. 7a: Jo et al., 1998). These two cytokine growth factors act through the same receptor complex, and therefore stimulate the same downstream signaling events. As in goldfish RGCs, CNTF-induced outgrowth in rat RGCs utilizes a purine-sensitive mechanism: outgrowth in rat RGCs was blocked by 6-TG and restored with inosine. By itself, inosine induced a small but significant amount of outgrowth (Fig. 7b: Benowitz et al., 1998). Although BDNF and certain other growth factors also enhanced the survival of rat RGCs as reported (Meyer-Franke et al., 1995), none of these induced the same extent of outgrowth as CNTF or LIF (Fig. 7c: Jo et al., 1998). Conditioned media obtained from either the rat sciatic nerve or optic nerve contained axon-promoting activity, which was neutralized with an anti-CNTF antibody. This would suggest that CNTF is a major endogenous growth-promoting factor for mature mammalian RGCs. Indeed, intravitreal injections of CNTF increase the ability of RGCs to regenerate their axons into a peripheral nerve graft (Cho et al., 1998). However, it seems unlikely that CNTF alone can account for the effects of implanting Schwann cells into the retina. Arguing against this is the fact that the optic nerve itself has among the highest levels of CNTF in the nervous system (Stockli et al., 1991), yet RGCs whose cut endings are exposed to the cellular environment of the optic nerve fail to regenerate their axons in the absence of additional factors provided by peripheral nerve Schwann cells.

Figure 6 Involvement of the MAP kinase and PI3 kinase signaling pathways in axon outgrowth from goldfish RGCs. To investigate whether two well-characterized signal transduction pathways are involved in outgrowth induced by AF-1 or inosine, RGCs were pretreated with PD 98059 (50 um), a specific inhibitor of MEK-1 and 2,LY 294002, an inhibitor of PI3 kinase signaling, or both, prior to being stimulated by AF-1 or inosine. Neither inhibitor by itself, blocked growth stimulated by AF-1, though both combined had some effect. In contrast, either inhibitor alone blocked c.50% of the growth induced by inosine and the two combined blocked all inosine-induced growth. b. In this schema, AF-1 acts upstream from N-kinase, since inhibiting the latter with 6-TG blocks all AF-1-induced growth. Inosine is proposed to be an agonist of N-kinase. By itself, inosine stimulates a lower level of growth than AF-1, which suggests that AF-1 stimulates additional pathways besides PKN. Inosine can compete with 6-TG to restore the full level of growth induced by AF-1. MAP kinase and PI3 kinase may not be on the direct signaling pathway activated by AF-1, since blockade of either alone has no effect on AF-1-induced growth. However, they may be constitutively activated in our cultures (e.g., by the insulin in the culture media), and contribute somewhat to growth. Blocking MAP kinase signaling with PD 980959, or the PI3 kinase signaling pathway with LY294002 inhibits the weaker growth induced by inosine, but has a lesser effect on growth stimulated by AF-1, since the latter may activate additional signaling pathways.

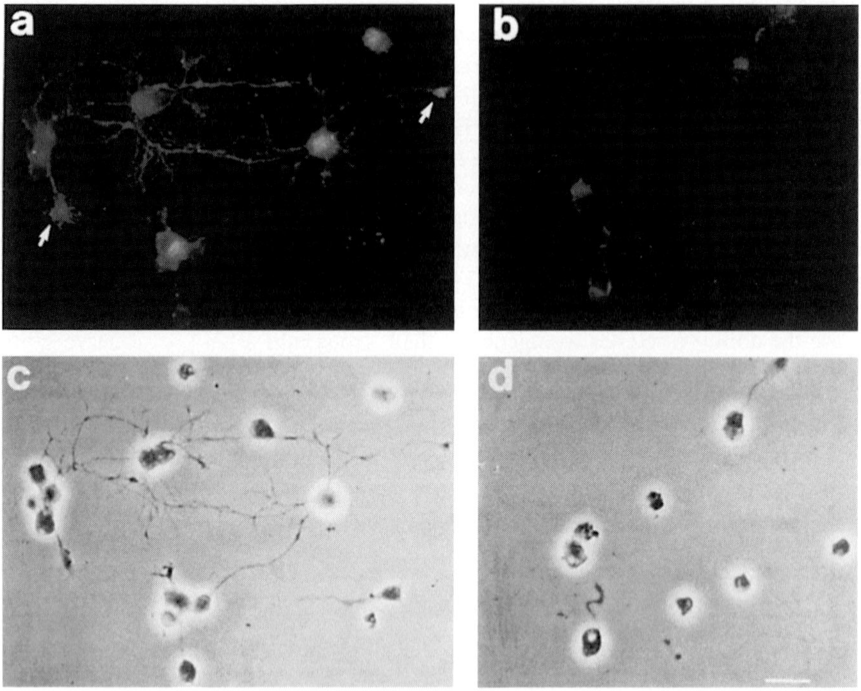

Figure 7 CNTF induces axon outgrowth and GAP-43 expression in rat RGCs. (a-d) Immunopurified RGCs from postnatal day 8 rat were cultured for 2 days in the absence (c,d) or presence (a,b) of CNTF (50 ng/ml). Cultures were fixed, immunostained with an anti-GAP-43 antibody (a,c) followed by a fluorescent secondary antibody, and visualized under fluorescence (a,c) or phase-contrast (b,d) illumination. Scale bar: 50 μm. (e,f) Effects of various trophic factors on axon outgrowth and survival. (e) CNTF and LIF, which both activate the same receptor complex, induced striking axonal outgrowth (defined as the fraction of RGCs extending an axon >5 cell diameter in length); NGF and aFGF showed only minor effects. (f) CNTF, LIF, BDNF, and aFGF all increased cell survival over controls. $^*p < 0.05$, $^{**}p < 0.01$, $^{***}p < 0.002$. (g) CNTF-induced outgrowth is mediated by a purine-sensitive mechanism. Cultured rat RGCs were maintained in defined media either alone, or with various combinations of inosine (25 μm), CNTF (5 ng/ml), and 6-thioguanine as shown. Inosine increased growth above baseline by 52% (*lane 2 vs lane 1,* $^{**}p < 0.01$); CNTF had a more pronounced effect (*lane 3,* $^{***}p < 0.001$) that was blocked by 6-TG (*lane 5)* but restored upon the addition of inosine ($^*p < 0.05$) (from Benowitz et al., 1998).

e. f. g.

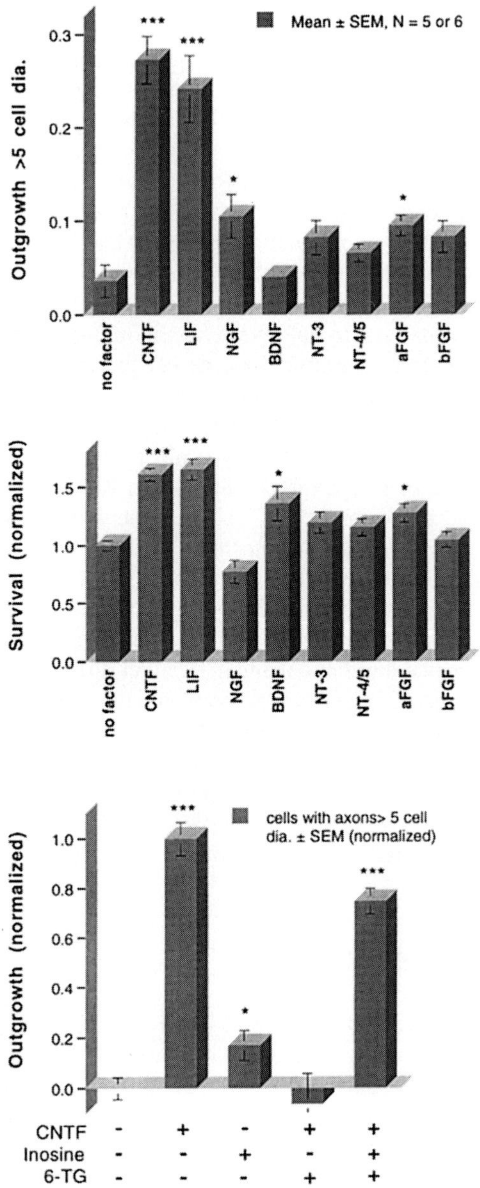
Mean ± SEM, N = 5 or 6
Outgrowth >5 cell dia.
0.0
0.1
0.2
0.3
no factor
CNTF
LIF
NGF
BDNF
NT-3
NT-4/5
aFGF
bFGF
Survival (normalized)
0.0
0.5
1.0
1.5
no factor
CNTF
LIF
NGF
BDNF
NT-3
NT-4/5
aFGF
bFGF
cells with axons> 5 cell dia. ± SEM (normalized)
Outgrowth (normalized)
0.0
0.2
0.4
0.6
0.8
1.0
CNTF - + - + +
Inosine - - + - +
6-TG - - - + +

To investigate whether CNTF or any other trophic agent can mimic the effect of Schwann cells in stimulating RGCs to regenerate their axons through the optic nerve, various factors were injected intravitreally into rats with optic nerve injury and no peripheral nerve grafts. Surprisingly, all groups with intravitreal injections, including controls with only a puncture wound to the posterior chamber, showed extensive axon growth past an injury site; as expected, controls with no intravitreal manipulations showed no growth at all. Thus, puncturing the sclera and retina is sufficient to set off events that activate RGCs' regenerative program. Similar puncture wounds have been shown to enhance RGC survival (Mansour-Robaey et al., 1994) and to be neuroprotective for photoreceptors (Faktorovich et al., 1992). These injuries lead to a delayed upregulation of CNTF and basic FGF mRNA (Wen et al., 1995). However, whether either of these mediates the effect of a puncture wound on axon regeneration is difficult to test, since the effect of an injection per se is such a powerful stimulus. In any event, these findings confirm the fact that RGC axons can regenerate through the optic nerve, and indicate that the inhibitory influences exerted by CNS myelin proteins, e.g. NI-250 (Nogo) or MAG (Li et al., 1996; McKerracher et al., 1994; Mukhopadhyay et al., 1994; Shafer et al., 1996) can be at least partly overcome (Berry et al., 1996). Identification of the cellular source and nature of the factor(s) that support RGC axon regeneration through the optic nerve are questions of considerable interest. One question raised by these findings is whether the enhancement of axonal regeneration past an injury site is secondary to increased cell survival. In agreement with others (Mansour-Robaey et al., 1994; Koeberle and Ball, 1998), we found that a puncture wound to the posterior chamber enhances cell survival in addition to axon regeneration. However, one indication that enhanced survival does not itself insure regeneration following optic nerve injury comes from studies in transgenic mice overexpressing the antiapoptotic gene bcl-2. Although bcl-2 overexpression almost completely prevents RGCs from undergoing cell death after optic nerve crush (Bonfanti et al., 1996), such animals show little or no axon growth past an optic nerve injury site, even when treated with antibodies to NI-250 (Nogo: Chierzi et al., 1998). Thus, additional factors must be responsible for inducing axon outgrowth.

VII. SUMMARY AND FUTURE DIRECTIONS

Regeneration of the optic nerve occurs spontaneously in lower vertebrates. This process appears to be triggered by molecules secreted by optic nerve glia, including the low molecular weight factor AF-1 and a polypeptide AF-3. Regeneration is marked by an upregulation of GAP-43 and other gene products required for the establishment of anatomically appropriate connections. Intracellularly, one of the key signal transduction steps involves a purine-sensitive kinase. Further details on the signal transduction cascade leading to axon regeneration and the expression of attendant gene products remain to be deciphered.

In mammals, although RGCs normally fail to regenerate injured axons, advances over the past 15 years indicate that this may not be insurmountable. Axon regeneration occurs readily through a peripheral nerve graft, and can even be stimulated to occur through the optic nerve itself when RGCs are exposed to appropriate signaling molecules. The identity of these factors is clearly an important question. However, with axon extension becoming more tractable, we will need to face another equally important question regarding axon guidance and target recognition during regeneration. Do the molecular signaling systems that enable RGC axons to find their correct targets get re-expressed after optic nerve injury? Some of the molecules likely to be important include cadherins (Riehl et al., 1996); L1-mediated axon guidance via FGF receptor signaling (Brittis et al., 1996); netrin-DCC interactions (Deiner et al., 1997); GAP-43 signaling in the ventral diencephalon (Kruger et al., 1998); ephrin-Eph receptor interactions that govern topographic organization in central targets (Nakamoto et al., 1996; Bähr and Wizenmann, 1996; Braisted et al., 1997; Frisén et al., 1998); and the machinery required for activity-dependent tuning of the retinal map upon its central targets, e.g., particular NMDA receptor subunits, growth factors and their receptors, and nitric oxide signaling mechanisms (Cramer et al., 1996; Shi et al., 1997; Schatz, 1997; Wu and Cline, 1998). While these all remain daunting questions, the possibility of restoring visual function after optic nerve injury seems considerably more possible than a decade ago.

ACKNOWLEDGMENTS: We are grateful to the National Eye Institute of NIH (NIH EY05690) and the Boston Neurosurgical Foundation who supported research from our group described in this chapter.

REFERENCES

Aguayo AJ, Rasminsky M, Bray GM, Carbonetto S, McKerracher L, Villegas-Perez MP, Vidal-Sanz M, Carter DA (1991) Degeneration and regeneration of injured neurons in the nervous system of adult mammals. Phil Trans Royal Soc London Ser B 331:337-343.

Alessi DR, Cuenda A, Cohen P, Dudley DT, Saltiel AR (1995) PD 098059 is a specific inhibitor of the activation of mitogen-activated protein kinase *in vitro* and *in vivo*. J Biol Chem 270:27489-27494.

Ballestero RP, Wilmot GR, Agranoff BW, Uhler MD (1997) gRICH68 and gRICH70 are 2',3' cyclic-nucleotide phosphodiesterases induced during goldfish optic nerve regeneration. J Biol Chem 272:11479-11486.

Bähr M, Wizenmann A (1996) Retinal ganglion cell axons recognize specific guidance cues present in the deafferented adult rat superior colliculus. J Neurosci 16:5106-5116.

Barres BA, Silverstein BE, Corey DP, Chun LLY (1988) Immunological, morphological, electrophysiological variation among retinal ganglion cells purified by panning. Neuron 1:791-803.

Bastmeyer M, Schlosshauer B, Stuermer CA (1990) The spatiotemporal distribution of N-CAM in the retinotectal pathway of adult goldfish detected by the monoclonal antibody D3. Development 108:299-311.

Batistatou A, Volonte C, Greene LA (1992) Nerve growth factor employs multiple pathways to induce primary response genes in PC12 cells. Molec Biol Cell 3:363-371.

Benowitz LI, Routtenberg A (1997) GAP-43: an intrinsic determinant of neural development and synaptic plasticity. Trends Neurosci 20:84-91.

Benowitz LI, Jing Y, Tabibiazar R, Jo SA, Petraush B, Stuermer CAO, Rosenberg PA, Irwin N (1998) Axon outgrowth is regulated by an intracellular purine-sensitive mechanism in retinal ganglion cells. J Biol Chem 273:29626-29634.

Benowitz LI, Lewis E (1983) Increased transport of 44-49,000 dalton acidic proteins during regeneration of the goldfish optic nerve, a 2-D gel analysis. J Neurosci 3:2153-2163.

Benowitz LI, Shashoua VE, Yoon MG (1981) Specific changes in rapidly-transported proteins during regeneration of the goldfish optic nerve. J Neurosci 1:300-307.

Bermingham-McDonogh O, McCabe KL, Reh TA (1996) Effects of GGF/Neuregulins on neuronal survival and neurite outgrowth correlates with erbB2/neu expression in developing rat retina. Development 122:1427-1438.

Bernhardt RR, Tongiorgi E, Anzini P, Schachner M (1998) Increased expression of specific recognition molecules by retinal ganglion cells and by optic pathway glia accompanies the successful regeneration of retinal axons in adult zebrafish. J Comp Neurol 376:353-364.

Berry M, Carlile J, Hunter A (1996) Peripheral nerve explants grafted into the vitreous body of the eye promote the regeneration of retinal ganglion cell axons severed in the optic nerve. J Neurocytol 25:147-170.

Blaugrund E, Sharma S, Schwartz M (1992) L1 immunoreactivity in the developing fish visual system. Brain Res 574:244-250.

Bormann P, Zumsteg VM, Roth LW, Reinhard E (1998) Target contact regulates GAP-43 and alpha-tubulin mRNA levels in regenerating retinal ganglion cells. J Neurosci Res 52:405-419.

Braisted JE, McLaughlin T, Wang HU, Friedman GC, Anderson DJ, O'Leary DD (1997) Graded and lamina-specific distributions of EphB receptor tyrosine kinases in the developing retinotectal system. Dev Biol 191:14-28.

Brittis PA, Silver J, Walsh FS, Doherty P (1996) Fibroblast growth factor receptor function is required for the orderly projection of ganglion cell axons in the development mammalian retina. Molec Cell Neurosci 8:120-128.

Burnstock G (1990) Purinergic mechanisms. Ann NY Acad Sci 603:1-617.

Carmignoto G, Maffei L, Candeo P, Canella R, Comelli C (1989) Effect of NGF on the survival of rat retinal ganglion cells following optic nerve section. J Neurosci 9:1263-1272.

Caroni P, Schwab M (1988a) Two membrane protein fractions from rat central myelin with inhibitory properties for neurite growth and fibroblast spreading. J Cell Biol 106:1281-1288.

Cho EYP, So KF (1992) Characterization of the sprouting response of axon-like processes from retinal ganglion cells after axotomy in adult hamters: a model using intravitreal implantation of a preripheral nerve. J Neurocytol 21:589-603.

Cohen A, Bray GM, Aguayo AJ (1994) Neurotrophin-4/5 (NT-4/5) increases adult rat retinal ganglion cell survival and neurite outgrowth in vitro. J Neurobiol 25:953-959.

Collis MG, Jacobson KA, Tomkins DM (1987) Apparent affinity of some 8-phenyl-substituted xanthines at adenosine receptors in guinea-pig aorta and atria. Brit J Pharmacol 92:69-75.

Cowley S, Paterson H, Kemp P, Marshall CJ (1994) Activation of MAP kinase is necessary and sufficient for PC12 cell differentiation and for transformation of NIH 3T3 cells. Cell 77:841-852.

Cramer KS, Angelucci A, Hahm JO, Bogdanov MB, Sur M (1996) A role for nitric oxide in the development of the ferret retinogeniculate projection. J Neurosci 16:7995-8004.

David S, Jackson DL, Kottis V, Dunn RJ, Braun PE (1994) Identification of myelin-associated glycoprotein as a major myelin- derived inhibitor of neurite growth. Neuron 13:805-811.

Deiner MS, Kennedy TE, Fazeli A, Serafini T, Tessier-Lavigne M, Sretavan DW (1997) Netrin-1 and DCC mediate axon guidance locally at the optic disc: loss of function leads to optic nerve hypoplasia. Neuron 19:575-589.

Doherty P, Smith P, Walsh FS (1996) Shared cell adhesion molecule (CAM) homology domains point to CAMs signaling via FGF receptors. Perspectives on Dev Neurobiol 4:157-168.

Doster SK, Lozano AM, Aguayo AJ, Willard MB (1991) Expression of the growth-associated protein GAP-43 in adult rat retinal ganglion cells following axon injury. Neuron 6:635-647.

Dowling JE (1987) The Retina: An Approachable Part of the Brain Belknap. Cambridge, MA.

Faktorovich EG, Steinberg RH, Yasumura D, Matthes MT, LaVail MM (1992) Basic fibroblast growth factor and local injury protect photoreceptors from light damage in the rat. J Neurosci 12:3554-3567.

Frisén J, Yates PA, McLaughlin T, Friedman GC, O'Leary DDM, Barbacid M (1998) Ephrin-A5 (AL-1/RAGS) is essential for proper retinal axon guidance and topographic mapping in the mammalian visual system. Neuron 20:235-243.

Glasgow E, Druger RK, Levine EM, Fuchs C, Schechter N (1992) Plasticin, a novel type III neurofilament protein from goldfish retina: increased expression during optic nerve regeneration. Neuron 9:373-381.

Glasgow E, Druger RK, Fuchs C, Lane WS, Schechter N (1994) Molecular cloning of gefiltin (ON1): serial expression of two new neurofilament mRNAs during optic nerve regeneration. EMBO J 13:297-305.

Grafstein, B (1986) The retina as a regenerating organ, In R. Adler D.B. Farber (Eds.), The Retina: A Model for Cell Biology Studies Part II. Academic Press, NY: 275-335.

Greene LA, Volonte C, Chalazonitis A (1990) Purine analogs inhibit nerve growth factor-promoted neurite outgrowth by sympathetic and sensory neurons. J Neurosci 10:1479-1485.

Greene LA, Kaplan DR (1995) Early events in neurotrophin signalling via Trk and p75 receptors. Curr Opin Neurobiol 5:579-587.

He Q, Dent EW, Meiri KF (1997) Modulation of actin filament behavior by GAP-43 (neuromodulin) is dependent on the phosphorylation status of serine 41, the protein kinase C site. J Neurosci 17:3515-3524.

Heacock AM, Agranoff B (1982) Protein synthesis and transport in the regenerating goldfish visual system. Neurochem Res 7:771-788.

Herdegen T, Bastmeyer M, Bahr M, Stuermer C, Bravo R, Zimmerman M (1993) Expression of jun, krox, and CREB transcription factors in goldfish and rat retinal ganglion cells following optic nerve lesion is related to axonal sprouting. J Neurobiol 24:528-543.

Hopkins JM, Ford-Holevinski TS, McCoy JP, Agranoff BW (1985) Laminin and optic nerve regeneration in the goldfish. J Neurosci 5:3030-3038.

Hull M, Bähr M (1994) Regulation of immediate-early gene expression in rat retinal ganglion cells after axotomy and during regeneration through a peripheral nerve graft. J Neurobiol 25:92-105.

Jacobson, M (1991) Developmental Neurobiology (3rd edition). Plenum Publishing, NY.

Jo SA, Wang E, Benowitz L (1999) CNTF is an endogenous axon regeneration factor for mammalian retinal ganglion cells. Neuroscience 89:579-591.

Johnson J, Barde YA, Schwab M, Thoenen H (1986) BDNF supports survival of cultured rat retinal ganglion cells. J Neurosci 6:3031-3038.

Jung M, Petrausch B, Stuermer CA (1997) Axon-regenerating retinal ganglion cells in adult rats synthesize the cell adhesion molecule L1 but not TAG-1 or SC-1. Molecular and Cellular Neurosciences 9:116-131.

Kimura K, Hattori S, Kabuyama Y, Shizawa Y, Takayanagi J, Nakamura S, Toki S, Matsuda Y, Onodera K, Fukui Y (1994) Neurite outgrowth of PC12 cells is suppressed by wortmannin, a specific inhibitor of phosphatidylinositol-3 kinase. J Biol Chem 269:18961-18967.

Kita Y, Kimura KD, Kobayashi M, Ihara S, Kaibuchi K, Kuroda S, Ui M, Iba H, Konishi H, Kikkawa U, Nagata S, Fukui Y (1998) Microinjection of activated phosphatidylinositol-3 kinase induces process outgrowth in rat PC12 cells through the Rac-JNK signal transduction pathway. J Cell Sci 111:907-915.

Koeberle PD, Ball AK (1998) Effects of GDNF on retinal ganglion cell survival following axotomy. Vis Res 38:1505-1515.

Kruger K, Tam AS, Lu C, Sretavan DW (1998) Retinal ganglion cell axon progression from the optic chiasm to initiate optic tract development requires cell autonomous function of GAP-43. J Neurosci 18:5692-5705.

Landreth GE, Agranoff BW (1976) Explant culture of adult goldfish retina: effect of prior optic nerve crush. Brain Res 118:299-303.

Landreth GE, Agranoff BW (1979) Explant culture of adult goldfish retina: a model for the study of CNS regeneration. Brain Res 161:39-53.

Lau KC, So KF, Tay D (1994) Intravitreal transplantation of a segment of peripheral nerve enhances axonal regeneration of retinal ganglion cells following distal axotomy. Exp Neurol 128:211-215.

Lavie Y, Dybowski J, Agranoff BW (1997) Wortmannin blocks goldfish retinal phosphatidylinositol-3 kinase and neurite outgrowth. Neurochem Res 22:373-378.

Li M, Shibata A, Li C, Braun PE, McKerracher L, Roder J, Kater SB, David S (1996) Myelin-associated glycoprotein inhibits neurite/axon growth and causes growth cone collapse. J Neurosci Res 46:404-414.

Mansour-Robaey S, Clarke DB, Wang Y-C, Bray GM, Aguayo A (1994) Effects of ocular injury and administration of brain-derived neurotrophic factor on survival and regrowth of axotomized retinal ganglion cells. Proc Natl Acad Sci (USA) 91:1632-1636.

McKerracher L, David S, Jackson DL, Kottis V, Dunn RJ, Braun PE (1994) Identification of myelin-associated glycoprotein as a major myelin-derived inhibitor of neurite outgrowth. Neuron 13:805-811.

McKerracher L, Roder J, Kater SB, David S (1996) Myelin-associated glycoprotein inhibits neurite/axon growth and causes growth cone collapse. J Neurosci Res 46:404-414.

Mey J, Thanos S (1993) Intravitreal injections of neurotrophic factors support the survival of axotomized retinal ganglion cells in adult rats in vivo. Brain Res 602:304-317.

Meyer RL, Miotke JA, Benowitz LI (1994) Injury induced expression of growth-associated protein-43 in adult mouse retinal ganglion cells in vitro. Neuroscience 63:591-602.

Meyer-Franke A, Laplan MR, Pfrieger FW, Barres BA (1995) Characterization of the signaling interaction that promotes the survival and growth of developing retinal ganglion cells in culture. Neuron 15:805-819.

Moya KL, Benowitz LI, Jhaveri S, Schneider GE (1988) Changes in rapidly-transported proteins in developing hamster retinofugal axons. J Neurosci 8:4445-4454.

Mukhopadhyay G, Doherty P, Walsh FS, Crocker PR, Filbin MT (1994) A novel role for myelin-associated glycoprotein as an inhibitor or axonal regeneration. Neuron 13:757-767.

Murray M, Grafstein B (1969) Changes in the morphology and amino acid incorporation in regenerating goldfish optic neurons. Exp Neurol 23:544-560.

Nakamoto M, Cheng H-J, Friedman GC, McLaughlin T, Hansen JJ, Yoon CH, O'Leary DDM, Flanagan JG (1996) Topographically specific effects of Elf-1 on retinal axon guidance in vitro and retinal mapping in vivo. Cell 86:755-766.

Neve RL, Coopersmith R, McPhie DL, Santeufemio C, Pratt KG, Murphy CJ, Lynn SD (1998) The neuronal growth-associated protein GAP-43 interacts with rabaptin-5 and participates in endocytosis. J Neurosci 18:7757-7767.

Ng TF, So KF, Chung S (1995) Influence of peripheral nerve grafts on the expression of GAP-43 in regenerating retinal ganglion cells in adult hamsters. J Neurocytol 24:487-496.

Ott H, Bastmeyer M, Stuermer CAO (1998) Neurolin, the goldfish homolog of DM-GRASP, is involved in retinal axon pathfinding to the optic disk. J Neurosci 18:3363-3372.

Paschke KA, Lottspeich F, Stuermer CAO (1992) Neurolin, a cell surface glycoprotein on growing retinal axons in the goldfish visual system is re-expressed during retinal axonal regeneration. J Cell Biol 117:863-875.

Perry GW, Burmeister DW, Grafstein B (1987) Fast axonally transported proteins in regenerating goldfish optic axons. J Neurosci 7:792-806.

Quitschke W, Schechter N (1983) Specific optic nerve proteins during regeneration of the goldfish retinotectal pathway. Brain Res 258:69-78.

Rabacchi SA, Ensini M, Bonfanti L, Gravina A, Maffei L (1994) Nerve growth factor reduces apoptosis of axotomized retinal ganglion cells in the neonatal rat. Neuroscience 63:969-973.

Ramon Y, Cajal S (1928) Degeneration and regeneration in the nervous system. Tr: J De-Filipe and EG Jones, Oxford University Press, NY, 1991.

Riehl R, Johnson K, Bradley R, Grunwald GB, Cornel E, Lilienbaum A, Holt CE (1996) Cadherin function is required for axon outgrowth in retinal ganglion cells in vivo. Neuron 17:837-848.

Rodriguez-Tebar A, Jeffrey PL, Thoenen H, Barde YA (1989) The survival of chick retinal ganglion cells in response to brain derived neurotrophic factor depends on their embryonic age. Dev Biol 136:296-303.

Schaden H, Stuermer CA, Bahr M (1994) GAP-43 immunoreactivity and axon regeneration in retinal ganglion cells of the rat. J Neurobiol 35:1570-1578.

Schafer M, Fruttiger M, Montag D, Schachner M, Martini R (1996) Disruption of the gene for the myelin-associated glycoprotein improves axonal regrowth along myelin in C57BL/Wlds mice. Neuron 16:1107-1113.

Schulte T, Paschke KA, Laessing U, Lottspeich F, Stuermer CA (1997) Reggie-1 and reggie-2, two cell surface proteins expressed by retinal ganglion cells during axon regeneration. Development 124(2):577-587.

Schulz M, Raju T, Ralston G, Bennett MR (1990) A retinal ganglion cell neurotrophic factor purified from the superior colliculus. J Neurochem 55:832-841.

Schwalb JM, Boulis NM, Gu M-F, Winickoff J, Jackson PS, Irwin N, Benowitz LI (1995) Two factors secreted by the goldfish optic nerve induce retinal ganglion cells to regenerate axons in culture. J Neurosci 15:5514-5525.

Schwalb JM, Gu M-f, Stuermer CAO, Bastmeyer M, Hu G-f, Boulis NM, Irwin N, Benowitz LI (1996) Optic nerve glia secrete a low molecular weight factor that stimulates retinal ganglion cells to regenerate axons in goldfish. Neuroscience 72:901-910.

Segal RA, Greenberg ME (1996) Intracellular signaling pathways activated by neurotrophic factors. Ann Rev Neurosci 19:463-489.

Shatz CJ (1997) Emergence of order in visual system development. Proc Natl Acad Sci (USA) 93:602-608.

Shi J, Aamodt SM, Constantine-Paton M (1997) Temporal correlations between functional and molecular changes in NMDA receptors and GABA neurotransmission in the superior colliculus. J Neurosci 17:6264-6276.

Skene JHP, Willard M (1981) Changes in axonally transported proteins during axon regeneration in toad retinal ganglion cells. J Cell Biol 89:86-95.

So KF, Aguayo AJ (1985) Lengthy regrowth of cut axons from ganglion cells after peripheral transplantation into the retina of adult rats. Brain Res 328:349-354.

Sperry RW (1963) Chemoaffinity in the orderly growth of nerve fiber patterns and connections. Proc Natl Acad Sci USA 50:703-710.

Strittmater SM, Frankhauser C, Huang PL, Mashimo H, Fishman MC (1995) Neuronal pathfinding is abnormal in mice lacking the neuronal growth cone protein GAP-43. Cell 80:445-452.

Thanos S, Bahr M, Barde YA, Vanselow J (1989) Survival and axonal elongation of adult rat retinal ganglion cells: in vitro effects of lesioned sciatic nerve and brain derived neurotrophic factor (BDNF). Eur J Neurosci 1:19-26.

Vielmetter J, Lottspeich F, Stuemer CA (1991) The monoclonal antibody E587 recognizes growing (new and regenerating) retinal axons in the goldfish retinotectal pathway. J Neurosci 11:3581-3593.

Volonte C, Rukenstein A, Loeb DM, Greene LA (1989) Differential inhibition of nerve growth factor responses by purine analogues: correlation with inhibition of a nerve growth factor-activated protein kinase. J Cell Biol 109:2395-2403.

Wen R, Song Y, Cheng T, Matthes MT, Yasumura D, LaVail MM (1995) Injury-induced upregulation of bFGF and CNTF mRNAs in the rat retina. J Neurosci 15:7377-7385.

Weibel D, Cadelli D, Schwab ME (1994) Regeneration of lesioned rat optic nerve fibers is improved after neutralization of myelin-associated neurite growth inhibitors. Brain Res 642:259-266.

Wigley CB, Berry M (1988) Regeneration of adult rat retinal ganglion cell processees in monolayer culture: comparisons between cultures of adult and neonatal neurons. Dev Brain Res 42:85-98.

Wilmot GR, Raymond PA, Agranoff BW (1993) The expression of the protein p68/70 within the goldfish visual system suggests a role in both regeneration and neurogenesis. J Neurosci 13:387-401.

Wu GY, Cline HT (1998) Stabilization of dendritic arbor structure in vivo by CaMKII. Science 279:222-226.

3

Regeneration of Axons in the CNS of Amphibians and Reptiles

Lynda D. Beazley
University of Western Australia, Nedlands, Australia

I. INTRODUCTION

This chapter concerns axonal regeneration in the central nervous system of amphibians and reptiles. It concentrates on the primary visual system and in particular on events in the retina, visual pathway and primary visual centers during optic nerve regeneration. Amphibians, both Urodeles (salamanders and newts) and Anurans (frogs and toads), have been popular experimental models for such studies since their capacity for optic nerve regeneration was first described (Matthey, 1925). Optic nerve regeneration takes place in some reptiles also but has been studied far less extensively than in amphibians and differs in some key respects. In contrast to the optic nerve, other parts of the amphibian and reptilian central nervous systems undergo little or no axonal regeneration. Examples in frog are tectal efferents (*Rana pipiens*: Lyon and Stelzner, 1987), the spinal cord (*Xenopus laevis*: Michel and Reier, 1979; Clarke et al., 1986) and dorsal root ganglia regenerating within the spinal cord (*X. laevis,* Katzenstein and Bohn, 1984). As exceptions, spinal cord regeneration takes place in premetamorphic frog (*X. laevis:* Beattie et al., 1990) and to a lesser extent in adult lizard (*Anolis carolinensis,* Simpson, 1968).

II. OVERVIEW OF OPTIC NERVE REGENERATION

A. The Lesion Procedure-*The type and location of the nerve lesion influence the outcome of regeneration. The most common procedure is extracranial nerve crush, severing all axons but leaving the nerve sheath intact as a conduit for regeneration.*

Axons are usually severed by crushing the optic nerve with forceps. Alternatives include cryosurgery (*Vipera aspis:* Rio et al., 1989) or cutting, a procedure that severs the nerve sheath as well as the axons allowing them to escape from the visual pathway (*Rana temporaria:* Gaze and Jacobson, 1963; *X. laevis:* Bohn et al., 1982; *R. pipiens*: Blanco and Orkand, 1996). As in mammals, necrosis within the distal nerve segment is probably more extensive after a cut than a crush (rat: Berkelaar et al., 1994).

Lesions are usually performed extracranially, approaching the nerve via the orbit or the roof of the mouth; for intracranial lesions, the approach is again via the mouth with the bone overlying the nerve being deflected or removed. The nerve sheath is tough extracranially; it survives nerve crush and acts as a conduit for regrowing axons. Intracranially, the thin nerve sheath is often torn by nerve crush, allowing axons to escape. As a result, regeneration is more reliable after extracranial than intracranial nerve crush (*R. temporaria:* Gaze and Jacobson, 1963; *Litoria (Hyla) moorei:* Humphrey and Beazley, 1982, 1983). Unlike mammals, in amphibians and reptiles, the ocular blood supply is external to the optic nerve and is readily avoided during surgery. Regeneration has also been studied after transection of the optic chiasm (*R. pipiens:* Waldeck and Gruberg, 1995) or optic tract (*X. laevis:* Bohn and Reier, 1982; Szaro et al., 1985). In Urodeles, optic nerve regeneration takes place even after destruction of the retina. A new retina is generated from the retinal pigment epithelium and optic axons regrow into the brain (*Triturus viridescens:* Burgen and Grafstein, 1962; Gaze and Watson, 1964; Cronly-Dillon, 1968).

B. Outcomes of Optic Nerve Regeneration-*Optic axons regenerate to visual centers and form a topographically ordered projection in frogs but not in lizards*

In amphibians severed optic axons regenerate along the visual pathway within 1-3 months. Axons reenter visual centers, reestablish topographically ordered projections and vision is restored (reviewed by Sperry, 1951; Gaze, 1960, 1970; Beazley 1984). Optic nerve regeneration in reptiles is less successful and seems to vary between species. For example, in the gecko *Nephrurus stellatus* axons do not regenerate beyond the lesion site (Beazley et al., 1999) and in the viper snake regeneration is protracted and limited in extent (*V. aspis:* Rio et al., 1989). By contrast, in a lizard, *Ctenophorus ornatus*, many optic axons regenerate to visual centers within 2 months of nerve crush. However, in the long term, the central projections lack topographic order and animals are functionally blind (Beazley et al., 1997; Stirling et al., 1999).

III. CELL SURVIVAL AND CELL DEATH

A. Ganglion Cell Death-*Many ganglion cells die after axotomy in frogs and lizard, apparently by apoptosis*

The early anatomical and behavioural studies of optic nerve regeneration in fish and amphibians (Matthey, 1925; Sperry, 1943, 1944) described substantial axonal regrowth into the brain. The robust regeneration observed, along with the restoration of vision, led to the assumption that the vast majority of ganglion cells survive axotomy and regenerate their axons. However, the retina and optic nerve were not studied in sufficient detail to address the issue. The assumption has proved to be true for goldfish (Murray et al., 1982) but not for frogs or lizards. The question of ganglion cell death induced by axotomy has yet to be addressed in Urodeles.

In other systems, both neural and nonneural, injured cells die by necrosis or apoptosis (Wyllie et al., 1980). Necrotic cells swell before death, due to the entry of water, whereas apoptotic cells become pyknotic. The appearance of dying ganglion cells after optic nerve lesion in frogs or lizards suggests that death is by apoptosis. DNA electrophoresis and DNA fragmentation using the TdT-dUTP terminal nick-end labelling (TUNEL) have yet to confirm that, in frogs and lizards, as in mammals (rat: Berkelaar et al., 1994; monkey: Quigley et al., 1995), axotomised ganglion cells die by apoptosis.

B. The Extent of Cell Survival and Cell Death-*In frogs, 30-60% of ganglion cells die after axotomy; about one third do so in lizards. By contrast, cell numbers remain stable in other retinal populations such as displaced amacrine cells and cells of the inner nuclear layer*

Retinal ganglion cell numbers, estimated from retinal wholemounts, usually fall by 30-60% within 2-3 months of optic nerve lesion in frogs (*X. laevis:* Beazley, 1981; Jenkins and Straznicky, 1986; *L. moorei:* Humphrey and Beazley, 1985; *R. pipiens:* Scalia et al., 1985; Beazley et al., 1986; Stelzner and Strauss 1986). In lizards, counts were undertaken in sectioned material due to the multi-layered nature of the ganglion cell layer. Values were found to be reduced by approximately one third at one year after nerve crush; shorter time intervals have yet to be examined (*C. ornatus:* Beazley et al., 1997).

It seems likely that the reductions observed represent the absolute extent of ganglion cell loss during optic nerve regeneration. Autoradiographic studies have shown that there is no compensatory generation of retinal ganglion cells in frogs to replace dying ganglion cells (*R. pipiens:* Gruberg and Stirling, 1974; *L. moorei:*

Pedalina and Beazley, 1986). Similarly, retinal cell generation is presumed to be absent from lizards during optic nerve regeneration. It can be assumed therefore that 40-70% of ganglion cells usually survive axotomy and regenerate their axons in frogs and lizard whilst the remainder die.

Although the vast majority of ganglion cell somata lie in the ganglion cell layer, in both amphibians and lizards as in other vertebrates studied (Ramon y Cajal, 1892), a small proportion lie in the inner nuclear layer (*R. pipiens:* Frank and Hollyfield, 1987; Singman and Scalia, 1990a; *L. moorei:* Dunlop et al., 1992; *C. ornatus:* Starac et al., 1996). These are termed Dogiel or displaced ganglion cells. In both frogs and lizards many Dogiel cells project to the basal optic nucleus, part of the accessory optic system (*R. pipiens*: Montgomery et al., 1981; *C. ornatus:* Dunlop and Beazley, unpublished observations). Retrograde transport of neuronal tracers in frogs and lizards has shown that comparable proportions of displaced and orthotopic ganglion cells survive optic nerve regeneration (*L. moorei:* Dunlop et al., 1992; *C. ornatus,* Dunlop and Beazley, unpublished observations).

Within other neural systems, cell death in one cell population can in turn trigger losses from cells afferent (Tong et al., 1982) and efferent to it (Cowan, 1973). However, unlike primates (Gills and Wadsworth, 1967), frogs or lizard do not display such changes as a result of ganglion cell death. Displaced amacrine cells are axonless cells with somata in the ganglion cell layer and processes contacting ganglion cells (Perry, 1981). Counts from retinal sections and wholemounts indicate that these interneurons, representing 10-20% of the cells in the ganglion cell layer of normal frogs and lizards, survive optic nerve regeneration (*L. moorei:* Humphrey and Beazley, 1985; *R. pipiens*: Singman and Scalia, 1990b; *C. ornatus*: Beazley et al., 1997). Moreover, cell counts of sectioned retinae in frogs suggest that the inner nuclear layer, the layer containing cells afferent to ganglion cells, also maintains a full cell complement (*L. moorei*: Darby et al., 1990). It is unclear whether depletion of the ganglion cell population during optic nerve regeneration leads anterogradely to the death of retinorecipient cells in primary visual centers of frogs or lizards.

C. Survival of Ganglion Cell Classes-*Ganglion cells of each class survive and undergo axonal regeneration in frogs*

Frogs, as with other vertebrates including mammals (cat: Wassle et al., 1981), possess several classes of ganglion cells each with distinct morphologies (plethodontid salamanders: Linke and Roth, 1989; *R. pipiens*: Pomeranz, 1971; Frank and Hollyfield, 1987; *X. laevis:* Sakuguchi et al., 1984; Straznicky and Straznicky, 1988; Toth and Straznicky, 1989) and electrophysiological properties (*R. temporaria:* Gaze et al., 1965; *R. pipiens*: Maturana et al., 1960). Moreover, ganglion cells can be defined as either 'on' or 'off' cells to reflect their center/surround response properties (cat: Famiglietti and Kolb,1976). The dendrites of 'on' ganglion cells terminate in the inner part of the inner plexiform layer, and those of 'off' cells in the outer part. In addition, distinct immuno-reactivities are seen amongst the ganglion cell population in frogs (*R. pipiens:* Kuljis and Karten, 1982; *L. moorei:* Humphrey et al., 1995) although the relationship to the classically defined classes is uncertain.

Electrophysiological recording of visual input to the optic tectum, the major primary visual center, has revealed that ganglion cells of each class survive regeneration (*R. temporaria*: Keating and Gaze, 1970). It is unclear whether they do so to comparable extents or whether the dendrites of 'on' and 'off' cells retain the characteristic sublaminar distributions in the inner plexiform layer (*R. pipiens:* Frank and Hollyfield 1987).

Ganglion cells with distinct immuno-reactivities survive regeneration (*L. moorei:* Humphrey et al., 1995). At one juncture, it seemed that in the frog *R. pipiens* ganglion cells with substance P-like immuno-reactivity survive optic nerve regeneration but those with other profiles such as bombesin and leucine-enkephalin do not (Kuljis and Karten, 1985). In reaching their conclusion, the authors compared the appearance of the tectum at 99 days after deafferentation (Kuljis and Karten, 1983) with that of 270 days after optic nerve crush. However, as discussed by Humphrey and his colleagues (1995), the findings of Kuljis and Karten (1985) agree with the study in *L. moorei* and indicate the survival of each immunocytochemically defined ganglion cell class. Kuljis and Karten had not allowed for the protracted survival to 99 days of disconnected distal segments of severed optic axons in the deafferented tectum (Section V.V; *R. esculenta:* Lazar, 1980, *R. pipiens:* Matsumoto and Scalia, 1981; *L. moorei:* Humphrey et al., 1992).

Little is known of ganglion cell classes or their responses during optic nerve regeneration in lizards.

IV. RETINAL RESPONSES DURING OPTIC NERVE REGENERATION

The retina responds to optic nerve lesion in several ways. Ganglion cells change their metabolism to initiate regeneration of a new distal axonal segment and retinal rewiring takes place to counteract the loss of ganglion cells. Coincidentally, transient changes take place within the retinal vasculature.

A. Metabolic Changes Within Ganglion Cells-*Axotomised ganglion cells undergo a cell soma reaction, indicating an increased protein synthesis. The appearance is transient in frogs but permanent in lizard. Most of the proteins synthesized are axonally transported.*

All axotomised ganglion cells in frogs (*R. pipiens*: Humphrey, 1988) and lizards (*C. ornatus:* Beazley et al., 1997) exhibit a cell soma reaction (Soreide, 1981), an appearance that is also termed chromatolysis and reflects increased protein synthesis. In frogs, the appearance persists for weeks or months, until optic axon regeneration is complete and stable connections are reestablished in visual brain centers

(Section **IX.A**). The retinal response differs in lizards, however, with ganglion cells continuing to exhibit an intense cell soma reaction even at the longest time interval studied, more than a year after nerve crush (*C. ornatus:* Beazley et al., 1997). Presumably ganglion cell somata continue to undertake abnormally high levels of protein synthesis to form new terminals that search for but do not recognise appropriate postsynaptic partners (Section **IX.A**).

The profile of protein synthesis during optic nerve regeneration is best understood for fish (goldfish: Grafstein, 1967; Barron et al., 1985) but has also been documented in frogs (*X. laevis:* Szaro et al., 1984, 1985). Proteins were labelled with ^{35}S-methionine injected into the eye and their transport tracked autoradiographically. In addition, two-dimensional gel separation identified proteins present in the regenerating but not in the normal nerve. Some of these proteins, which may correspond to ones found in the regenerating optic nerve of goldfish (Benowitz et al., 1981), were in the fastest transported group but others were components of the intermediate and slow groups. No comparable studies have yet been undertaken for reptiles. The production of cytoskeletal proteins is discussed in Section **V.B.**

B. Long-term Structural Changes in the Ganglion Cell Population- *Reflecting ganglion cell losses, densities of surviving cells are reduced across the retina. Somata are hypertrophied and dendritic trees are remodelled.*

The ganglion cell layer of frogs and lizards is abnormal in several respects after optic nerve regeneration. One change is that the layer contains abnormally few ganglion cells. These cells are usually identified by retrograde labelling or by their characteristic morphology. Analyses of wholemounted and sectioned retinae have shown that surviving ganglion cells are present at reduced densities across the retina (*R. pipiens*: Scalia et al., 1985; Stelzner and Strauss, 1986; Beazley et al., 1986; *L. moorei*: Humphrey and Beazley, 1985; *C. ornatus:* Beazley et al., 1997). Another abnormality is that, although chromatolysis is transient in frogs, the surviving ganglion cells remain somewhat enlarged in the long term (*R. pipiens*: Humphrey, 1988; Stelzner and Strauss, 1988). Presumably the increased size reflects the greater metabolic demands placed on each ganglion cell within the depleted population. In lizards, ganglion cells remain chromatolysed in the long term, a further indication that regeneration does not reach a stable endpoint (Section **IX.A**).

In the frog *R. pipiens,* the somata of about 5% of the surviving ganglion cells become displaced towards the inner plexiform layer during optic nerve regeneration (*R. pipiens:* Scalia et al., 1985; Singman and Scalia, 1990a). The displacement is thought to involve migration of the nucleus and some somal contents rather than cell motility and is presumably linked at least in part to the removal of dying ganglion cells. It seems likely that the change is most marked in species, such as *R. pipiens,* that undergo particularly extensive ganglion cell death.

The surviving ganglion cells in both frogs and lizards are presumed to undergo dendritic hypertrophy to compensate for their depleted numbers. The change has been quantified only for large ganglion cells in frogs (*X. laevis:* Straznicky, 1988). Changes in retinal wiring may also extend to axons. It is unclear whether in frogs and lizards optic axons form intraretinal collateral sprouts following optic nerve lesion as have been demonstrated in goldfish by filling individual cells with fluorescent dye (Becker and Cooke, 1990). However, the frog *X. laevis* develops a permanent swirl of neuritic processes around the optic nerve head after section of the optic nerve or tract (Bohn and Reier, 1982). The ultrastructural appearance suggests the swirl is comprised of axon collaterals; their functional impact is unknown. Equivalent investigations have yet to be carried out in lizard.

C. Nonneural Changes–*A transient episode of retinal neovascularisation takes place in frog, presumably triggered by the degeneration of ganglion cells and their axons.*

Retinal changes after optic nerve lesion are not confined to neurons. In frog, the retina receives a vascular bed via the hyaloid artery. A transient neovascularisation of the bed after optic nerve crush has been demonstrated by transcardial perfusion of India ink (*L. moorei:* Tennant et al., 1993). The time course of the neovascularisation matches that of ganglion cell death, suggesting that angiogenesis is triggered by the dying cells themselves or the phagocytosing cells attracted to them. Thus the transient vessels are most numerous in areas with the greatest numbers of dying ganglion cell somata and of axons, namely the area centralis and the optic nerve head respectively. The abnormal vasculature is likely to lead to a breakdown of the blood-retinal barrier. The importance of this abnormality on the survival or death of ganglion cells is unknown. The retinal vasculature in lizards is contained within a *conus capillaris*; its response to optic nerve lesion has yet to be investigated although macroscopically it appears unchanged (*C. ornatus:* Beazley et al., 1997; *N. stellatus:* Beazley et al., 1999).

Changes within the macroglial population of the retina after axotomy have yet to be studied in amphibians or reptiles. However, the beds of microglia present in the inner and outer plexiform layers appear to remain unchanged throughout optic nerve regeneration in frogs (*R. pipiens,* L.D. Beazley and V.H. Perry unpublished observations).

V. THE REGENERATING AXON

During optic nerve regeneration, axonal sprouts form at the lesion site or elsewhere and one or more sprouts per axon regrow into the brain. To do so, new membrane and cytoskeletal proteins must be produced. If regeneration is to reach completion, excess sprouts must be lost and axons that were previously myelinated must become remyelinated.

A. Axonal Sprouting-*Extensive axonal sprouting takes place transiently in some species of frog but not others. Sprouting is thought to persist in lizards.*

During regeneration of the optic nerve in goldfish (Murray, 1982) and in mammalian peripheral nerves (Perry et al., 1987), each regenerating axon produces several sprouts. In the long term, only one sprout survives, enlarging to become the regenerated portion of the axon. Similarly, large numbers of axonal sprouts are present in the regenerating optic nerve of the frog *R. pipiens* (Scott and Foote, 1981). Counts of these axonal profiles indicate that sprouts form both between the eye and the crush site and to an even greater extent at and beyond it (*R. pipiens*: Stelzner and Strauss, 1986). Excess sprouts are removed only at a stage when projections have consolidated in primary visual centers.

However, a recent study of optic nerve regeneration in the frog *L. moorei* suggests a different sequence of events in this species. Counts of axonal profiles and of retrogradely labelled ganglion cells, as well as an analysis of the morphology of individual axons, suggests that there are few if any excess sprouts at any point along the visual pathway (Dunlop et al., submitted for publication). Rather, it seems that each severed axon that regenerates forms a growth cone close to the crush site and the single process regenerates into the brain. Reasons for the differing results in the two species are as yet unclear.

In lizards the extent of axonal sprouting throughout optic nerve regeneration has yet to be documented. Preliminary findings from our laboratory suggest that growth associated protein (GAP)-43, an indicator of axon growth, is limited to the crush site at early stages of regeneration (Bartlett et al., in preparation). The result suggests that axons regrow from the crush site and do not sprout extensively further back towards the eye. In the long term, numbers of axon profiles between the crush site and the brain exceed the numbers of ganglion cells and of axons behind the eye by one third (*C. ornatus:* Beazley, 1997). Presumably at least some of the excess profiles represent long persisting axonal sprouts arising at or beyond the crush site.

B. Regeneration-Associated Protein Expression-*Expression of membrane proteins is upregulated during optic nerve regeneration. There is also increased expression of neurofilament proteins to build a new cytoskeleton. In frogs the expression is progressive and is probably coordinated by cues along the visual pathway. In lizards, expression of the neurofilament protein gefiltin is upregulated permanently.*

The regenerating axon must produce new membranes as it grows. In a study of the *X. laevis* tadpoles, a monoclonal antibody (Mab5) specific to the neuronal cell surface protein neuropilin (formerly referred to as A5) was used to detect expression of the protein during optic nerve regeneration. As in early stages of development, the protein is present in optic axons during regeneration; levels fall again as regeneration reaches completion (Fujisawa et al., 1996). The protein may be involved during development in neuronal cell interactions (Satoda et al., 1995) and/or neuronal recognition (Fujisawa et al., 1989) but its role during regeneration is uncertain.

Axonal regrowth also requires the production of a new cytoskeleton. Immuno-cytochemical studies using antibodies characterised in Western blots of the optic nerve in the frog *X. laevis* have revealed a progressive pattern of expression of the neurofilament proteins XNIF, NF-L, NF-H and NF-M. The regenerative sequence is reminiscent of, but not identical to, that found during development (*X. laevis:* Charnas et al., 1992; Zhao and Szaro, 1994, 1995). Moreover, certain phosphorylated forms are expressed only after regenerating axons reach the tectum. The result suggests that cues along the pathway coordinate neurofilament expression.

The possibility of such coordination has been supported by further studies of these neurofilament proteins and of another, xefiltin, present in *X. laevis*. Xefiltin (Zhao and Szaro, 1997a) is found in growth cones and is closely related to α-internexin and an intermediate filament present in goldfish, namely gefiltin (Glasgow et al., 1994). The expression of xefiltin (Zhao and Szaro, 1995, 1997b) is virtually identical to that of the neurofilament proteins described previously (Zhao and Szaro, 1994). Moreover, the expression of these neurofilament proteins was examined in two abnormal pathways, the retinoretinal projection (Section **VII. B**) and optic axons deprived of their major target by bilateral tectal ablation (Zhao and Szaro, 1995, 1997b). Expression of xefiltin, NF-H and the phosphorylated form of NF-M, was found to be reduced in the retinoretinal pathway; their expression was delayed by tectal ablation. The results indicate that, as in goldfish (Glasgow et al., 1994), separate parts of the pathway modify components of the cytoskeleton in ways that may be associated with choosing targets and stabilising projections.

Recent immuno-cytochemical and *in situ* hybridisation studies have examined the expression of gefiltin during optic nerve regeneration in lizards (*C. ornatus:* Rodger et al., 1998). As in goldfish (Glasgow et al., 1994), gefiltin expression in ganglion cells rises during optic axon regrowth. However, in goldfish, the expression falls when retinotopic projections have stabilised in visual centers. By contrast, in lizards levels remain high for at least one year after nerve crush. The sustained expression presumably reflects a continuing remodelling of axon terminals as the unstable regenerated projection searches unsuccessfully for appropriate target cells (Section **IX.A**).

Plasticin is another neurofilament protein that is expressed in the goldfish retina and optic nerve during optic nerve regeneration (Glasgow et al., 1992, Fuchs et al., 1994). Plasticin has been visualised using polyclonal antibodies raised to a plasticin fusion protein. Whereas normally immuno-reactivity is most prominent in newly generated ganglion cell somata and their axons, during optic nerve regeneration the entire population of somata becomes positive along with its dendrites in the inner plexiform layer and axons proximal to the crush site. Peak intensity is seen 20 days after lesion. It is not clear whether plasticin is present in frogs but studies suggest that it is absent from lizards (*C.ornatus:* Rodger et al., 1998).

C. Demyelination/Remyelination-*Amphibian and lizard optic nerves are partially myelinated. After regeneration in frogs the percentage of myelination returns to normal levels. In lizards the optic nerve is largely demyelinated after regeneration.*

Ultrastructural analysis reveals that amphibian and reptilian optic nerves are only partially myelinated (1-9% lungless salamanders: Linke and Roth, 1990; 2-3% *R. pipiens:* Stelzner and Strauss, 1986; *L. moorei:* Playford and Dunlop, 1993; 11% *X. laevis:* Dunlop et al., 1984; 83% *V. aspis*: Rio et al., 1989; 21% *C. ornatus:* Beazley et al., 1997). Electrophysiological recording and morphological analyses have suggested that myelination in the frog visual pathway is restricted to large calibre axons of the dimming detector class (*R. pipiens:* Maturana et al., 1960). This suggestion is supported by a study in which individual ganglion cells were recorded electrophysiologically and then labelled with an axonal tracer (*R. pipiens:* Stirling and Merrill, 1987).

The sequence and extent of remyelination after optic nerve regeneration has been described ultrastructurally in frogs (*R. pipiens*: Stelzner and Strauss, 1986; *L. moorei:* Dunlop et al., submitted for publication). The segment between the eye and the lesion does not undergo extensive demyelination. Beyond the lesion, all regenerating axon sprouts are initially unmyelinated. Remyelination takes place only after projections are stabilised in the brain and any excess sprouts are lost (*R. pipiens*: Stelner and Strauss, 1986; *L. moorei:* Dunlop et al., submitted for publication). At this stage regenerated axons presumably first reach a threshold diameter for remyelination (Rushton, 1951). In the long term, the percentage of myelinated axons matches that in the normal animal although, as a consequence of ganglion cell death (Section **III.A**), the absolute number is reduced. An immunocytochemical study distinguished oligodendrocytes from astrocytes by a lack of intermediate filaments in *X. laevis* tadpoles. Counts of oligodendrocytes fell, presumably matching the reduction in the number of ganglion cells and therefore of optic axons requiring remyelination (Runnger-Brandle et al., 1995).

Ultrastructural examination has indicated that, unlike the regenerated optic nerves in frogs, those in snakes and lizards undergo demyelination and do not become remyelinated to a substantial extent (*V. aspis*: Rio et al., 1989; *C. ornatus:* Beazley et al., 1997). Moreover, the segment of the optic nerve between the eye and the crush site in lizards undergoes retrograde demyelination. Eventually only 3-5% of axons are myelinated along the length of the regenerated nerve.

There are several possible reasons why percentage myelination remains low in lizards. The low levels are likely to be linked to the inability of most regenerated axons to form stable central projections (Section **IX.A**), remove their excess axonal sprouts (Section **V.A**) and return to their normal dimensions. Alternatively, all ganglion cells that are myelinated in the normal animal may die, leaving only the unmyelinated population to regenerate. However, this explanation seems unlikely since, after regeneration, electrophysiological recording reveals the return of responses to dimming light (*C. ornatus:* Stirling et al., 1999); in frogs (*R. pipiens:* Stirling and Merrill, 1987) and presumably in lizards also, ganglion cells with this property are normally myelinated. A third possibility is that all regenerated axons remain unmyelinated and the myelinated axons in a regenerated optic nerve represent an efferent projection from the brain to the eye; such a projection has been reported in other reptiles (Reperant et al., 1989).

VI. THE VISUAL PATHWAY DURING OPTIC NERVE REGENERATION

There are molecular and structural changes to the vascular, glial and neuronal components within the visual pathway after optic nerve lesion.

A. An Environment Permissive for Axonal Regeneration-*Neural cell adhesion molecules are present during optic nerve regeneration in frogs. The role of myelin during regeneration in amphibians and reptiles is not well understood. It may be that, as in fish, the components of myelin are inhibitory to axonal regeneration immediately after lesion but become permissive within a few days.*

Neural cell adhesion molecules (NCAMs) mediate adhesive interactions between growing axons and their environment and are implicated as recognition molecules in the tectum during development in salamanders and frogs (*Pleurodeles waltl, Discoglossus pictus:* Becker et al., 1993) and optic nerve regeneration in zebrafish (Bernhardt et al., 1996). Antibodies to NCAM have indicated that NCAMs are also present in the visual pathway of salamanders during optic nerve regeneration (*Pleurodeles waltl:* Becker et al., 1993). During development in the salamander, NCAM seems to be associated with polysialic acid, a posttranslational modification that weakens the strength of NCAM-NCAM binding and other cell substrate interactions facilitating exploratory axonal pathfinding (Acheson et al., 1991; Rutishauser and Landmesser, 1991). By contrast, polysialic acid is not associated with NCAM during optic nerve regeneration, compatible with regenerating axons making navigational errors.

A further demonstration of the role of NCAMs during optic nerve regeneration in frogs was provided by the effect of tectal implants of agarose containing antibodies to NCAM (*X. laevis:* Fraser et al., 1988). The morphology of individual axons labelled with horseradish peroxidase (HRP), along with enlarged receptive fields as assessed electrophysiologically, indicated a disruption to the growth and retraction of terminal arbors. Similar issues have yet to be addressed in reptiles.

The presence of certain components of myelin may influence the success, or otherwise of regeneration. It is well-established that some myelin subunits inhibit axonal regeneration in mammals (Bastmeyer et al., 1991). Moreover, the application of masking monoclonal antibody IN-1 can reduce the inhibitory effect. In the goldfish optic nerve (Bastmeyer et al., 1993), and to a lesser extent in the spinal cord (Sharma et al., 1993), axonal regeneration is successful, apparently because fish myelin does not contain the inhibitors of axonal growth or expresses them at low levels. More recent studies indicate that optic nerve myelin in fish may be inhibitory to axonal regeneration immediately after lesion but becomes permissive to it within a few days (goldfish: Sivron et al., 1994, Wanner et al., 1995).

A similarly permissive environment presumably is present or comes about in the amphibian optic nerves after lesion. An *in vitro* study in frogs examined the regenerative response of the growth cones of optic axons in the presence of oligodendrocytes extracted from either the spinal cord or optic nerve *(X. laevis:* Lang et al., 1995). The results indicated that optic axons regenerate in the presence of myelin from the optic nerve, but not the spinal cord. Moreover, application of the masking molecule IN-1 encouraged optic axons to grow on spinal cord oligodendrocytes, a result confirming that local conditions are critical for optic axon regeneration.

A study in the lizard *Gallotia galloti* examined whether the optic nerve regeneration observed in this species takes place because axons encounter a growth promoting environment (Lang et al., 1998). It was found that *in vitro* axons of rat dorsal root ganglia were unable to regenerate when challenged with lizard myelin or oligodendrocytes. The result suggests the environment is a nonpermissive substrate but that lizard axons are relatively insensitive to growth inhibiting components of optic nerve myelin and oligodendrocytes.

A yet more recent study of the salamander *P. waltl* has assessed immunocytochemically the levels of tenascin-R during optic nerve regeneration (Becker et al., 1999). This extracellular matrix molecule is known to be inhibitory to neurite outgrowth and appears concomitantly with myelination during metamorphosis. Levels were found to fall to undetectable levels within 8 days of nerve crush, along with a reduction in the level of myelin-associated glycoprotein. Since regenerated axons were first seen distal to the lesion at 9 days, the authors concluded that the removal of inhibitory molecules correlated with axonal regeneration.

Nevertheless, the immediate environment cannot be the sole factor governing axonal regeneration in frog. Innate differences between cell populations must also be important. Thus when both optic axons and tectal efferents are severed by optic tract lesion, they presumably experience the same environment at their cut ends. Nevertheless, optic axons regenerate but the tectal efferents do not (*R. pipiens*: Lyon and Stelzner, 1987).

B. Vascular Changes/Blood-brain barrier-*Neovascularisation is seen within 1 day at and beyond the crush site in frog; it may be the site of the observed transient breach of the blood-brain barrier.*

Neovascularisation is one is the most immediate structural changes yet documented after optic nerve crush in frogs. A light and electron microscopy study has revealed new intraparenchymal vessels at and distal to a nerve crush in the normally avascular nerve as early as 24 hours after lesion. The vessels persist to the latest stage yet examined, namely 8 days (*R. pipiens*: Liuzzi and Miller, 1990).

The new vessels presumably lack a blood-brain barrier. The finding is compatible with the results of a study in which rhodamine B-isocyanate conjugated to bovine serum albumin was perfused transcardially in frogs at various stages of optic nerve regeneration (*L. moorei:* Tennant and Beazley, 1992). As in goldfish (Kiernan and Contestabile, 1980), a breakdown of the blood-brain barrier takes place. The region lacking such a barrier is seen to move sequentially along the length of the visual pathway and across the tectum, coincident with the front of regenerating axons. If axonal regeneration is prevented by nerve ligation, a breakdown of the barrier along the visual pathway is not observed. The result indicates that a breach of the blood-brain barrier is triggered by regenerating axons but not by degenerating ones. The significance of the breakdown in terms of macromolecules gaining access to the front of regenerating axons is unknown.

Neovascularisation and the integrity of the blood-nerve barrier within the visual pathway during optic nerve regeneration have yet to be addressed in reptiles.

C. Macrophages and Microglia

In frogs, coincident with neovascularisation and axon outgrowth, massive numbers of granulocytes, macrophages and microglia invade the lesion site and distal nerve (*R. pipiens:* Liuzzi and Miller, 1990; *X. laevis:* Goodbrand and Gaze, 1991; Wilson et al., 1992; *L. moorei:* Dunlop et al., submitted for publication). Both ultrastructural and immuno-cytochemical studies reveal that the invasion matches that seen in goldfish (Battisti et al., 1995; Nona et al., 1998) with peak numbers of macrophage-like cells being present during the first week after crush. The cells are presumed to phagocytose cellular debris resulting from the lesion. However, macrophage-like cells may also enhance axonal regrowth, as demonstrated in the mammalian peripheral nervous system (mouse: Perry et al., 1987).

In lizards, preliminary studies suggest that macrophages are present at the crush site 1 week after crush but their numbers are already reduced by 2 weeks. Unlike frogs, lizard macrophages are not found in large numbers elsewhere in the visual pathway (*C. ornatus:* Bartlett et al., in preparation). The result supports other findings that suggest a protracted removal of debris from the pathway (Section **VI.E**).

D. Astrocytes

Changes take place within the resident astrocyte population after optic nerve lesion in frogs and lizards. Whereas in mammals the formation of an astrocytic scar is thought to inhibit axonal regeneration (McKeon et al., 1991), this is not the case in frog. Axons regenerate through astrocytic material, even penetrating grafts of scar tissue produced by extensive damage to the optic nerve (*X. laevis:* Reier and Webster, 1974, Reier, 1979).

In a recent immuno-cytochemical study (*X. laevis:* Rungger-Brandle et al., 1995), astrocytes were identified by their expression of cytokeratin. The identification was used since in frogs, as in goldfish (Nona et al., 1989; Giordano et al., 1989, 1990) but unlike mammals, astrocytes lack glial fibrillary acidic protein (GFAP). Astrocytes were seen to invade the lesion site within 1 day of crush, apparently providing a temporary scaffold for regenerating axons. Similarly, in lizards GFAP-positive cells are present in the crush site by 1 week (*C. ornatus:* Bartlett et al., in preparation). Detailed studies have yet to be undertaken in amphibians or reptiles to reveal whether, as in fish spinal cord (Nona and Stafford, 1995; Nona, 1998) and the optic nerve of goldfish and rat (Blaugrund et al., 1997;), axons precede astrocytes into the lesion.

In addition to changes at the lesion site, astrocytic cytoplasm can be seen ultrastructurally to undergo long term hypertrophy throughout the regenerating optic nerve of frogs and lizards (*L. moorei:* Humphrey and Beazley, 1985; *C. ornatus*: Beazley et al., 1997). Zonulae adherentes between astrocytic processes also become more prominent, presumably providing mechanical stability. Changes in the electrical properties of astrocytes after regeneration have yet to be addressed. However, after retinal ablation *in situ* glial voltage dependent membrane properties have been assessed and shown to depend on interactions between astrocytes and neighbouring axons (*R. pipiens:* Blanco et al., 1993).

E. Degenerating Axons-*Some disconnected distal segments of severed axons persist along the visual pathway and in visual centers throughout regeneration.*

In adult frogs, the disconnected distal segments of myelinated axons disappear from the optic nerve within a few days or weeks of lesion, leaving only myelin debris. However, the distal segments of some unmyelinated axons display an unusually slow degeneration (*R. temporaria:* Manteifel and D'yachkova, 1970; *R. esculenta:* Lazar 1980; *R. pipiens:* Matsumoto and Scalia, 1981; Blanco and Orkand, 1993; *L. moorei:* Humphrey et al., 1992), a feature more marked at post-metamorphic and at larval stages (*X. laevis:* Wilson et al., 1992). For 3-6 months, the segments retain a normal appearance, perform axonal transport and conduct action potentials if electrically stimulated. Moreover, an anterograde tracing study in which the tracer HRP was applied in separate animals to either side of the crush site confirmed that regeneration is essentially complete before the disconnected distal segments disappear (*L. moorei:* Humphrey et al., 1992).

The limited evidence available for reptiles suggests that removal of disconnected segments of severed axons may be even more protracted, at least in alligators and crocodiles, than in amphibians (*Alligator mississippiensis, Caiman crocodilus:* Kruger and Maxwell, 1969). The significance of this longevity is not known. It may be that the slow degenerating segments interfere with the successful restoration and consolidation of regenerated visual projections (Section **VIII**) by continuing to occupy most postsynaptic sites.

VII. AXONAL NAVIGATION

Given the changes that take place within the visual pathway that awaits regenerating axons, axonal navigation is unlikely to be perfect. However, such precision is not a prerequisite for successful regeneration. It is sufficient for axons to navigate to appropriate brain centers, a feat achieved in frogs and to a large extent in lizards.

A. Regenerating Axons Within the Visual Pathway-*Axons favour the periphery of the optic nerve at early stages of regeneration in frogs but later invade its core. In lizards, a peripheral location is maintained throughout. Within the optic tract, axons stay superficial in frogs but line its entire borders in lizards. Axon order is lost.*

Regenerating optic axons are present in large numbers in the distal segment of the optic nerve of amphibians and lizards. However, the distribution of axons is abnormal. In newts and frogs, ultrastructural and axon tracing studies have shown that regrowing axons initially favour the periphery of the optic nerve but later also invade its core (*P. waltl:* Becker et al., 1999; *X. laevis:* Wilson et al., 1992). In a study of the early stages of regeneration in frogs (*L. moorei:* Dunlop et al., submitted for publication), degenerating and regenerating axons were labelled with different carbocyanine dyes. Regenerating axons were seen to grow around the periphery of the nerve initially, largely avoiding the disconnected distal segments of severed axons (Section **VI.E**); only later do regenerating axons invade the core. By contrast, in lizards, axonal tracing with carbocyanine dyes has shown that regenerated axons tend to retain a peripheral location in the optic nerve throughout regeneration (*C. ornatus:* Dunlop, submitted for publication, b).

Axon trajectories are also abnormal in the optic tract of both frogs and lizards throughout regeneration. In frogs, most regenerating axons adopt a superficial location (*X. laevis:* Gaze and Grant, 1978) and in lizards line the entire borders of the tract (*C. ornatus:* Dunlop, submitted for publication, b). Presumably in both cases, regenerating axons are avoiding the disconnected distal segments of severed axons. A second factor may be involved in frogs. Retinal ganglion cells are generated in adult life in frogs and their ingrowing axons grow superficially along the optic tract presumably following navigational cues (*X. laevis:* Grant and Gaze, 1978; *R. pipiens:* Reh et al., 1983). It is possible that these cues are read also by regenerating axons. Since in lizards retinal ganglion cells are not generated in adulthood (*C. ornatus*: Beazley et al., 1998), cues would presumably no longer be available to encourage regenerating axons into a superficial location.

As in other vertebrates, optic axons in amphibians and lizards are ordered along the visual pathway. Order reflects both the retinal location of the parent cell body (*R. pipiens:* Scalia and Arango, 1983; Montgomery and Fite, 1989; *C. ornatus*: Beazley et al., 1997) and the stage at which it was generated (*R. pipiens:* Reh et al., 1983). After regeneration in newts, frogs and lizards, as in goldfish (Bernhardt and Easter, 1988, Springer et al., 1990), little or no axon order is apparent in either the optic nerve or tract (*R. pipiens:* Udin, 1978; *X. laevis:* Fawcett and Gaze, 1981; *Cynops pyrrogaster:* Fujisawa, 1981; Fujisawa et al., 1982; *C. ornatus:* Beazley et al., 1997).

As an exception, in the frog *X. laevis,* regenerating axons demonstrate some selective navigation at the division of the optic brachia. Normally, axons from dorsal and ventral retina enter the tectum via the lateral and medial optic brachia respectively (*X. laevis:* Straznicky et al., 1979). If an eye composed solely of ventral retina is constructed early in life, a so-called double ventral compound eye, optic axons enter the tectum only via the medial brachium. During optic nerve regeneration, the axons again favour this route. The explanation may be that regenerating axons prefer to enter the brachium containing debris of the severed axons (Section **VI.E**) rather than a 'virgin' one.

B. Pathway Selection/Axonal Misrouting–*in frogs and lizards some axons become misrouted at the chiasm to form an enhanced projection to the ipsilateral side of the brain. A retinoretinal projection via the chiasm to the opposite eye forms transiently in frogs but is permanent in lizards. Regenerating axons stay exclusively within the visual pathway in frogs but in lizards a minority deviate from it.*

In both frogs and lizards some regenerating axons become misrouted at the optic chiasm. One consequence is an abnormally heavy input into the ipsilateral optic tract (*X. laevis:* Glastonbury and Straznicky, 1978, Straznicky et al., 1980; *R. pipiens:* Stelzner et al., 1981; *L. moorei:* Humphrey and Beazley, 1985; *C. ornatus:* Tran et al., 1996; Beazley et al., 1997; Dunlop et al., 2000). It is thought that in frogs, unlike goldfish (Sharma and Tsai, 1991), the ipsilaterally projecting regenerated axons are axons in their own right and not collateral branches of contralaterally projecting ones (*R. pipiens:* Stelzner and Strauss, 1986).

Other regenerating axons, on reaching the chiasm, are misdirected away from the brain. As in developing mammals (rat: Bunt and Lund, 1981), some regenerating axons in frogs and lizards enter the opposite optic nerve and grow into the other eye (*R. pipiens:* Bohn and Stelzner, 1981a-c; *L. moorei:* Tennant et al., 1993; *C. ornatus:* Beazley et al., 1997; Dunlop et al., 2000). Retrograde labelling from the opposite eye indicates that the retinoretinal projection is formed by approximately 5% and 1% of ganglion cells in the frogs *R. pipiens* (Bohn and Stelzner, 1981a) and *L. moorei* (Tennant et al., 1993) respectively. Moreover, up to 80% of retinoretinal axons were found to be collateral branches of axons growing along the optic tract (*R. pipiens:* Bohn and Stelzner, 1981a; Stelzner and Strauss, 1986). Quantitative studies of the retinoretinal projection have yet to be carried out in lizards.

During optic nerve regeneration in frogs the retinoretinal projection is transient and disappears when projections to visual centers become consolidated. The long term accumulation of the retrograde tracer diamidino yellow in retinal ganglion cells that form the transient retinoretinal projection indicates that the parent cells do not die. Presumably after withdrawal of the retinoretinal branch, the cells are maintained by sustaining collaterals to visual brain centers (*L. moorei:* Tennant et al., 1993). In contrast to frogs, the lizard forms a permanent retinoretinal projection (*C. ornatus:* Dunlop submitted for publication, b). It is further evidence that in lizards regenerating axons cannot recognise and respond to inappropriate targets (Section **VIII.B**).

Anterograde tracing studies demonstrate that regenerating optic axons stay almost exclusively within the optic tract in frogs (*R. pipiens*: Stelzner et al., 1981) and probably also in snakes (*V. aspis:* Rio et al., 1989). The confinement persists in frogs even when areas adjacent to the optic tract, such as the nucleus rotundus, are denervated by axon transection at the isthmal level (*R. pipiens:* Bohn and Stelzner, 1980). Despite the proximity of extensive terminal degeneration, the regenerating optic axons do not deviate from the optic tract.

A recent study in lizards traced regenerated projections with carbocyanine dyes. Most regenerating axons remain within the optic tract and projections are more pronounced at an intermediate stage of regeneration, namely 4-6 months, than at earlier or later stages. However, throughout regeneration some axons deviate into secondary visual nuclei such as the nucleus rotundus and isthmic nucleus whilst others follow highly aberrant paths, for example, to the olfactory bulb (*C. ornatus:* Dunlop et al., 2000).

VIII. THE SEARCH FOR VISUAL CENTERS

In amphibians and lizards, most optic axons regenerate to the tectum; minor primary visual centers are also reinnervated. In lizard, optic axons terminate also in secondary visual and nonvisual centers.

A. Tectal Innervation-*Axons reinnervate the superficial retino-recipient tectal layers. Although the projection is more pronounced contralaterally, the ipsilateral input is abnormally heavy and in some species is electrically silent.*

In newts, frogs and lizards, most optic axons reinnervate the contralateral optic tectum (*T. viridescens*: Sperry 1943; *R. pipiens*: Singman and Scalia, 1990b, 1991; *C. ornatus*: Beazley et al., 1997). An ultrastructural study in frogs has shown that regenerating axons tend to form synapses *de novo* rather than occupying long-persisting vacant sites. The number of synapses returns to normal levels (*X. laevis:* Ostberg and Norden, 1979). Presumably, hypertrophy of axonal arbors and an increased synaptic complement per terminal compensates for a reduced ganglion cell number (Section **II. A**). There is little or no invasion of the denervated tectum as a result of sprouting across the mid-line by axons from the other eye to the opposite tectum (*R. pipiens:* Stelzner, 1979).

Most regenerating axons regain their location in the superficial retino-recipient tectal layers in both amphibians and lizards. In frogs, regenerated axons continue to occupy the retinorecipient layers of the contralateral tectum even if forced to compete for territory with a regenerating mandibular nerve grafted onto the rostrodorsal surface of the tectum (*R. pipiens:* Kaplan and Clemente, 1985). By HRP labelling of either the mandibular or optic inputs, it was clear that the two inputs interact with the tectal substrate independently. The growth pattern of the mandibular input is highly segregated and disordered whereas that of the optic ingrowth is fascicular and ordered.

The specificity extends also to ganglion cell classes. Thus, electrophysiological recording and immuno-cytochemistry have demonstrated that the characteristic depth distribution of terminal arbors of different ganglion cell classes is restored in the contralateral tectum after regeneration (*R. temporaria:* Keating and Gaze, 1970; *L. moorei:* Humphrey et al., 1995). The issue has yet to be addressed in lizards.

Innervation to the ipsilateral tectum is abnormally pronounced in both amphibians and lizards after optic nerve crush (*R. pipiens:* Singman and Scalia, 1990b, 1991; *C. ornatus:* Tran et al., 1996; Beazley et al., 1997; Dunlop et al. 2000) or complete chiasmal transection (*R. pipiens:* Waldeck and Gruberg, 1995). Although the projection extends throughout the retino-recipient tectal layers in amphibians, in lizards it tends to lie mostly in the deepest part. We do not yet understand the significance of this localisation. Possibly the ganglion cell class that normally projects to this sublamina does so after regeneration and no other ganglion cell classes are represented. However, the density of the regenerated projection suggests that regrowing axons are unable to displace the resident input from the partner eye and 'build up' at the inner border of the retinorecipient region.

Unlike Ranid frogs (*R. temporaria:* Gaze and Jacobson, 1963), the frog *X. laevis* (Straznicky et al., 1980) and the lizard (*C. ornatus*: Beazley et al., 1997, Stirling et al., 1999) regenerate a projection to the ipsilateral tectum that is undetectable electrophysiologically and presumably therefore is nonfunctional. It seems that the regenerated projection cannot compete for terminal sites with the resident population of optic axons from the unoperated partner eye. If this population is removed by severing the intact optic nerve in the frog, the regenerated ipsilateral projection becomes electrophysiologically active within 2-4 weeks (*X. laevis*: Straznicky et al., 1980).

B. Minor Visual Centers and Nonstandard Targets-*Minor visual centers become reinnervated in frogs and lizards. Nonstandard targets are also innervated in lizards.*

In addition to the tectum, minor primary visual centers are also reinnervated during optic nerve regeneration in frogs and lizards (*R. pipiens:* Stelzner et al., 1981; *L. moorei*: Humphrey and Beazley, 1985; *C. ornatus:* Beazley et al., 1997, Dunlop et al., 2000). A study in frogs using ^{3}H-proline autoradiography suggested that nuclei in the anterior thalamus became reinnervated only several weeks after those in posterior thalamus and the tectum (*R. pipiens:* Stelzner et al., 1981). However, using the more sensitive tracer HRP, Scalia reported that axons escaping from an optic nerve deflected into the telencephalon reinnervated thalamic and pretectal regions before the tectum (*R. pipiens:* Scalia, 1987). In lizards, carbocyanine dyes have demonstrated that during optic nerve regeneration, as in development (Rodger et al., in preparation), diencephalic nuclei are reinnervated before the tectum (Dunlop et al., 2000).

It would be interesting to determine whether ganglion cells of different classes selectively reinnervate appropriate minor visual nuclei after optic nerve regeneration as in normal animals. The question could be addressed by examining whether the basal optic nucleus regains input from displaced ganglion cells (*R. pipiens:* Montgomery et al., 1981; *C. ornatus:* Dunlop and Beazley in preparation). However, it is known that, as in normal frogs, only ganglion cells from temporoventral retina reinnervate ipsilateral diencephalic nuclei after optic nerve regeneration (*X. laevis:* Hoskins and Grobstein, 1985). The issue has yet to be addressed in lizards. Moreover, it is unclear whether, as in normal animals (*R. pipiens:* Stirling and Merrill, 1987), some ganglion cells projecting to the tectum form collateral branches to a minor visual center.

There is one major difference between optic nerve regeneration in frogs and lizards in terms of targets innervated. In frogs, the regenerated projections extend exclusively to primary visual centers and radical procedures are required before regenerating optic axons can be induced to innervate nonstandard targets. Thus, after complete ablation of one optic tectum (*R. pipiens:* Cantore and Scalia, 1987), regenerating axons labelled with HRP have been shown by light and electron microscopy to enter the lateral thalamic neuropil and in some frogs also the isthmic nucleus; these regions are normally innervated by the tectum. The result suggests that regenerating axons respond to signals that are present in these regions but are normally suppressed by their tectal input. The synapses formed ultrastructurally in the nonstandard targets resemble those formed in the tectum. Similarly, regenerated axons will terminate and form synapses in the olfactory cortex if forced to regenerate into the forebrain (*R. pipiens:* Scalia, 1987).

By contrast to the specificity of target recognition displayed in frogs, in lizards even one year after crush some regenerated axons innervate secondary visual centers such as the nucleus rotundus. Yet other axons project to non-visual areas including the olfactory bulb (*C. ornatus:* Dunlop et al., 2000).

IX. SELECTING POSTSYNAPTIC CELLS: RETINOTOPY OF REGENERATED PROJECTIONS

For successful regeneration, axonal arbors must reform retinotopically appropriate arrays (*R. pipiens:* Scalia and Fite, 1974) in visual centers and transmit input to postsynaptic cells. Thereby a spatially appropriate representation of visual space is relayed to the brain and vision restored. The feat is achieved in amphibians but not in lizard.

A. Formation and Stability of Topographic Projections-*In amphibians regenerating optic nerves reestablish and stabilise topographic maps in the tectum and vision is restored. In lizard a transient low fidelity map is formed but thereafter all order is lost; as a consequence blindness persists.*

In salamanders, anterograde labelling reveals that individual axon terminals extend widely through the superficial layers of the contralateral tectum (*C. pyrrogaster:* Fujisawa, 1981; Fujisawa et al., 1982). Compatible with this observation, electrophysiological recording has shown that projections are initially diffuse. Retinotopic order has been found to become progressively more pronounced over a period of weeks, approaching the precision found in normal newts and frogs (*R. pipiens:* Maturana et al., 1959; *T. viridescens*: Cronly-Dillon et al., 1968; *L. moorei:* Humphrey and Beazley, 1982, 1985).

From the initial stage, visual input is transmitted to postsynaptic cells irrespective of whether it is topographic or nontopographic. To demonstrate this connectivity, electrophysiological recordings were made of the regenerated input to the contralateral tectum and the secondary projection from this tectum to the opposite one via the isthmic nucleus (*R. pipiens*: Adamson et al., 1984). The indirect pathway was found to respond to visual stimuli in appropriate and in inappropriate locations.

The return of visual function in frogs after optic nerve regeneration also confirms that the regenerated input is transmitted to post-synaptic cells. Good monocular vision is regained (*R. pipiens:* Singman and Scalia, 1991) although there is some impairment of binocular tasks such as prey capture and avoidance of obstacles after unilateral optic nerve regeneration (*L. moorei:* Dunlop et al., 1997). The impairment probably reflects at least in part the inferior quality of the visual input via a reduced complement of ganglion cells in the experimental eye (Section II.I).

Retinotopy is restored in frogs even if a size disparity is introduced between retina and tectum. Thus optic input from a surgically-created half retina can be shown by electrophysiological recording to project retinotopically over an entire tectum (*X. laevis:* Straznicky et al., 1978). In the converse experiment, if the optic nerve is crushed and the caudal half of the contralateral tectum is removed, electrophysiological recording demonstrates that, as in fish (goldfish: Schmidt, 1978), the entire retina is represented retinotopically but in a compressed form across the remaining rostral half (*R. pipiens:* Udin, 1977). However in frogs, unlike fish, compression does not occur if the optic nerve remains intact. Rather nasal retina when deprived of caudal tectum projects in a disorganized fashion to the caudal border of the remaining rostral half tectum. Presumably the regenerating axons cannot compete successfully with an established projection in the remaining half tectum but can do so if axons from both hemiretinae regenerate simultaneously.

The regenerated projection is also retinotopically ordered to the ipsilateral as well as the contralateral tectum. In Ranid frogs electrophysiological recording and behavioural studies have demonstrated that the regenerated projection is mirror symmetric to that within the opposite tectum (*R. temporaria:* Gaze and Jacobson, 1963; *R. pipiens:* Singman and Scalia, 1990b, 1991; Waldeck and Gruberg, 1995). If the optic nerve in its entirety is relocated to force it to regenerate into the ipsilateral side of the brain field, the aberrant innervation can be shown to compete with the resident one from the other eye. Behavioural assessment suggested that with time functional connections are formed but are the mirror-image of those to the other tectum (*R. pipiens:* Misantone and Stelzner, 1974).

Unlike amphibians, in lizards, optic nerve regeneration does not lead to the restoration of ordered functional projections. Recently the retinotectal projections have been mapped electrophysiologically using an *in vitro* isolated eye-cup, optic nerve and midbrain preparation (Stirling et al., 1998, 1999). Between 2 and 4.5 months no order is present amongst the inconstant, rapidly fatiguing responses. However, between 4.5 and 6-7 months, a low-fidelity map is present; at this stage, projections are most pronounced anatomically (Stirling et al., 1999; Dunlop et al., 2000). The order is imperfect but is most apparent along the ventrotemporal to dorsonasal axis of the retina, projecting along the rostrocaudal tectal axis. However, unlike the amphibians or fish, a process of consolidation does not take place. Rather, the low-fidelity map is permanently lost beyond 6-7 months, confirming our anatomical evidence for lack of topography at one year (*C. ornatus*: Beazley et al., 1997).

The visual behaviour of lizards during optic nerve regeneration suggests that the non-retinotopic input is transmitted to postsynaptic cells. The lizards are at first unresponsive to stimuli such as live prey presented exclusively to the visual field of the experimental eye. At later stages, however, some lizards orient to moving prey, indicating visual input has reached postsynaptic sites. However, at no stage do lizards strike at prey using the experimental eye. Moreover, in some animals, the regenerated input seems intolerable. If a cover is placed over the unoperated partner eye, the lizards close the experimental eye until the cover is removed (*C. ornatus:* Stirling et al., 1999). Preliminary electrophysiological evidence also suggests that retinotectal input reaches postsynaptic cells in lizards. The light evoked spike activity recorded from both normal eyes and those with regenerated optic nerves is reversibly blocked by kynurenic, a glutamate receptor blocker (Stirling et al., submitted for publication).

B. Mechanisms of Map Formation-*Cytochemical cues, probably arranged in gradients and possibly involving ephrins, may set up the initial low-fidelity map. An activity-dependent mechanism involving NMDA receptors is thought to then refine and stabilize the projection. It seems that the activity-dependent mechanism is insufficient to stabilize the transient map in lizards.*

Map restoration seems to be a two-step process during optic nerve regeneration in amphibians as in fish (goldfish: Schmidt, 1990, 1993). In lizards the first step probably takes place but not the second.

The first step is a search for appropriate cytochemical cues. Although regenerating axons may be substantially misdirected when they exit the optic tract and reenter the optic tectum (Section **IV.A**), they have been shown in salamanders to search extensively for retinotopically appropriate sites (C. *pyrrogaster:* Fujisawa, 1981; Fujisawa et al., 1982). The family of Eph tyrosine kinase receptors and their ligands, the ephrins, are present as complementary gradients within the eye and tectum during development and have been implicated in map formation (Flanagan et al., 1998). Studies are currently in progress in our laboratory to determine if ephrins are upregulated during optic nerve regeneration in frog. However, preliminary evidence for lizards suggests that ephrin A2 is upregulated and expressed as a gradient in the lizard tectum during optic nerve regeneration (*C.ornatus:* Rodger et al., 1999). By contrast, ephrin A5 is absent from the regenerating system. Both ephrin A2 and A5 are expressed during development at the time the map is being put in place (Rodger et al., in preparation). The results imply that, during optic nerve regeneration in lizards, ephrin A2 may be involved in setting up the low fidelity map and that an absence of ephrin A5 and/or other synapse consolidating molecules play a role in its demise.

In addition, the remains of the disconnected distal segments of severed axons (Section **VI.E**) may provide local signals to regenerating axons. An ultrastructural reconstruction of a regenerating growth cone in frogs revealed that it was associated with the disconnected distal segment of a myelinated axon (*R. pipiens:* Scalia and Matsumoto, 1985). It may be that in frogs, as in fish (goldfish: Sharma and Romeskie, 1977), degenerating debris can influence map restoration. For example, a projection compresses immediately into a partial tectum but only if a sufficient period of time has elapsed to allow for the removal of degenerating debris (Section **VI.E**; goldfish: Sharma and Romeskie, 1977). In reptiles, disconnected distal segments of severed axons probably persist for exceedingly long periods. It may be that the slow degenerating segments interfere with the successful restoration and consolidation of regenerated visual projections by continuing to occupy many postsynaptic sites.

The second stage of map restoration is an activity-dependent process whereby, as during development (cat: Meister et al., 1991), axons that 'fire together, wire together'. Thus adjacent regions of retina produce similar volleys of electrical activity and those axon terminals adjacent to one another in the tectum will be reinforced; conversely, adjacent terminals receiving input from distant retinal locations will be downgraded. Evidence from studies of goldfish indicates that the activity-dependent mechanism involves the n-methyl-D-asparate (NMDA) family of receptors (Schmidt, 1990, 1993). Reinforcing this possibility, a recent study has shown that immuno-reactivity for a sub-unit 1 of the NMDA receptor is expressed during optic nerve regeneration in frog (*R.pipiens*: Janusonis and Fite, 1997). The immuno-reactivity is present bilaterally in thalamic and pretectal nuclei as well as the tectum. However, levels remain particularly high in the misrouted axons that innervate the ipsilateral tectum (Section **VIII.B**). The result suggests that these misrouted axons continue to use an activity-dependent mechanism as they compete with the resident optic axon population from the other eye to re-establish synaptic connections.

Mechanisms in the postsynaptic cells presumably also play a part in stabilising the developing connections. Thus mRNAs for nicotinic acetylcholine receptors found in frogs (*R. pipiens:* Sargent et al., 1989) at the retino-tectal synapse are presumably upregulated during restoration of visual maps in frogs as has been reported in goldfish (Hieber et al., 1992). Equivalent studies have yet to be undertaken in lizards.

X. REASONS FOR GANGLION CELL DEATH IN FROGS AND LIZARD

A study in frogs suggests that ganglion cells do not fall into two categories in terms of their viability after axotomy with 'fish-like' ones that survive and 'mammal-like' ones that do not (*L. moorei*: Beazley and Darby, 1993). The extents of ganglion cell survival were estimated from cell counts in wholemounted retinae for frogs in which the optic nerve had regenerated once and those in which the regenerated nerve was recrushed and allowed to regenerate a second time. Had there been two categories of ganglion cell, all the 'mammal-like' ones would have been eliminated during the first episode of regeneration and no subsequent death would have occurred during the second. The finding of similar proportions of ganglion cell loss on each occasion suggest that, during each episode of regeneration, ganglion cells enter a lottery with only a percentage surviving. The factors influencing the outcome could be located within the retina, at the lesion site or elsewhere along the visual pathway and/or within visual centers. Factors leading to ganglion cell death in reptiles remain largely unexplored.

A. Events In The Retina and Proximal Visual Pathway-*Ganglion cells die if their axons fail to reenter and cross the lesion site.*

Ganglion cells start to die in frog before regenerating axons reach the visual centers, implying that peripheral events precipitate at least some ganglion cell loss (*L. moorei*: Humphrey and Beazley, 1985; *R. pipiens*: Stelzner and Strauss, 1986). However, events in the retina do not seem to be crucial. In frogs and lizards, the comparable extents of ganglion cell survival for the displaced and orthotopic ganglion cells suggest that events within the retinal ganglion cell layer do not induce ganglion cell death (Section **III.B**; *L. moorei:* Dunlop et al., 1992; *C. ornatus:* Dunlop and Beazley, unpublished observations). Moreover, the proportional loss of ganglion cells is comparable across the retina suggesting factors such as cell crowding (Section **IV.B**) or localised transient neovascularisation (Section **VI.B**) are not crucial.

It seems more likely that events within the visual pathway up to and including the lesion site are crucial for ganglion cell survival. Counts of retrogradely labelled ganglion cells and of optic axons on either side of the lesion in the frog *L. moorei* suggest that in this species events at the lesion site are the major determinant of ganglion cell survival (Dunlop et al., 2000). The findings suggest that the entire complement of optic axons is represented between the eye and the crush site but the number of axons regenerating beyond it matches the number of long-term survivors. The findings indicate that ganglion cells survive if their axons regenerate across the lesion but eventually die if their attempts fail, presumably by denying them long-term access to trophic factors (Jacobson, 1991) within the distal visual pathway or visual centers. The proposal is supported by the finding of more extensive ganglion cell death if the lesion extends over a greater length of nerve (*L. moorei*: Tennant and Beazley, 1992).

Moreover, events between the eye and crush site probably underlie the greater extent of ganglion cell survival in *L moorei*, at around 70% (Humphrey and Beazley, 1985), as compared to *R. pipiens* at 40-50% (Scalia et al., 1985; Beazley et al., 1986; Stelzner and Strauss, 1986). It seems likely that the extent of axonal sprouting during optic nerve regeneration varies between frogs, being far more pronounced in *R. pipiens* than in *L. moorei* (Section **VI.A**). The result suggests that in *R. pipiens,* but not in *L. moorei,* axons withdraw from the lesion before starting to regrow and presumably thereby reduce their chances of reaching and penetrating the lesion site and thus of surviving in the long term.

B. Events Distal to the Lesion-*Failure to follow normal visual pathways or form projections in visual centers does not precipitate ganglion cell death in frogs or lizards.*

Another reason for ganglion cell death during optic nerve regeneration in frogs might be that regenerating axons go astray en route to the visual brain centers. However, this possibility seems to be unlikely. Some regenerating axons enter the opposite optic nerve (Section **VII.B**) but survive, withdrawing the misdirected axon and forming an appropriate connection in the brain (*L. moorei*: Tennant et al., 1993). Moreover, even totally misrouted axons seem to survive in the long term. Examples are axons deflected to enter the midbrain via the third nerve route (*X. laevis:* Beazley and Lamb, 1979) or the forebrain via the telencephalon (*R. pipiens*: Scalia 1987); in lizards, ganglion cells survive even if their axons spontaneously follow abnormal pathways (Section **VIII.B**).

It also seems unlikely that events in visual brain centers precipitate ganglion cell death. For example, competition for terminal space does not seem to be critical during optic nerve regeneration as it is during development (rat: O'Leary et al., 1986). Application of tetrodotoxin to the retina throughout optic nerve regeneration in frogs, to abolish sodium-mediated action potentials, does not reduce the extent of ganglion cell loss (*L. moorei*: Sheard and Beazley, 1988). Moreover, a failure to consolidate retinotopic projections in lizards (Section **IX.A**) does not lead to extensive ganglion cell death.

XI. OPTIC NERVE REGENERATION: IMPLICATIONS FOR OTHER VERTEBRATE CLASSES

There is a spectrum of responses to optic nerve section amongst the vertebrate phylum with the amphibians and reptiles at key transition points. An understanding of the factors at work after optic nerve lesion in these vertebrate classes will help to define those aspects of regeneration that will be necessary to encourage a successful outcome in mammals including man.

A. Continued Retinal Neurogenesis and Optic Nerve Regeneration- *Continued retinal ganglion cell generation is not a prerequisite for axonal regeneration but may be necessary for the consolidation of retinotopic maps.*

In fish and amphibians (goldfish: Meyer 1978; *X. laevis*: Straznicky and Gaze, 1971; *Limnodynastes dorsalis*: Coleman et al., 1984), retinal ganglion cells are generated and added to the established population in adult life. The entire population retains the capacity to undergo successful axonal regeneration. By contrast, in birds and mammals, retinal neurogenesis is complete early in life (chicken: Kahn 1974; cat: Walsh and Polley, 1985; quokka wallaby: Harman and Beazley, 1989) and shortly thereafter the capacity for optic nerve regeneration is lost (Kiernan, 1979; Keirstead et al.1992). It has therefore been suggested that axonal regeneration takes place spontaneously after lesion only in systems with continued neurogenesis (Holder and Clarke, 1988). The hypothesis has been refuted in lizards and aged *X. laevis.* In both, optic nerve regeneration is extensive despite an absence of retinal ganglion cell generation (*X. laevis*: Taylor et al., 1989; *C. ornatus*: Beazley et al., 1998).

However, it may be that the ability to reform topographic projections, rather than undergo axonal regeneration *per* se, is linked to continued neurogenesis. Presumably, whilst new axons continue to arrive at visual centers, the target cells might retain cues to allow the new arrivals to find and consolidate appropriate connections. When axonal ingrowth is complete, such signals would no longer be required and map consolidation would be precluded. We do not yet know if retinotopy is restored during optic nerve regeneration in aged *X. laevis*. In lizard, a low fidelity map forms at early stages of regeneration but is not stabilised thereafter (Section **IX.A**). The study is compatible with continued generation of retinal ganglion cells being linked to the capacity to stabilise and consolidate retinotopic projections.

B. Prevention of Ganglion Cell Death-*Application of growth factors protects mammalian ganglion cells after axotomy. Modification of the lesion and the distal nerve, including masking particular myelin subunits, will be necessary to induce optic axon regeneration in mammals.*

It is unclear whether, given sufficient support, all ganglion cells could survive axotomy in any vertebrate class other than fish. Studies in which nerve growth factor (NGF) was applied to the lesioned optic nerve in frogs did not influence either the cell soma reaction or rate of axonal regeneration (*R. pipiens:* Humphrey, 1987, 1988). The result contrasts with the findings of an enhanced cell body reaction and faster regeneration in the presence of NGF in newts (*T. viridescens*: Turner and Glaze, 1977). The possible protective and/or regeneration enhancing actions of other growth factors have yet to be tested. However, ligation of the nerve does delay the death of some ganglion cells in frogs (*L. moorei:* Humphrey et al., 1989) suggesting that the neuroma formed proximal to the ligature provides transient trophic support that is retrogradely transported to the ganglion cell somata.

It is likely that survival of axotomised ganglion cells can be encouraged by modifying the lesion site to render it permissive of regenerating axons. The ability of optic axons to regenerate readily along a grafted peripheral nerve (rat: Vidal-Sanz et al., 1987; Thanos et al., 1997) demonstrates that many ganglion cells retain the potential for axonal regeneration. Moreover, optic axon regeneration, albeit modest in extent, was observed in rats when monocytes cultured along with segments of sciatic or optic nerve were transplanted into the lesion site (Lazarov-Spiegler et al., 1996).

Having negotiated the lesion, the local environment of the distal optic nerve must be modified to render it permissive to regenerating axons. Particular subunits of mammalian myelin are likely to be inhibitory factors that must be masked to allow regeneration (rat spinal cord: Schnell and Schwab, 1990). However, myelin is not the sole agent inhibiting optic axon regeneration. The Browman-Wyse rat mutant lacks myelin from patches of the optic nerves, yet axons will not regenerate through the myelin-free zones (Berry et al., 1992). As an alternative to masking inhibitory factors it may be possible to protect regenerating optic axons en route to the brain by Schwann cells or olfactory ensheathing cells, as have been demonstrated recently in the rat spinal cord (Li et al., 1997).

C. Restoration of Organized Projections-*Regenerated axons must form terminals that search widely in visual centers to form and consolidate a retinotopic projection.*

Studies in frogs and lizards suggest that, if factors inhibitory to axonal regeneration are removed or masked in mammals, many optic axons will regain access to visual centers. However, it will then be necessary to induce regenerating axons in mammals to search widely within these centers for partner postsynaptic cells. When optic axons reenter visual centers via a peripheral nerve graft in rat, they remain 'clumped' near the point of entry (Thanos et al., 1997). Moreover, the axons retain the retinotopy, an inappropriate one for visual centers, present in the nerve. Presumably it will be necessary to protect terminals from factors, similar to those along the visual pathway, that inhibit the axonal growth and thus prevent searching within target regions.

However, a second step will then be required. Findings of a transient low fidelity map in lizards (Section **IX.A**) imply that the presence of putative map-making molecules, such as ephrins, in visual centers may be insufficient to form an organized projection term. It may be necessary to induce additional factors, possibly within the NMDA system, to consolidate a map. Only at this stage, will axons reach a critical diameter to allow them to be remyelinated and thus restore a system approaching normality.

XII. SUMMARY

In this chapter I have argued that the amphibians and reptiles represent 'half-way houses' amongst the vertebrate phylum in terms of their capacity for optic nerve regeneration. Just as these classes are phylogenetically intermediate between the fish and the birds and mammals, so their capacities for optic nerve regeneration are reduced as compared to that of fish but exceed the abortive response of birds and mammals. As a consequence, studies of optic nerve regeneration in amphibians and reptiles provide insights into the factors associated with successful or unsuccessful central nerve regeneration in all vertebrates including man. Moreover, differences between optic nerve regeneration in amphibians and reptiles may provide insights into the prerequisites for the restoration and stabilisation of topographic projections in the brain.

REFERENCES

Acheson, A., J.L. Sunshine, U. Rutishauser (1991) NCAM polysialic acid can regulate both cell-cell and cell-substrate interactions. *Journal of Cell Biology* 114: 143-153.

Adamson, J., J. Burke and P. Grobstein (1984) Recovery of the ipsilateral oculotectal projection following nerve crush in the frog: Evidence that retinal afferents make synapses at abnormal tectal locations. *Journal of Neuroscience* 4: 2635-2649.

Barron, K.D., C.M. McGuinness, L.J. Misantone, M.F. Zanakis, B. Grafstein and M. Murray (1985) RNA content of normal and axotomized retinal ganglion cells of rat and goldfish. *Journal of Comparative Neurology* 236: 265-273.

Bastmeyer, M., M. Bahr and C.A.O. Stuermer (1993) Fish optic nerve oligodendrocytes support axonal regeneration of fish and mammalian retinal ganglion cells. *Glia* 8: 1-11.

Bastmeyer, M., M. Beckmann, M.E. Schwab and C.A.O. Stuermer (1991) Growth of regenerating goldfish axons is inhibited by rat oligodendrocytes and CNS myelin but not by goldfish optic nerve tract oligodendrocyte-like cells and fish CNS myelin. *Journal of Neuroscience* 11: 626-640.

Battisti, W.P., J. Wang, K. Bozek and M. Murray (1995) Macrophages, microglia and astrocytes are rapidly activated after crush injury of the goldfish optic nerve: A light and electron microscopic analysis. *Journal of Comparative Neurology* 354: 306-320.

Beattie, M.S., J.C. Bresnahan and G. Lopate (1990) Metamorphosis alters the response to the spinal cord transection in *Xenopus laevis* frogs. *Journal of Neurobiology* 21: 1108-1122.

Beazley, L.D. (1981) Retinal ganglion cell death and regeneration of abnormal retinotectal projections after removal of a segment of optic nerve in *Xenopus* tadpoles. *Developmental Biology* 85: 164-170.

Beazley, L.D. (1984) Formation of specific nerve connections in the visual system of lower vertebrates. *Current Topics In Research In Synapses* 1: 55-117.

Beazley, L.D., J.E. Darby and V.H. Perry (1986) Cell death in the retinal ganglion cell layer during optic nerve regeneration in the frog *Rana pipiens*. *Vision Research* 26: 543-556.

Beazley, L.D., J.E. Darby (1993) A second episode of ganglion cell death takes place when an optic nerve regenerates a second time in the frog. *Visual Neuroscience*. 10: 297-301.

Beazley, L.D. and A.H. Lamb (1979) Rerouted optic axons in *Xenopus* tadpoles form normal visuotectal projections. *Brain Research* 179: 373-378.

Beazley, L.D., P.W. Sheard, M. Tennant, D. Starac and S.A. Dunlop (1997) Optic nerve regenerates but does not restore topographic projections in the lizard *Ctenophorus ornatus*. *Journal of Comparative Neurology* 377: 105-120.

Beazley, L.D., M. Tennant, T.M. Stewart and S.D. Anstee (1998) Optic nerve regeneration in the adult lizard *Ctenophorus ornatus* shows that neurogenesis is not obligatorily linked to axonal regeneration but may be a pre-requisite for map restoration. *Vision Research* 316: 789-793.

Beazley, L.D., A. Barber, P. Runham, R.V. Stirling and S.A. Dunlop (1999) Failure of optic nerve regeneration in the gecko *Nephrusus stellatus*. *Neurosci.Abs.* 29: 194.22.

Becker, C.G., T. Becker, G. Roth (1993) Distribution of NCAM180 and polysialic acid in the developing tectum mesencephali of the frog *Discoglossus pictus* and the salamander *Pleurodeles waltl*. *Cell Tissue Research* 289-301.

Becker, C.G., T. Becker, R.L. Meyer and M. Schachner (1999) Tenascin-R inhibits the growth of optic fibers *in vitro* but is rapidly eliminated during nerve regeneration in the Salamander *Pleurodeles waltl*. *Journal of Neuroscience* 19: 813-827.

Becker, C.G., T. Becker and G. Roth (1993) Distribution of NCAM-180 and polysialic acid in the developing tectum mesencephali of the frog *Discoglossus pictus* and the salamander *Pleurodeles waltl*. *Cell Tissue Research* 272: 289-301.

Becker, D.L. and J.E. Cook (1990) Changes in goldfish retinal ganglion cells during axonal regeneration. *Proceedings of the Royal Society of London, Series B* 241: 73-77.

Benowitz, L.I., V.E. Shashoua and M.G. Yoon (1981) Transported proteins in the regenerating optic nerve: regulation by interactions with the optic tectum. *Science* 222: 185-188.

Berkelaar, M., D.B. Clarke, Y.C. Wang, G.M. Bray and A.J. Aguayo (1994) Axotomy results in delayed death and apoptosis of retinal ganglion cells in adult rats. *Journal of Neuroscience* 14: 4343-4368.

Bernhardt, R.R. and S.S. Easter (1988) Regenerated optic fibres in goldfish reestablish a crude sectoral order in the visual pathway. *Journal of Comparative Neurology* 277: 403-419.

Bernhardt, R.R., E. Tongiorgi, P. Anzini and M. Schachner (1996) Increased expression of specific recognition molecules by retinal ganglion cells and by optic pathway glia accompanies the successful regeneration of retinal axons in adult zebrafish. *Journal of Comparative Neurology* 376: 253-264.

Berry, M., S. Hall, L. Rees, J. Carlile and J.P.H. Wyse (1992) Regeneration of axons in the optic nerve of the adult Browman-Wyse (BW) mutant rat. *Journal of Neurocytology* 21: 426-448.

Blanco, R.A., H. Marrero, P.M. Orkand and R.K. Orkand (1993) Changes in ultrastructure and voltage-dependent currents at the glia limitans of the frog optic nerve following retinal ablation. *Glia* 8: 97-105.

Blanco, R.E. and P.M. Orkand (1996) Astrocytes and regenerating axons at the proximal stump of the severed frog optic nerve. *Cell Tissue Research* 286: 337-345.

Blaugrund, E., V. Lavie, I. Cohen, A. Solomon, D.J. Schreyer and M. Schwartz (1993) Axonal regeneration is associated with glial migration: Comparison between the injured optic nerves of fish and rats. *Journal of Comparative Neurology* 330: 105-112.

Bohn, R.C. and P.J. Reier (1982) Anomalous axonal outgrowth at the retina caused by injury to the optic nerve or tectal ablation in adult *Xenopus*. *Journal of Neurocytology* 11: 211-234.

Bohn, R.C., P.J. Reier and E.B. Sourbeer (1982) Axonal interactions with connective tissue and glial substrata during optic nerve regeneration in *Xenopus* larvae and adults. *American Journal of Anatomy* 165: 397-419.

Bohn, R.C. and D.J. Stelzner (1980) Denervation of non-optic brain areas along the course of the optic tract does not affect the success of optic nerve regeneration in frogs. *Journal of Comparative Neurology* 190: 763-779.

Bohn, R.C. and D.J. Stelzner (1981a) The aberrant retino-retinal projection during optic nerve regeneration in the frog. I. Time course of formation and cells of origin. *Journal of Comparative Neurology* 196: 605-620.

Bohn, R.C. and D.J. Stelzner (1981b) The aberrant retino-retinal projection during optic nerve regeneration in the frog: II. Anterograde labelling with horseradish peroxidase. *Journal of Comparative Neurology* 196: 621-632.

Bohn, R.C. and D.J. Stelzner (1981c) The aberrant retino-retinal projection during optic nerve regeneration in the frog: III. Effects of crushing both nerves. *Journal of Comparative Neurology* 196: 633-643.

Bunt, S.M. and R.D. Lund (1981) Development of a transient retino-retinal pathway in hooded and albino rats. *Brain Research* 211: 399-404.

Burgen, A.S.V. and B. Grafstein (1962) Retinotectal connections after retinal regeneration. *Nature* 196: 898-899.

Cantore, W.A. and F. Scalia (1987) Ultrastructural evidence of the formation of synapses by retinal ganglion cell axons in two nonstandard targets. *Journal of Comparative Neurology* 261:137-147.

Charnas, L.R., B.G. Szaro and H. Gainer (1992) Identification and developmental expression of a novel low molecular weight neuronal intermediate filament protein expressed in *Xenopus laevis*. *Journal of Neuroscience* 12: 3010-3024.

Clarke, J.D.W., D.A. Tonge and N.H.K. Holder (1986) Stage-dependent restoration of sensory dorsal columns following spinal cord transection in anuran tadpoles. *Proceedings of the Royal Society London, Series B* 227: 67-82.

Coleman, L.A., S.A. Dunlop and L.D. Beazley (1984) Patterns of cell division during visual streak formation in the frog *Limnodynastes dorsalis*. *Journal of Embryology and Experimental Morphology* 83: 119-135.

Cowan, W.M. (1973) Neuronal death as a regulative mechanism in the control of cell number in the nervous system. *Development and aging of the nervous system.* Academic Press: 19-41.

Cronly-Dillon, J. (1968) Pattern of retinotectal connections after retinal regeneration. *Journal of Neurophysiology* 31: 547-577.

Darby, J.E., R.A. Carr and L.D. Beazley (1990) Retinal ganglion cell death during regeneration of the frog optic nerve is not accompanied by appreciable cell loss from the inner nuclear layer. *Anatomy and Embryology* 182: 487-492.

Dunlop, S.A. and L.D. Beazley (1984) A morphometric study of the retinal ganglion cell layer and optic nerve from metamorphosis in *Xenopus laevis*. *Vision Research* 24: 417-427.

Dunlop, S.A., M.F. Humphrey and L.D. Beazley (1992) Displaced retinal ganglion cells in normal frogs and those with regenerated optic nerves. *Anatomy and Embryology* 185: 431-438.

Dunlop, S.A., J.D. Roberts, K.N. Armstrong, S.J. Edwards, S.J. Reynolds, M.D. Thom and L.D. Beazley (1997) Impaired vision for binocular tasks after unilateral optic nerve regeneration in the frog *Litoria moorei*. *Behavioural Brain Research* 84:195-201.

Dunlop, S.A., W.M. Ross, A. Shimada and C.R.Braekevelt (submitted for publication) Retinal ganglion cell death is associated with a failure of axons to cross the lesion site during optic nerve regeneration in the frog *Litoria moorei*.

Dunlop, S.A., N. Tran, J. Papadimitriou, N.Tran and L.D. Beazley (2000). Retinal projections throughout optic nerve regeneration in the ornate dragon lizard *Ctenophorus ornatus*. *J. Comp. Neurol.*, 416: 188-2000.

Famiglietti, E.V. and H. Kolb (1976) Structural basis for ON- and OFF-center responses in retinal ganglion cells. *Science* 194:193-195.

Fawcett, J.W. and R.M. Gaze (1981) The organisation of regenerating axons in the *Xenopus* optic nerve. *Brain Research* 229: 487-490.

Flanagan, J.G. and P. Vanderhaegen (1998) The ephrins and eph receptors in neural development. *Annual Review of Neursocience* 21: 309-345.

Frank, B.D. and J.G. Hollyfield (1987) Retinal ganglion cell morphology in the frog, *Rana pipiens*. *Journal of Comparative Neurology* 266: 413-434.

Fraser, S.E., M. Scott Carhart, B.A. Murray, C.M. Chuong and G.M. Edelman (1988) Alterations in the *Xenopus* retinotectal projection by antibodies to *Xenopus* N-CAM. *Developmental Biology* 129: 217-230.

Fuchs, C., E. Glasgow, P.F. Hitchcock and N. Schechter (1994) Plasticin, a newly identified neurofilament protein, is preferentially expressed in young retinal ganglion cells of adult goldfish. *Journal of Comparative Neurology* 350: 452-462.

Fujisawa, H., T Otsuki, S. Takagi and T. Tsuji (1989) An aberrant retinal pathway and visual centres in *Xenopus* tadpoles share a common cell surface molecule, A5 antigen. *Developmental Biology* 135: 27-37.

Fujisawa, H. (1981) Retinotopic analysis of fiber pathways in the regenerating retinotectal system of the adult newt *Cynops pyrrohogaster. Brain Research* 206: 43-57.

Fujisawa, H., N. Tani, K. Watanabe and Y. Ibata (1982) Branching of regenerating retinal axons and preferential selection of appropriate branches for specific neuronal connection in the newt. *Developmental Biology* 90: 43-57.

Fujisawa, H., S. Takagi and T. Hirata (1995) Growth-Associated expression of a membrane protein, neuropilin, in *Xenopus* optic nerve fibers. *Developmental Neuroscience* 17: 343-349.

Gaze, R.M. (1960) Regeneration of the optic nerve in amphibia. *International Review of Neurobiology* 2: 1-40.

Gaze, R.M. (1970) Formation of nerve connections. New York: Academic Press.

Gaze, R.M. and P. Grant (1978) The diencephalic course of regenerating retinotectal fibres in *Xenopus* tadpoles. *Journal of Embryology and Experimental Morphology* 44:201-216.

Gaze, R.M., M. Jacobson and G. Szekely (1965) "Convexity-detectors" in the frog's visual system. *Journal of Physiology* 169: 1-3.

Gaze, R.M. and M. Jacobson (1963) A study of the retinotectal projection during regeneration of the optic nerve in the frog. *Proceedings of the Royal Society London, Series B* 157: 420-448.

Gaze, R.M. and W.E. Watson (1968) Cell division and migration in the brain after optic nerve lesions. "*Growth of the Nervous System" Ciba Foundation Symposium*: 53-67.

Gills, J-P and J.A.C. Wadsworth (1967) Retrograde trans-synaptic degeneration in the inner nuclear layer of the retina. *Investigative Ophthalmology and Visual Science*-6: 437-448.

Giordano, S., E. Glasgow, P. Tesser and N. Schechter (1989) A type II keratin is expressed in glial cells of the goldfish visual pathway. *Neuron* 2:1507-1516.

Giordano, S., C. Hall, W. Quitschke, E. Glasgow and N. Schechter (1990) Keratin 8 of simple epithelia is expressed in glia of the goldfish nervous system. *Differentiation* 44:163-172.

Glagow, E., R.K. Druger, E.M. Levine, C. Fuchs and N. Schechter (1992) Plasticin, a novel type III neurofilament protein from goldfish retina: Increased expression during optic nerve regeneration. *Neuron* 9: 373-381.

Glasgow, E., R.K. Druger, C. Fuchs, W.S. Lane and N. Schechter (1994) Molecular cloning of gefiltin (ON1): serial expression of two neurofilament mRNAs during optic nerve regeneration. *European Molecular Biology Organisation Journal* 13: 297-305.

Glastonbury, J. and K. Straznicky (1978) Aberrant ipsilateral retinotectal projection following optic nerve section in *Xenopus. Neuroscience Letters* 7: 67-72.

Goodbrand, I.A. and R.M. Gaze (1991) Microglia in tadpoles of *Xenopus laevis*: normal distribution and response to optic nerve injury. *Anatomy and Embryology* 184: 71-82.

Grafstein, B. (1967) Transport of protein by goldfish optic nerve fibres. *Science* 157: 196-198.

Gruberg, E.R. and R.V. Stirling (1974) An autoradiographic study of the changes in the frog tectum after cutting the optic nerve. *Brain Research* 76: 359-362.

Harman, A.M. and L.D. Beazley (1989) Generation of retinal ganglion cells in the wallaby *Setonix brachyurus. Neuroscience* 28: 219-232.

Heiber, V., B.W. Agranoff and D. Goldman (1992) Target-Dependent regulation of retinal nicotinic acetylcholine receptor and tubulin RNAs during optic nerve regeneration in goldfish. *Journal of Neurochemistry* 58: 1009-1015.

Hirsch, S., M.A. Cahill and C.A.O. Stuermer (1995) Fibroblasts at the transection site of the injured goldfish optic nerve and their potential role during retinal axonal regeneration. *Journal of Comparative Neurology* 360: 599-611.

Holder, N. and J.W.D. Clarke (1988) Is there a correlation between continuous neurogenesis and directed axon regeneration in the vertebrate nervous system? *Trends in Neuroscience* 11: 94-99.

Hoskins, S.G. and P. Grobstein (1985) 1. Retinal distribution of ipsilaterally projecting cells in normal and experimentally manipulated frogs. *Journal of Neuroscience* 5: 911-919.

Humphrey, M.F. (1987) Effect of different optic nerve lesions on retinal ganglion cell death in the frog *Rana pipiens*. *Journal of Comparative Neurology* 266: 209-219.

Humphrey, M.F. (1988) A morphometric study of the retinal ganglion cell response to optic nerve severance in the frog *Rana pipiens*. *Journal of Neurocytology* 17: 293-304.

Humphrey, M.F. and L.D. Beazley (1982) An electrophysiological study of early retinotectal projection patterns during optic nerve regeneration in *Hyla moorei*. *Brain Research* 239: 595-602.

Humphrey, M.F. and L.D. Beazley (1983) An electrophysiological study of early retinotectal projection patterns during regeneration following optic nerve crush inside the cranium in *Hyla moorei*. *Brain Research* 269: 153-158.

Humphrey, M.F. and L.D. Beazley (1985) Retinal ganglion cell death during optic nerve regeneration in the frog *Hyla moorei*. *Journal of Comparative Neurology* 236: 382-402.

Humphrey, M.F., J.E. Darby and L.D. Beazley (1989) Retinal ganglion cell death is transiently delayed when optic nerve regeneration is prevented in the frog *Hyla moorei*. *Journal of Comparative Neurology* 279:187-198.

Humphrey, M.F., S.A. Dunlop, A. Shimada and L.D. Beazley (1992) Disconnected optic axons persist in the visual pathway during regeneration of the retino-tectal projection in the frog. *Experimental Brain Research* 90: 630-634.

Humphrey, M.F., G.M.C. Renshaw, P.D. Kitchener and L.D. Beazley (1995) Substance P, bombesin and leucine-enkephalin immunoreactivities are restored in the frog tectum after optic nerve regeneration. *Journal of Comparative Neurology* 354: 295-305.

Jacobson, M. (1991) Developmental Neurobiology. Plenum Press, New York, London.

Janusonis, S. and K.V. Fite (1997) NMDAR1-like immunoreactive fibers appear in the ipsilateral optic tract during optic nerve regeneration in *Rana pipiens*. *Neuroscience Letters* 236: 1-4.

Jenkins, S. and C. Straznicky (1986) Naturally occurring and induced ganglion cell death. A retinal whole-mount autoradiographic study in *Xenopus*. *Anatomy and Embryology* 174: 59-66.

Kahn, A.J. (1974) An autoradiographic study of the time of appearance of neurons in the developing chick neural retina. *Developmental Biology* 38: 30-40.

Kaplan, E.I. and C.D. Clemente (1985) Peripheral nerve grafts to the frog optic tectum: A morphological study of foreign axon regeneration in the central nervous system. *Journal of Comparative Neurology* 235: 395-415.

Katzenstein, M.B. and R.C. Bohn (1984) Regeneration of transected dorsal root ganglion cell axons into the spinal cord in adult frogs (*Xenopus laevis*). *Brain Research* 300: 188-191.

Keating, M.J. and R.M. Gaze (1970) The depth distribution of visual units in the contralateral optic tectum following regeneration of the optic nerve in the frog. *Brain Research* 21: 197-206.

Keirstead, H.S., S.J. Hasan, G.D. Muir and J.D. Steeves (1992) Suppression of the onset of myelination extends the permissive period for the functional repair of embryonic spinal cord. *Proceedings of the National Academy of Science, USA* 89:11664-11668.

Kiernan, J.A. (1979) Hypothesis concerned with axonal regeneration in the mammalian nervous system. *Biological Reviews* 54, 155-197.

Kiernan, J.A. and A. Contestabile (1980) Vascular permeability associated with axonal regeneration in the optic system of the goldfish. *Acta Neuropathologica* (Berlin) 51: 39-45.

Kruger, L. and D.S. Maxwell (1969) Wallerian degeneration in the optic nerve of a reptile: An electron microscopic study. *American Journal of Anatomy* 125: 247-270.

Kuljis, R.O. and H.J. Karten (1982) Laminar organisation of the peptide-like immunoreactivity in the anuran optic tectum. *Journal of Comparative Neurology* 212:188-201.

Kuljis, R.O. and H.J. Karten (1983) Modifications in the laminar organisation of peptide-like immunoreactivity in the anuran optic tectum following retinal deafferentation. *Journal of Comparative Neurology* 217: 239-251.

Kuljis, R.O. and H.J. Karten (1985) Regeneration of peptide-containing retinofugal axons into the optic tectum with reappearance of a substance P-containing lamina. *Journal of Comparative Neurology* 240:1-15.

Kuljis, R.O., J.E. Krause and H.J. Karten (1984) Peptide-like immunoreactivity in anuran optic nerve fibers. *Journal of Comparative Neurology* 226: 222-237.

Lang, D.M., M. Monzon-Mayor, C.E. Bandtlow and C.A.O. Stuermer (1998) Retinal axon regeneration in the lizard *Gallotia galloti* in the presence of CNS myelin and oligodendrocytes. *Glia* 23: 61-74.

Lang, D.M., B.P. Rubin, M.E. Schwab and C.A.O. Stuermer (1995) CNS myelin and oligodendrocytes of the Xenopus spinal cord - but not optic nerve - are nonpermissive for axon growth. *Journal of Neuroscience* 15: 99-109.

Lazar, G. (1980) Long-term persistence, after eye-removal, of unmyelinated fibres in the frog visual pathway. *Brain Research* 199: 219-224.

Lazarov-Spiegler, O., A.S. Solomon, A.B. Zeev-Brann, D.L. Hirschbert, V. Lavie and M. Schwartz (1996) Transplantation of activated macrophages overcomes central nervous system regrowth failure. *The FASEB Journal* 10:1296-1302.

Li, Y., P.M. Field and G. Raisman (1997) Repair of adult rat corticospinal tract by transplants of olfactory ensheathing cells. *Science* 277:2000-2002.

Linke, R. and G. Roth (1989) Morphology of retinal ganglion cells in lungless salamanders (Fam. Plethodontidae): an HRP and Golgi study. *Journal of Comparative Neurology* 289: 361-374.

Linke, R. and G. Roth (1990) Optic nerves in plethodontid salamanders (amphibia, urodela): neuroglia, fiber spectrum and myelination. *Anatomy and Embryology* 181: 37-48.

Liuzzi, F.J. and R.H. Miller (1990) Neovascularization occurs in response to crush lesions of adult frog optic nerves. *Journal of Neurocytology* 19: 224-234.

Lyon, M.J. and D.J. Stelzner (1987) Tests of the regenerative capacity of tectal efferent axons in the frog, *Rana pipiens*. *Journal of Comparative Neurology* 255: 511-525.

Manteifel, Y.B. and L.N. D'Yachkova (1970) Ultrastructure and functional characteristics of the optic nerve of *Rana temporaria L.* in the normal and during regeneration. *Neirofiziol* 2: 627-635.

Matsumoto, D.E. and F. Scalia (1981) Long-term survival of centrally projecting axons in the optic nerve of the frog following destruction of the retina. *Journal of Comparative Neurology* 202:135-155.

Matthey, R. (1925) Recuperation de la vue apres resection des nerfs optiques chez le triton. *Comptes Rendus de Seance Societe de Biologie* 93: 904-906.

Maturana, H.R., J.Y. Lettvin and W.S. McCulloch (1960) Anatomy and physiology of vision in the frog *Rana pipiens*. *Journal of General Physiology* 43:129-175.

Maturana, H.R., J.Y. Lettvin, W.S. McCulloch and W.H. Pitts (1959) Evidence that cut nerve fibers in a frog regenerate to their proper places in the tectum. *Science* 130:1709-1710.

McKeon, R.J., R.C. Schreiber, J.S. Rudge and J. Silver (1991) Reduction of neurite outgrowth in a model of glial scarring following CNS injury is correlated with the expression of inhibitory molecules on reactive astrocytes. *Journal of Neuroscience* 11: 3398-3411.

Meister, M., R. Wong, D. Baylor and C. Shatz (1991) Synchronous bursts of action potentials in ganglion cells of the developing mammalian retina. *Science* 252: 939-943.

Meyer, R.L. (1978) Evidence from thymidine labelling for continuing growth of the retina and tectum in juvenile goldfish. *Experimental Neurology* 59: 99-111.

Michel, M.E. and P.J. Reier (1979) Axonal-ependymal associations during early regeneration of the transected spinal cord in *Xenopus laevis* tadpoles. *Journal of Neurocytology* 8: 529-548.

Misantone, L.J. and D.J. Stelzner (1974) Behavioural manifestations of competition of retinal endings for sites in doubly innervated frog optic tectum. *Experimental Neurology* 45: 364-376.

Montgomery N., and K.V. Fite (1989) Retinotopic organization of central optic projections in Rana pipiens. *Journal of Comparative Neurology* 283:526-540.

Montgomery, N., K.V. Fite and L. Bengston (1981) The accessory optic system of *Rana pipiens*. Neuroanatomical connections and intrinsic organisation. *Journal of Comparative Neurology* 236: 382-402.

Murray, M. (1982) A quantitative study of regenerative sprouting by optic axons in goldfish. *Journal of Comparative Neurology* 209: 352-362.

Murray, M., S.C. Sharma, and M.E. Edwards (1982) Target regulation of synaptic number in the compressed retinotectal projection of the goldfish. *Journal of Comparative Neurology* 209: 374-385.

Nona, S.N. (1998) Repair in goldfish central nervous system. *Restorative Neurology and Neuroscience* 12: 1-11.

Nona, S.N.and C.A. Stafford (1995) Glial repair at the lesion site in regenerating goldfish spinal cord: An immunohistochemical study using species specific antibodies. *Journal of Neuroscience Research* 42: 350-356.

Nona, S.N., S.A.S. Shehab, C.A. Stafford and J.R. Cronly-Dillon (1989) Glial fibrillary acidic protein (GFAP) from goldfish: Its localisation in the visual pathway. *Glia* 2: 189-200.

Nona, S.N., A.M. Tomlinson and C.A. Stafford (1998) Temporary colonisation of the site of lesion by macrophages is a prelude to the arrival of regenerated axons in injured goldfish optic nerve. *Journal of Neurocytology* 27: 791-803.

O'Leary, D.D.M, D. Crespo, J.W. Fawcett and W.M. Cowan (1986) The effect of intraocular tetrodotoxin on the postnatal reduction in the numbers of optic axons in the rat. *Developmental Brain Research* 30: 96-103.

Ostberg, A. and J. Norden (1979) Ultrastructural study of degeneration and regeneration in the amphibian tectum. *Brain Research* 168: 441-455.

Playford, D.E. and S.A. Dunlop (1993) A biphasic sequence of myelination in the developing optic nerve of the frog. *Journal of Comparative Neurology*. 333: 83-93.

Pedalina, R. and L.D. Beazley (1986) A tritiated thymidine study of cell division in the retina during optic nerve regeneration for the frog *Hyla moorei*. *Neuroscience Letters* 23: 70.

Perry, V.H. (1981) Evidence for an amacrine cell system in the ganglion layer of the rat retina. *Neuroscience* 6: 931-944.

Perry, V.H., M.C. Brown and S.C. Gordon (1987) The macrophage response to central and peripheral nerve injury - a possible role of macrophages in regeneration. *Journal of Experimental Medicine* 165:1218-1223.

Pomeranz, B. (1971) Metamorphosis of frog vision: Changes in ganglion cell physiology and anatomy. *Experimental Neurology* 34:187-199.

Quigley, H.A., R.W. Nickells, L.A. Kerigan, M.E. Pease, D.J. Thibault and D.J. Zack (1995) Retinal ganglion cell death in experimental glaucoma and after axotomy occurs by apoptosis. *Investigative Ophthalmology and Visual Science* 36: 69-78.

Ramon, Y. Cajal, S.R. (1892) La retinae des vertibres. English translation: The structure of the retina (compiled and translated by Thorpe S.A and Glickstein, M.) Thomas, Springfield, III. In *La Cellule*. 9:17-257.

Reh, T.A., E. Pitts and M. Constantine-Paton (1983) The organisation of fibers in the optic nerve of normal and tectum-less *Rana pipiens*. *Journal of Comparative Neurology* 218: 282-296.

Reier, P.J. (1979) Penetration of grafted astrocytic scars by regenerating optic nerve axons in *Xenopus* tadpoles. *Brain Research* 164: 61-68.

Reier, P.J. and H.D. Webster (1974) Regeneration and remyelination of *Xenopus* tadpole optic nerve fibres following transection or crush. *Journal of Neurocytology* 3: 591-618.

Reperant, J., D. Miceli, N.P. Vesselkin and S. Molotchnikoff (1989) The centrifugal visual system of vertebrates: A century old search reviewed. *International Review of Cytology* 118: 115-171.

Rio, J.P., J. Reperant, R. Ward, J. Peyrichoux and N. Vesselkin (1989) A preliminary description of the regeneration of optic nerve fibers in a reptile, *Vipera aspis*. *Brain Research* 479: 151-156.

Rodger, J., C. Bartlett, L.D. Beazley and S.A. Dunlop (1999) Ephrin A2 is re-expressed in a rostro-caudal gradient across the optic tectum during optic nerve regeneration in the lizard *C. ornatus*. *Neurosci Abs.*,29, 194.21.

Rodger, J., S.A. Dunlop, J.M. Papadimitriou and L.D. Beazley (1998) The neurofilament protein gefiltin is persistently upregulated following optic nerve crush in the lizard *Ctenophorus ornatus*. *American Neuroscience Society* 24: 420.19.

Rungger-Brandle, E., C. Alloid, B. Fouquet and M.M. Messerli (1995) Behaviour of macroglial cells, as identified by their intermediate filament complement, during optic nerve regeneration of *Xenopus* tadpole. *Glia* 13: 255-271.

Rushton, W.A.H. (1951) A theory of the effects of fibre size in medullated nerve. *Journal of Physiology* 115:101-122.

Rutishauser, U. (1984) Developmental biology of a neural cell adhesion molecule. *Nature* 310: 549-554.

Sakaguchi, D.S., R.K. Murphey, R.K. Hunt and R. Tompkins (1984) The development of retinal ganglion cells in a tetraploid strain of *Xenopus laevis*: A morphological study utilizing intracellular dye injection. *Journal of Comparative Neurology* 224: 231-251.

Sargent, P.B., S.H. Pike, D.B. Nadel and J.M. Lindstrom (1989) Nicotinic acetylcholine receptor-like molecules in the retina, retinotectal pathway, and optic tectum of the frog. *Journal of Neuroscience* 9: 565-573.

Satoda, M., S. Takagi, K. Ohta, T. Hirata and H. Fujisawa (1995) Differential expression of two cell surface proteins, neuropilin and plexin in *Xenopus* olfactory axon sub-classes. *Journal of Neuroscience* 15: 942-955.

Scalia, F. (1987) Synapse formation in the olfactory cortex by regenerating optic axons: ultrastructural evidence for polyspecific chemoaffinity. *Journal of Comparative Neurology* 263: 497-513.

Scalia, F. and V. Arango (1983) The anti-retinotopic organisation of the frog's optic nerve. *Brain Research* 266:121-126.

Scalia, F., V. Arango and E.L. Singman (1985) Loss and displacement of ganglion cells after optic nerve regeneration in adult *Rana pipiens*. *Brain Research* 344: 267-280.

Scalia, F. and K.V. Fite (1974) A retinotopic analysis of the central connections of the optic nerve in the frog. *Journal of Comparative Neurology* 158: 455-478.

Scalia, F. and D.E. Matsumoto (1985) The morphology of growth cones of regenerating optic nerve axons. *Journal of Comparative Neurology* 231: 323-338.

Schmidt, J.T. (1978) Retinal fibers alter tectal markers during expansion of the half retinal projection in goldfish. *Journal of Comparative Neurology* 177: 279-300.

Schmidt, J.T. (1990) Long-term potentiation and activity-dependent retinotopic sharpening in the regenerating retinotectal projection of goldfish: common sensitive period and sensitivity to NMDA blockers. *Journal of Neuroscience* 10: 233-246.

Schmidt, J.T. (1993) Activity-driven mechanisms for sharpening retinotopic projections: Correlated activity, NMDA receptors, calcium entry and beyond. *Formation and Regeneration of Nerve Connections,* ed. Sharma S.C. & Fawcett J.W. pp185-204.

Schnell L. and M.E. Schwab (1990) Axonal regeneration in the rat spinal cord produced by an antibody against myelin-associated neurite growth inhibitors. *Nature* 343: 269-272.

Scott, T.M. and J. Foote (1981) A study of degeneration, scar formation and regeneration after section of the optic nerve in the frog *Rana pipiens*. *Journal of Anatomy* 133: 213-225.

Sharma, S.C. and M. Romeskie (1977) Immediate compression of the goldfish retinal projection to a tectum devoid of degenerating debris. *Brain Research* 133: 367-370.

Sharma, S.C. and C. Tsai (1991) Retention of retinal axon collateral is responsible for induced ipsilateral retinotectal projections in adult goldfish. *Vision Research* 31: 499-505.

Sharma, S.C., A.G. Jadhao and P.D. Prasada Rao (1993) Regeneration of supraspinal neuron projection in the adult goldfish. *Brain Research* 620: 221-228.

Sheard, P.W. and L.D. Beazley (1988) Retinal ganglion cell death is not prevented by application of tetrodotoxin during optic nerve regeneration for the frog *Hyla moorei*. *Vision Research* 28: 461-470.

Simpson, S.B. (1968) Morphology of the regenerated spinal cord in the lizard, *Anolis carolinensis*. *Journal of Comparative Neurology* 134: 193-210.

Singman, E.L. and F. Scalia (1990a) Further study of the outward displacement of retinal ganglion cells during optic nerve regeneration, with a note on the normal cells of Dogiel in the adult frog. *Journal of Comparative Neurology* 301: 80-92.

Singman, E.L. and F. Scalia (1990b) Quantitative study of the tectally projecting retinal ganglion cells in the adult frog: I. The size of the contralateral and ipsilateral projections. *Journal of Comparative Neurology* 302: 792-809.

Singman, E.L. and F. Scalia (1991) Quantitative study of the tectally projecting retinal ganglion cells in the adult frog. II. Cell survival and functional recovery after optic nerve transection. *Journal of Comparative Neurology* 307: 351-369.

Sivron, T., M.E. Schwab and M. Schwartz (1994) Presence of growth inhibitors in fish optic nerve myelin: Postinjury changes. *Journal of Comparative Neurology* 343: 237-246.

Soreide, A.J. (1981) Variations in the axon reaction after different types of nerve lesion. Light and electron microscopic studies on the facial nucleus of the rat. *Acta Anatomica* 110:173-188.

Sperry, R.W. (1943b) Visuomotor coordination in the newt (*Triturus viridescens*) after regeneration of the optic nerve. *Journal of Comparative Neurology*. 79: 33-55.

Sperry, R.W. (1944) Optic nerve regeneration with return of vision in anurans. *Journal of Neurophysiology* 7: 57-69.

Sperry, R.W. (1951) Mechanisms of neural maturation. *Handbook of Experimental Psychology*. Wiley, New York pp 236-280.

Springer, A.D., K.D. Morel and B.R. Wilson (1990) Topographic disorganisation of the optic tracts following long-term optic nerve regeneration: A quantitative image analysis study. *Journal of Comparative Neurology* 298: 458-471.

Starac, D., S.A. Dunlop and L.D. Beazley (1996) Displaced retinal ganglion cells in the lizard *Ctenophorus ornatus*. *Proceedings of the Australian Neuroscience. Society* 7: 48.

Stelzner, D.J. (1979) Evidence of collateral sprouting in the frog visual system. *Brain Research* 168: 382-387.

Stelzner, D.J., R.C. Bohn and J.A. Strauss (1981) Expansion of the ipsilateral retinal projection in the frog brain during optic nerve regeneration: Sequence of reinnervation and retinotopic organisation. *Journal of Comparative Neurology* 201: 299-317.

Stelzner, D.J. and J.A. Strauss (1986) A quantitative analysis of frog optic nerve regeneration: Is retrograde ganglion cell death or collateral axonal loss related to selective reinnervation? *Journal of Comparative Neurology* 245: 83-106.

Stelzner, D.J. and J.A. Strauss (1988) Increase in ganglion cell size after optic nerve regeneration in the frog, *Rana pipiens*. *Experimental Neurology* 100: 210-215.

Stirling, R.V., S.A. Dunlop and L.D. Beazley (1998) An *in vitro* technique to map retinotectal projections in reptiles. *Journal of Neuroscience Methods* 81: 85-89.

Stirling, R.V, S.A. Dunlop and L.D. Beazley (1999) Electrophysiological evidence for transient topographic organisation during optic nerve regeneration in the lizard *Ctenophorus ornatus*. *Visual Neuroscience* 16: 682-693.

Stirling, R.V., S.A. Dunlop and L.D. Beazley (submitted for publication) Visually evoked extracellular spikes recorded from the lizard optic tectum *in vitro* are postsynaptic.

Stirling, R.V. and E.G. Merrill (1987) Functional morphology of frog retinal ganglion cells and their central projections: The dimming detectors. *Journal of Comparative Neurology* 258: 477-495.

Straznicky, C. (1988) On the dendritic arbors of retinal ganglion cells. *Neuroscience. Letters (Supplement)* 30: 539.

Straznicky, K. and R.M. Gaze (1971) The growth of the retina in *Xenopus laevis*: An autoradiographic study. *Journal of Embryology and Experimental Morphology* 26: 67-79.

Straznicky, K., D. Tay and C. Lunam (1978) Changes in retinotectal projection in adult *Xenopus* following partial retinal ablation. *Neuroscience Letters* 8: 105-111.

Straznicky, C., R.M. Gaze and T.J. Horder (1979) Selection of appropriate medial branch of the optic tract by fibres of ventral retinal origin during development and regeneration:

An autoradiographic study in *Xenopus*. *Journal of Embryology and Experimental Morphology* 50: 253-267.

Straznicky, C., D. Tay and J. Glastonbury (1980) Regeneration of an abnormal ipsilateral visuotectal projection in *Xenopus* is delayed by the presence of optic fibres from the other eye. *Journal of Embryology and Experimental Morphology* 57: 129-141.

Straznicky, C. and I.T. Straznicky (1988) Morphological classification of retinal ganglion cells in adult *Xenopus laevis*. *Anatomy and Embryology* 178: 143-153.

Szaro, B.G., L.A. Faulkner, R.K. Hunt and Y. Peng Loh (1984) Axonal transport of [^{35}S] methionine labeled proteins in *Xenopus* optic nerve: Phases of transport and the effects of nerve crush on protein patterns. *Brain Research* 297: 337-355.

Szaro, B.G., Y.P. Loh and R.K. Hunt (1985) Specific changes in axonally transported proteins during regeneration of the frog (*Xenopus laevis*) optic nerve. *Journal of Neuroscience* 5: 192-208.

Taylor, J.S.H., J.L. Lack and S.S. Easter (1989) Is the capacity for optic nerve regeneration related to continuous retinal ganglion cell production in the frog? A test of the hypothesis that neurogenesis and axon regeneration are obligatorily linked. *European Journal of Neuroscience* 1: 626-638.

Tennant, M. and L.D. Beazley (1992) Dimensions of the lesion site influence the extent of retinal ganglion cell death during optic nerve regeneration in the frog *Litoria (Hyla) moorei*. *Proceedings of Australian Neuroscience Society* 3: 97.

Tennant, M. and L.D. Beazley (1992) A breakdown of the blood-brain barrier is associated with optic nerve regeneration in the frog. *Visual Neuroscience* 9: 149-155.

Tennant, M., S.R. Bruce and L.D. Beazley (1993) Survival of ganglion cells which form the retino-retinal projection during optic nerve regeneration in the frog. *Visual Neuroscience* 10: 681-686.

Tennant, M., S.R. Moore and L.D. Beazley (1993) Transient neovascularisation of the frog retina during optic nerve regeneration. *Journal of Comparative Neurology* 336:605-612.

Thanos, S., R. Naskar, P. Heiduschka (1997) Regenerating ganglion cell axons in the adult rat establish retinofugal topography and restore visual function. *Experimental Brain Research* 114: 483-491.

Tong, L., P.D. Spear, R.E. Kalil and E. Callahan (1982) Loss of retinal X-cells in cats with neonatal or adult visual cortex damage. *Science* 217: 72-75.

Toth, P. and C. Straznicky (1989) Dendritic morphology of identified retinal ganglion cells in *Xenopus laevis*: A comparison between the results of Horseradish Peroxidase and Cobaltic-Lysine retrograde labelling. *Archives of Histology and Cytology* 52: 87-93.

Tran, N., S.A. Dunlop, J.M. Papadimitriou, and L.D. Beazley (1996) Time course of optic nerve regeneration in the lizard *Ctenophorus ornatus*. *American Neuroscience Abstracts* 26: 591.1.

Turner, J.E. and K.A. Glaze (1977) The early stages of Wallerian degeneration in the severed optic nerve of the newt (*Triturus viridescens*). *Anatomical Record* 187: 291-310.

Udin, S.B. (1977) Re-arrangements of the retinotectal projection in *Rana pipiens* after unilateral caudal half-tectum ablation. *Journal of Comparative Neurology* 173: 561-582.

Udin, S.B. (1978) Permanent disorganisation of the regenerating optic tract in the frog. *Experimental Neurology* 58: 455-470.

Vidal-Sanz, M., G.M. Bray, M.P. Villegas-Perez, S. Thanos and A.J. Aguayo (1987) Axonal regeneration and synapse formation in the superior colliculus by retinal ganglion cells in the adult rat. *Journal of Neuroscience*. 7: 2894-2909.

Waldeck, R.F. and E.R. Gruberg (1995) Regrowth of optic fibers and behavioural recovery after optic chiasm transection. *Experimental Neurology* 132: 229-238.

Walsh, C. and E.H. Polley (1985) The topography of ganglion cell production in the cat's retina. *Journal of Neuroscience* 5: 741-750.

Wanner, M., D.M. Lang, C.E. Bandtlow, M.E. Schwab, M. Bastmeyer and C.A.O. Stuermer (1995) Re-evaluation of the growth-permissive substrate properties of goldfish optic nerve myelin and myelin proteins. *Journal of Neuroscience* 15: 7500-7508.

Wassle, H., B.B. Boycott and R.-B. Illing (1981) Morphology and mosaic of on and off-beta cells in the cat retina and some functional considerations. *Proceedings of the Royal Society London, Series B* 212:177-195.

Wilson, M.A., R.M. Gaze, I.A. Goodbrand and J.S.H. Taylor (1992) Regeneration in the *Xenopus* tadpole optic nerve is preceded by a massive macrophage/microglial response. *Anatomy and Embryology* 186: 75-89.

Wyllie, A.H., J.F.R. Kerr and A.R. Currie (1980) Cell death: The significance of apoptosis. *International Review of Cytology* 68: 251-306.

Zhao, Y. and B.G. Szaro (1994) The return of phosphorylated and non-phosphorylated epitopes of neurofilament proteins to the regenerating optic nerve of *Xenopus laevis*. *Journal of Comparative Neurology* 343: 158-172.

Zhao, Y. and B.G. Szaro (1995) The optic tract and tectal ablation influence the composition of neurofilaments in regenerating optic axons on *Xenopus laevis*. *Journal of Neuroscience* 15: 4629-4640.

Zhao, Y. and B.G. Szaro (1997a) Xefiltin, a new low molecular weight neuronal intermediate filament protein of *Xenopus laevis*, shares sequence features with goldfish gefiltin and mammalian alpha-internexin and differs in expression of XNIF and NF-L. *Journal of Comparative Neurology* 377: 158-172.

4

Axonal and Synaptic Regeneration by Salamander Photoreceptors

Ellen Townes-Anderson
University of Medicine and Dentistry New Jersey Medical School, Newark, New Jersey

Michele Nachman-Clewner
Joan and Sanford I. Weill Graduate School of Medical Sciences of Cornell University, New York, New York

I. INTRODUCTION

The most feared disability, compared to the loss of memory, hearing, speech, and limb movement, is the loss of vision (National Advisory Eye Council, 1994). Many of the causes of blindness are a result of retinal disease. In the retina, it is the photoreceptor cell which is particularly sensitive to insult and a common denominator among retinal disorders is the degeneration and death of photoreceptor cells. After the loss of the primary sensory neurons, however, 20-75% of the retinal ganglion cells, and even a larger percentage of inner retinal neurons, remain (Stone et al., 1992; Humayun et al., 1999). There has been interest, therefore, in trying to transplant healthy photoreceptor cells back into degenerate retinas in order to restore sight. Although transplanted photoreceptors, whether from adult, embryonic or fetal sources, survive for long periods of time in the subretinal space in animal models, there is little evidence of synaptic integration with the host retina (Gouras et al., 1991, 1994; Lazar and Del Cerro, 1992; Silverman and Hughes, 1989; Silverman et al., 1992). Thus, there is a need to better understand synaptogenesis by photoreceptor cells in general and regeneration of the axonal fiber and terminal in the case of adult cells.

Recently there have also been demonstrations that the synaptic connectivity between photoreceptor cells and second order neurons, the horizontal and bipolar cells, can change in retinal disease and that these changes precede observable degeneration of the photoreceptor cell. Most of these changes occur in rod cell axons and include; retraction of the axon terminal towards the cell body, in a cat model of retinal detachment (Erickson et al., 1983; Lewis et al., 1998); increase in the number of synaptic active zones, in mice with genetic or light-produced retinal degenerations (Jansen and Sanyal, 1984, 1987, 1992); and neuritic process outgrowth, in human retinas afflicted with retinitis pigmentosa (Li et al., 1995; Milam et al., 1996). On the one hand, these structural alterations give hope that the photoreceptor terminal, in particular the rod terminal, is capable of regenerative growth and synapse formation. On the other hand, these changes indicate that inappropriate plasticity and sprouting are possible and that the mechanisms involved in axonal maintenance need to be determined in order to harness the apparent regenerative potential.

This chapter will review what is known about axonal plasticity and synaptogenesis by adult salamander (*Ambystoma tigrinum*) photoreceptors and discuss possible implications for regeneration of functional synapses by mammalian rod and cone cells.

II. THE PHOTORECEPTOR SYNAPSE: NORMAL STRUCTURE

In common with all vertebrate retinas, salamander rod and cone cells make ribbon synapses and basal junctions with second order neurons (Fig. 1). Their terminals, which are wide and contain multiple active zones, are also called pedicles. The presynaptic terminal of the ribbon synapse is characterized by the presence of thin, electron dense plaques, the so-called ribbons. In the salamander rod cell there is an average of 7.3 ribbons per terminal (Townes-Anderson et al., 1985). The ribbons are attached to the cytoplasmic face of the plasma membrane and occur along invaginations of the terminal surface, along relatively flat regions of the terminal, and along basal processes or telodendria which extend from the body of the terminal. Other than the ribbon, the principal intracellular organelle in the axon terminal is the small clear synaptic vesicle; probably more than 100,000 vesicles fill the terminal (see Pierantoni and McCann, 1981). The vesicles are densest around the synaptic ribbons and each ribbon is coated with vesicles which attach by molecules as yet unidentified. The ribbon, therefore, serves to aggregate large numbers of vesicles at the active zone. In response to depolarization, vesicular exocytosis causes the release of the excitatory amino acid, glutamate (Copenhagen and Jahr, 1989). Exocytosis is Ca^{++}-dependent and occurs on either side of the attachment site of the ribbon to the plasma membrane. In the salamander, one ribbon active zone can be presynaptic to 1-3 postsynaptic processes (a monad, dyad, or triad respectively) (Lasansky, 1973). Additional intracellular components in the rod ending include elements of smooth endoplasmic reticulum (presumably endo-

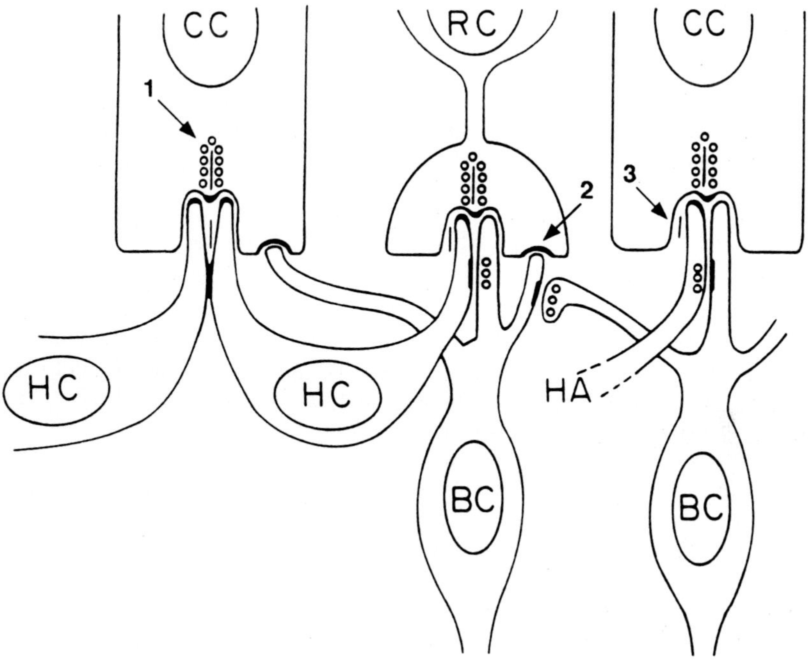

Figure 1 Synaptic interactions by rod and cone cells in the outer synaptic layer of the salamander retina. 1: Photoreceptors form ribbon synapses with the processes of horizontal and bipolar cells. Although there are many ribbon synapses made by a single rod or cone terminal only one ribbon per terminal is illustrated here. 2: Basal junctions occur between photoreceptors and bipolar cells. 3: Distal junctions are found in some cold blooded vertebrate retinas including the salamander. They occur between photoreceptors and horizontal cells. Note that the rod cell has a short axonal fiber whereas the cone cell terminal is broadly continuous with the cell body. CC, cone cell; RC, rod cell; HC, horizontal cell; BC, bipolar cell; HA, horizontal cell axon. (Based on the work of Lasansky, 1973).

somes and calcisomes), coated vesicles, dense-cored vesicles which probably contain melatonin, multivesicular bodies, lysosomes and cytoskeletal elements; mitochondria, however, are not present. Cone cell pedicles are structurally similar. The most noticeable difference between the two terminals is the presence of a short axonal fiber, about 15 μm in length, between the terminal and cell body in the rod cell and the absence of any fiber between the cone pedicle and cell body. In salamander rod photoreceptors, moreover, there can be more than one axon per cell and more than one axon terminal per axon (Lasansky, 1973; Mandell et al., 1993). In general, ribbon synapses are molecularly similar to conventional chemical synapses with three notable differences: 1) ribbon synapses contain no synapsins (Mandell et al., 1990); 2) rod axons and terminals contain no tau or neurofilaments but instead contain the embryonic forms of two microtubule-associated proteins, MAP2c and MAP5, a homolog of MAP1B (Dräger, 1983; Tucker and Matus, 1988); and 3) transmitter release is controlled by L-type, as opposed to N- and P/Q-type, voltage-gated Ca^{++} channels (Rieke and Schwartz, 1994, 1996; Schmitz and Witkovsky, 1997). Recent evidence suggests that in rod cell terminals L-type channels cluster at the ribbon active zone in strips or small spots (Nachman-Clewner et al., 1999).

III. PHOTORECEPTORS CAN BE ISOLATED FROM THE ADULT RETINA

Since the early seventies it has been possible to isolate morphologically identifiable rod and cone cells from vertebrate retina (Lam, 1972). Culture of adult photoreceptors, however, was not feasible until the development of adhesive substrates. Adult central nervous system neurons do not adhere to standard cell culture substrates like laminin and collagen (Townes-Anderson et al., 1988). This may be a result of the very low levels of extracellular matrix normally present in adult central nervous system tissue. The adhesive substrate developed for salamander neurons was a monoclonal antibody raised against retinal cell membranes (MacLeish et al., 1983). Application of the antibody to the culture surface produced immediate neuronal adhesion with no evidence of neurotoxicity.

Using enzymatic digestion followed by mechanical trituration, isolated salamander photoreceptors are obtained in varying states of intactness (Fig. 2). The photoreceptor cell contains several distinct regions: the cell body where the nucleus is located, the inner segment which contains synthetic organelles and the mitochondria, the outer segment which is the photosensitive portion of the cell, and the synaptic terminal. After retinal dissociation, rod and cone cells can retain or lose their outer segment. Rod cells can also either retain or lose their axon and axon terminal; cone cells, on the other hand, always retain their axon terminal since it is broadly continuous with the cell body.

Isolated photoreceptors have been examined with a variety of techniques to assess whether or not normal functions are retained *in vitro*. At the electron microscopic level, all intracellular organelles appear healthy (Townes-Anderson et al., 1985). In the presynaptic terminal, when present, there continues to be a high density of synaptic vesicles; with immunocytochemistry this results in bright immunostaining of the axon terminal for synaptic vesicle membrane proteins such as SV2 and synaptophysin. In addition, 73% of synaptic ribbons remain attached to the plasmalemma and invaginations of the surface continue to be present even though all postsynaptic processes have been removed. However, when the outer segment is retained, an interesting alteration occurs between the inner and outer segments of the rod cell. The outer segment contains membranous disks loaded with photopigment, rhodopsin. Opsin (the protein component of the photopigment) is abundant in the plasma membrane as well as the disks of the outer segment. The outer segment is normally separated from the inner segment, the exten-

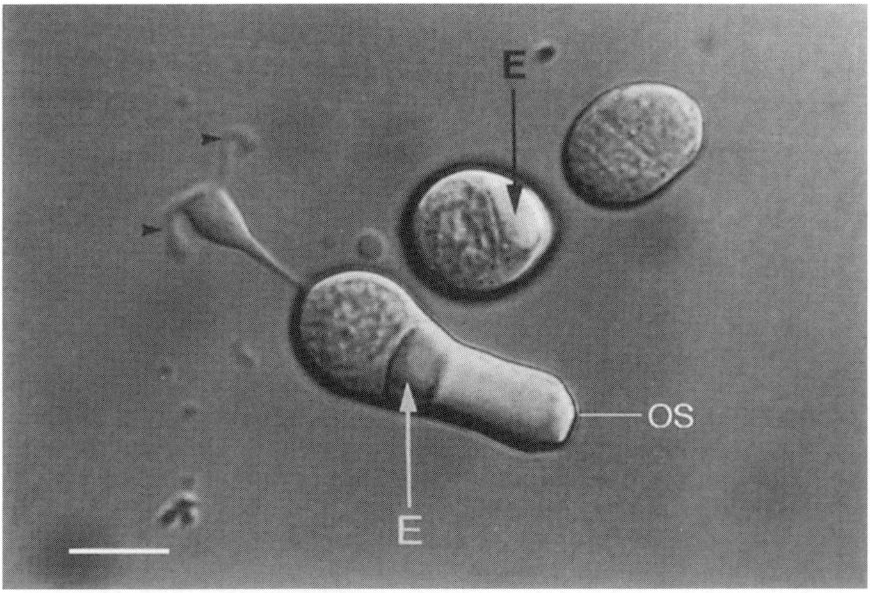

Figure 2 Freshly isolated salamander rod cells. Photoreceptors occur in varying states of intactness. Here, two rod cells are identified by the presence of an aggregation of mitochondria in the inner segment, called the ellipsoid (E), a characteristic feature of amphibian photoreceptors. One cell retains its outer segment (OS), its axon and axonal terminal, and even basal processes (arrowheads). The other cell has lost both the outer segment and axon. Bar = 10 μm.

sion of the cell body which contains the cytoplasmic organelles, by a thin connecting cilium. After isolation, the inner and outer segments become fused. This may allow abnormal exchange of molecules between these two cell regions.

Similar fusion between the inner and outer segments has been seen in intact retina (Richardson, 1969; Townes-Anderson, 1995). Its effect on photoreceptor cell biology remains to be determined. Immunocytochemistry, however, has demonstrated that opsin is present in relatively equal intensity in the plasma membrane of the inner and outer segments when inner / outer segment fusion occurs (Mandell et al., 1993) suggesting that the normal barrier to opsin diffusion between these two cell regions no longer exists. With electrophysiological techniques, isolated rod and cone cells which retain their outer segment have been shown to have normal hyperpolarizing responses to light (MacLeish et al., 1982). There is also the expected uptake of tracer into coated vesicles, endosomes and synaptic vesicles during depolarization when electron dense tracers are applied to cells which retain their axon terminal (Fig. 3) (Townes-Anderson et al., 1985) indicating that synaptic vesicle exocytosis and vesicle recycling have occurred. Membrane capacitance measurements have additionally shown that vesicle fusion is calcium dependent (Rieke and Schwartz, 1996).

Thus, many characteristic cell activities remain after cell isolation. Indeed, confidence in the functional integrity of isolated photoreceptors has produced numerous studies on ion currents, membrane receptors, Ca^{++} homeostasis, etc. (e.g. Bader et al., 1982; Townes-Anderson and Vogt, 1987; Wilkinson and Barnes, 1996; Rieke and Schwartz, 1996) using these cells.

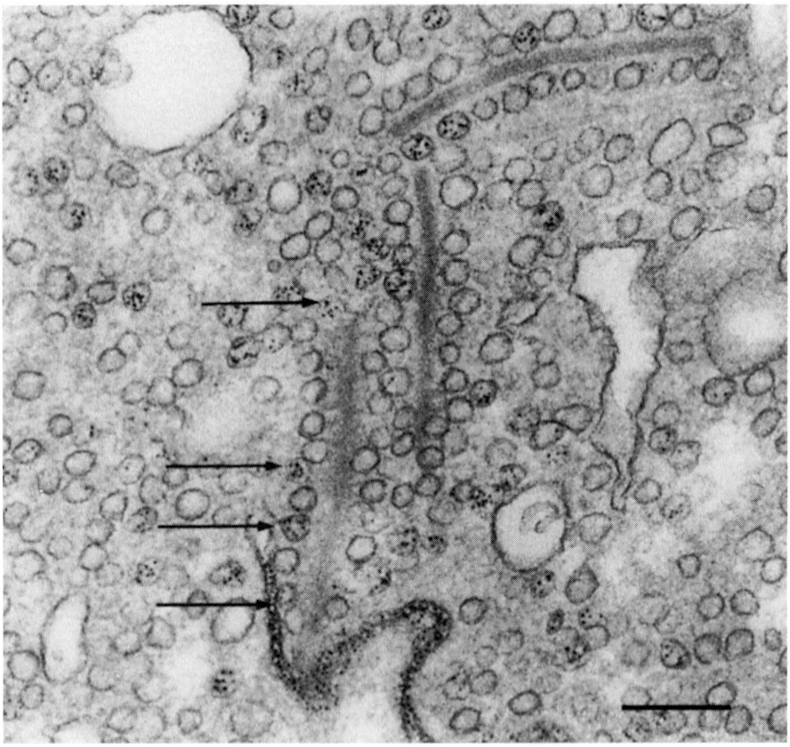

Figure 3 Synaptic uptake of tracer by isolated rod cells during depolarization. Cationic ferritin, applied to cultures in the presence of 50 mM KCl for 30 minutes, appears in synaptic vesicles. Some of the vesicles are attached to synaptic ribbons (arrows). This indicates that vesicle exo- and endocytosis have occurred in response to a depolarizing stimulus. Bar = 0.2μm.

IV. PHOTORECEPTORS IN CULTURE CAN REGENERATE AXONS AND PRESYNAPTIC VARICOSITIES

When salamander rod and cone cells are maintained in culture, dramatic growth occurs (Mandell et al., 1993); this growth is observed in all photoreceptors receptors regardless of their state of intactness. The increase in the number of new processes is most rapid during the first 3 days in culture and levels off after 1 week. Two types of processes are produced. First, filopodia filled with actin appear; subsequently, some of the processes thicken, fill with microtubules, and become neurites. Concomitant with the appearance of neuritic processes, there is formation of varicosities which are filled with synaptic vesicles as seen with electron microscopy and light microscopic immunocytochemistry for SV2 and synaptophysin. These varicosities have the ability to recycle synaptic vesicles in response to depolarization, thus we have called them synaptic or presynaptic varicosities (Fig. 4). Nocodazole, a microtubule depolymerizing agent, reversibly blocks varicosity development (Mandell et al., 1993). Polymerization of microtubules, therefore, is necessary not only for development of neurites but also for formation of synaptic varicosities. Although filopodial processes can sometimes extend for 80 μm, the maximum length of neuritic processes is 20 μm. Cells which produce neurites, usually have more than one. For rods, the average number of synaptic varicosities per cell is 1.6 with a few cells making as many as 9 varicosities. In the retina, adult rod cells can have multiple axons and terminals; on average, therefore, the neuritic processes *in vitro* recreate an axonal arborization that is within the range of what has been observed for normal adult photoreceptors. Cone cells have consistently fewer varicosities than rod cells. They also have broader, lamellar-like processes, and comparatively high levels of cell body staining for synaptic vesicle membrane protein. This too may relate to the *in vivo* situation since multiple axons are not present in the cone cell and the cone terminal appears as a broad cytoplasmic extension with synaptic vesicles present in close proximity to the nucleus.

The growth observed *in vitro* is not dependent on unknown serum factors since it can occur in a defined medium (Mandell et al., 1993). Normally insulin and thyroxine are added to the medium, however, qualitatively similar growth also occurs in a simple Ringer's solution. Growth is also not dependent on culture substrate. The antibody substrate which is routinely used insures survival of an overwhelming majority of photoreceptors. With concanavalin A or uncoated plastic as a substrate, a smaller number of cells survive but similar outgrowth occurs. Finally, growth is not dependent on the presence of other cells. By successive dilution, wells with a single photoreceptor can be obtained. Over a period of 7 days, these cells produce both filopodia and varicosity-bearing neurites. The lack of dependence on environmental conditions suggests that the observed growth is an intrinsic property of the cell. The initial stimulus for the growth may be injury incurred during retinal dissociation or perhaps disinhibition due to removal of postsynaptic cells and surrounding glia.

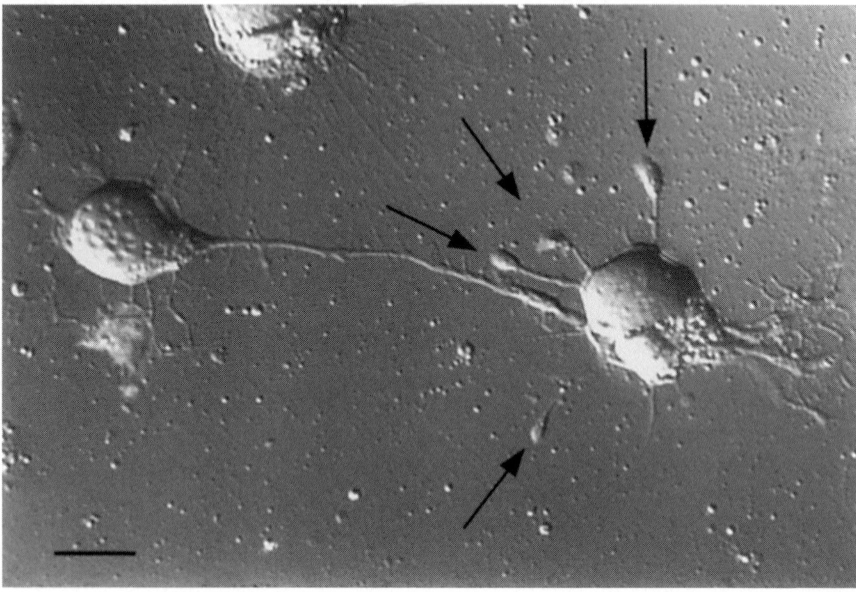

Figure 4 Growth of varicosity-bearing neurites. Over time in culture, rod and cone cells produce new neurites. This photoreceptor has formed several neurites each terminating in a single synaptic varicosity (arrows). A multipolar cell has also extended a process towards the photoreceptor. Bar = 10μm.

The site for initiation of outgrowth from the cell body depends on the type of process involved. Filopodia can radiate as a corona circumferentially around the cell; some cells, however, have several thick filopodia arising from the apical pole of the cell (Fig. 5). In photoreceptors there are fine processes known as calycal processes filled by actin bundles which normally arise from the apical surface of the inner segment to surround the base of the outer segment. The actin in the calyces originates from bundles of actin fibers just underneath the plasma membrane of the inner segment; the actin bundles form longitudinal stripes in labeled cells (Fig. 5) similar to what has been observed in other species (Vaughan and Fisher, 1987; Del Priore et al., 1987). The longest and most prominent filopodia, therefore, are likely to originate from former calyces. The microtubule-containing neurites can also arise from anywhere along the cell surface but originate more frequently from the apical and basal poles of the photoreceptors. In quantitative analyses (Townes-Anderson and Sherry, unpublished data), approximately 60% of all regenerated neurites arose from within 30 degrees of the apical and basal poles, regardless of whether or not the rod cell retained its outer segment. For the particular case of rod cells which had lost their outer segment, close to half of the neurites grew from the basal pole, the pole from which the axon fiber originates, whereas less than a fifth of the processes arose from the apical pole. Isolated cells, therefore, even after loss of both the outer segment and axon fiber, retain some normal polarity with respect to the origin of the regenerative neuritic growth.

In rod cells, there are significant differences in the rate of outgrowth depending on whether or not the original pedicle is present after cell isolation (Nachman-Clewner and Townes-Anderson, 1996). Cells with an axon are considered detargeted because of the removal of postsynaptic processes; cells without an axon and terminal are axotomized. This axotomy usually occurs at or very close to the cell body. When cells with and without an axon were identified immediately after plating and followed for 1-2 days in culture, it was discovered that those with an axon had 80% more processes and 4 times as many synaptic varicosities compared to cells without an axon. Analyzing cell growth with video time lapse photography helped explain these results. Time lapse studies revealed a dramatic structural plasticity in the original axon fiber and terminal within the first 48 hours of culture (Fig. 6). Initially the axon and its terminal are retracted towards the cell body forming a hump or cap on the basal pole of the cell; the axon terminal then flattens and forms a prominent lamellipodium (referred to as the axonal lamellipodium); filopodia arise from the axonal lamellipodium as well as from the cell body and calycal processes; finally, neuritic processes are formed, primarily from filopodia extending from the axonal lamellipodium at the posterior pole, and varicosities appear.

Due to the rapidity of the process and the retention of prominent synaptic vesicle membrane immunostaining in the axonal processes throughout this restructuring (Nachman-Clewner and Townes-Anderson, 1996), it has been proposed that components of the original axon, like the synaptic vesicles and cytoskeletal elements, are reutilized to quickly reform new presynaptic structures (Fig. 6). Reutilization of preexisting neuronal proteins has been previously proposed for other nerve cell types during regeneration (Matthews et al., 1976; Cotman and Nadler, 1978). Moreover, synaptic vesicles represent a pool of potential presynaptic membrane. Indeed, the rod cell terminal may be particularly flexible structurally because of the abundance of synaptic vesicles: in cat rod cells, ~130 vesicles are docked at the active zone and ~640 vesicles are tethered to the ribbon ready to reload docking sites compared to the average of ~50 docked vesicles at the active zone of a conventional synapse (Rao-Mirotznik et al., 1995). It is al ready known that the photoreceptor ribbon presynaptic terminal in the intact retina can expand and retract in dark and light respectively; changes in area and/or surface contour have been reported for turtle, chick, and rat retina (Schaeffer and Raviola, 1978; Cooper and McLaughlin, 1982; Case and Plummer, 1993). This plasticity is due in part to vesicle exo- and endocytosis. Vesicle exocytosis, and thus membrane addition, predominates in the dark when the photoreceptor cell is depolarized, and membrane retrieval, endocytosis, predominates in light conditions when the cell is hyperpolarized. During the retraction and regrowth of neur-

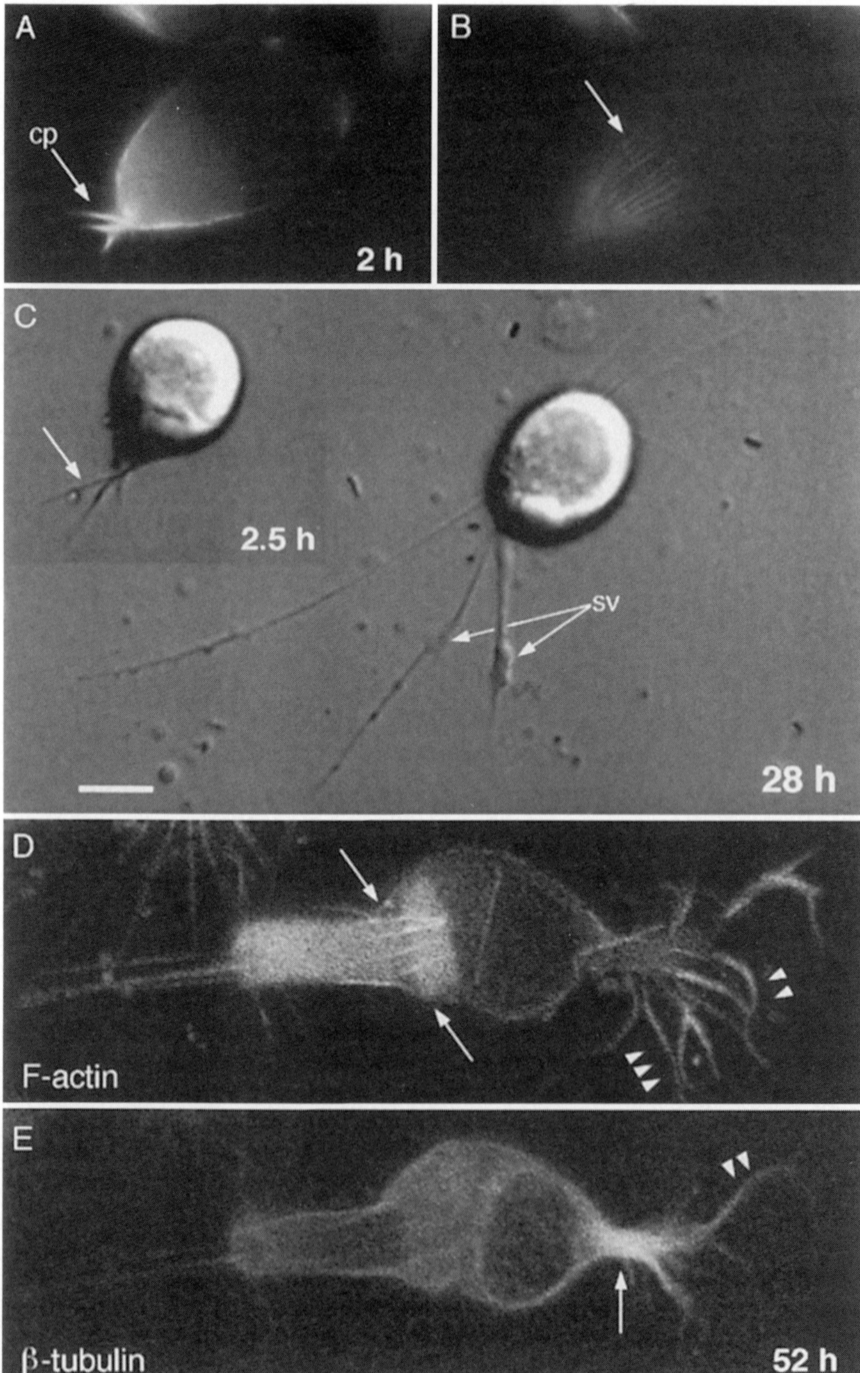
A
cp
2 h
B
C
2.5 h
sv
28 h
D
F-actin
E
β-tubulin
52 h

ites observed in culture similar changes in the relative rates of exo- and endocytosis could accompany cytoskeletal rearrangements of actin and microtubules and produce filopodia, lamellipodia, and new neurites. Vesicles in newly formed varicosities are capable of depolarization-induced synaptic vesicle recycling even in the absence of synaptic ribbons (Mandell et al., 1993). Additionally, at 2 days *in vitro*, synaptic vesicles in axonal lamellipodia take up tracer added to the cultures without depolarization. This uptake, in the absence of stimuli, indicates that constitutive synaptic vesicle recycling occurs during the restructuring of axonal processes (Fig.7) (Nachman-Clewner and Townes-Anderson, unpublished data). Such constitutive synaptic vesicle recycling has also been reported for growing neurites in developing hippocampal neurons (Matteoli et al., 1992).

If original components are reutilized, there may be no need for upregulation of synthesis of cytoskeletal and presynaptic elements for regeneration to occur. There is some evidence that synthesis of the synaptic vesicle membrane proteins SV2 and synaptophysin is not upregulated for many days after cell isolation (Nachman-Clewner and Townes-Anderson, 1996). Synaptic vesicle membrane proteins are not present, at levels detectable by immunocytochemistry, in the Golgi apparatus 1-48 hours after cell plating; in contrast, opsin is present in the Golgi at all times and is probably constitutively expressed. After 7 days *in vitro*, synaptic vesicle membrane protein and rab 6, a marker used for the *trans* Golgi, colocalize in all photoreceptors. At this time, the total amount of synaptophysin protein in rod cells which had an original axon and those which had lost their axon

---

Figure 5 Cytoskeleton of regenerating photoreceptors. Process growth was followed with time-lapse video microscopy and analyzed by labeling for actin and tubulin at selected times *in vitro*. A: Freshly isolated photoreceptor labeled with fluorescein phalloidin, a toxin that binds to filamentous actin (F-actin). Actin bundles are present in multiple calycal processes (cp) which project from the apical surface of the cell. B: At a different focal plane, the bundles can be seen to extend into the inner segment where they appear as longitudinal stripes (arrow). C: Calycal processes present at the time of plating (arrow) form filopodia as well as synaptic varicosity (sv) bearing neurites after 1 day *in vitro*. D and E: Rod cell which retained its outer segment and axon, after 2 days *in vitro*; double labeled with phalloidin and anti-β-tubulin and viewed in 1 μm confocal section. Longitudinal bundles of actin persist in the inner segment (D, arrows) and are continuous with actin filaments in newly regenerated filopodia at the cell's apical pole. At the basal pole, actin-filled filopodia (D, arrowheads) arise from the main body of the axonal lamellipodium which is devoid of actin but loaded with β-tubulin (E, arrow), a pattern previously described for growth cone lamellipodia. Tubulin labeled neurites have also formed from the axonal lamellipodium (E, arrowheads). Since the original axon and terminal contain tubulin and actin, it is possible that original cytoskeletal elements are reutilized and reorganized during axonal regeneration. Bar = 10μm.

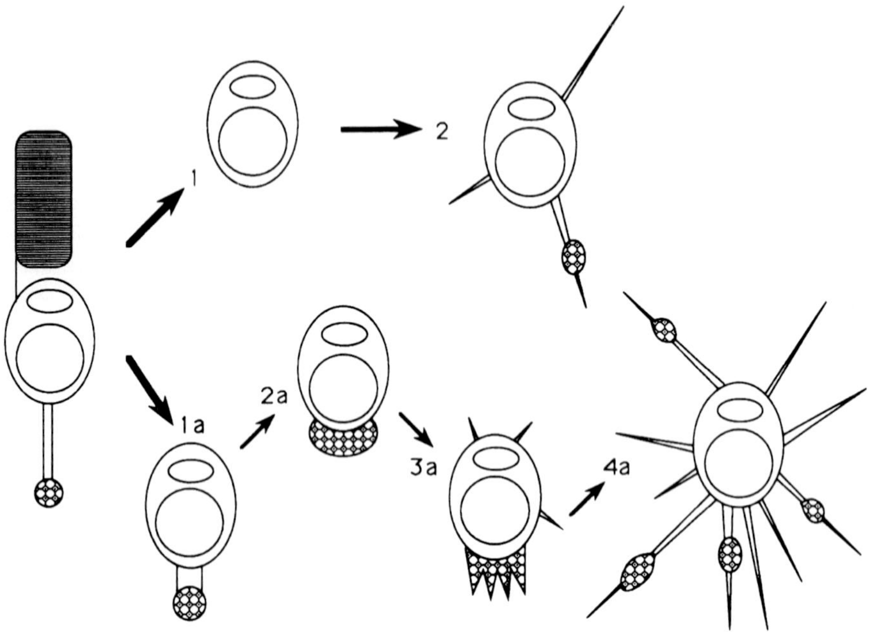

Figure 6 Differences in regeneration between detargeted and axotomized rod cells. This diagram illustrates axonal remodeling and the hypothesized reutilization of axonal components. A fully intact rod photoreceptor is shown at left with its outer segment (shaded), axon, and axon terminal (stippled pattern represents accumulation of synaptic vesicles). Pathway 1a depicts a detargeted rod cell, i.e. a cell which has retained its original axon; axotomized neurons are represented in pathway 1. As the axon retracts (1a), forming a cap (2a) and axonal lamellipodium (3a), pre-existing synaptic vesicles are redistributed for reuse in the formation of numerous presynaptic varicosities (4a), prior to the onset of new synaptic protein synthesis. In contrast, axotomized cells have lost more of their axonal components (1) and consequently, regenerate relatively fewer processes and varicosities (2) during early stages. (From Nachman-Clewner and Townes-Anderson, 1996.)

is the same, based on quantitative immunocytochemistry. This is significant because cells which lose their axons lose the majority of their synaptic vesicle membrane protein staining. In addition, at 7 days, there is no longer any statistical difference in the number of processes in these two cell populations. Thus, sometime after 48 hours increased synthesis of synaptic vesicle constituents occurs and, by one week, differences in regenerative growth between axotomized and detargeted (i.e. not axotomized) rod cells no longer exist.

How does photoreceptor process regeneration differ from the better known axonal regeneration of a projection neuron? The photoreceptor axon terminal is only tens of microns or less away from the cell body. The time to complete axonal regeneration is therefore expected to be significantly shorter than for projection (Golgi type I) neurons. In addition, photoreceptor process elongation does not occur via a growth cone, unlike development of long axonal and dendritic processes; rather, neuritic processes form by the thickening of selected filopodia.

Observation of cells in culture has also demonstrated that in rod photoreceptors, axotomy, which occurs at the cell body, does not cause cell death in contrast to results in other nerve cell types (Lieberman, 1974; Fishman and Parks, 1998). Whether mechanisms of regenerative growth in photoreceptors are in other ways unique is unknown. It is also not known if photoreceptor regeneration mimics the process regeneration of local (Golgi type II) neurons since little is known about how short axons are reformed. With respect to reutilization and reorganization of synaptic constituents after removal of postsynaptic partners, as discussed, this may occur in other neurons and conceivably is prominent where robust sprouting after denervation has been reported (e.g. Cotman et al., 1981).

V. AXONAL REGENERATION LEADS TO SYNAPTIC REGENERATION

Adult salamander photoreceptors make functional synapses with other retinal neurons in culture. About 11% of the photoreceptors make contact, through their regenerated neurites and presynaptic varicosities, with the processes or cell bodies of other neurons (Sherry et al., 1996). Interestingly, photoreceptors which make contacts produce statistically more presynaptic varicosities than photoreceptors which do not contact other cells; this suggests that cell contact enhances regeneration. The first functional synapses appear after 10 days *in vitro* (MacLeish and Townes-Anderson, 1988). New photoreceptor synapses contain one or more synaptic ribbons and both clear and dense-cored synaptic vesicles (Fig. 8) (MacLeish and Townes-Anderson, 1988; Sherry et al., 1996). Contact is with a single postsynaptic cell; dyads and triads have not been observed.

A quantitative analysis of the preferences of photoreceptors for synaptic partners yielded unexpected results (Sherry et al., 1996). Whereas *in situ,* rod and cone cells synapse with horizontal and bipolar cells, in culture, photoreceptors showed a significant preference for multipolar (amacrine and ganglion) cells as synaptic partners. Analysis of the amino acid neurotransmitter contained by the preferred cells showed that photoreceptors sought out GABA (gamma aminobutyric acid)-ergic multipolar cells. Based on the known transmitter content of amacrine and ganglion cells, it is most likely that the postsynaptic GABAergic cell forming synapses with photoreceptors is an amacrine cell.

GABA is one of many neurotransmitters that can effect neurite outgrowth (Mattson and Kater, 1989). It is present early in developing retina and has been proposed to play a role in rabbit photoreceptor synaptic development (Osborne et al., 1986; Spoerri, 1988; Messersmith and Redburn, 1990; Redburn, 1992). Horizontal cells, which in amphibians and mammals are the first cells to form synaptic contact with photoreceptors (Blanks et al., 1974; Chen and Witkovsky, 1978;

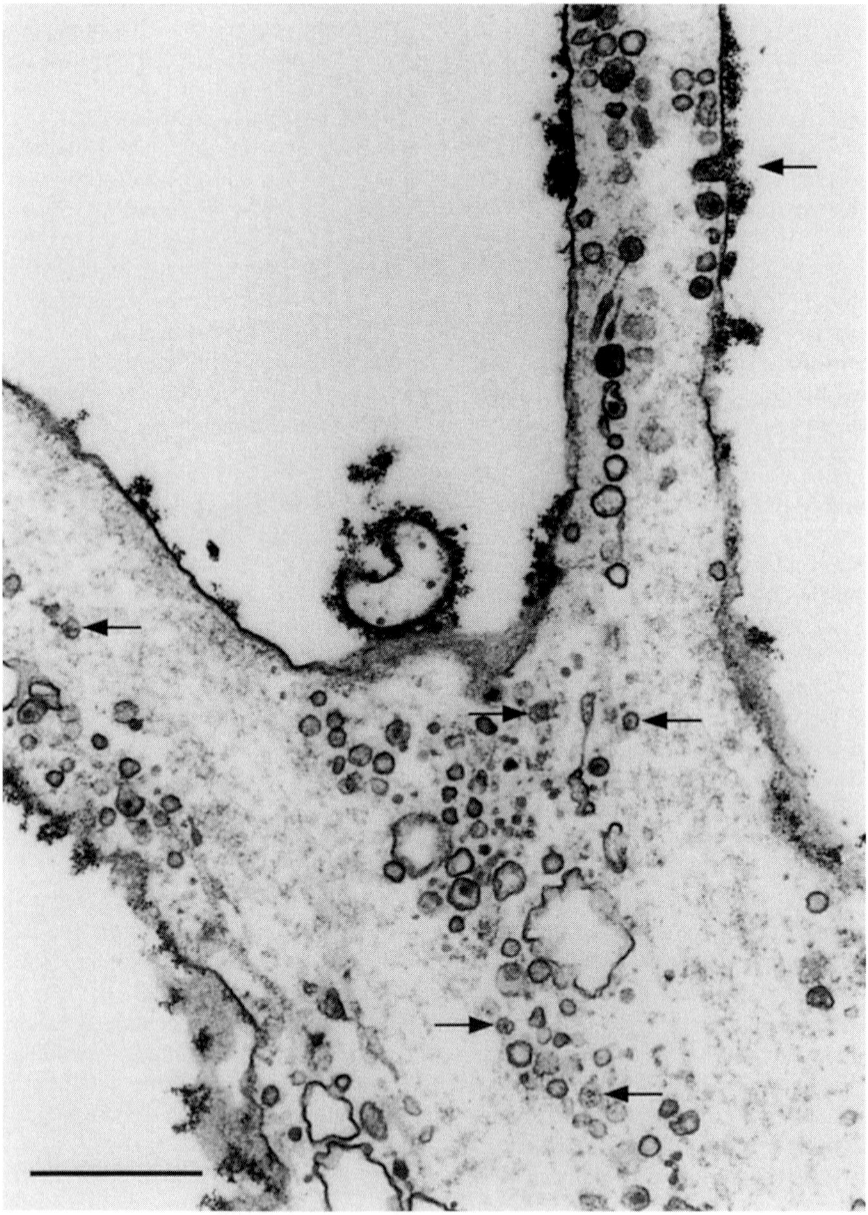

Figure 7 Evidence of constitutive vesicular recycling during axonal restructuring. Cationic ferritin was applied to cultures for 30 minutes *without* depolarization. In freshly isolated cells, no uptake of the tracer into vesicles was observed. But here, in a cell cultured for 48 hours, endocytic pits and labeled vesicles (arrows) are present in processes growing from the axonal lamellipodium. Bar = 0.5μm.

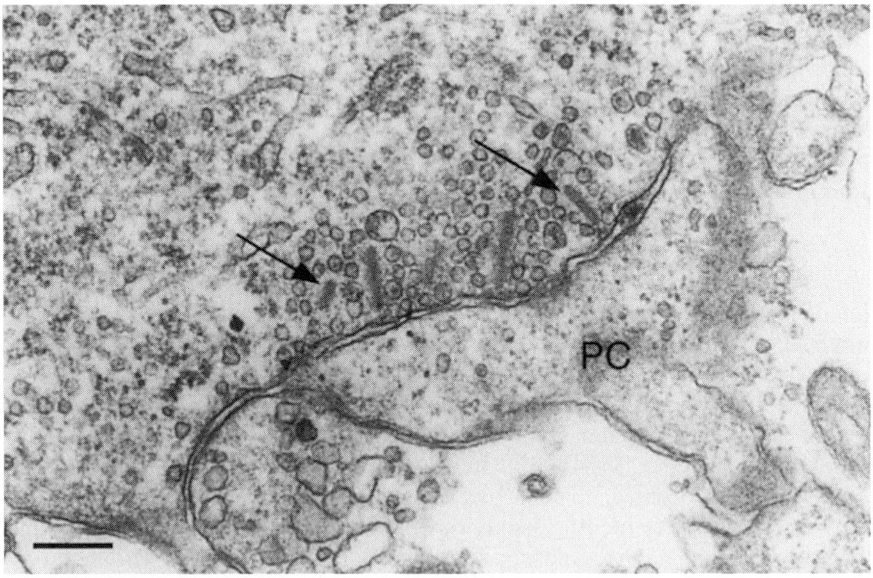

Figure 8 Regeneration of the ribbon synapse. After one to two weeks in culture, contacts form between photoreceptors and other retinal neurons. Here, a cone cell is contacting a postsynaptic cell (PC); multiple synaptic ribbons (arrows) line the presynaptic plasma membrane. Bar = 0.5μm.

Morrison, 1978; Maslim and Stone, 1986), are GABAergic. Thus, contact with GABAergic cells is a feature of developmental synaptogenesis. In ferret retinal development, however, there is convincing evidence of photoreceptor processes in the inner retina (Johnson et al., 1999). And in human retina afflicted with retinitis pigmentosa, new neuritic growth from rod cells extends into the inner retina (Li et al., 1995). Contact with amacrine cells, therefore, may not be entirely novel for photoreceptors. It remains unclear, however, whether photoreceptor/amacrine synapses occur during development and, therefore, whether contact preferences seen in culture during synaptic regeneration are or are not recapitulating a developmental stage. Considering the myriad of factors which must be in place to guide axonal outgrowth and synaptogenesis during embryonic development, it would not be surprising for regenerative synaptogenesis to exhibit its own particular characteristics.

VI. FUTURE DIRECTIONS: THE FULL SCOPE OF THE REGENERATIVE POTENTIAL OF PRIMARY VISUAL NEURONS REMAINS TO BE DISCOVERED

An *in vitro* system of adult amphibian retinal neurons has provided the opportunity to examine the regeneration of axons and functional synapses by photoreceptors. Both rod and cone cells in this system are capable of process outgrowth and formation of new synaptic connections. Moreover, plasticity of detargeted cells *in vitro* mirrors the axonal changes observed in photoreceptors in animal models and human retinal disease. The retinal cell culture should allow the continued elucidation of the mechanisms involved in photoreceptor regeneration. Recent work, for instance, indicates that calcium influx through L-type Ca^{++} channels is necessary for axonal retraction and also plays a role in neurite extension (Nachman-Clewner et al., 1999). A similar dependency on the activity of L-type channels for process growth has been observed in embryonic and postnatal central nervous system neurons (Suarez-Isla et al., 1984; Williams et al., 1994; Ramakers et al., 1998). Assessment of factors known to contribute to synaptic plasticity and axonal growth in other systems, such as the Rho family of GTPases, Gap-43, neurotransmitters and neurotrophins, and axonal guidance signals, will also be possible. The final outcome may be complex. Some aspects of photoreceptor regenerative growth appear to recapitulate developmental processes while others appear to be unique to adult neurons. Furthermore, since ribbon synapses and their associated axon fibers have some special molecular characteristics, some of the signals and mechanisms for regeneration will probably be distinct from those observed in projection neurons such as retinal ganglion cells.

Evidence from amphibian and mammalian cells suggests that regeneration by rods and cones will be somewhat different as well. Already it has been reported that salamander cones produce fewer presynaptic varicosities in culture (Mandell et al., 1993). Cones also produce fewer processes, have a significantly higher density of synaptophysin immunoreactivity per unit area than rod cells after 7 days in culture (Nachman-Clewner and Townes-Anderson, unpublished data), and contain more synaptic vesicles in the cell body (Mandell et al., 1993). *In vivo*, in human and mammalian retina, rods are more sensitive to degenerative disease than cones (Schmidt, 1985; Curcio et al., 1993) and the structural synaptic plasticity of rods in affected retinas has been reported to be different than that of cone cells: in mouse retinal degenerations, synaptic growth occurs only in rod terminals (Jansen and Sanyal, 1984); in retinitis pigmentosa, neuritic growth into the inner retina is by rod cells and not cones (Li et al., 1995; Milam et al., 1996). Differences between the molecular palettes of rod and cone terminals are beginning to emerge. For instance, salamander cone but not rod cells have cyclic GMP dependent Ca^{++} channels in the presynaptic membrane (Rieke and Schwartz, 1994) whereas comparison of the data from a predominantly cone (Tucker et al., 1988) and a predominantly rod retina (Tucker and Matus, 1988) suggests that there are differences in cytoskeletal elements. In addition to the salamander culture system, which contains rod and cone cells, there are several proven culture systems from warm blooded and mammalian animals which can be used to test synaptic development and regeneration by specific photoreceptor cell classes, e.g. embryonic chick cone cells (Adler et al., 1984), fetal mouse rod cells (Kljavin and Reh, 1991), and adult primate rod and cone cells (O'Malley and MacLeish, 1993). Understanding the differences in regenerative potential and mechanisms of synaptogenesis between the photoreceptor cell types will be important in treating degenerative retinal disease and in producing successful photoreceptor transplants.

A central problem for regeneration in the central nervous system is the presence of inhibitory factors which prevent otherwise capable nerve cells from successful regeneration. Even in amphibia, where nerve cells are well known to regenerate more vigorously than mammalian cells, there are some neurons which fail to regrow (Lyon and Stelzner, 1987). An underlying concern, therefore, is that the retina expresses inhibitory factors which, under normal circumstances, may help preserve fine point-to-point resolution by limiting synaptic connectivity, but which, during attempts at graft/host synaptic integration, may prevent new synapses from forming between photoreceptors and second order neurons. Already, *in vitro* work suggests that encouraging interactions between photoreceptors and third order retinal neurons (amacrine cells) may be more productive than trying to reestablish the normal interactions between photoreceptors and second order neurons. One might speculate that these repulsive factors are elements of laminar specificity, established after retinal layers, especially synaptic layers, have developed. Many parameters of photoreceptor synaptic regeneration, including possible inhibitory factors, remain to be discovered.

ACKNOWLEDGMENTS

The authors gratefully acknowledge the support of NIH grants EY06135 and EY12031 during the course of their studies on photoreceptors.

REFERENCES

Adler R, Lindsey JD, Elsner CL (1984) Expression of cone-like properties by chick embryo neural retina cells in glial-free monolayer cultures. J Cell Biol 99:1173-1178.

Bader CR, Bertrand D, Schwartz EA (1982) Voltage-activated and calcium-activated currents studied in solitary rod inner segments from the salamander retina. J Physiol 331:253-284.

Blanks JC, Adinolfi AM, Lolley RN (1974) Synaptogenesis in the photoreceptor terminal of the mouse retina. J Comp Neurol 156:81-94.

Case CP, Plummer CJ (1993) Changing the light intensity of the visual environment results in large differences in numbers of synapses and in photoreceptor size in the retina of the young adult rat. Neuroscience 55:653-666.

Chen F, Witkovsky P (1978) The formation of photoreceptor synapses in the retina of larval Xenopus. J Neurocytol 7:721-740.

Cooper NGF, McLaughlin BJ (1982) Structural correlates of physiological activity in chick photoreceptor synaptic terminals: Effects of light and dark stimulation. J Ultrastruct Res 79:58-73.

Copenhagen DR, Jahr CE (1989) Release of endogenous excitatory amino acids from turtle photoreceptors. Nature 341:536-539.

Cotman CW, Nieto-Sampedro M, Harris EW (1981) Synapse replacement in the nervous system of adult vertebrates. Physiol Rev 61:684-784.

Curcio CA, Millican CL, Allen KA, Kalina RE (1993) Aging of the human photoreceptor mosaic: Evidence for selective vulnerability of rods in central retina. Invest Ophthalmol Vis Sci 34:3278-3296.

Del Priore LV, Lewis A, Tan S, Carley WW, Webb WW (1987) Fluorescence light microscopy of F-actin in retinal rods and glial cells. Invest Ophthalmol Vis Sci 28:633-639.

Dräger UC (1983) Coexistence of neurofilaments and vimentin in a neurone of adult mouse retina. Nature 303:169-172.

Du J, Gouras P, Kjeldbye H, Kwun R, Lopez R (1992) Monitoring photoreceptor transplants with nuclear and cytoplasmic markers. Exp Neurol 115:79-86.

Erickson PA, Fisher SK, Anderson DH, Stern WH, Borgula GA (1983) Retinal detachment in the cat: The outer nuclear and outer plexiform layers. Invest Ophthalmol Vis Sci 24:927-942.

Fishman PS, Parks DA (1998) Death of transcallosal neurons after close axotomy. Brain Res 779:231-239.

Gouras P, Du J, Kjeldbye H, Kwun R, Lopez R, Zack DJ (1991) Transplanted photoreceptors identified in dystrophic mouse retina by a transgenic reporter gene. Invest Ophthalmol Vis Sci 32:3167-3174.

Gouras P, Du J, Kjeldbye H, Yamamoto S, Zack DJ (1994) Long-term photoreceptor transplants in dystrophic and normal mouse retina. Invest Ophthalmol Vis Sci 35:3145-3153.

Humayun MS, Prince M, de Juan Jr E, Barron Y, Moskowitz M, Klock IB, Milam AH (1999) Morphometric analysis of the extramacular retina from postmortem eyes with retinitis pigmentosa. Invest Ophthalmol Vis Sci 40:143-148.

Jansen HG, Sanyal S (1984) Development and degeneration of retina in rds mutant mice: Electron microscopy. J Comp Neurol 224:71-84.

Jansen HG, Sanyal S (1987) Synaptic changes in the terminals of rod photoreceptors of albino mice after partial visual cell loss induced by brief exposure to constant light. Cell Tissue Res 250:43-52.

Jansen HG, Sanyal S (1992) Synaptic plasticity in the rod terminals after partial photoreceptor cell loss in the heterozygous rds mutant mouse. J Comp Neurol 316:117-125.

Johnson PT, Williams, RR, Cusato, K, Reese,BE (1999) Rods and cones project to the inner plexiform layer during development. J. Comp Neurol 414:1-12.

Kljavin IJ, Reh TA (1991) Müller cells are a preferred substrate for *in vitro* neurite extension by rod photoreceptor cells. J Neurosci 11:2985-2994.

Lam DMK (1972) Biosynthesis of acetylcholine in turtle photoreceptors. Proc Nat Acad Sci USA 69:1987-1991.

Lasansky A (1973) Organization of the outer synaptic layer in the retina of the larval tiger salamander. Phil Trans R Soc Lond B 265:471-489.

Lazar E, del Cerro M (1992) A new procedure for multiple intraretinal transplantation into mammalian eyes. J Neurosci Methods 43:157-169.

Lewis GP, Linberg KA, Fisher SK (1998) Neurite outgrowth from bipolar and horizontal cells after experimental retinal detachment. Invest Ophthalmol Vis Sci 39:424-434.

Li Z-Y, Kljavin IJ, Milam AH (1995) Rod photoreceptor neurite sprouting in retinitis pigmentosa. J Neurosci 15:5429-5438.

Lieberman AR (1974): Some factors affecting retrograde neuronal responses to axonal lesions. In: Essays on the nervous system (Bellairs R, Gray EG eds), pp 71-105. Oxford: Clarendon Press.

Lipton SA, Kater SB (1989) Neurotransmitter regulation of neuronal outgrowth, plasticity and survival. Trends Neurosci 12:265-270.

Lyon MJ, Stelzner DJ (1987) Tests of the regenerative capacity of tectal efferent axons in the frog, Rana pipiens. J Comp Neurol 255:511-525.

MacLeish P, Tachibana M, Townes-Anderson E (1982): Morphological and electrophysiological properties of dissociated retinal neurons. In: Advances in pharmacology and therapeutics II, Volume 2 (Yoshida H, Hagihara Y, Ebashi S eds), pp 245-253. New York: Pergamon Press.

MacLeish PR, Barnstable CJ, Townes-Anderson E (1983) Use of a monoclonal antibody as a substrate for mature neurons *in vitro*. Proc Nat Acad Sci USA 80:7014-7018.

MacLeish PR, Townes-Anderson E (1988) Growth and synapse formation among major classes of adult salamander retinal neurons *in vitro*. Neuron 1:751-760.

Mandell JW, MacLeish PR, Townes-Anderson E (1993) Process outgrowth and synaptic varicosity formation by adult photoreceptors *in vitro*. J Neurosci 13:3533-3548.

Mandell JW, Townes-Anderson E, Czernik AJ, Cameron R, Greengard P, De Camilli P (1990) Synapsins in the vertebrate retina: Absence from ribbon synapses and heterogeneous distribution among conventional synapses. Neuron 5:19-33.

Maslim J, Stone J (1986) Synaptogenesis in the retina of the cat. Brain Res 373:35-48.

Matteoli M, Takei K, Perin MS, Südhof TC, De Camilli P (1992) Exo-endocytotic recycling of synaptic vesicles in developing processes of cultured hippocampal neurons. J Cell Biol 117:849-861.

Matthews DA, Cotman C, Lynch G (1976) An electron microscopic study of lesion-induced synaptogenesis in the dentate gyrus of the adult rat. II. Reappearance of morphologically normal synaptic contacts. Brain Res 115:23-41.

Messersmith EK, Redburn DA (1990) Kainic acid lesioning alters development of the outer plexiform layer in neonatal rabbit retina. Int J Devl Neuroscience 8:447-461.

Milam AH, Li Z, Cideciyan AV, Jacobson SG (1996) Clinicopathologic effects of the Q64ter rhodopsin mutation in retinitis pigmentosa. Invest Ophthalmol Vis Sci 37:753-765.

Morgans CW, Brandstätter JH, Kellerman J, Betz H, Wässle H (1996) A SNARE complex containing syntaxin 3 is present in ribbon synapses of the retina. J Neurosci 16:6713-6721.

Morrison JD (1978) Development of photoreceptor and bipolar cell terminals in kitten retina. J Physiol 284:118P-119P.

Nachman-Clewner M, St.Jules R, Townes-Anderson E (1999) L-type calcium channels in the photoreceptor ribbon synapse: Localization and role in plasticity. J. Comp Neurol 415:1-16.

Nachman-Clewner M, Townes-Anderson E (1996) Injury-induced remodelling and regeneration of the ribbon presynaptic terminal *in vitro*. J Neurocytol 25:597-613.

National Advisory Eye Council (1994) Vision research - A national plan:1994-1998. National Institutes of Health Publication No. 93-3186.

O'Malley MB, MacLeish PR (1993) Monoclonal antibody substrates facilitate long-term regenerative growth of adult primate retinal neurons. J Neuro Methods 47:61-71.

Osborne NN, Patel S, Beaton DW, Neuhoff V (1986) GABA neurones in retinas of different species and their postnatal development in situ and in culture in the rabbit retina. Cell Tissue Res 243:117-123.
Pierantoni RL, McCann GD (1984): A quantitative study on synaptic ribbons in the photoreceptors of turtle and frog. In: Photoreceptors (Borsellino A, Cervetto L eds), pp 255-283. New York : Plenum Press.
Ramakers GJA, Winter J, Hoogland TM, Lequin MB, van Hulten P, van Pelt J, Pool CW (1998) Depolarization stimulates lamellipodia formation and axonal but not dendritic branching in cultured rat cerebral cortex neurons. Dev Brain Res 108:205-216.
Rao-Mirotznik R, Harkins AB, Buchsbaum G, Sterling P (1995) Mammalian rod terminal: Architecture of a binary synapse. Neuron 14:561-569.
Redburn DA (1992) Development of GABAergic neurons in the mammalian retina. Prog Brain Res 90:133-147.
Richardson TM (1969) Cytoplasmic and ciliary connections between the inner and outer segments of mammalian visual receptors. Vision Res 9:727-731.
Rieke F, Schwartz EA (1994) A cGMP-gated current can control exocytosis at cone synapses. Neuron 13:863-873.
Rieke F, Schwartz EA (1996) Asynchronous transmitter release: control of exocytosis and endocytosis at the salamander rod synapse. J Physiol 493:1-8.
Schaeffer SF, Raviola E (1978) Membrane recycling in the cone cell endings of the turtle retina. J Cell Biol 79:802-825.
Schmidt SY (1985): Retinal degenerations. In: Handbook of Neurochemistry, Vol.10 (Lajthe A ed), pp 461-507. New York: Plenum Press.
Schmitz Y, Witkovsky P (1997) Dependence of photoreceptor glutamate release on a dihydropyridine-sensitive calcium channel. Neuroscience 78:1209-1216.
Sherry DM, St.Jules RS, Townes-Anderson E (1996) Morphologic and neurochemical target selectivity of regenerating adult photoreceptors *in vitro*. J Comp Neurol 376:476-488.
Silverman MS, Hughes SE (1989) Transplantation of photoreceptors to light-damaged retina. Invest Ophthalmol Vis Sci 30:1684-1690.
Silverman MS, Hughes SE, Valentino TL, Liu Y (1992) Photoreceptor transplantation: Anatomic, electrophysiologic, and behavioral evidence for the functional reconstruction of retinas lacking photoreceptors. Exp Neurol 115:87-94.
Spoerri PE (1988) Neurotrophic effects of GABA in cultures of embryonic chick brain and retina. Synapse 2:11-22.
Stone JL, Barlow WE, Humayun MS, de Juan Jr E, Milam AH (1992) Morphometric analysis of macular photoreceptors and ganglion cells in retinas with retinitis pigmentosa. Arch Ophthalmol 110:1634-1639.
Suarez-Isla BA, Pelto DJ, Thompson JM, Rapoport SI (1984) Blockers of calcium permeability inhibit neurite extension and formation of neuromuscular synapses in cell culture. Dev Brain Res 14:263-270.
Townes-Anderson E (1995) Intersegmental fusion in vertebrate rod photoreceptors. Rod cell structure revisited. Invest Ophthalmol Vis Sci 36:1918-1933.
Townes-Anderson E, Dacheux RF, Raviola E (1988) Rod photoreceptors dissociated from the adult rabbit retina. J Neurosci 8:320-331.
Townes-Anderson E, MacLeish PR, Raviola E (1985) Rod cells dissociated from mature salamander retina: Ultrastructure and uptake of horseradish peroxidase. J Cell Biol 100:175-188.

Townes-Anderson E, Mandell JW, MacLeish P (1992) Effect of the outer segment on the formation of synaptic varicosities by adult rod cells *in vitro*. Invest Ophthalmol Vis Sci 33:S1059 (Abstract).

Tucker RP, Binder LI, Matus AI (1988) Differential localization of the high- and low-molecular weight variants of MAP2 in the developing retina. Develop Brain Res 38:313-318.

Tucker RP, Matus AI (1988) Microtubule-associated proteins characteristic of embryonic brain are found in the adult mammalian retina. Devel Biol 130:423-434.

Vaughan DK, Fisher SK (1987) The distribution of F-actin in cells isolated from vertebrate retinas. Exp Eye Res 44:393-406.

Wilkinson MF, Barnes S (1996) The dihydropyridine-sensitive calcium channel subtype in cone photoreceptors. J Gen Physiol 107:621-630.

Williams EJ, Walsh FS, Doherty P (1994) The production of arachidonic acid can account for calcium channel activation in the second messenger pathway underlying neurite outgrowth stimulated by NCAM, N-cadherin, and L1. J Neurochem 62:1231-1234.

5

Cues from Developmental Models of Spinal Cord Regeneration for the Repair of the Injured Adult CNS

John D. Steeves
University of British Columbia, Vancouver, British Columbia, Canada

I. INTRODUCTION AND RATIONALE FOR NEURODEVELOPMENT PROVIDING A DISCOVERY PATH TO ADULT CNS REPAIR

As will be discussed below and in other chapters of this volume, there is evidence that the immature or developing central nervous system (CNS) has an enhanced capacity for anatomical regeneration, accompanied by functional recovery, that is not as evident within the injured mature or adult CNS. In fact, the term regeneration implies a recapitulation, of at least some, of the initial developmental events.

When compared to a "warm-blooded" vertebrate (i.e. bird or mammal), the enhanced spontaneous repair of the injured adult CNS by a "cold-blooded" vertebrate (i.e. fish, amphibian or reptile) has been partially attributed to the indeterminate pattern of growth (i.e. continued development) which is maintained throughout their entire adult life. This situation is not as prevalent within "warm-blooded" vertebrates. Nevertheless, the recent advances in understanding particular molecular and cellular aspects of CNS development have already provided a few of the "tools" to recreate some of the appropriate developmental conditions within the mature CNS of birds and mammals that can facilitate at least partial repair after traumatic injury.

Broadly speaking, the goals for adult CNS repair can be defined as:

1. Contain the amount of primary damage, as well as limit the degree of secondary cell damage and cyst cavity formation.

2. Bridge lost tissue with transplanted cells and promote the expression of factors, as well as 'developmental' programs, that facilitate axonal regeneration.
3. Block endogenous mechanisms within the adult CNS that suppress axonal regeneration and functional reconnection.
4. Stimulate appropriate sensorimotor activity to enhance functional plasticity within surviving circuits, as well as functionally consolidate any induced anatomical repair.

With primary emphasis on repair after injury of the spinal cord in higher vertebrates, I will first outline some examples in developing birds and mammals where anatomical repair and/or functional recovery has been observed after traumatic injury. I will then summarize some of the current understanding about the identified differences between the immature and mature nervous system that may underlie the enhanced repair of CNS injuries during development.

II. EXAMPLES OF ENHANCED REPAIR AND RECOVERY AFTER INJURY OF THE DEVELOPING AVIAN OR MAMMALIAN SPINAL CORD

A. Spinal Lesions of the Neonatal and Weanling Mammalian Cord

Clemente and Chambers, in William Windle's book (Windle, 1955), summarized developmental spinal cord injury studies during the first half of the 20th centrury (see also Guth, 1975). Starting in the 1970's, Dennis Stelzner and his colleagues examined the effects of subtotal spinal cord injuries as well as spinal transection in neonatal and weanling rats (Stelzner et al., 1975; Weber and Stelzner, 1977; Stelzner et al., 1979; Bernstein et al., 1981; Bernstein and Stelzner, 1983). They noted little gliosis or scar formation surrounding a neonatal lesion (postnatal day, P0 to P5), whereas a lesion on P21 to P26 resulted in significant gliosis. Another interesting, age related, difference between neonatal and weanling transects was the reduced degree of demyelination evident some weeks after spinal transection in a neonatal rat. This could be explained by the reduced amount of myelination at neonatal stages of rat spinal cord development, with myelinating events being arrested as a result of spinal injury. Using the tract tracing methods available at that time, there was little, if any, evidence for axonal growth across a transection, regardless of the age of injury.

Spinal injured neonates exhibited better locomotor recovery than animals injured as weanlings which was attributed to enhanced neonatal "plasticity" within the intrinsic spinal cord circuits, caudal to the level of injury. It has been known since the early part of the century that the isolated mammalian cord can exhibit some functional recovery after a spinal transection, even when there is no anatomical reconnection (c.f. Sherrington, 1910; Brown, 1911; Muir and Steeves,

1997). These behavioral improvements have sometimes led researchers to conclude inaccurately that there was functional axonal regeneration.

More recently, there have been several published studies on behavioral recovery and anatomical repair after a spinal transection in neonatal rats (Iwashita et al., 1994; Miya et al., 1997; Asada et al., 1998) or neonatal kittens (Howland et al., 1995a,b). At the time of transection, some of these studies also incorporated either fetal spinal cord tissue or peripheral nerve transplants into the injury site. The rigor of the behavioral and morphological analyses varied and it is always a challenge to demonstrate that any improved functional recovery is due to enhanced anatomical regeneration (see below). Nevertheless, in comparison to control animals, neonatal transects and especially neonatal transects with tissue transplants showed improved motor function and increased morphological continuity after injury.

Most importantly, the authors of these studies were careful in their speculation on the possible mechanisms underlying the improved recovery of neonatal transects. For example, both Barbara Bregman and her colleagues (Howland et al., 1995) and Marion Murray and her colleagues (Miya et al., 1997) discuss the possibility that a neonatal tissue transplant could serve as a source of trophic/tropic support for nearby injured neurons, as well as either a bridge (i.e. substrate) for regenerating axons across the injury site, or as a relay station where regenerating axons could synapse with neurons within the transplant which then project out of the graft to target neurons on the other side. Compensation (i.e. plasticity) within the lumbar cord is also mentioned as a potential contributor to any improved function. Finally, differences in the overall state of CNS development (e.g. relative expression of growth factors) and/or the response to injury (e.g. relative state of myelination or astrogliotic response) are always worthy of consideration when comparing CNS repair in an immature situation with that in a more mature CNS.

B. Anatomical Differentiation Between Regenerating Axons and Late Developing Axons as the Mediators of Functional Recovery After Injury of the Immature CNS

If we accept that the immature CNS has at least some enhanced capacity for functional repair after injury, then identifying the cellular mechanisms underlying this improved recovery becomes important to defining possible strategies for the injured adult CNS. In the studies cited above (Iwashita et al., 1994; Howland et al., 1995; Howland et al., 1995; Miya et al., 1997; Asada et al., 1998), retrograde and anterograde tract tracing, as well as serotonin (5-HT) and noradrenergic (NA) immunocytochemistry, were used to characterize the degree of axonal growth through or around a spinal cord lesion. After injury of the immature CNS, two basic axonal growth responses are possible. First, axonal growth could be due to subsequent axonal outgrowth from late developing neurons, uninjured by the CNS lesion. Second, at least some of the observed axonal outgrowth could result from "true" regeneration of previously severed projections. This discussion assumes that sprouting from uninjured (i.e. surviving) projections does not substantially contribute to the observed anatomical repair (not that this possibility might be a major contributor to recovery after an adult CNS injury).

The primary evidence for regeneration of severed axons has relied on the use of two distinguishable, retrogradely-transported, fluorescent dyes. These experiments are technically difficult and require the animal to survive at least two and often three separate surgeries. In the simplest configuration, the first dye is injected into the cord a few days prior to transection and the second dye is injected into the cord some time after the transection (usually 3-4 weeks later). Upon analysis, neurons labeled with only the first dye are indicative of cells that were projecting through the spinal cord at the time of the transection. Neurons labeled with only the second dye are potentially late developing projections that were not present at the time of transection and are therefore uninjured. Only those neurons labeled with both dyes are potential regenerating neurons (Fig. 1).

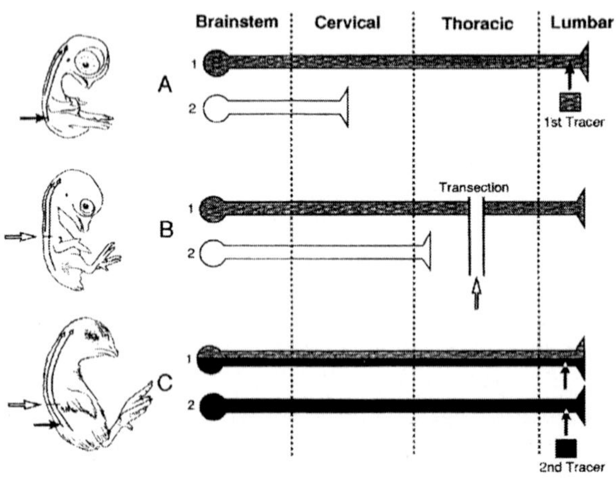

Figure 1 Schematic representation of experimental procedure for retrograde double labeling of axotomized brainstem-spinal neurons in the developing chick. ***A***, On embryonic day (E) E3-E15, of the 21 day *in ovo* development period, the lumbar spinal cord was injected with the first fluorescent tract-tracing dye. Note: hypothetical neuron #1 has already extended an axon to the level of the lumbar cord, but the hypothetically late-developing neuron (#2) has yet to project an axon as far as the site of the dye injection. Thus, neuron #1 becomes labeled with the first retrograde dye, whereas neuron #2 remains unlabeled. ***B***, The low cervical to mid-thoracic cord was fully transected 1-2 days later, thereby severing the axon of neuron #1, but leaving the axon of neuron #2 undamaged (as it has yet to descend to the level of the transection injury). ***C***, After an additional 7-10 days of recovery, a second retrograde dye that is distinguishable from the first dye is injected into the lumbar cord (several segments caudal to the transection site). Note: since both neuron #1 and #2 have now completed axonal development and reached the lumbar cord, they both become labeled with the second retrograde tract-tracing dye. However, neuron #1 is double-labeled, having been previously labeled with the first retrograde dye. Modified from Hasan et al., (1993).

There are two important criteria that must be satisfied in this type of protocol. One is the first dye can only remain viable for retrograde transport for a limited time, otherwise any late developing fibers could incorporate and retrogradely transport both dyes simultaneously, leading to a false-positive interpretation that axonal regeneration had occurred. In addition, the second dye must be confined to a region of the spinal cord that is some distance from the injury site (i.e. the second dye cannot have directly diffused to or across the lesion level). If this were to happen, axons that grew towards (but not across) the lesion could incorporate the second dye and once again lead to an incorrect interpretation of axonal regeneration.

To protect against these possible errors, some investigators have removed the first dye (e.g. fast blue) after a few days, via aspiration of the injected spinal tissue, creating a spinal lesion at the same time. Others (Hasan et al., 1993), have used another control to check for the temporal viability of the first dye (e.g. rhodamine conjugated to dextran amine or "fluoro ruby"). For example, the embryonic spinal cord was transected at the time of first dye injection, just rostral to the dye location. This blocked any retrograde labeling of descending brainstem-spinal neurons by the first dye. One to two weeks later, following the injection of the second dye, none of the second labeled neurons contained the first dye. This indicated that the first dye did not remain viable for co-transport. Finally, all investigators have examined the maximum extent of diffusion for the second dye to assure that the second dye injections were placed sufficiently far from the spinal lesion (usually caudally by at least 2-3 spinal segments) to avoid diffusion to the level of the lesion.

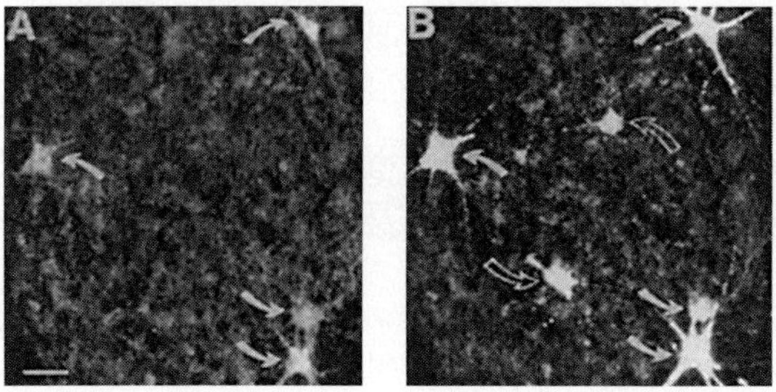

Figure 2 Photomicrographs of retrograde labeled reticulospinal neurons within the ventromedial reticular formation of the caudal pons in an E20 embryo that had its thoracic cord transected on E11. ***A***, Retrograde labeling by first dye (fluorescein conjugated to dextran amine, 0.1 μl, injected on E9). ***B***, same field as in ***A***, but now photograph is taken with a fluorescent filter that enables the visualization of the second dye (rhodamine conjugated to dextran amine or fluoro ruby, 0.3 μl, injected on E18). The presence of double labeled reticulospinal neurons (solid arrows) indicates regeneration of previously axotomized fibers, whereas the presence of single-labeled neurons (open arrows) indicates subsequent axonal projections from late developing reticulospinal neurons. For color plates of double labeling data, see Hasan et al., (1993). Modified from Hasan et al., (1993).

Using these double-labeling protocols, evidence for regenerating axons contributing to the observed neuroanatomical repair, after injury of the immature CNS, have been reported for a number of species, including embryonic chick (Keirstead et al., 1992; Hasan et al., 1993), neonatal opossum (Xu and Martin, 1991), and neonatal rat (Bates and Stelzner, 1993; Bernstein-Goral and Bregman, 1993). In all cases the best evidence for anatomical regeneration was observed in those animals where the spinal cord was injured at a younger age and/or fetal grafts were implanted into the injured region. The results vary, but up to 30% of the descending brainstem-spinal neurons were double labeled (Fig. 2).

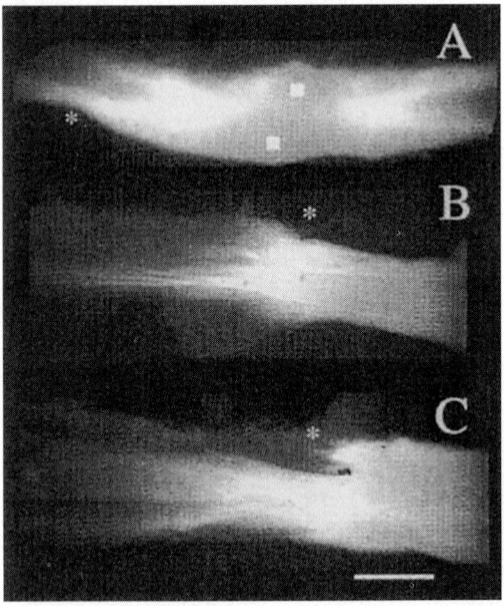

Figure 3 Anterograde tract tracing evidence for regrowth of descending spinal projections through an E9 low cervical transection (indicated by *) of three different embryonic chick spinal cords. DiI crystals were placed several segments above the transection (indicated by filled boxes in **A,** out of field, but to the right in **B** and **C**) in paraformaldehyde fixed cords after physiological recordings (on E14-E15) indicated functional coupling across the previously severed cord. Scale bar, 1 mm in **A**, 0.5 mm in **B** and **C**. Modified from Sholomenko and Delaney, 1998.

Most authors agree that these percentage estimates are crude approximations, but always represent an underestimate, since, for some unexplained reason, injection of both retrograde dyes (simultaneously or sequentially) into the uninjured immature spinal cord only resulted in approximately 30% of the descending neurons being double labeled (Hasan et al., 1993). In short, one cannot assure that each dye is taken up by all axons or transported in an equally efficient manner. Anterograde tracing has also been used (Sholomenko and Delaney, 1998) to follow the extent of axonal regeneration after spinal transection of the developing chick (Fig. 3). Using a different technology, time-lapse video microscopy, axonal regeneration from injured brainstem-spinal neurons was directly observed within the *in vitro* neonatal opossum spinal cord. (Varga et al., 1996).

C. Electrophysiological Evidence for Functional Recovery After Injury of the Immature CNS

Most examinations of functional or behavioral recovery after a spinal cord injury have relied on analyses of behavioral abilities, usually locomotor, because most animals, if they have the capacity, will attempt to move, either spontaneously or in a "goal-directed" manner. Over the years, these analyses have become more standardized and rigorous in their design, evaluation and interpretation (e.g., Basso et al., 1995). Another method for examining functional recovery, albeit technically more demanding, is to use controlled forms of electrical stimulation on one side of the lesion, combined with discrete types of recording from target cells on the other side of the lesion. This evoked response analysis has been accomplished after spinal injury of the embryonic chick (Hasan et al., 1993; Sholomenko and Delaney, 1998) and neonatal opossum (Varga et al., 1995; Varga et al., 1996).

In the case of the chick, focal electrical stimulation (50 μA) of a functionally defined "locomotor" region within the ventromedial pontomedullary reticular formation of the brainstem was combined with electromyographic (EMG) recording from various leg muscles after a high to midthoracic transection of the spinal cord. Each animal was surgically decerebrated under inhalation anesthetic, prior to stimulation trials, to eliminate the necessity for continued anesthesia which would have made it impossible to record any evoked limb responses. Decerebration is a classical surgical procedure to study the isolated brainstem and spinal cord and removes the perception of any pain by the animal. The effective spread of current from the stimulating electrode tip was no more than a couple of hundred micrometers and therefore confined to the brainstem (at least 10-20 millimeters from the spinal transection site). The "locomotor" region that was activated within the reticular formation is known to have direct reticulospinal projections to the lumbar spinal cord and was one of the regions within the chick brainstem exhibiting double labeled neurons after spinal transection (Hasan et al., 1993). Only upon stimulation did the animal commence rhythmic alternating stepping movements which ceased when the stimulation was terminated. The only possible avenue for transmission of these low intensity stimulation signals was across the previously transected thoracic cord as a result of functional reconnection of descending reticulospinal signals during the intervening recovery period. It is possible that both reticulospinal regeneration and propriospinal regeneration may have mediated this functional recovery.

Sholomenko and Delaney (1998) have used highly sophisticated voltage-sensitive dyes, as well as intracellular recording to document the extent of func-

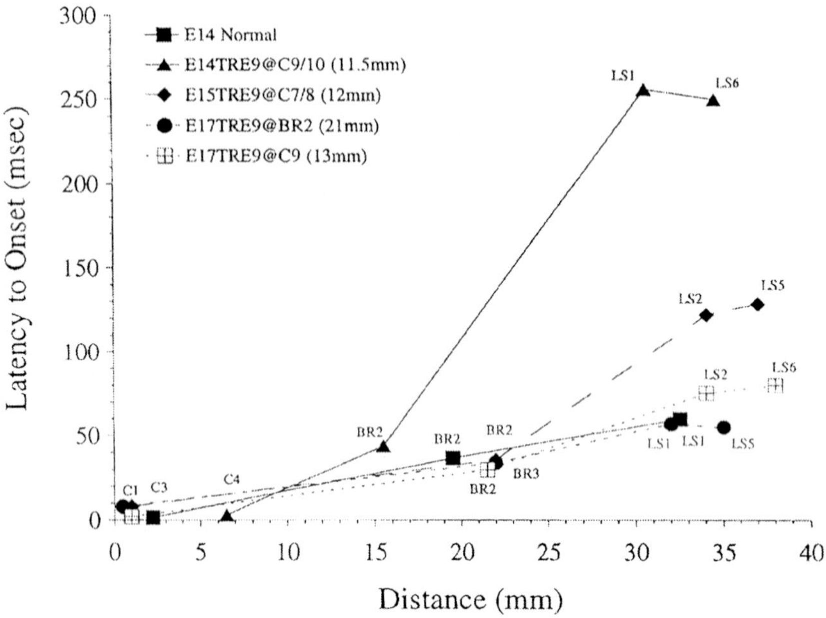

Figure 4 Recovery of connections with increasing time after transection of the embryonic chick spinal cord. Relationship between the averaged latencies to the onset of evoked motor activity (EMA) and distance from the stimulating electrode for different levels of the spinal cord in one uninjured (normal) and 4 transected spinal preparations. The uninjured preparation (E14 Normal – filled squares) shows the short latency to onset and the linear relationship between the latency and distance traversed by the signal along the spinal cord. After 5 days of recovery (E14 transected on E9 – filled triangles) demonstrates a considerably longer latency for EMSs at caudal (lumbosacral) levels of recording. A further day of recovery (E15 transected on E9 – filled diamonds) shows somewhat shorter latencies at all levels of recording. However, it is only after 8 days of recovery (two E17 animals transected on E9 – filled circles and open boxes) that the latency to distance relationship approaches the uninjured (normal) spinal cord transmission situation. Abbreviations: TR = transected, C = rostral cervical cord, BR = brachial cord (equivalent to caudal cervical cord), LS = lumbosacral cord). Modified from Sholomenko and Delaney, 1998.

tional recovery after transection of the embryonic chick spinal cord. The extent of axonal growth across the transection was greater the longer the recovery time after embryonic injury. Both propriospinal and descending brainstem-spinal projections contributed to the motor responses and intracellular postsynaptic potentials that could be evoked (Fig. 4) in response to stimulation on the opposite side of the injury site (re-lesion blocked subsequent signal transmission).

For the isolated and cultured opossum spinal cord (Varga et al., 1995; Varga et al., 1996), stimulation of a dorsal root 5 days after damage, caudal to a complete crush injury of the spinal cord, was paired with recording from a ventral root on the opposite side of the lesion (Fig. 5). Alternatively, stimulation of a dorsal root on the same side of a previous hemisection injury was combined with recording from a ventral root rostral to and on the same side of the lesion (just prior to stimulation and recording trials, the opposite side of the spinal cord was hemisected to prevent transmission of signals along these pathways). Ventral root responses were only evoked during dorsal root stimulation, presumably via regenerated ascending projections from dorsal root ganglion (DRG) cells (for review, see Nicholls and Saunders, 1996).

When combined with the anatomical data, this electrophysiological evidence provides a compelling argument that regenerating axons can acquire functionally appropriate targets. Whether these neurons are reacquiring the identical targets that would normally be acquired during development is unknown, In addition, the degree of functional plasticity, or "rewiring" within the damaged immature cord may be greater than that within the injured adult cord.

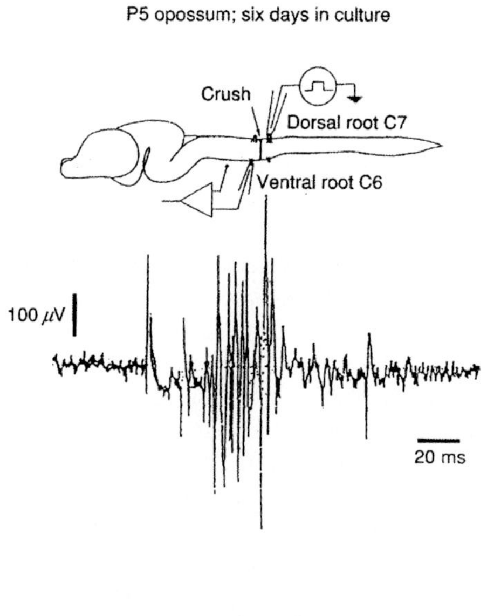

Figure 5 Five days after a spinal cord crush injury of the P5 (developing) opossum cord, stimulation of dorsal root ganglion (DRG) fibers gave rise to evoked activity in ventral roots on the opposite side of a spinal crush injury. These results suggest that DRGs can regenerate across the injured cord to (monosynaptically or polysynaptically) reconnect with motoneurons in adjacent spinal segments. Modified from Nicholls and Saunders, 1996.

III. POTENTIAL DEVELOPMENTAL FACTORS AND MECHANISMS THAT MAY CONTRIBUTE TO ENHANCED REPAIR OF THE MATURE INJURED SPINAL CORD

Perhaps the most important reason for evaluating the repair of the immature CNS is the possibility that an increased understanding of traumatic situations during development will identify potential therapeutic targets for improving the degree of recovery after an adult spinal cord or brain injury. Such studies enable us to test more directly which developmental events are more critical to adult CNS regeneration and functional repair. Many of the other chapters in this volume deal with specific aspects of this puzzle. Here, I will briefly summarize what has been uncovered, to date, in developing models of CNS injury, as well as try to identify which aspects have not been adequately addressed.

A. Developmental Transition Point between Permissive and Restrictive Stages for Functional Regeneration

If it is accepted that there is a period during development when functional regeneration can occur, then it follows that at some point during an animal's ontogeny it loses this capacity and adopts the highly limited repair abilities of the mature CNS. When this transition from permissive to restrictive states occurs is important to define, as are the developmental changes that accompany this transition point. The main question becomes what factors and mechanisms are present early in development that favor the regeneration of neurons in comparison to what is occurring as the CNS concludes development that may repress adult repair (i.e. late developmental events that "stabilize" primary neuronal projections and connections). The potential list is varied and includes changes in the expression pattern and phenotype of: genes for axonal outgrowth, growth factors, cellular substrates, "supporting" glial cells, and the immune system.

To determine the developmental transition point for CNS repair requires examination of CNS repair at numerous stages of development. For higher vertebrates, this has only been practical in species that complete a substantial amount of their neural development externally. To date, attempts to transect the mammalian spinal cord *in utero* and then examine repair processes have been without success. For many reasons, such surgical interventions are extremely difficult, not the least of which is the often induced abortion of the fetus. Instead, two other "warm-blooded" vertebrate groups have been extensively examined, the oviparous chicken (c.f. Steeves et al., 1994) and the marsupial opossum (c.f. Nicholls and Saunders, 1996), although there has also been some study of the isolated (i.e. *in vitro*) developing fetal rat spinal cord (Saunders et al., 1992).

The developing chicken requires 21 days to complete *in ovo* development and hatch. The hatchling chick is a precocial animal, immediately capable of most mature behaviors (e.g. locomotion), which underscores the need for neural development to be accelerated and virtually complete upon leaving the egg. Ungulate animals (e.g. horse) are another precocial group of hoofed mammals that also complete the majority of neurodevelopment prior to birth.

Studies of the developing chick have revealed that neurogenesis within the brainstem and spinal cord is virtually complete by E5 (McConnell and Sechrist, 1980). In the meantime descending axonal projections by reticulospinal neurons enter the cervical cord on E3 (Glover, 1993), with the first functional synaptic connections between descending neurons and spinal motoneurons appearing on E6 (Sholomenko and O'Donovan, 1995). All descending projections have been completed around E11(Okado and Oppenheim, 1985; Glover, 1993), with spinal cord myelination beginning on E13 (Keirstead et al., 1997) (Fig. 6). Anatomical and functional examination for the repair of the injured spinal cord at different stages of development suggests that functional regeneration occurred after transection up to and including E12, but diminishes dramatically after a transection on or after E13 (Shimizu et al., 1990; Hasan et al., 1991; Hasan et al., 1993; Sholomenko and Delaney, 1998). After E13, the transected chick spinal cord showed no evidence of axonal regeneration or functional recovery and the animal was as compromised as the mature/adult avian or mammalian spinal cord (Hasan et al., 1993).

For the marsupial opossum, whether the studies were undertaken in the South American (Mondelphis) or North American (Didelphis) species, transections of the developing spinal cord at early stages of development (e.g. P4-P11 in Didelphis) resulted in greater regeneration than those undertaken at later stages of development (e.g. P19-P32 in Didelphis) (Nicholls and Saunders, 1996).

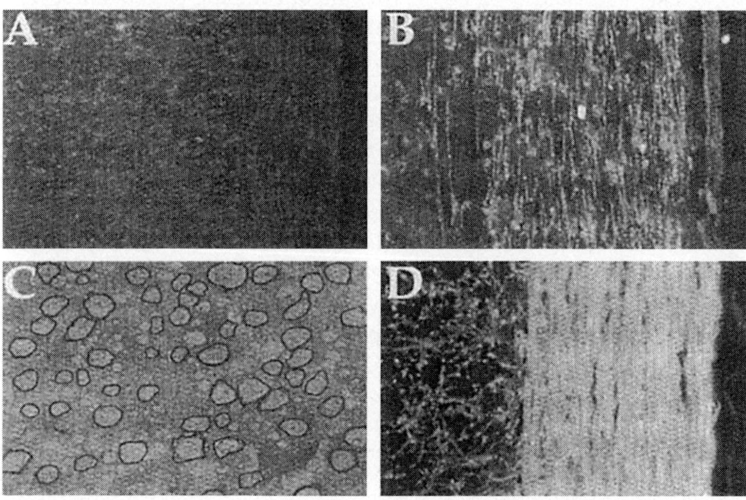

Figure 6 Developmental pattern of myelination in the chick thoracic spinal cord. **A**, Lack of MBP immunofluorescence in a parasagittal section from a normal E12 chick, indicating that spinal cord myelination has yet to commence (external margin of white matter is on right). **B**, MBP immunofluorescence in a parasagittal section from a normal E13 chick, indicating the onset of initial MBP immunoreactivity as cord myelination begins. **C**, Electron micrograph of a transverse section of a normal E15 spinal cord showing the cross-sectional profile of myelinated axons. **D**, MBP immunofluorescence pattern in a parasagittal section from a normal P5 spinal cord showing a mature pattern of MBP immunofluorescence. Modified from Keirstead et al., (1997) .

B. CNS Myelin

Identification of the transition point, between a permissive period for functional regeneration and the subsequent restrictive period that extends throughout adult life, facilitates the investigation of what cellular and molecular changes correlate at this developmental stage. Numerous candidates require screening, but in the chick, E13 corresponds to the onset of spinal cord myelination. An immunological protocol was developed that enabled spinal cord myelination to be delayed to later stages of development (Keirstead et al., 1992).

The immunological treatment consisted of the combined direct intraspinal injection of two components. The first is a myelin-specific antibody that binds to an antigen on the external surface of oligodendrocytes or myelin (e.g. Galactocerebroside, GalC), with the further specification that the antibody have a high affinity (e.g. an IgG) for binding (or fixing) serum complement proteins, the second component. The GalC antibody marks the developing oligodendrocyte and/or newly formed myelin for destruction by the serum complement proteins. Injection of this immunological cocktail into the thoracic cord of a developing chick on E10-E11, effectively suppresses myelin formation within the thoracic cord until approximately E17 (Fig. 7). If the appearance of spinal myelin was a contributing factor to the lack of functional axonal regeneration after an E13 transection, then the delay in spinal myelin development should extend the permissive period for repair to later stages of development. This situation was examined in an experimentally "myelin-suppressed" animal after an E15 thoracic cord transection (i.e. within the normal restrictive period for regeneration). The degree of anatomical regeneration (Fig. 8) and functional recovery (Fig. 9) was equivalent to that of an embryo transected prior to the onset of spinal cord myelin development (i.e. prior to E13).

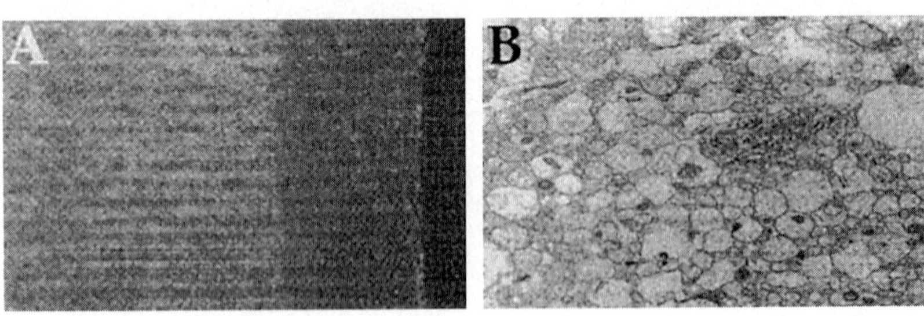

Figure 7 Developmental myelin suppression in the thoracic spinal cord of the embryonic chick. ***A***, MBP immunofluorescence staining in a parasagittal section from an E15 animal that has been transiently myelin suppressed via an E11 intraspinal injection of heterologous serum complement proteins along with a myelin-specific antibody (e.g. GalC). ***B***, Electron micrograph of a transverse section from an E15 thoracic cord that has been previously myelin suppressed (as described in ***A*** and in the text); note the absence of myelinated axons. Modified from Keirstead et al., (1997).

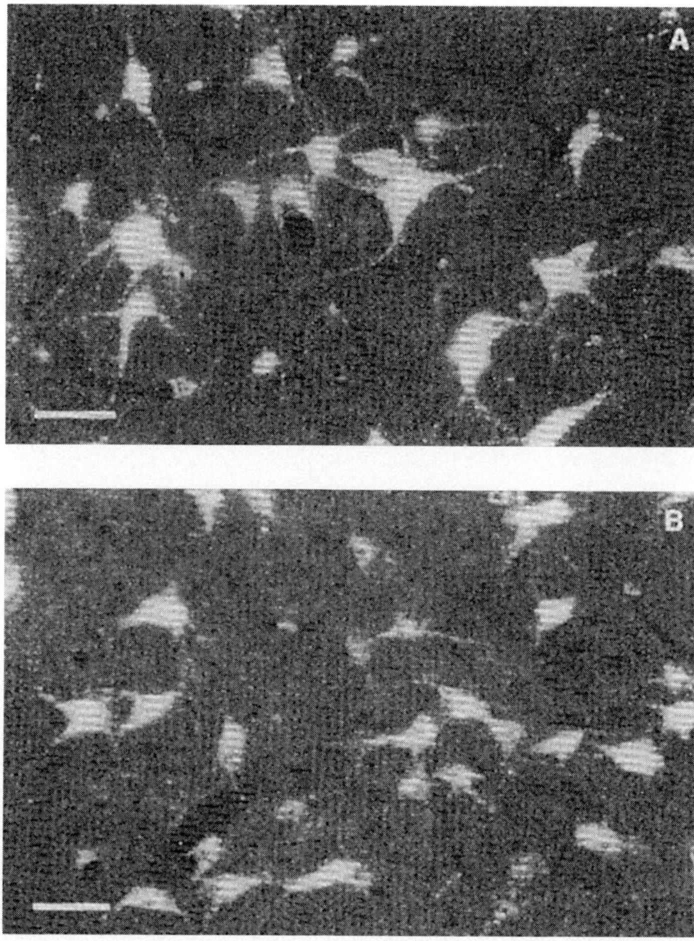

Figure 8 Photomicrographs of retrograde labeled reticulospinal neurons within transverse sections of the ventromedial reticular from the caudal pons in P4 chicks. Brainstem-spinal neurons were labeled by the injection of "fluoro ruby" fluorescent dye into the lumbar cord on P2. ***A***, The distribution and pattern of reticulospinal neurons within a normally myelinated, untransected (control) hatchling. ***B***, The distribution and pattern of labeling of reticulospinal neurons within an experimental animal where myelination within the thoracic cord had been immunologically suppressed on E10, prior to transection of the thoracic cord on E15. Note the similar number and distribution of retrograde labeled reticulospinal neurons. Comparable anatomical repair was evident for other brainstem-spinal projections (e.g. vestibulospinal, raphé-spinal) Scale bar, 50 μm for ***A*** and ***B***. Modified from Keirstead et al., (1992).

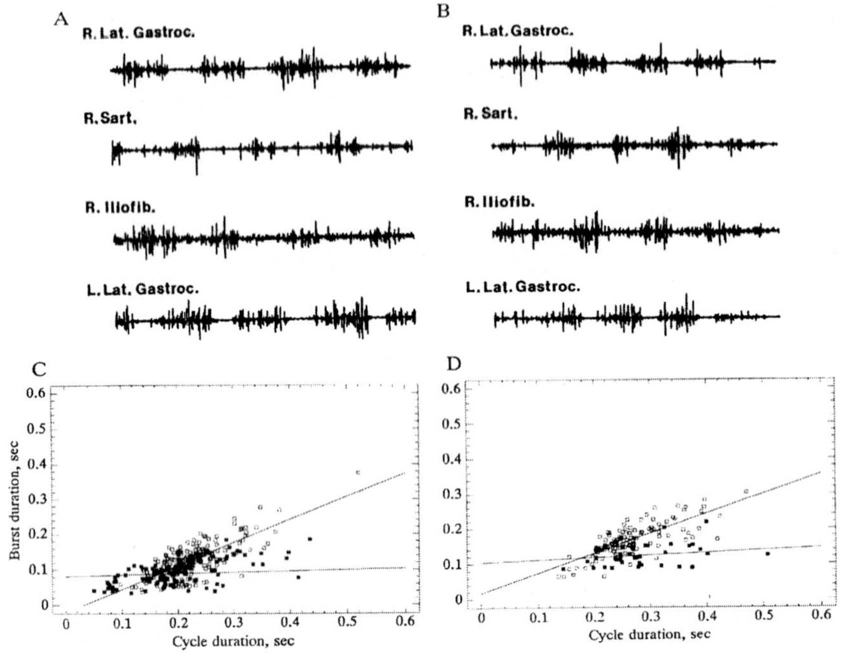

Figure 9 ***A*** and ***B***, Simultaneous electromyographic (EMG) recordings from four leg muscles during spontaneous (open-field) over-ground walking by a normally myelinated, untransected (control) P3 chick (***A***) and a myelin-suppressed, E15 transected chick (***B***). The myelin-suppressed, E15 transected chicks showed the same muscle activity patterns as the normal control animals and were visually indistinguishable from the controls. ***C*** and ***D***, regression of muscle activity (burst) duration versus step cycle duration for the lateral gastrocnemius (open boxes) and sartorius muscles (filled boxes) during walking. As expected of an ankle extensor muscle, the burst duration of the lateral gastrocnemius increased with increasing cycle duration, and equally expected was the relatively constant burst duration of the hip flexor sartorius muscle burst duration as cycle duration increased. Both normal controls (***C***) and experimental (***D***) exhibited similar slopes for regression lines (P,0.05). The coefficients of determination (r^2) for the lateral gastrocnemius and sartorius are 0.58 and 0.04 in ***C*** and 0.59 and 0.08 in ***D***. Modified from Keirstead et al., (1997).

John Nicholls, Norman Saunders and their colleagues have also observed that the isolated developing spinal cord of the South American opossum (Monodelphis) shows extensive functional regeneration, *in vitro* (Nicholls and Saunders, 1996). CNS tissue can be removed from the neonatal animal on P1-P18 and maintained in culture for periods exceeding 7 days. During this time, axonal outgrowth after a crush injury can be directly viewed with time lapse video microscopy of carbocyanine-filled neurons (e.g. DiI or DiO).

Axonal regeneration is quite robust up to the developmental stage when myelination normally begins within the cord (approximately P12). A similar *in vivo* transition point for the repair of spinal cord injuries has been observed for neonatal opossums still attached to their mothers (Saunders et al., 1995; Saunders et al., 1998). The permissive period for axonal regeneration can be extended to later stages of development (i.e. > P12) through the application of the IN-1 antibody to the injured cord (Fig. 10); (Varga et al., 1995a,b; Varga et al., 1996). IN-1 is known to suppress the inhibition of axonal outgrowth produced by some CNS myelin proteins (e.g. NI35/250; Schwab and Bartholdi, 1996)) This and other data collected from adult animals (McKerracher et al., 1994; Mukhopadhyay et al., 1994; Keirstead and Steeves, 1998) suggests that the developmentally late appearance of CNS myelin, hypothesized to stabilize the pattern of previously formed CNS projections, also has the additional effect of suppressing any substantial outgrowth by injured adult CNS axons (c.f. Keirstead and Steeves, 1998). Indeed, the suppression of adult myelin inhibitory actions within the mature or adult CNS also facilitates improved axonal regeneration and functional recovery (Bregman et al., 1995; Keirstead et al., 1995; Dyer et al., 1998). Nevertheless, the degree of CNS regeneration in the mature or adult CNS does not approach the robust percentages observed in the developing CNS (Keirstead et al., 1995), suggesting that factors or mechanisms other than myelin are contributing to the failure of adult CNS regeneration.

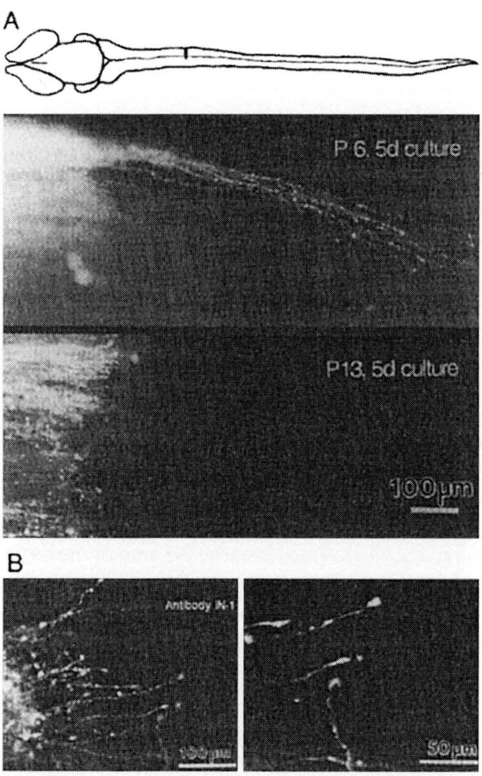

Figure 10 Transition from permissive to restrictive periods for opossum spinal cord regeneration and its prolongation by application of myelin-specific antibodies. ***A***, DiI labeled axonal outgrowth of fibers occurs after a hemisection cervical cord spinal crush at P6, but not after a crush injury on P13. The developmental transition point for axonal regeneration occurs around P12. ***B***, Application of the IN-1 antibody to the P13 cultured opossum spinal cord enabled some fibers to grow into and across the lesion site. The IN-1 antibody blocks the axonal growth inhibitory effects of some myelin-associated proteins. Modified from Nicholls and Saunders (1996).

C. CNS Astrocytes

But what other changes within the developing CNS might also contribute to the functional regeneration observed within the embryonic or early neonatal spinal cord? The observations in the spinal injured embryonic chick (Fig. 11); (Hasan et al., 1991), fetal rat (Saunders et al., 1992), early neonatal rat (Bates and Stelzner, 1993) and developing opossum (Varga et al., 1995a,b; Varga et al., 1996) are all in agreement that there is very little astrogliotic scarring when the spinal injury is performed early in development. Recent studies have also observed that some adult neurons can overcome the postulated inhibitory actions of CNS myelin (Davies et al., 1997; Li et al., 1998), if the lesion is limited in size or the neurons are provided with a permissive substrate for growth (e.g. olfactory ensheathing cells). These and other studies suggested that factors associated with the extracellular matrix and/or astrocytes may be equally important. Please see other chapters in this volume for further discussion of these issues.

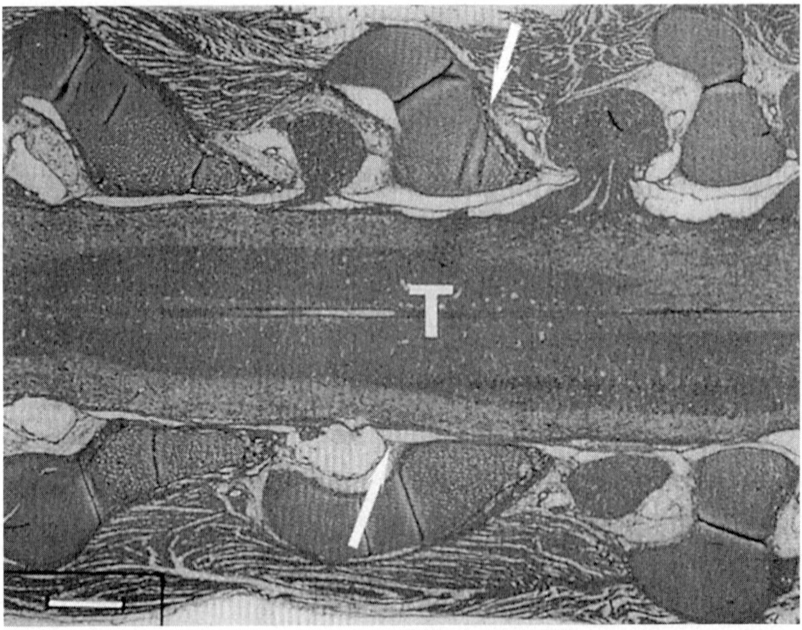

Figure 11 Photomicrograph of a toluidine blue-stained parasagittal section through the thoracic spinal cord of an E20 chick where the transection was performed on E10 (within the permissive period for spinal cord regeneration). The transection site was between the 2 white arrowheads. If a chick embryonic spinal cord was completely severed (transected) prior to E13, there was usually little evidence of subsequent glial scarring. Scale bar, 400 μm. Modified from Hasan et al., (1991).

In terms of the E13 transition point between the permissive and restrictive periods for regeneration in the embryonic chick, the expression patterns of proteoglycans (normally associated with astrocytes) also shift within the developing spinal cord environment. Heparan sulphate proteoglycan (HSPG) is predominantly expressed during the permissive period, whereas chondroitin sulphate proteoglycan (CSPG) is more highly expressed during the restrictive period (Dow et al., 1994). From E9 through to E19, the observed 50% decrease in the HSPG:CSPG ratio was a product of both a decreased synthesis of HSPGs and an increased synthesis of CSPGs. A high HSPG:CSPG ratio may account for the robust neurite growth promoting activity within chick DRG explant cultures grown on E9 proteoglycan fractions immobilized on a laminin substrate. Conversely around E13, CSPG synthesis increases as HSPG expression decreases and these changes may mask the neurite growth promoting effects of HSPG. E17 proteoglycan fractions were inhibitory to DRG neurite outgrowth, but the removal of the influence of CSPGs (by Chondroitinase digestion) in E17 proteoglycan extracts enabled DRG neurites to grow on a poly-D-lysine substrate (to the same magnitude as that observed on a laminin substrate). Heparinase pretreatment of an E17 proteoglycan fraction did not remove the neurite inhibitory activity (Dow et al., 1994).

Proteoglycans are produced by astrocytes and they are composed of a protein core with attached sugar moieties called glycosaminoglycans and are characterized as chondroitin sulfate, heparan sulfate, keratan sulfate, and dermatan sulfate (Margolis and Margolis, 1993; Margolis et al., 1996). Chondroitin sulfate proteoglycans are one category of molecules that increase and persist within the extracellular matrix following traumatic cord injury, often associated with the glial scar and the subsequent formation of a cyst cavity (Fitch and Silver, 1997; Fitch and Silver, 1997). What is now required is an experimental intervention that would reduce the level of CSPG expression after spinal injury to ascertain whether this treatment reduces CNS damage and/or facilitates neural repair.

D. CNS Cell Death

The center of a spinal cord injury may be predominantly characterized by necrotic death (Balentine, 1978); whereas, the surrounding tissue forms a region which may be analogous to the penumbra of focal ischemic lesions in the brain where active or apoptotic cell death (ACD) may predominate (Choi, 1996). Several mechanisms may contribute to this phenomenon, including: anoxia, excitotoxicity, free radical generation, proteases released from neighboring necrotic cells, inflammatory responses and macrophage invasion. The secondary degeneration induced by this process may also exacerbate the formation of cyst cavities (Dusart and Schwab, 1994).

Neuronal death after axonal injury has been reported in a variety of neuronal systems which may differ in their extent, time course and possibly in the underlying molecular triggers. Some of the differences appear to relate to the age of the animal, the distance of the axonal injury from the parent cell body and the specific neuronal phenotype (please see other chapters in this volume for continued discussion). For example, cell death occurs within a few days after axonal injury of motoneurons (Sendtner et al., 1992) or after axonal injury of corticospinal neurons within the postnatal (but not adult) rodent spinal cord (Giehl and Tetzlaff, 1996; Giehl et al., 1998). In general, the degree of ACD after axonal injury is greater in developing nervous systems, than that observed after an adult nervous system injury.

In support of this statement, very little death is seen in descending spinal projection neurons when they are axotomized late in the development of the chick (e.g. E17, McBride and Steeves, unpublished observations) or in adult rats (Barron et al., 1988; Kobayashi et al., 1997), unless the axonal injury site is very close to the cell body, such as in root avulsions of spinal motoneurons (Wu et al., 1994) or in subcortical lesions of adult corticospinal neurons (Giehl and Tetzlaff, 1996).

While injuries that induce either acute or protracted periods of cell death are both characterized by ACD (Villegas-Perez et al., 1993; Rossiter et al., 1996), protracted forms are poor models to quantify molecular changes, since very few dying cells are detectable at any given time point. In comparison to the mature injured CNS, the enhanced ACD surrounding an injury within the developing CNS should enable a more quantitative assessment of *in vivo* strategies to reduce ACD (e.g. inhibition of caspase enzymes).

Massive glial cell death has also been reported after neurotrauma. For example, large numbers of apoptotic oligodendrocytes have been quickly detected (within days) following spinal cord injury in the embryonic and mature chick (McBride and Steeves, in preparation), adult rat (Crowe et al., 1997) and monkey (Crowe et al., 1997). This death appears to occur in regions of axonal degeneration as well as within regions of the proximal axons, and is seen several segments distant from the injury site. This suggests it is not a direct response to the injury but an active response to the changing condition within injured axons. The fact that it occurs within such a short time span also suggests that the spinal demyelination, often associated with Wallerian degeneration, may be initiated before the distal axon has actually degenerated (i.e. it is not a passive response). Thus, even after an incomplete spinal cord injury, diminished functional recovery, may be partially attributed to the slowing or cessation of action potential conduction as a consequence of oligodendrocyte ACD triggering demyelination of spared axons (Blight, 1985) .

E. CNS Growth Factors

The myriad of growth factors that have been identified over the past couple of decades is impressive and continues to grow in number. The challenge is to match these molecules to specific influences on the developing and mature CNS, as well as to identify their roles in mediating functional repair after injury. Here I will focus on some of our initial findings directed toward elucidating the roles of growth factors on a few of the identified neuronal targets for spinal cord repair. A contusion or penetrating injury of the spinal cord can axotomize numerous populations of neurons, including: descending (e.g. brainstem-spinal and corticospinal pathways), ascending (e.g. dorsal column pathways) and propriospinal neurons.

As mentioned above, there is both necrotic and apoptotic cell death surrounding the site of CNS injury. The loss of local neurons and glial cells is unquestioned, but it has been noted in both the developing and mature CNS that neurons originating some distance from the site of injury will survive axotomy of their primary axon. This phenomenon is distance dependent. The farther the axotomy is from the originating neuronal cell body, the better the survival and reduction of subsequent atrophy of the neuronal cell body. These surviving neurons are therefore available as the potential "engines" of functional regeneration. Nevertheless, these surviving, injured neurons may require appropriate trophic support to mount a regenerative response.

Application of the appropriate trophic factors can ameliorate adult CNS neuronal atrophy resulting from an axotomy, with the concomitant upregulation of growth-associated genes thought to be important for axonal regeneration. This was recently demonstrated by Tetzlaff and colleagues (Kobayashi et al., 1997) for axotomized rubrospinal neurons with the direct infusion of brain derived neurotrophic factor (BDNF) near the red nucleus. Since little is known about the trophic sensitivities of other brainstem-spinal populations, studies have been initiated in an effort to identify mechanisms for improving axonal regeneration and functional repair after a spinal cord injury.

In vitro assays of brainstem-spinal neurons have been developed (Pataky and Steeves, in preparation) that are based on prior *in vivo* retrograde labeling from within the developing spinal cord. The developing chick embryo is ideally suited to these experiments because the organization of descending projections is similar to mammalian brainstem-spinal pathways (Steeves et al., 1987; Webster et al., 1990; Webster and Steeves, 1991) and it offers easy access to retrogradely label developing brainstem-spinal neurons prior to culturing.

Dissociated cultures were initially prepared from the entire hindbrain (pons and medulla) of animals previously subjected to a carbocyanine dye (DiI) retrograde tracing protocol, resulting in *in vitro* assays containing raphespinal, reticulospinal, coeruleospinal and vestibulospinal DiI-labeled neurons. The effect on survival of DiI-labeled neurons was determined for astrocyte-conditioned medium and several members of the fibroblast growth factor (FGF) family known to be synthesized by astrocytes, FGF-1 and FGF-2 (Hatten et al., 1988). The technique can be refined to allow the study of an additional paramater, neurite outgrowth, using explants of particular DiI-labeled brainstem-spinal populations. For example, microdissection from the hindbrain of the vestibulospinal nucleus produced assays for survival and neurite outgrowth, respectively measured using dissociated or explant cell cultures. To assess whether the FGFs can act directly on brainstem-spinal neurons, the expression of FGF receptors was also examined.

On E8, dissociated cultures containing labeled neurons were prepared from the brainstem. Astrocyte-conditioned medium (ACM) promoted the survival of brainstem-spinal neurons derived from whole hindbrain dissociates. Astrocytes synthesize a variety of trophic factors, including FGFs, and FGF-2 application to the serum free culture medium (but not FGF-1) also stimulated survival. As expected, if the FGF effects were stimulating non-neuronal cells (e.g. astrocytes) to release another (as yet) unidentified factor, FGF-2 function blocking antibodies would not and did not suppress ACM-promoted survival, nor were FGF-2 levels elevated in ACM, as detected by ELISA.

These *in vitro* assays can be refined to produce dissociated (survival assay) or explant (neurite outgrowth assay) cultures from specific brainstem-spinal nuclei, such as vestibulospinal neurons. Once again, FGF-2 promoted both survival and neurite outgrowth of identified vestibulospinal neurons. Interestingly, FGF-1 promoted neurite outgrowth, but not survival; the converse was true of FGF-9. Vestibulospinal neurons did not express fibroblast growth factor receptor mRNA, once again suggesting an indirect mechanism for the FGF effects. Thus the differential effects of specific growth factors on survival and/or neurite outgrowth of distinct brainstem-spinal phenotypes can be distinguished, and it suggests that specific descending and ascending spinal populations should be individually studied to identify which trophic factors will be beneficial for *in vivo* application after an adult spinal cord injury.

Several investigators are already experimentally using specific trophic factors *in vivo* to stimulate improved repair after an adult spinal cord injury. Of particular relevance to the present discussion is the report that FGF-1 application to the severed adult rat spinal cord facilitated increased brainstem-spinal and propriospinal regeneration when combined with directed peripheral nerve bridges across the site of injury (Cheng et al., 1996). Our *in vitro* findings also suggest that FGF-1 has a distinct role in promoting brainstem-spinal neurite outgrowth.

A second *in vivo* study reported that after adult spinal cord hemisection, the application of neurotrophin-3 (NT-3) at the site of injury enhances reticulospinal and rubrospinal axon elongation into a peripheral nerve transplant, but not raphe-spinal, vestibulospinal or coeruleospinal growth (Ye and Houle, 1997). Our preliminary *in vitro* data suggests NT-3 does not promote brainstem-spinal neuron survival in whole brainstem dissociated cultures, but it does stimulate neurite outgrowth from isolated *in vitro* explants containing reticulospinal neurons. Thus, the application of the appropriate factor(s) after an adult spinal cord injury may improve the repair of severed brainstem-spinal projections, especially when combined with treatments to neutralize the axonal growth inhibition that is apparent within the injured adult CNS.

IV. FUTURE CONSIDERATIONS

A. Extracellular Matrix Molecules

There has been an exponentially increasing body of knowledge about the identity and possible developmental functions of molecules associated with the extracellular matrix (Tessier-Lavigne and Goodman, 1996). For example, in the developing CNS, laminin is associated with astrocytes (Stichel and Muller, 1994), glial limitans (Luckenbill-Edds et al., 1995) and newly formed blood vessels, along with their integrin receptors, and there is substantial down-regulation of laminin expression in adult life. It is well acknowledged that laminin can serve as a highly permissive substrate for *in vitro* CNS axonal outgrowth and can readily associate with HSPGs. Along with NCAM (Saffell et al., 1992), N-Cadherin, and an ever growing list of extracellular matrix molecules, laminin expression may be another underlying factor for the relatively robust nature of CNS regeneration in developing animals. To extensively review extracellular matrix molecules is beyond the scope of this review. Instead, I will briefly review a fast "developing" field (pun intended) concerned with the recently discovered netrin, semaphorin and ephrin families.

Netrin-1 and Netrin-2 were isolated biochemically from embryonic chicken brain using an *in vitro* outgrowth/attraction assay of commissural neurons (Kennedy and Tessier-Lavigne, 1995). Subsequent *in vitro* studies established their role as chemoattractants of commissural neurons as well as chemorepellents for trochlear neurons (Serafini et al., 1996). Netrins are the mammalian homologue of UNC-6, a protein in the nematode C. elegans that directs ventral and dorsal axonal guidance and cell migration (Hedgecock and Norris, 1997). Thus, netrins can exert a dual function, attraction or repulsion, which appears to be dependent on the type of receptor expressed by the neuron. Two rat homologues of UNC-5, a receptor for UNC-6 in the nematode worm, have recently been cloned (UNC5H1 and UNC5H2; Leonardo et al., 1997). UNC5H receptors are expressed in the developing rat ventral spinal cord, DRG, cortex, optic cup, hippocampus, and cerebellum as well as parts of the brainstem, midbrain and diencephalon. Substantial UNC5H1 expression is still seen in the cortex, hippocampus and cerebellum in the 10 day old rat (Leonardo et al., 1997). A vertebrate orthologue of another nematode receptor (UNC 40) was also identified. This receptor had been previously discovered to play a role in another vertebrate situation and has a highly descriptive name, Deleted in Colorectal Cancer (DCC). DCC acts as a vertebrate netrin receptor mediating directed outgrowth of commissural axons towards a nearby floorplate *in vitro* (Keino-Masu et al., 1996). While UNC-5 and its vertebrate counterparts have been presumed to mediate the repulsive affect of Netrin, there are lines of evidence that suggest DCC may also play a role (de la Torre et al., 1997). Both of these responses can be blocked with antibodies that recognize DCC (de la Torre et al., 1997).

Consistent with the widespread expression of netrin receptors in the developing brain, the involvement of netrins in the guidance of various types of CNS axons, as well as cell migration, has become increasingly evident. For example, the netrin response of cranial motoneurons varies depending on their projection patterns, i.e. whether the axons leave the brainstem ventrally or dorsally, netrin mediated guidance may act as a repellent or attractant. Moreover there is now evidence that netrins play a role in the guidance of a variety of neurons, including Xenopus and mouse retinal ganglion cell axons (de la Torre et al., 1997), efferent projections from the mouse cerebral cortex (Metin et al., 1997), commissural and longitudinal projections of the mouse and chick brain and spinal cord (Fazeli et al., 1997; MacLennan et al., 1997) and striatal and nigral projections (Livesey and Hunt, 1997). In short, netrins may have diverse roles in neuronal migration and axonal guidance during development. They appear to be bifunctional molecules, with the type of response dependent on the receptor-type expressed by the neuron.

The Semaphorin family of glycoproteins has been implicated in repulsive axonal guidance (Kolodkin and Ginty, 1997). This structurally diverse secreted and transmembrane family of proteins is characterized by a 500 amino acid Semaphorin domain that is highly conserved between vertebrates and invertebrates (Kolodkin et al., 1993). The first member of the Semaphorin family identified was Grasshopper Semaphorin I (G-Sema I), originally named fasciclin IV (Kolodkin et al., 1992). Soon after the initial cloning of G-Sema I, other Semaphorins were identified in vertebrates and invertebrates, leading to the generation of a number of subclasses of Semaphorins. These included Sema II, an invertebrate secreted form found in drosophila and Sema III, a vertebrate secreted form found in mouse and human. Independently, Luo et al. (Luo et al., 1995) cloned a growth cone collapsing molecule called Chick Collapsin 1, which turned out to be an orthologue of Human Sema III. A number of other Semaphorin molecules have now been identified and presently 6 classes of Semaphorins have been distinguished. While the number of Semaphorins continues to grow, the majority of the functional work has concentrated on the secreted Semaphorins, particularly in the subfamilies Sema II and III. Experiments from a variety of systems has shown these Semaphorins to be inhibitory for neurite outgrowth (Kolodkin and Ginty, 1997). In contrast the transmembrane Semaphorin, Sema I, may be attractive or inhibitory for neurite outgrowth (Wong et al., 1997).

In mouse, Sem D (Sema III subfamily) was found to be highly expressed in the developing ventral spinal cord and has been shown *in vitro* to selectively inhibit growth of NGF-responsive, but not NT-3-responsive, DRG neurons. A comprehensive *in situ* hybridization and immunohistochemical analysis of the expression of Semophorin III/D in the developing rat nervous system showed that Sema III/D is widely expressed. Among the regions identified were the ventral spinal cord, layer V of the neocortex and reticular neurons of the brainstem (Giger et al., 1996). Given the apparent developmental role and developmental regulation of semaphorins it is conceivable that at least some members of the Semaphorin family are reexpressed after axonal injury, e.g. Sema III/D. While it will be important to examine whether Semaphorins are repulsive to spinal cord projection axons it may be equally important to analyze the injured neurons for the expression of the semaphorin receptors, the neuropilins.

Neuropilin (neuropilin-1) was previously recognized as neuronal surface antigen A5, and has recently been identified as a receptor for Semaphorin III/D (He and Tessier-Lavigne, 1997). Neuropilin-1 is a transmembrane protein. A second related receptor (neuropilin-2) has also been cloned and shown to be the receptor for Sem E and Sema IV but not Sema III/D. Its expression is largely non-overlapping with neuropilin-1. Neuropilin-1 was shown to be transiently expressed in embryonic mouse spinal cord motoneurons (E11.5-13.5) and expressed from E11.5 until birth in dorsal root and cranial ganglia. Neuropilin-1 was localized mainly on axons during the phase of active growth, including spinal nerve roots, optic nerve fibers and olfactory nerve fibers. Interestingly, it appears to persist within the olfactory system into adulthood which is consistent with maintained olfactory cell migration and axonal projection in growth. Even more interesting, neuropilin-1 is reexpressed by successfully regenerating retinal ganglion cell axons in Xenopus (Fugisawa et al., 1996). Thus, the analysis of both SemIII/D and its receptor within spinal cord projection neurons after a spinal cord injury should be of great interest.

The Eph receptor family, named after the first member discovered in a erythropoietin-producing hepatocellular carcinoma cell line, is the largest known receptor tyrosine kinase family with at least 14 members. It has been implicated in a variety of patterning events during embryonic development, particularly in the nervous system. Eph members appear to play a role in axonal guidance and topographic map formation of neural projections (for review see Holland et al., 1996). The ligands of these receptors, the Ephrins, are typically membrane bound, which underscores their probable roles in contact-mediated cell-to-cell interaction. A recent nomenclature committee agreed to refer to the ligands as ephrin-A or ephrin-B depending on whether they are linked to the membrane by a glycosylphophatidyl-inositol (GPI) linker (ephrin-A1-5) or via a transmembrane domain (ephrin-B1-3). Those receptors that interact primarily with the ephrin-A family are referred to as EphA receptors (EphA1 to EphA8) and those that interact primarily with the ephrin-B family are the EphB receptors (EphB1 to EphB6), with the exception of ephrinB3 binding to EphA4. Within each subclass there is some promiscuity among the A receptors and the A ligands and their relative affinities may vary considerably.

The involvement of Ephrins in axonal guidance and in cell migration was first demonstrated in the development of the retino-tectal projection (Drescher et al., 1995). Ganglion cells of the retina express gradients of EphA3, EphA4, EphA5 and EphB2 receptors, which are also complemented by gradients of ligand expression within the tectum (Ephrin A2 and A5) (Drescher et al., 1997). Disturbance of this expression pattern or the ectopic overexpression of ligands within the tectum produced a marked disruption of the retinotectal projection. Ephrins also play a role in the development of a variety of other areas in the CNS, for example they play a role in hindbrain segmentation, brain commissure formation, forebrain patterning, neural crest cell migration and *in vitro* axon bundling (Drescher, 1997).

It has been proposed that Ephrins provide inhibitory cues to axonal growth cones. It is therefore conceivable that this ligand receptor system also plays a role in adult CNS regeneration failure. Presently (and this may rapidly change), there are no reports on the expression of Eph receptors in spinal cord projection neurons of adults. Extremely relevant for this discussion is the finding by Winzenmann et al. (Wizenmann et al., 1993) that the retinotectal neural guidance cues which appear to be responsible for the retinotopic innervation are lost during adulthood but are reexpressed following optic nerve injury and tectal denervation.

In summary, many of these molecules appear to serve dual roles, acting as repulsive signals for some neuronal growth cones, while attracting other growth cones. Their roles in the mechanisms that guide developing axons are becoming established and thus, they have strong potential for being involved in therapeutic solutions for facilitating and directing appropriate axonal regrowth after an adult CNS injury. However, most of the available data on the expression patterns and/or roles of these molecules have only been collected from the intact developing nervous system or from *in vitro* cell culture analysis. To date, little information has been gathered about alterations in their expression patterns that correlate with the pathological changes of spinal cord or brain injury, especially during development.

The continued study of guidance molecules is an obvious direction for future research that will undoubtedly bring new insight to understanding traumatic injury of the adult CNS. These examinations are on the near horizon and only await the further characterization of these extracellular matrix molecules and the design of techniques to alter their expression after either a developmental or adult CNS injury.

B. Immune System Responses to CNS Injury

It is generally thought that both microglia and peripherally derived monocytes respond to injury in various proportions depending on the type and severity of the lesion. The severity and molecular components of the immune response after CNS injury, as well as the timing in the recruitment of immune reactions, may also influence any potential beneficial or detrimental outcomes. Presently, clinical care of human spinal cord injury involves the rapid administration of high dose steroids, such as methylprednisolone, and it is unquestioned that this treatment affects the immune system.

It is far from clear whether the inflammatory response to injury exacerbates or limits the initial mechanical trauma. Recent studies suggest that certain immune reactions, be it the addition of specific anti-inflammatory agents (Guth, et al., 1994), cytokines (e.g. Klusman and Schwab, 1997) or the transplantation of activated macrophages (Lazarov-Spiegler et al., 1996; Rabchevsky and Streit, 1998; Rapalino et al., 1998) into the site of spinal injury may facilitate repair. The immune system is another complex control network that is only beginning to be examined for its potential roles in ameliorating CNS neurotrauma injuries. Characterizing the immune reactions to CNS damage in both developing and mature animals may provide important directions in the design of the necessary therapeutic interventions .

In conclusion, it is widely acknowledged that functional recovery after human spinal cord injury will not rely on the application of one type of treatment, but will involve the application of a combination of approaches in the appropriate sequence. Thus for the student of functional CNS regeneration, there are a number of unexplored avenues for future investigation and it is assured that information gathered from the developing nervous system will be central to continued progress.

ACKNOWLEDGEMENTS

The past and present support of various agencies has been essential to my research. I am grateful to the Medical Research Council (Canada), the Neuroscience Network (Canada), the Neurotrauma Fund (Canada), and the Paralyzed Veterans of America. I am also indebted to my colleagues in the CORD (Collaboration On Repair Discoveries) research group at the University of British Columbia. CORD Internet site: (http://cord.ubc.ca).

REFERENCES

Asada Y, Kawaguchi S, Hayashi H, Nakamura T (1998) Neural repair of the injured spinal cord by grafting: Comparison between peripheral nerve segments and embryonic homologous structures as a conduit of CNS axons. Neuroscience Research 31:241-249.

Balentine JD (1978) Pathology of experimental spinal cord trauma. II. Ultrastructure of axons and myelin. Laboratory Investigation 39:254-266.

Barron KD, Dentinger MP, Popp AJ, Mankes R (1988) Neurons of layer Vb of rat sensorimotor cortex atrophy but do not die after thoracic cord transection. Journal of Neuropathology & Experimental Neurology 47:62-74.

Basso DM, Beattie MS, Bresnahan JC (1995) A sensitive and reliable locomotor rating scale for open field testing in rats. Journal of Neurotrauma 12:1-21.

Bates CA, Stelzner DJ (1993) Extension and regeneration of corticospinal axons after early spinal injury and the maintenance of corticospinal topography. Experimental Neurology 123:106-117.

Bernstein DR, Bechard DE, Stelzner DJ (1981) Neuritic growth maintained near the lesion site long after spinal cord transection in the newborn rat. Neuroscience Letters 26:55-60.

Bernstein DR, Stelzner DJ (1983) Plasticity of the corticospinal tract following midthoracic spinal injury in the postnatal rat. Journal of Comparative Neurology 221:382-400.

Bernstein-Goral H, Bregman BS (1993) Spinal cord transplants support the regeneration of axotomized neurons after spinal cord lesions at birth: a quantitative double labeling study. Experimental Neurology 123:118-132.

Blight AR (1985) Delayed demyelination and macrophage invasion: a candidate for secondary cell damage in spinal cord injury. Central Nervous System Trauma 2:299-315.

Bregman BS, Kunkel-Bagden E, Schnell L, Dai HN, Gao D, Schwab ME (1995) Recovery from spinal cord injury mediated by antibodies to neurite growth inhibitors. Nature 378:498-501.

Brown TG (1911) The intrinsic factors in the act of progression in the mammal. Proceedings of the Royal Society 84:308-319.

Cheng H, Cao Y, Olson L (1996) Spinal cord repair in adult paraplegic rats: partial restoration of hind limb function. Science 273:510-513.

Choi D (1996) Ischemia-induced neuronal apoptosis. Current Opinion in Neurobiology 6:667-672.

Crowe MJ, Bresnahan JC, Shuman SL, Masters JN, Beattie MS (1997) Apoptosis and delayed degeneration after spinal cord injury in rats and monkeys [published erratum appears in Nat Med 1997 Feb;3(2):240]. Nature Medicine 3:73-76.

Davies SJ, Fitch MT, Memberg SP, Hall AK, Raisman G, Silver J (1997) Regeneration of adult axons in white matter tracts of the central nervous system. Nature 390:680-683.

de la Torre JR, Hopker VH, Ming GL, Poo MM, Tessier-Lavigne M, Hemmati-Brivanlou A, Holt CE (1997) Turning of retinal growth cones in a netrin-1 gradient mediated by the netrin receptor DCC. Neuron 19:1211-1224.

Dow KE, Ethell DW, Steeves JD, Riopelle RJ (1994) Molecular correlates of spinal cord repair in the embryonic chick: heparan sulfate and chondroitin sulfate proteoglycans. Experimental Neurology 128:233-238.

Drescher U (1997) The Eph family in the patterning of neural development. Current Biology: R799-R807.

Drescher U, Bonhoeffer F, Muller BK (1997) The Eph family in retinal axon guidance. Current Opinion in Neurobiology 7:75-80.

Drescher U, Kremoser C, Handwerker C, Loschinger J, Noda M, Bonhoeffer F (1995) In vitro guidance of retinal ganglion cell axons by RAGS, a 25 kDa tectal protein related to ligands for Eph receptor tyrosine kinases. Cell 82:359-370.

Dusart I, Schwab ME (1994) Secondary cell death and the inflammatory reaction after dorsal hemisection of the rat spinal cord. European Journal of Neuroscience 6:712-724.

Dyer JK, Bourque JA, Steeves JD (1998) Regeneration of brainstem-spinal axons after lesion and immunological disruption in adult rat. Experimental Neurology 154:12-22.

Fazeli A, Dickinson SL, Hermiston ML, Tighe RV, Steen RG, Small CG, Stoeckli ET, Keino-Masu K, Masu M, Rayburn H, Simons J, Bronson RT, Gordon JI, Tessier-Lavigne M, Weinberg RA (1997) Phenotype of mice lacking functional Deleted in colorectal cancer (DCC) gene. Nature 386:796-804.

Fitch MT, Silver J (1997) Activated macrophages and the blood-brain barrier: inflammation after CNS injury leads to increases in putative inhibitory molecules. Experimental Neurology 148:587-603.

Fitch MT, Silver J (1997) Glial cell extracellular matrix: boundaries for axon growth in development and regeneration. Cell & Tissue Research 290:379-384.

Fugisawa H, Takagi S, Hirata T (1996) Growth-associated expression of a membrane protein, neuropilin, in Xenopus optic nerve fibers. Developmental Neuroscience 17:343-349.

Giehl KM, Schutte A, Mestres P, Yan Q (1998) The survival-promoting effect of glial cell line-derived neurotrophic factor on axotomized corticospinal neurons in vivo is me-

diated by an endogenous brain-derived neurotrophic factor mechanism. Journal of Neuroscience 18:7351-7360.
Giehl KM, Tetzlaff W (1996) BDNF and NT-3, but not NGF, prevent axotomy-induced death of rat corticospinal neurons in vivo. European Journal of Neuroscience 8:1167-1175.
Giger RJ, Wolfer DP, De Wit GM, Verhaagen J (1996) Anatomy of rat semaphorin III/collapsin-1 mRNA expression and relationship to developing nerve tracts during neuroembryogenesis. Journal of Comparative Neurology 375:378-392.
Glover JC (1993) The development of brainstem projections to the spinal cord in the chicken embryo. Brain Research Bulletin 30:265-271.
Guth L (1975) History of central nervous system regeneration research. Experimental Neurology 48:3-15.
Hasan SJ, Keirstead HS, Muir GD, Steeves JD (1993) Axonal regeneration contributes to repair of injured brainstem-spinal neurons in embryonic chick. Journal of Neuroscience 13:492-507.
Hasan SJ, Nelson BH, Velenzuela JI, Keirstead HS, Shull SE, Ethell DW, Steeves JD (1991) Functional repair of transected spinal cord in embryonic chick. Restorative Neurology and Neuroscience 2:137-154.
Hatten ME, Lynch M, Rydel RE, Sanchez J, Joseph-Siverstein J, Moscatelli D, Rifkin DB (1988) In vitro neurite extension by granule neurons is dependent upon astroglial-derived fibroblast growth factor. Developmental Biology 125:280-289.
He Z, Tessier-Lavigne M (1997) Neuropilin is a receptor for the axonal chemorepellent Semaphorin III. Cell 90:739-751.
Hedgecock EM, Norris CR (1997) Netrins evoke mixed reactions in motile cells. Trends in Genetics 13:251-253.
Holland SJ, Gale NW, Mbamalu G, Yancopoulos GD, Henkemeyer M, Pawson T (1996) Bidirectional signalling through the EPH-family receptor Nuk and its transmembrane ligands. Nature 383:722-725.
Howland DR, Bregman BS, Tessler A, Goldberger ME (1995a) Development of locomotor behavior in the spinal kitten. Experimental Neurology 135:108-122.
Howland DR, Bregman BS, Tessler A, Goldberger ME (1995b) Transplants enhance locomotion in neonatal kittens whose spinal cords are transected: a behavioral and anatomical study. Experimental Neurology 135:123-145.
Iwashita Y, Kawaguchi S, Murata M (1994) Restoration of function by replacement of spinal cord segments in the rat. Nature 367:167-170.
Keino-Masu K, Masu M, Hinck L, Leonardo ED, Chan SS, Culotti JG, Tessier-Lavigne M (1996) Deleted in colorectal cancer (DCC) encodes a netrin receptor. Cell 87:175-185.
Keirstead HS, Dyer JK, Sholomenko GN, McGraw J, Delaney KR, Steeves JD (1995) Axonal regeneration and physiological activity following transection and immunological disruption of myelin within the hatchling chick spinal cord. Journal of Neuroscience 15:6963-6974.
Keirstead HS, Hasan SJ, Muir GD, Steeves JD (1992) Suppression of the onset of myelination extends the permissive period for the functional repair of embryonic spinal cord. Proceedings of the National Academy of Sciences of the United States of America 89:11664-11668.
Keirstead HS, Pataky DM, McGraw J, Steeves JD (1997) In vivo immunological suppression of spinal cord myelin development. Brain Research Bulletin 44:727-734.

Keirstead HS, Steeves JD (1998) CNS myelin: Does a stabilizing role in neurodevelopment result in inhibition of neuronal repair after injury. The Neuroscientist 4:273-284.

Kennedy TE, Tessier-Lavigne M (1995) Guidance and induction of branch formation in developing axons by target-derived diffusible factors. Current Opinion in Neurobiology 5:83-90.

Klusman I, Schwab ME (1997) Effects of pro-inflammatory cytokines in experimental spinal cord injury. Brain Research 762:173-184.

Kobayashi NR, Fan DP, Giehl KM, Bedard AM, Wiegand SJ, Tetzlaff W (1997) BDNF and NT-4/5 prevent atrophy of rat rubrospinal neurons after cervical axotomy, stimulate GAP-43 and Talpha1-tubulin mRNA expression, and promote axonal regeneration. Journal of Neuroscience 17:9583-9595.

Kolodkin AL, Ginty DD (1997) Steering clear of semaphorins: neuropilins sound the retreat. Neuron 19:1159-1162.

Kolodkin AL, Matthes DJ, Goodman CS (1993) The semaphorin genes encode a family of transmembrane and secreted growth cone guidance molecules. Cell 75:1389-1399.

Kolodkin AL, Matthes DJ, O'Connor TP, Patel NH, Admon A, Bentley D, Goodman CS (1992) Fasciclin IV: sequence, expression, and function during growth cone guidance in the grasshopper embryo. Neuron 9:831-845.

Lazarov-Spiegler O, Solomon AS, Zeev-Brann AB, Hirschberg DL, Lavie V, Schwartz M (1996) Transplantation of activated macrophages overcomes central nervous system regrowth failure. FASEB Journal 10:1296-1302.

Leonardo ED, Hinck L, Masu M, Keino-Masu K, Ackerman SL, Tessier-Lavigne M (1997) Vertebrate homologues of C. elegans UNC-5 are candidate netrin receptors. Nature 386:833-838.

Li Y, Field PM, Raisman G (1998) Regeneration of adult rat corticospinal axons induced by transplanted olfactory ensheathing cells. Journal of Neuroscience 18:10514-10524.

Livesey FJ, Hunt SP (1997) Netrin and netrin receptor expression in the embryonic mammalian nervous system suggests roles in retinal, striatal, nigral, and cerebellar development. Molecular & Cellular Neurosciences 8:417-429.

Luckenbill-Edds L, Kaiser CA, Rodgers TR, Powell DD (1995) Localization of the 110 kDa receptor for laminin in brains of embryonic and postnatal mice. Cell & Tissue Research 279:371-377.

Luo Y, Shepherd I, Li J, Renzi MJ, Chang S, Raper JA (1995) A family of molecules related to collapsin in the embryonic chick nervous system [published erratum appears in Neuron 1995 Nov;15(5):following 1218]. Neuron 14:1131-1140.

MacLennan AJ, McLaurin DL, Marks L, Vinson EN, Pfeifer M, Szulc SV, Heaton MB, Lee N (1997) Immunohistochemical localization of netrin-1 in the embryonic chick nervous system. Journal of Neuroscience 17:5466-5479.

Margolis RK, Margolis RU (1993) Nervous tissue proteoglycans. Experientia 49:429-446.

Margolis RK, Rauch U, Maurel P, Margolis RU (1996) Neurocan and phosphacan - two major nervous tissue-specific chondroitin sulfate proteoglycans. Perspectives on Developmental Neurobiology 3:273-290.

McConnell JA, Sechrist J (1980) Identification of early neurons in the brainstem and spinal cord: an autoradiographic study in the chick. Journal of Comparative Neurology 192:769-783.

McKerracher L, David S, Jackson DL, Kottis V, Dunn RJ, Braun PE (1994) Identification of myelin-associated glycoprotein as a major myelin-derived inhibitor of neurite growth. Neuron 13:805-811.

Metin C, Deleglise D, Serafini T, Kennedy TE, Tessier-Lavigne M (1997) A role for netrin-1 in the guidance of cortical efferents. Development 124:5063-5074.

Miya D, Giszter S, Mori F, Adipudi V, Tessler A, Murray M (1997) Fetal transplants alter the development of function after spinal cord transection in newborn rats. Journal of Neuroscience 17:4856-4872.

Muir GD, Steeves JD (1997) Sensorimotor stimulation to improve locomotor recovery after spinal cord injury. Trends in Neurosciences 20:72-77.

Mukhopadhyay G, Doherty P, Walsh FS, Crocker PR, Filbin MT (1994) A novel role for myelin-associated glycoprotein as an inhibitor of axonal regeneration. Neuron 13:757-767.

Nicholls J, Saunders N (1996) Regeneration of immature mammalian spinal cord after injury. Trends in Neurosciences 19:229-234.

Okado N, Oppenheim RW (1985) The onset and development of descending pathways to the spinal cord in the chick embryo. Journal of Comparative Neurology 232:143-161.

Rabchevsky AG, Streit WJ (1998) Role of microglia in postinjury repair and regeneration of the CNS. Mental Retardation & Developmental Disabilities Research Reviews 4:187-192.

Rapalino O, Lazarov-Spiegler O, Agranov E, Velan GJ, Yoles E, Fraidakis M, Solomon A, Gepstein R, Katz A, Belkin M, Hadani M, Schwartz M (1998) Implantation of stimulated homologous macrophages results in partial recovery of paraplegic rats. Nature Medicine 4:814-821.

Rossiter JP, Riopelle RJ, Bisby MA (1996) Axotomy-induced apoptotic cell death of neonatal rat facial motoneurons: time course analysis and relation to NADPH-diaphorase activity. Experimental Neurology 138:33-44.

Saffell JL, Ashton SV, Walsh FS, Doherty P (1992) The changing role of NCAM as a neurite outgrowth-promoting molecule during development. Biochemical Society Transactions 20:410-412.

Saunders NR, Balkwill P, Knott G, Habgood MD, Mollgard K, Treherne JM, Nicholls JG (1992) Growth of axons through a lesion in the intact CNS of fetal rat maintained in long-term culture. Proceedings of the Royal Society of London - Series B: Biological Sciences 250:171-180.

Saunders NR, Deal A, Knott GW, Varga ZM, Nicholls JG (1995) Repair and recovery following spinal cord injury in a neonatal marsupial (Monodelphis domestica). Clinical & Experimental Pharmacology & Physiology 22:518-526.

Saunders NR, Kitchener P, Knott GW, Nicholls JG, Potter A, Smith TJ (1998) Development of walking, swimming and neuronal connections after complete spinal cord transection in the neonatal opossum, Monodelphis domestica. Journal of Neuroscience 18:339-355.

Schwab ME, Bartholdi D (1996) Degeneration and regeneration of axons in the lesioned spinal cord. Physiological Reviews 76:319-370.

Sendtner M, Holtmann B, Kolbeck R, Thoenen H, Barde YA (1992) Brain-derived neurotrophic factor prevents the death of motoneurons in newborn rats after nerve section. Nature 360:757-759.

Serafini T, Colamarino SA, Leonardo ED, Wang H, Beddington R, Skarnes WC, Tessier-Lavigne M (1996) Netrin-1 is required for commissural axon guidance in the developing vertebrate nervous system. Cell 87:1001-1014.

Sherrington CS (1910) Remarks on the reflex mechanism of the step. Brain 33:1-25.

Shimizu I, Oppenheim RW, O'Brian M, Schneiderman A (1990) Anatomical and functional recovery following spinal cord transection in the chick embryo. Journal of Neurobiology 21:918-937.

Sholomenko GN, Delaney KR (1998) Restitution of functional neural connections in chick embryos assessed in vitro after spinal cord transection in ovo. Experimental Neurology 154:430-451.

Sholomenko GN, O'Donovan MJ (1995) The development and characterization of pathways descending to the spinal cord in the isolated embryonic chick brainstem/spinal cord preparation. Journal of Neurophysiology 733:1223-1233.

Steeves JD, Keirstead HS, Ethell DW, Hasan SJ, Muir GD, Pataky DM, McBride CB, Petrausch B, Zwimpfer TJ (1994) Permissive and restrictive periods for brainstem-spinal regeneration in the chick. Progress in Brain Research 103:243-262.

Steeves JD, Sholomenko GN, Webster DM (1987) Stimulation of the pontomedullary reticular formation initiates locomotion in decerebrate birds. Brain Research 401:205-212.

Stelzner DJ, Ershler WB, Weber EB (1975) Effects of spinal transection in neonatal and weanling rats: survival and function. Experimental Neurology 46:156-177.

Stelzner DJ, Weber EB, Prendergast JN (1979) A comparison of the effect of mid-thoracic spinal hemisection in the neonatal or weanling rat on the distribution and density of dorsal root axons in the lumbosacral cord of the adult. Brain Research 172:407-426.

Stichel CC, Muller HW (1994) Relationship between injury-induced astrogliosis, laminin expression and axonal sprouting in the adult rat brain. Journal of Neurocytology 23:615-630.

Tessier-Lavigne M, Goodman CS (1996) The molecular biology of axon guidance. Science 274:1123-1133.

Varga ZM, Bandtlow CE, Erulkar SD, Schwab ME, Nicholls JG (1995a) The critical period for repair of CNS of neonatal opossum (Monodelphis domestica) in culture: correlation with development of glial cells, myelin and growth-inhibitory molecules. European Journal of Neuroscience 7:2119-2129.

Varga ZM, Fernandez J, Blackshaw S, Martin AR, Muller KJ, Adams WB, Nicholls JG (1996) Neurite outgrowth through lesions of neonatal opossum spinal cord in culture. Journal of Comparative Neurology 366:600-612.

Varga ZM, Schwab ME, Nicholls JG (1995b) Myelin-associated neurite growth-inhibitory proteins and suppression of regeneration of immature mammalian spinal cord in culture. Proceedings of the National Academy of Sciences of the United States of America 92:10959-10963.

Villegas-Perez MP, Vidal-Sanz M, Rasminsky M, Bray GM, Aguayo AJ (1993) Rapid and protracted phases of retinal ganglion cell loss follow axotomy in the optic nerve of adult rats. Journal of Neurobiology 24:23-36.

Weber EB, Stelzner DJ (1977) Behavioral effects of spinal cord transection in the developing rat. Brain Research 125:241-255.

Webster DM, Rogers LJ, Pettigrew JD, Steeves JD (1990) Origins of descending spinal pathways in prehensile birds: do parrots have a homologue to the corticospinal tract of mammals? Brain, Behavior & Evolution 36:216-226.

Webster DM, Steeves JD (1991) Funicular organization of avian brainstem-spinal projections. Journal of Comparative Neurology 312:467-476.

Windle WF. 1955. *Regeneration in the Central Nervous System.* Charles C. Thomas Publishers, Springfield.

Wizenmann A, Thies E, Klostermann S, Bonhoeffer F, Bahr M (1993) Appearance of target-specific guidance information for regenerating axons after CNS lesions. Neuron 11:975-983.

Wong JT, Yu WT, O'Connor TP (1997) Transmembrane grasshopper Semaphorin I promotes axon outgrowth in vivo. Development 124:3597-3607.

Wu W, Han K, Li L, Schinco FP (1994) Implantation of PNS graft inhibits the induction of neuronal nitric oxide synthase and enhances the survival of spinal motoneurons following root avulsion. Experimental Neurology 129:335-339.

Xu XM, Martin GF (1991) Evidence for new growth and regeneration of cut axons in developmental plasticity of the rubrospinal tract in the North American Opossum. Journal of Comparative Neurology 313:103-112.

6

Intrinsic Control of Regeneration and the Loss of Regenerative Ability in Development

James W. Fawcett
Cambridge University, Cambridge, England

I. INTRODUCTION

Adult mammalian CNS axons generally do not regenerate when cut. However, regeneration in the mammalian PNS occurs rapidly, even amongst motor neurons which have their cell bodies in the CNS, and these axons can reconnect to appropriate targets and restore function. The immature mammalian CNS also has considerable powers of axon regeneration, and most CNS axons will regenerate if cut early enough in development. In the rodent spinal cord, for instance, the corticospinal tract and other descending tracts will regenerate up to several days after birth, particularly if a graft is inserted into the injury site to provide a bridge to allow the axons to cross the site of injury and get to the host cord beyond the lesion (Kalil, Reh, 1982; Bregman et al., 1993). After approximately 7 days postnatally, spinal cord and other CNS lesions result in very limited or absent axon regeneration. What is the reason for loss of CNS regeneration in mammals? In principle the loss of regenerative ability during development could be due to changes in the neurons and axons themselves, which make them unable to respond to axotomy with a vigorous regenerative response, or it could be due to changes in the CNS environment which might develop the ability to block the axonal regenerative response. This chapter examines this question, and shows evidence that both axon and environment change with development in ways which result in blocking the regenerative response.

II. LOSS OF AXON REGENERATION - AXON OR ENVIRONMENT?

A. *In vivo* experiments suggest intrinsic neuronal limitations

If one wished to decide whether the major changes that limit regeneration are glial or neuronal in origin, how would one do it? There are two main types of *in vivo* experiment that can address this issue. The first type of experiment is age mismatch, in which an embryonic environment is apposed to elderly neurons or vice versa. The second type of experiment is to look for temporal correlations between changes in neurons and changes in the environment and see whether these always correlate with loss of regeneration, or whether there are instances when the usual correlations are absent, yet the behavior persists.

Many types of age mismatch experiments have been done in many parts of the CNS. In general these have involved grafting embryonic tissue into the adult CNS, because adult CNS tissue seldom survives transplantation, and grafting into embryos is technically difficult to achieve.

If adult neurons have lost some of their axonal growth potential relative to embryonic ones, it should be possible to see differences when both are placed in the same environment. Thus, embryonic neurons placed into the adult nervous system might be able to grow axons in an environment in which regeneration of adult axons fails. The results of such experiments obviously depend on many types of molecular interaction, some of which are discussed below, but the basic observation is that embryonic neurons grafted into the adult will often grow axons into the host CNS for a considerable distance. For example retina at a range of ages has been grafted into host brains in many positions. The results depend to some extent on the position into which the transplant is placed, but the overall result is that embryonic retina has a considerable ability to extend axons into the host brain and make connections, but this abilty declines with age (Hankin & Lund, 1992). Transplants of cortex, hippocampus, spinal cord and other parts of the CNS show similar results; axon outgrowth from transplants is greatest when the tissue is taken at a particular age, and then declines with increasing age. The region of the nervous system that has probably been transplanted the most is the substantia nigra, because of its relevance to Parkinson's disease. Transplants of embryonic substantia nigra placed in the striatum, which is the normal target area for the nigral dopaminergic neurons, will grow axons into the host brain in a halo of connections stretching for several millimeters around the transplant, and these axons will form functional synaptic connections with appropriate host neurons. However, this only happens if the nigral transplant tissue is taken from a donor embryo of precisely the right age. In rats this is embryonic day 14 (E14), which is about midway through the period during which the nigral dopaminergic neurons are undergoing their final cell divisions (Brundin et al., 1988). The transplanted tissue therefore consists of a mixture of cells at different developmental stages. There are dopaminergic neurons that are postmitotic, starting to differentiate, and beginning to grow their axons. Also present are neuronal progenitor cells that have yet to become postmitotic. Following transplantation all the surviving dopaminergic neurons in the grafts are cells that were postmitotic before transplantation-none of the precursors differentiate into dopaminergic neurons (Sinclair et al., 1999). This places a limit on the earliest age at which this neuronal population can be transplanted, since transplants taken at a time when all the dopaminergic neurons are in the form of precursors will generate no dopaminergic neurons after transplantation. However there is also a late limit, because cells that are transplanted after embryonic day 18 will survive very poorly, and those few cells that survive transplantation will not grow axons into the host CNS (Bjorklund, 1992) There is therefore a very narrow time window for dopaminergic neurons, and the same applies to other neuronal types, during which transplanted neurons will grow axons into and innervate an adult host CNS. This time corresponds to the time when a particular neuronal type has just undergone its final cell division, and is growing its axon to its target. At this time it is reasonable to assume that the neuron must be expressing a genetic program that is appropriate for growing axons to a target.

If the time over which neurons are expressing this axon growth genetic program could be prolonged would axons be able to grow further into an adult host CNS? This question has not been addressed explicitly, but it is likely that experiments in which human embryonic CNS tissue is implanted into a rodent host are relevant to this issue. The reason is that human embryonic development is much slower than that of rodents, and the period during which axons are growing from many types of neuron is therefore more prolonged. In the nigral dopaminergic system grafts of human embryonic ventral mesencephalon, removed at the time when the dopaminergic neurons are about halfway through their period of development, have been grafted into rat hosts. When rat ventral mesencephalic transplants are placed orthotopically in the lesioned substantia nigra they grow axons for very limited distances of less that a hundred microns. However, human ventral mesencephalic transplants will grow axons for distances of a centimetre or more, with processes being seen throughout the host forebrain, and even extending down towards the spinal cord. Growth is not completely random, since there is preferential innervation of structures that would normally receive dopaminergic innervation (Wictorin et al., 1992). Similar experiments with other transplants of human CNS tissue have produced similar results.

The probable interpretation of these various results is that at the time when they have just undergone their final cell division and started to grow an axon, neurons express a genetic program that is appropriate to growing axons for considerable distances through CNS tissue. The ability to grow axons through CNS tissue is lost with increasing developmental age in most neuronal types, so it is reasonable to assume that this genetic program is not reactivated in its entirety following axonal damage, and this is therefore probably a reason for the lack of an effective regenerative response in injured adult CNS axons.

However, one experiment which may provide a counter example to the conclusion that adult neurons are unable to mount an effective regenerative response is one in which adult sensory neurons have been implanted into adult rat white matter. Provided this is done with minimal local trauma, these neurons are able to regenerate their axons for long distances through this environment (Davies et al., 1997). However, it may be relevant that these are neurons that are from outside the CNS that are able to mount a vigorous regenerative response to axotomy in peripheral nerves. Also, these neurons continue to express in adulthood some growth associated genes that are turned off in most CNS neurons (see below).

The other main type of experiment which addresses the issue of whether the cessation of axon growth in mammalian CNS is environmental or neuronal in origin comes from examining correlations between the time when regeneration ceases in particular pathways and the events going on in the glial environment. Axon regeneration in the CNS of mammalian and avian embryos is well documented, and in most of these animals, regeneration ceases at roughly the same time in all the axonal tracts throughout the CNS. This time correlates with the onset of myelination and various changes in astrocytes, changes in proteoglycan expression, adhesion molecule expression and many other things. It is therefore difficult to disentangle neuronal and environmental influences. However, loss of regenerative ability and glial maturation are not nearly so closely correlated in marsupials. Marsupials tend to be born at a relatively immature stage and hence much of their CNS development is postnatal. Both retinal and spinal neurons are capable of regeneration in these immature systems. Regenerating axons in immature marsupials have the ability to renavigate through the CNS in order to reach their correct targets and make accurate connections; behavioral assessments show that these regenerated axons can restore normal function. However, for each type of axon there is a so called critical period: before that time axon regeneration occurs rapidly and accurately; after that period and on into adulthood, neurons that are axotomised do not regenerate. What happens to end this regenerative critical period? Changes in the glial environment cannot be the only answer, because the end of the critical period differs for different pathways, and this does not always correlate with the glial changes that happen at the same time as regeneration ceases in eutherian mammals. Two examples are seen in the visual system and in the spinal cord. In the axons of retinal ganglion cells regeneration ceases in the opossum by day 14, two weeks before the first evidence of the onset of myelination and the other associated glial changes (Maclaren, Taylor, 1997; Maclaren, Taylor, 1995; Maclaren, 1996). The downregulation of regenerative ability is seen in all parts of the optic pathway, including the nonmyelinated part of the axonal pathway in the retina. The onset of the critical period has been examined in various axonal projections in the spinal cord. Some of these pathways cease to regenerate at much the same time, and this correlates with the onset of myelination, but other tracts lose their regenerative ability much earlier. The last tracts to lose their regenerative ability are the descending pathways from the red nucleus and the raphe and reticular nuclei, but the descending projections from the other supraspinal nuclei lose their ability to regrow after axotomy earlier (Wang et al., 1998). However, despite this apparent lack of correlation between critical period and glial maturation there is evidence that myelin-related molecules may be involved in the inhibition of axon regeneration in the marsupial CNS. Nicholls and his collaborators have developed a method for keeping the CNS of newborn marsupials alive in culture long enough for them to go through their critical period. Application of the IN-1 antibody, which blocks the inhibitory effects of the myelin inhibitory molecule NI-250 allows some regeneration of descending axons in the cord after the normal critical period (Varga et al., 1995). There is no completely consistent universal change that has yet been demonstrated in the glial response to injury which correlates with the time of the critical period in marsupials. In the retina the Muller glial cells do show a reaction to injury, but this does not appear to alter at the end of the critical period nor result in production of proteoglycans or an obviously inhibitory scar. Nor is the immediate microglial response different before and after the critical period (Maclaren, Taylor, 1995; Maclaren, 1996). The conclusion of these experiments must be that in both spinal cord and retina there is some change in the intrinsic response of neurons to axotomy that is independent of glial maturation and the glial response to injury, and which greatly decreases the regenerative response of the axons after the critical period.

While the experiments above show clearly that there must be intrinsic neuronal changes that affect the regenerative response of cut axons, there are of course also major changes in the CNS environment that lead to the presence of a large number of inhibitory molecules in regions of CNS damage. These include the myelin-related molecules NI-250, MAG and tenascin-R, inhibitory molecules made by astrocytes which are predominantly the proteoglycans neurocan, phosphacan and brevican, and the inhibitory proteoglycan NG2 which is made by oligodendrocyte precursors. These changes are discussed below and in greater detail in subsequent chapters in this volume.

B. *In vitro* experiments support intrinsic neuronal limitations

Apart from the *in vivo* experiments discussed above, the other major tool for examining the developmental changes that affect axon regeneration are *in vitro* experiments. These give the opportunity of matching adult or embryonic neurons with various environments. The simplest type of experiment is to match neurons with environments that consist of a single type of molecule. A laminin substratum provides a surface over which almost all axonal types will grow to some extent. Thus neurons derived from the embryonic nervous system will almost without exception grow axons profusely on laminin surfaces. Do adult neurons have the same ability? This question is harder to answer, because rather few types of adult neuron can be maintained alive in tissue culture. Of those whose properties have been studied, dorsal root ganglion neurons provide an example of an adult cell which will grow axons robustly *in vitro* (Lindsay, 1988). However, these neurons are able to mount a vigorous regenerative response in adulthood *in vivo* after peripheral nerve damage, and continue to express various growth associated genes into adulthood. One major CNS neuronal type that will survive in culture and has some ability to grow axons is the retinal ganglion cell. As with most embryonic neuronal types, embryonic retinal ganglion cells, whether in explants or as dissociated cells, grow their axons profusely on a variety of surfaces including laminin (Cohen et al., 1986). Adult retinal ganglion cells have been studied mostly in explant cultures, in which a small square of retina about 0.5mm across is placed on the culture surface. These explants will grow axons over a laminin substratum, but the axons are rather few in number, thin, and slow growing . There is an enormous difference in the overall vigour of growth between embyonic and adult retinal explants. Single dissociated retinal ganglion cells behave similarly (Ford-Holevinski et al., 1986; Johnson et al., 1988; Wigley, Berry, 1988; Meyer, Miotke, 1990).

More lifelike experiments *in vitro* involve combining neurons with various types of CNS glial cell or CNS tissue. Most of the main CNS inhibitory molecules are made either by oligodendrocytes or by astrocytes. In both cases there is a developmental change in the ability of neurons to grow their axons in association with these cell types. Astrocytes produce as their main inhibitory molecules a variety of proteoglycans, of which the major types are neurocan, phosphacan and brevican (see below) (Margolis et al., 1996; Snyder et al., 1996; Yamada et al., 1997, Asher et al. 1998). These molecules are soluble and not attached to the cell surface, so they float away into the medium from monolayers of astrocytes, which therefore provide a poor assay for most of the astrocyte inhibitory molecules. However three dimensional astrocyte cultures do not suffer from this problem, since the soluble proteoglycans are trapped in the intercellular spaces, and these cultures are inhibitory to the growth of many types of regenerating axon (Fawcett et al., 1989). Adult retina and postnatal dorsal root ganglion axons regenerate very poorly through these astrocyte tissues. However, their embryonic equivalents are not so inhibited, and embryonic dorsal root ganglion and retinal axons will grow profusely through three-dimensional astrocyte cultures. In the case of oligodendrocytes many axonal types will not grow over oligodendrocytes, due to the presence of NI-250, MAG, tenascin-R and other molecules (Schwab et al., 1993; McKerracher et al., 1994; Tang et al., 1997; Pesheva et al., 1993; Becker et al., 1999). The behavior when axon meets glial cell is that the axonal growth cone undergoes a collapse and withdrawal reaction, mediated by G-protein linked calcium release from internal calcium stores within the axon (Fawcett et al., 1989; Bandtlow et al., 1990; Bandtlow et al., 1993). Again, there is a difference in the response of embryonic and older neurons to oligodendrocytes, with those embryonic neuronal types that have been tested showing little or no growth cone collapse when the axon meets a mature oligodendrocyte. Similarly embryonic sensory neurons from dorsal root ganglia show growth on cryostat sections through the adult dorsal root entry zone, whereas older neurons do not (Shewan et al., 1995). This critical influence of neuronal age has also been explored in two organ co-culture systems. Entorhinal cortex projects to hippocampus, and entorhinal explants will also grow axons into hippocampal explants in co-cultures. However,

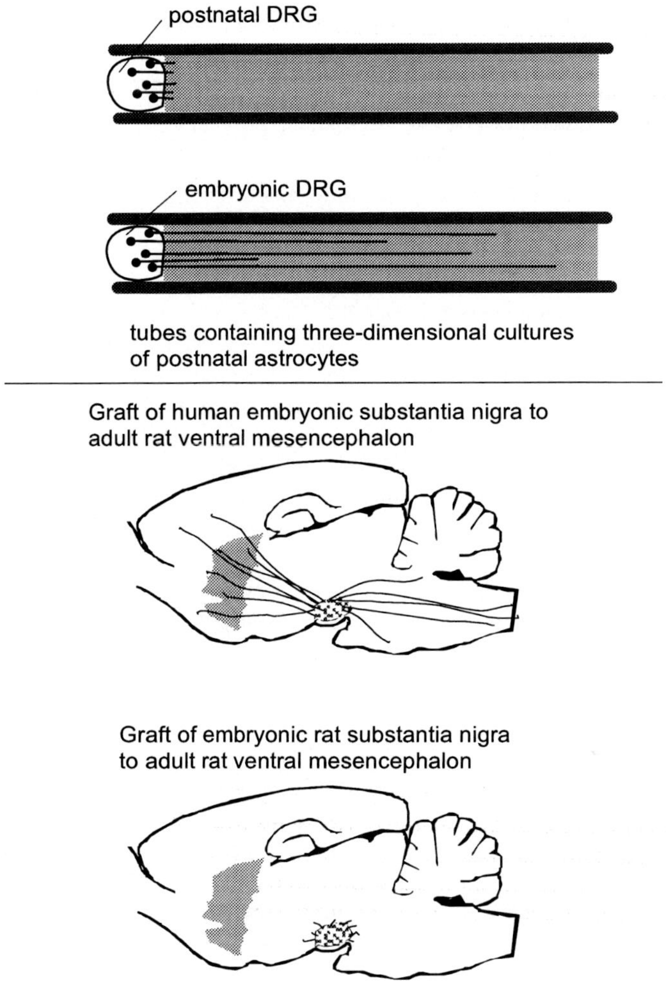

Figure 1 Two examples of intrinsic neuronal control of regeneration. The upper diagram illustrates experiments from Fawcett et al. 1989. Axons regenerating from a postnatal sensory ganglion are unable to penetrate a three-dimensional tissue of astrocytes. However axons from embryonic sensory ganglia can grow through this tissue. The lower diagram illustrates the experiments of Wictorin et al. 1992. Grafts of embyronic rat ventral mesencephalon placed orthtopically in the adult brain grow axons for very small distances. However human embryonic neurons are able to grow their axons much further.

the determinant of whether the axons grow is the age of the entorhinal explant. The age of the target hippocampal tissue makes no difference. Similarly, in co-cultures of retina and superior colliculus the extent of retinal axon growth is largely the age of the retina, not the age of the target tissue (Li et al., 1995; Chen et al., 1997). Illustrations of possible mechanisms of intrinsic neuronal control of regeneration are shown in Fig. 1and discussed further below.

III. THE GLIAL ENVIRONMENT CHANGES WITH DEVELOPMENT

A large number of experiments show that the environment of the damaged adult CNS is inhibitory to axon growth. However, axon growth clearly occurs in the embryonic nervous system, and axons continue to grow in the mammalian CNS up to the perinatal period. Is the loss of the ability of axons to grow in the CNS simply because the axons themselves become less vigorous in their growth, as described above, or is there a change in the permissiveness of the CNS environment? Again, the way to answer this question comes from time mismatch experiments, in which different ages of axons are matched against different ages of glial environment. In order to answer the question "is the embryonic glial environment more permissive to axon growth than the adult environment?" it is necessary to look at the ability of adult CNS axons to regenerate into embryonic tissue. This can be achieved by transplanting embryonic CNS tissue into the adult CNS. This has been done with many different CNS regions, with the overall conclusion that many types of adult CNS axons will regenerate into embryonic grafts. However, there have been few systematic studies into the effects of graft age, mainly because the time window for successful grafting of embryonic tissue is very narrow. Embryonic grafts to the cerebellum demonstrate the basic principle that host axons will regenerate into embryonic environments. However, they also reveal another important principle, because some axons, the climbing fibers from the inferior olive, will regenerate into the grafts, but Purkinje cell axons show no regenerative response: different neurons in the adult CNS show different levels of regenerative response (Rossi et al., 1995).

IV. CNS NEURONS DIFFER IN THE VIGOUR OF THEIR REGENERATIVE RESPONSE

The above example shows that when the axons of Purkinje cells and the climbing fibers are cut, and both are presented with the same permissive environment in the shape of embryonic CNS tissue, only the climbing fibers will regenerate. The same is found when Schwann cells are placed around the cut ends of the axons instead of embryonic CNS tissue; climbing fibers grow into the graft, Purkinje cell axons do not (Bravin et al., 1997). This type of phenomenon is not restricted to the cerebellum; there are other parts of the CNS where transplants of permissive tissue attract regenerating axons from some neuronal types, few from others. Peripheral nerve grafts placed in the thalamus, for instance, attract large numbers of axons from the thalamic reticular nucleus, but few axons from other neuronal types. Grafts of permissive tissue placed in the striatum attract many dopaminergic axons from the substantia nigra, but fewer from other neurons (Morrow et al., 1993;

Woolhead et al., 1998). These results show that different CNS axons differ in the vigour of their regenerative response to axotomy. The regenerative response can differ even within different branches of the same axon. This is demonstrated by the response to axotomy of the central and peripheral branches of sensory neurons. Sensory neurons have two axonal branches, one passing peripherally to form sensory endings in the skin and muscles, one passing via the dorsal root into the spinal cord to terminate on neurons in the dorsal horn or sensory nuclei. When the peripheral branch is damaged there is a vigorous regenerative response, which can lead to the regeneration of axons back to their target areas. However, when the central branch is damaged in the dorsal root the regenerative response is much less. Thus, if a peripheral nerve graft is attached to the peripheral branch, many axons regenerate into it. If a graft is placed on the dorsal root, rather few axons grow into it. However, damage to the peripheral branch of the axon increases the regenerative vigour of the central branch, such that it will now regenerate many axons into nerve grafts attached to the dorsal root (Chong et al., 1994; Chong et al., 1996). The practical conclusion of these findings is that if one wishes to induce regeneration of CNS axons in order to repair lesions, it is not sufficient just to make the environment permissive. Positive steps are necessary to induce regeneration of some types of axon.

V. THE REGENERATIVE RESPONSE IS DEPENDENT ON THE POSITION OF AXOTOMY

In the seminal experiments from the Aguayo laboratory in which peripheral nerve segments grafted to the spinal cord were shown to induce regeneration of CNS axons, it was noted that only neurons close to the insertion point of the grafts had regenerated their axons into them (David and Aguayo, 1981). In further experiments it turned out to be rare to see regeneration of axons from long tracts that had been cut far from their cell body, but common to see regeneration of axons cut close to their cell body. As described in more detail elsewhere in this volume, it is now apparent that this is a general principle. In the CNS the regenerative response of axons depends on where they are cut, with axons cut close to the soma usually showing a prompt and vigorous regenerative response, while axotomy further from the soma results in little or no regeneration even into the most permissive environments. This is in contrast to axons in peripheral nerves, which show a strong regenerative response wherever they are cut, even if the axons originated in the CNS from motor neurons.

VI. POSSIBLE MECHANISMS FOR THE REGULATION OF THE REGENERATIVE RESPONSE OF CNS AXONS

The three factors identified above that govern the neuronal regenerative response to axotomy are neuronal age, neuronal type, and position of axotomy. What might be the mechanism behind these differences? In order to find a way of identifying possible molecules the three obvious strategies are: 1) to look for molecules that are upregulated in neurons that can regenerate successfully but not in those that fail, 2) to look for differences between molecules expressed in regenerating axons and axons growing during devopment, and 3) to look for molecules that are upregulated when axons are damaged close to the cell body but not upregulated when the axon is damaged further away. If a molecule fits all these criteria, and if there is a biologically plausible mechanism by which it might affect axon growth then it is likely to be important in the regulation of the axonal regenerative response. Several molecules and mechanisms have been identified that are candidates. These can be divided, somewhat artificially, into molecules on the cell surface which directly mediate interactions with molecules in the environment, and molecules inside axons that affect the processes of growth cone advance and axon building.

A. GAP-43 and c-jun

GAP-43 is found on the inside of the growth cone membrane. Its role is not completely defined, but it plays a part in modulating the effect of cell surface molecules, such as adhesion molecules, on axon growth. It is a major target for phosphorylation in the growth cone, particularly by PKC which is present in large amounts in the growth cone, and phosphorylation or dephosphorylation probably modulates its action and affects cytoskeletal dynamics such as actin polymerization. Other GAP-43 like molecules such as CAP-23 exist, and may have similar functions (Caroni, 1997; Wiederkehr et al., 1997; Benowitz, Routtenberg, 1997; Meiri et al., 1998). GAP-43 fits most of the criteria set out above, because it is present during embryonic axon growth, reduced in most neurons in adultood, yet upregulated massively in succesfully regenerating axons. As far as we are aware no axon has been shown to regenerate for significant distances in the absence of GAP-43 expression. A crucial event in regeneration must therefore be the re-expression of this and associated proteins. There is a close correlation between GAP-43 expression and the regenerative efforts of axons. Thus, in several CNS neuronal types, particularly retinal ganglion cells and rubrospinal neurons it has been shown that there is strong upregulation of GAP-43 expression when axons are cut close to the cell body causing a vigorous regenerative response, but an absent or weaker response when the cut is more distal and there is little regeneration. On the other hand sensory and motor axons, which regenerate wherever they are cut, upregulate GAP-43 equally well after proximal or distal lesions (Doster et al., 1991; Tetzlaff et al., 1994; Kobayashi et al., 1997). In sensory neurons, whose central branch regenerates less well than the peripheral one, it has been found that crushing the peripheral branch leads to GAP-43 upregulation, while crushing the central branch leads to little or no upregulation. Moreover crushing the peripheral branch in order to induce GAP-43, increases subsequent regeneration of axons by the central branch into a nerve graft (Chong et al., 1996). It appears that there is an intrinsic response to axotomy which stimulates the axogenic response, and GAP-43 expression certainly correlates with this regenerative response as does c-jun expression. However possession of GAP-43 does not in itself guarantee that a neuron will regenerate its axon. Cerebellar Purkinje cells do not reexpress GAP-43 when their axons are cut, and those axons will not regenerate. However, when GAP-43 expression was targetted to these neurons in transgenic animals they were still not able to regenerate, although there was an increase in sprouting (Buffo et al., 1997). However GAP-43 overexpression does cause an increase in terminal growth at the neuromuscular junction and in the hippocampus (Aigner et al., 1995).

It is unlikely that GAP-43 is upregulated alone, and there is probably a group of genes whose expression changes at the same time, which may exert a joint effect on regenerative potential. Immediate early genes may be important in regulating this neuronal response to axotomy. C-jun in particular is upregulated after axotomy of peripheral and other axons and stays up until regenerating axons reach their targets.

B. Cytoskeletal proteins

Most of the patterns of expression of cytoskeletal genes that are seen during axonogenesis in embryos are recapitulated in regeneration. For instance one tubulin isoform, Talpha1 is expressed during axogenesis in embryos, and is re-expressed during axon regeneration (Miller et al., 1989). However this is not the case for the microtubule-associated proteins (MAPs). Axonal MAPs change during development, with the replacement in most CNS axons of MAP1b with MAP1a, with a change in the form of MAP2, and in the peripheral nervous system, tau changes to a large molecular weight form. These changes are not reversed in regeneration, which therefore occurs with a different complement of MAPs to initial development (Fawcett et al., 1994; Nothias et al., 1995). Transgenic knockout experiments have shown that to some extent MAPs are able to substitute for one another's function, but with some functional loss, so MAP1a in regenerating axons may not be fully replacing the function of the MAP1b that is present during development, and it is possible that the combination of MAPs present in regenerating growth cones is suboptimal for axon growth. MAP function is also modulated by complicated patterns of phosphorylation, some developmentally regulated, these phosphorylation patterns may recur in regeneration. However, adult neurons may in principle be capable of re-expressing embryonic MAPs as is shown by the upregulation of MAP1b in retinal axons regenerating *in vitro* (although they still continue to contain MAP1a). The intermediate filaments neurofilament and peripherin also do not revert to embryonic type during regeneration (Bates, Meyer, 1993; Bates et al., 1993).

C. Adhesion and other cell surface molecules

In order to subserve axon extension and to enable responses to guidance cues, axons must have the correct complement of cell surface molecules. Again there is clear evidence for a recapitulation of part of the developmental program, but other important molecules differ between development and regeneration. In regenerating peripheral nerve, integrins and several cell adhesion molecules are re-expressed during nerve regeneration. In regenerating axons in general at least some of the molecules needed for axonal guidance must be present since regenerating axons are able to respond to some guidance cues. For instance, adult retinal axons regenerating *in vitro* respond appropriately to axon guidance cues (Maclaren, Taylor, 1997; Bähr, Wizenmann, 1996; Wizenmann, Bähr, 1997). However, there are many significant differences in cell surface molecules between development and regeneration. One example is the splice variant of N-CAM found on adult neurons. This contains the exon VASE which is not found in embryogenesis. Expression of this molecule, or exogenous application of VASE peptide inhibits the axon growth response to N-CAM, possibly through interference with CAM signaling through the FGF receptor and may therefore be an intrinsic property that impedes regeneration (Doherty et al., 1992). There are also subtle changes in the adhesion molecules responsible for interaction with the extracellular matrix. There are developmental changes in retinal ganglion cell responses to laminin with age, but both embryonic and adult rodent ganglion cells will grow axons on laminin substrata. However, while growth from embryonic retina is β1 integrin dependent and embryonic axons are heavily stained by β1 integrin antibodies, growth from adult retina is not inhibited by β1 integrin antibodies, and there is little β1 on the axons (Bates, Meyer, 1997). Even in goldfish, in which CNS axons readily regenerate back to their correct targets (this volume, chapters by Stuermer and Leppert and and Benowitz, et al.,), several axonal cell surface molecules differ between initial outgrowth and regeneration.

D. Interactions with inhibitory molecules

Axons from embryonic neurons are able to grow over oligodendrocytes and through three-dimensional astrocyte cultures, both of which have inhibitory properties for regenerating axons. In order to do so the axons must lack receptors for the inhibitory molecules, or they must disregard the signals from them, or they must degrade the inhibitory molecules in their path. In the case of growth over oligodendrocytes there is evidence that either the receptors or the signaling pathways in the neuron differ between embryonic and postnatal periods. On exposure to myelin, there is a prolonged rise in calcium in the growth cones of postnatal sensory axons, and this calcium peak is involved in the ensuing growth cone collapse. However, in embryonic axons, which do not suffer growth cone collapse on exposure to myelin, the calcium peak is much smaller and shorter (Schwab et al., 1999). The main inhibitory molecules produced by astrocytes are proteoglycans, and it is probable that they exert their effects by blocking the growth promoting effects of laminin and possibly other extracellular matrix molecules. Why embryonic axons should be able to overcome these effects is not clear. It may be that they have different receptors for growth permissive matrix molecules, or it may be that they are able to produce proteases which can degrade the inhibitory proteoglycans and thereby increase the availability of permissive molecules. Inhibitory proteoglycans are certainly sensitive to proteolysis, and degrading them can make the growth environment more permissive (Zuo et al., 1998; Muir et al., 1998).

E. Bcl-2

The proto-oncogene Bcl-2 may play a key role in controlling the switching from the embryonic growth program to the adult pattern. Bcl-2 has been shown to play at least two roles in the regenerative response. It is a protective agent that counters the effects of neurotrophin withdrawal both during normal development and following axotomy (Takahashi et al., 1999). In the visual system, the loss of its expression coincides temporally with the end of the neonatal critical period for regeneration in mice. Furthermore overexpression of Bcl-2, in addition to protecting axotomised retinal ganglion cells from apoptosis, has been shown to prolong the time during which retinal ganglion cells can mount an effective regenerative response (Chen et al., 1995). Ideally, to achieve the maximal regeneration there needs to be a way to exploit the delicate balance between an apoptotic and regenerative response and BCl-2 over-expression may provide this.

VII. FACTORS IN THE ENVIRONMENT AFFECT REGENERATION

Inhibitory molecules have been identified on most types of glial cell. In some cases it is known that these are absent in the embryonic nervous system.

A. Molecules on oligodendrocytes

Since oligodendrocytes only appear perinatally in most parts of the CNS, by definition any inhibitory molecules on their surface must be absent during initial axon growth. In most regions of the CNS the time of myelination corresponds closely to the cessation of axon regeneration, although, as described above, not in all the tracts of the marsupial CNS. The major oligodendrocyte inhibitory molecules NI-250, MAG and tenascin-R have been described elsewhere in this volume (Schwab et al., 1993; McKerracher et al., 1994; Tang et al., 1997; Pesheva et al., 1993, Becker et al. 1999). A recent finding may provide insight into why some adult neurons have greater regenerative responses than others. One extreme in this respect is the Purkinje cell, which shows no regenerative response either in terms of axon sprouting or in terms of upregulating growth associated proteins after axotomy, even when presented with a permissive environment. The antibody IN-1 blocks the inhibitory effects of the myelin molecule NI-250. When this antibody was applied to the lesioned cerebellum there was an upregulation within Purkinje cells of two growth associated proteins, c-jun and CAP-23 (Zagrebelsky et al., 1998). The suggestion from this observation is that myelin inhibitory molecules might play a role in downregulating the regenerative responses of CNS axons, and that some neurons might be more affected by these molecules than others.

B. Molecules on astrocytes

The astrocytic response to CNS injury changes at roughly the same time as axon regeneration ceases, although in some pathways in marsupials this correlation does not hold completely. Before about 10 days of age, injury to the CNS produces little astrocyte response as assessed by changes in astrocyte morphology, increases in production of the astrocyte intermediate filament molecules GFAP and vimentin, and increases in production of proteoglycan glycosaminglycans. However, after that time any CNS injury results in astrocytic proliferation and massive upregulation of these factors (Smith et al., 1986; Allcutt et al., 1984). Astrocytes produce molecules inhibitory to axon growth, and most of these are proteoglycans. Astrocytes in CNS lesions produce several inhibitory proteoglycans, particularly phosphacan, brevican, neurocan and NG2 (Snyder et al., 1996; Plant et al., 1998; Grill et al., 1998, Asher et al. 1998). Any discussion on what makes them inhibitory is complicated by the fact that the inhibitory properties of at least some of them are modulated by the amount of glycosaminoglycan chain attached to the protein core, and by the extent of its sulphation (Smith-Thomas et al., 1994; Smith-Thomas et al., 1995). Inhibitory proteoglycans also have several modes of action, with direct interactions with adhesion molecules via the protein core, and rather less specific interactions with other matrix molecules. Some of these inhibitory interactions are affected by removal of glycosaminoglycan chains or inhibition of sulphation, while others are not. Neurocan and phosphacan are present in the embryonic CNS, but the degree to which they are inhibitory is not clear (Sakurai et al., 1996; Snyder et al., 1996; Engel et al., 1996; Sakurai et al., 1996; Asher et al., 1998). Brevican is upregulated after birth, as is NG2, which is found mainly on oligodendrocyte precursors (see below). While the position as regards specific proteoglycans is not clear, the general proteoglycan response to injury changes shortly after birth. In the newborn, CNS injury causes little change in immunostaining with antibodies that detect the glycosaminoglycan part of proteoglycans, while later there is a large increase in staining around any CNS lesion. Astrocytes removed from the injured CNS on pieces of filter material grafted into the brain are inhibitory to axon regeneration if taken later than 10 days after birth, and much of this inhibition can be removed by enzymatic removal of the glycosaminoglycan chains, but astrocytes removed earlier do not have inhibitory proteoglycans (McKeon et al., 1991; McKeon et al., 1995). These various pieces of evidence together suggest that the cessation of axon regeneration corresponds with the time when astrocytes develop the ability to produce inhibitory proteoglycans and to add to them sulphated glycosaminoglycan chains. These molecules are presumably upregulated by cytokines released at the injury site (Asher et al., 1998).

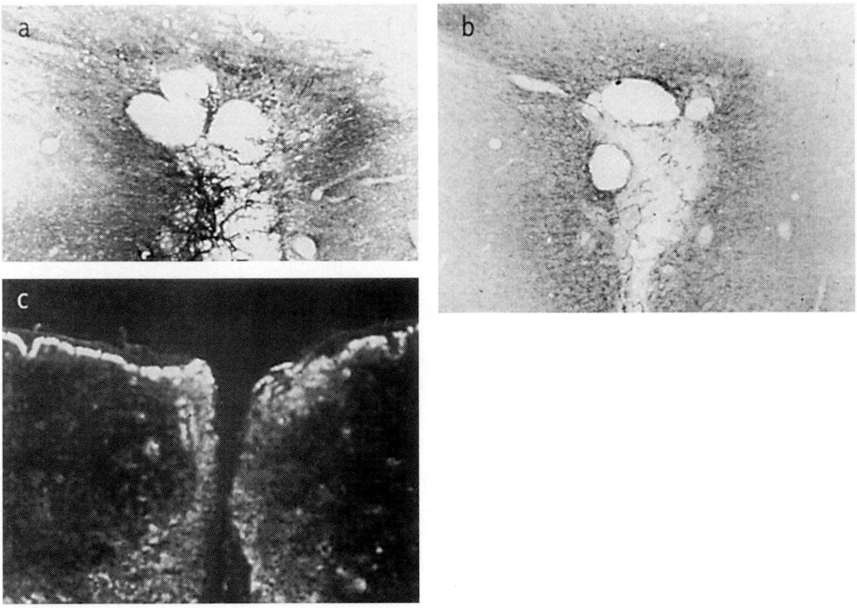

Figure 2 Expression of proteoglycans in CNS injuries. A) shows a lesion of the nigrostriatal tract, stained with the antibody CS56 which binds to the glycosaminoglycan chains of chondroitin sulphate proteoglycans. B) shows a similar lesion, stained with an antibody to the NG2 proteoglycan, showing the many small oligodendrocyte precursors that collect around CNS injuries. C) shows a cortical stab wound stained with an antibody to neurocan, showing local upregulation in the edges of the injury.

C. Oligodendrocyte precursors

Oligodendrocyte precursors first appear in the CNS around the time when axon growth is approaching completion, and then increase greatly in number during the period of myelination in the perinatal period. Adult oligodendrocyte precursors are present throughout the normal adult CNS. All forms of CNS injury result in a rapid and massive recruitment of these cells to the site of injury within a few days. The recruitment of oligodendrocyte precursors to CNS injury therefore, corresponds fairly precisely to the cessation of axon regeneration in the CNS. The significance of this is that these cells express the proteoglycan NG2, which is very inhibitory to axon growth, and that NG2 immunostaining of the cells increases greatly in CNS injuries (Levine, 1994; Dou, Levine, 1994; Levine, Nishiyama, 1996).

D. Meningeal cells

Any CNS injury that penetrates the meninges results in the migration of meningeal cells into the wound cavity, and these cells participate in the formation of a new glia limitans within the injury. In injuries of the spinal cord, where there is often much menigeal damage, there may be large numbers of meningeal cells within the glial scar that forms. Meningeal cells stimulate astrocytes to increase their production of matrix molecules including proteoglycans, and meningeal cells themselves produce the inhibitory proteoglycan NG2 and other protoglycans. These cells may therefore be responsible for some of the inhibition in CNS injuries, but it is not known how this might vary with development (Abnet et al., 1991; Levine, Nishiyama, 1996; Ness, David, 1997).

E. Neurotrophins and neurotrophin receptors

A crucial factor in determining the regenerative response may be the expression of neurotrophin receptors on the neuronal surface, and the availability of neurotrophins in the environment. Where there is a match there may be a regenerative response to axotomy but otherwise the response may be apoptosis. The requirement for specific neurotrophins is determined by the receptor array expressed by the particular neurons, and this not only differs between different neuron types, but also changes over time. The role of neurotrophins in the regenerative response can perhaps best be considered in the visual system and appears to be a critical balance between the enactment of the apoptotic or regenerative response. Retinal ganglion cells express the trk-B receptor and are known to be sensitive to BDNF from the time that they innervate their target cells in the superior colliculus and lateral geniculate, which are in turn known to express BDNF. If the retinal axons are severed it is assumed that there is a loss of the target derived neurotrophin and that most (90%) of the cells undergo apoptosis. Lesions close to the soma produce a rapid apoptotic response, whereas if a long length of axon is left intact, the response is slower. For RGCs application of BDNF directly to the vitreous provides sufficient trophic support to rescue cells from apoptosis (Klöcker et al., 1998) and therefore would allow for a regenerative response. Such a response has been shown after injections of BDNF and NT4/5 into the eye, following which there is extensive growth of axons in the retina itself, although these axons are unable to penetrate the astrocytic plug of the optic disc (Sawai et al., 1996). However, extensive regeneration of retinal ganglion cell axons in the retina and in the optic nerve has been seen after grafting lengths of peripheral nerve into the anterior chamber of the eye (Berry et al., 1996; Lau et al., 1994). These presumably secrete a variety of neurotrophic molecules, increasing the regenerative response of the ganglion cells and allowing their axons to overcome the inhibitory terrain of the crushed optic nerve. In the rubro-spinal pathway neurotrophins have also been shown to modulate the regenerative response. Normally rubro-spinal neurons upregulate GAP-43 and will regenerate into peripheral nerve grafts if axotomized close to the cell body, but not if lesioned more distally. However, application of the neurotrophins CNTF or BDNF to the cell bodies can enable GAP-43 expression and regeneration following distal lesions, as well as partially reversing neuronal atrophy (Kobayashi et al., 1997). The expression of neurotrophins in the environment surrounding axons can also greatly increase their ability to regenerate. Thus grafts of fibroblasts secreting NGF or NT-3 can attract regenerating axons, and injection of neurotrophins into the spinal cord can allow regenerating axons to cross the boundary from Schwann cell grafts back into CNS tissue. Grafts of fibroblasts secreting BDNF can elicit regenerative growth by rubrospinal axons through and adjacent to the graft and caudally in the lateral funniculus for distances up to 10 segments (Liu et al., 1999). All this suggests that there is a multifactorial response to axotomy, first preventing cell death and then initiating the appropriate gene transcription to promote axogenesis.

VIII. LESSONS FOR REPAIR IN THE CNS

If spinal cord injuries and other forms of CNS damage are to be repaired a first step has to be to induce axon regeneration. From the contents of this chapter and the other chapters in this volume it is clear that there is no single reason why axon regeneration fails in the adult CNS. Instead there are many reasons, some due to the poor regenerative response of adult CNS neurons, some due to the inhibitory nature of the damaged adult CNS. The combination of these factors leads to regenerative failure. In order to induce regeneration, therefore, there are many different ways in which one might intervene. The overall aim must be to alter the balance between the regenerative response of the axons and the permissiveness of the environment. In principle an axon with a very good regenerative response should be able to grow through even very inhibitory environments, while a highly permissive environment will induce regeneration of even very unwilling axons. In reality, it is unlikely that the regenerative response or the environment can be changed sufficiently to induce regeneration by themselves, so it will be necessary to combine several treatments. To increase the ability of axons to regrow, infusion of trophic factors and upregulation of the expression of growth-associated proteins and proteinases should be effective. To make the environment more permissive, it will be necessary to block inhibitory molecules on oligodendrocytes, and to take measures to degrade proteoglycans or prevent their upregulation in injuries. As detailed elsewhere in this book, several of these treatments by themselves have been partially successful.

IX. A DEVELOPMENTAL PERSPECTIVE

For the various reasons detailed above, and perhaps for other reasons we do not yet understand, mammals lose the ability to regenerate their axons shortly after birth. While we now understand many of the detailed mechanisms behind the loss of regenerative ability, it is possible that we have missed a fundamental change that underlies this. The reason for believing this is that regeneration is not lost just in the CNS in the perinatal period, regeneration is lost more or less at the same time in the entire body. Embryos are able to regenerate not just CNS axons, but also other body parts such as limbs. A similar switch is seen in evolution, with animals more primitive than frogs being able to regenerate CNS axons and other CNS parts, limbs, fins, tails and more. However, the ability to regenerate all these elements is lost at the same evolutionary point. Even in those amphibia which do not regenerate, premetamorphic larvae are regenerators but regeneration is lost with metamorphosis. From these considerations it is easy to argue that there might be a basic developmental switch that is thrown to turn off regeneration in the CNS and elsewhere at the end of mammalian development and that this same switch might have evolved in the frogs during evolution. However, this does not really fit with the detailed mechanisms outlined above, which do not seem to include a plausible mechanism for the inhibition of regeneration outside the CNS

Why should regeneration be turned off at the end of development, and why is it lost during evolution? In the absence of any firm data, there are various speculative hypotheses. 1) There is probably no evolutionary advantage in CNS regeneration, since regeneration takes a considerable amount of time, and by the time it is complete it is unlikely that the disabled animal will be alive. It is possible therefore that regeneration has been lost by accident as a result of being linked to a useful mutation that has nothing to do with regeneration. 2) It may be important in a complex brain to prevent excessive axonal sprouting and plasticity, and the inhibition of axon regeneration may be a result of the inhibitory milieu that has evolved for this purpose. 3) Inflammation, particularly the passage of large inflammatory cells such as neutrophils and macrophages, is probably very damaging to a complex tissue such as the CNS, and may result in derangement of the huge number of minute synaptic contacts. It is extremely difficult to induce a normal inflammatory response in the mammalian CNS, but many more macrophages appear in lower vertebrate CNS after damage. It may be that some of the inhibitory mechanisms may have evolved to exclude inflammatory cells.

X. FUTURE DIRECTIONS

Research into axonal regeneration in the CNS is entering a mature phase. We now know many of the inhibitory molecules in the environment of the damaged CNS, and we have methods for neutralizing some of them. We understand some of the ways in which the axons mount a regenerative response, and the signaling pathways behind them. Many of the pieces are therefore coming into place which will be needed for CNS repair. Research will therefore start to split into two main lines. One line will be the beginning of practical attempts to induce regeneration of CNS axons in animal models that are directly relevant to the treatment of human spinal cord injuries and other types of CNS trauma, and the first attempts at CNS repair in humans. The other line of research will be the continuation of investigation into the basic mechanisms of axon regeneration.

REFERENCES

Abnet K, Fawcett JW, Dunnett SB (1991) Interactions between meningeal cells and astrocytes in vivo and in vitro. Dev.Brain Res. 53:187-196.

Aigner L, Arber S, Kapfhammer JP, Laux T, Schneider C, Botteri F, Brenner HR, Caroni P (1995) Overexpression of the neural growth-associated protein GAP- 43 induces nerve sprouting in the adult nervous system of transgenic mice. Cell 83:269-278.

Allcutt D, Berry M, Sievers J (1984) A qualitative comparison of the reactions of retinal ganglion cell axons to optic nerve crush in neonatal and adult mice. Brain.Res. 318:231-240.

Asher RA, Fidler PS, Rogers JH, Fawcett JW (1998) TGFbeta stimulates neurocan synthesis in cultured rat astrocytes. Soc.Neurosci.Abstr. 24:56

Bandtlow C, Zachleder T, Schwab ME (1990) Oligodendrocytes arrest neurite growth by contact inhibition. J.Neurosci. 10:3837-3848.

Bandtlow CE, Schmidt MF, Hassinger TD, Schwab ME, Kater SB (1993) Role of intracellular calcium in NI-35-evoked collapse of neuronal growth cones. Science 259:80-83.

Bates CA, Meyer RL (1993) The heavy neurofilament protein is expressed in regenerating adult but not embryonic mammalian optic fibers *in vitro*. Exp.Neurol. 119:249-257.

Bates CA, Meyer RL (1997) The neurite-promoting effect of laminin is mediated by different mechanisms in embryonic and adult regenerating mouse optic axons in vitro. Developmental Biology 181:91-101.

Bates CA, Trinh N, Meyer RL (1993) Distribution of microtubule-associated proteins (MAPs) in adult and embryonic mouse retinal explants: Presence of the embryonic map, MAP5/1B, in regenerating adult retinal axons. Dev.Biol. 155:533-544.

Bähr M, Wizenmann A (1996) Retinal ganglion cell axons recognize specific guidance cues present in the deafferented adult rat superior colliculus. J.Neurosci. 16:5106-5116.

Becker CG, Becker T, Meyer RL, Schachner M (1999) Tenascin-R inhibits the growth of optic fibers *in vitro* but is rapidly eliminated during nerve regeneration in the salamander *Pleurodeles waltl* . Journal Of Neuroscience 19:813-827.

Benowitz LI, Routtenberg A (1997) GAP-43: An intrinsic determinant of neuronal development and plasticity. Trends Neurosci. 20:84-91.

Berry M, Carlile J, Hunter A (1996) Peripheral nerve explants grafted into the vitreous body of the eye promote the regeneration of retinal ganglion cell axons severed in the optic nerve. J.Neurocytol. 25:147-170.

Bjorklund A (1992) Dopaminergic transplants in experimental parkinsonism: cellular mechanisms of graft induced functional recovery. Curr.Opin.Neurobiol. 2:683-689.

Bravin M, Savio T, Strata P, Rossi F (1997) Olivocerebellar axon regeneration and target reinnervation following dissociated Schwann cell grafts in surgically injured cerebella of adult rats. Eur.J.Neurosci. 9:2634-2649.

Bregman BS, Kunkel-Bagden E, Reier PJ, Dai HN, McAtee M, Gao D (1993) Recovery of function after spinal cord injury: Mechanisms uniderlying transplant-mediated recovery of function differ after spinal cord injury in newborn and adult rats. Exp.Neurol. 123:3-16.

Brundin P, Barbin G, Strecker RE, Isacson O, Prochiantz A, Bjorklund A (1988) Survival and function of dissociated rat dopamine neurons grafted at different developmental stages or after being cultured in vitro. Dev.Brain Res. 39:233-243.

Buffo A, Holtmaat AJ, Savio T, Verbeek JS, Oberdick J, Oestreicher AB, Gispen WH, Verhaagen J, Rossi F, Strata P (1997) Targeted overexpression of the neurite growth-associated protein B-50/GAP-43 in cerebellar Purkinje cells induces sprouting after axotomy but not axon regeneration into growth-permissive transplants. J.Neurosci. 17:8778-8791.

Caroni P (1997) Intrinsic neuronal determinants that promote axonal sprouting and elongation. Bioessays 19:767-775.

Chen DF, Jhaveri S, Schneider GE (1995) Intrinsic changes in developing retinal neurons result in regenerative failure of their axons. Proc.Natl.Acad.Sci.USA 92:7287-7291.

Chen DF, Schneider GE, Martinou JC, Tonegawa S (1997) Bcl-2 promotes regeneration of severed axons in mammalian CNS. Nature 385:434-439.

Chong MS, Reynolds ML, Irwin N, Coggeshall RE, Emson PC, Benowitz LI, Woolf CJ (1994) GAP-43 expression in primary sensory neurons following central axotomy. J.Neurosci. 14:4375-4384.

Chong MS, Woolf CJ, Turmaine M, Emson PC, Anderson PN (1996) Intrinsic versus extrinsic factors in determining the regeneration of the central processes of rat dorsal root ganglion neurons: the influence of a periperal nerve graft. J.Comp.Neurol. 370:97-104.

Cohen J, Burne JF, Winter J, Bartlett P (1986) Retinal ganglion cells lose response to laminin with maturation. Nature 322:465-467.

David S, Aguayo AJ (1981) Axonal elongation into peripheral nervous system bridges after central nervous system injury in adult rats. Science 241:931-933.

Davies SJA, Fitch MT, Memberg SP, Hall AK, Raisman G, Silver J (1997) Regeneration of adult axons in white matter tracts of the central nervous system. Nature 390:680-684.

Doherty P, Moolenaar CECK, Ashton SV, Michalides RJAM, Walsh FS (1992) The VASE exon downregulates the neurite growth-promoting activity of NCAM 140. Nature 356:791-793.

Doster SK, Lozano AM, Aguayo AJ, Willard MB (1991) Expression of the growth-associated protein GAP-43 in adult rat retinal ganglion cells following axon injury. Neuron 6:635-647.

Dou C-L, Levine JM (1994) Inhibition of neurite growth by the NG2 chondroitin sulfate proteoglycan. J.Neurosci. 14:7616-7628.

Engel M, Maurel P, Margolis RU, Margolis RK (1996) Chondroitin sulfate proteoglycans in the developing central- nervous- system .1. cellular sites of synthesis of neurocan and phosphacan. Journal Of Comparative Neurology 366:34-43.

Fawcett JW, Housden E, Smith-Thomas L, Meyer RL (1989) The growth of axons in three dimensional astrocyte cultures. Dev.Biol. 135:449-458.

Fawcett JW, Mathews G, Housden E, Goedert M, Matus A (1994) Regenerating sciatic nerve axons contain the adult rather than the embryonic pattern of microtubule associated proteins. Neurosci. 61:789-804.

Fawcett JW, Rokos J, Bakst I (1989) Oligodendrocytes repel axons and cause axonal growth cone collapse. J.Cell Sci. 92:93-100.

Ford-Holevinski TS, Hopkins JM, McCoy JP, Agranoff BW (1986) Laminin supports neurite outgrowth from explants of axotomized adult rat retinal neurons. Brain.Res. 393:121-126.

Grill RJ, Stallcup WB, Tuszynski MH (1998) Temporal upregulation and spatial distribution of putative inhibitory and growth permissive substrate molecules in the injured adult rat spinal cord. Soc.Neurosci.Abstr. 24:1054

Johnson AR, Wigley CB, Gregson NA, Cohen J, Berry M (1988) Neither laminin nor prior optic nerve section are essential for the regeneration of adult mammalian retinal ganglion cell axons in vitro. J.Neurocytol. 17:95-104.

Kalil K, Reh T (1982) A light and electron microscopic study of regrowing pyramidal tract fibers. J.Comp.Neurol. 211:265-275.

Klöcker N, Cellerino A, Bähr M (1998) Free radical scavenging and inhibition of nitric oxide synthase potentiates the neurotrophic effects of brain-derived neurotrophic factor on axotomized retinal ganglion cells *in vivo*. J.Neurosci. 18:1038-1046.

Kobayashi NR, Fan DP, Giehl KM, Bedard AM, Wiegand SJ, Tetzlaff W (1997) BDNF and NT-4/5 Prevent Atrophy of Rat Rubrospinal Neurons after Cervical Axotomy, Stimulate GAP-43 and T1-Tubulin mRNA Expression, and Promote Axonal Regeneration. J.Neurosci. 17:9583-9595.

Lau KC, So KF, Tay D (1994) Intravitreal transplantation of a segment of peripheral nerve enhances axonal regeneration of retinal ganglion cells following distal axotomy. Exp.Neurol. 128:211-215.

Levine JM (1994) Increased expression of the ng2 chondroitin-sulfate proteoglycan after brain injury. Journal Of Neuroscience 14:4716-4730.

Levine JM, Nishiyama A (1996) The NG2 chondroitin sulfate proteoglycan: a multifunctional proteoglycan associated with immature cells. Perspect.Dev.Neurobiol. 3:245-259.

Li D, Field PM, Raisman G (1995) Failure of axon regeneration in postnatal rat entorhino-hippocampal slice coculture is due to maturation of the axon, not that of the pathway or target. European Journal Of Neuroscience 7:1164-1171.

Lindsay RM (1988) Nerve growth factors (NGF, BDNF) enhance axonal regeneration but are not required for survival of acult sensory neurons. J.Neurosci. 8:2394-2405.

Liu Y, Kim D, Hines BT, Chou S, Schallert T, Murray M, Tessler, A, Fischer, I (1999) Transplants of fibroblasts genetically modified to express BDNF promote regeneration of adult rat rubrospinal axons and recovery of limb function. J. Neurosci. 19:4370-4387.

Maclaren RE (1996) Expression of myelin proteins in the opossum optic nerve: late appearance of inhibitors implicates an earlier non-myelin factor in preventing ganglion cell regeneration. J.Comp.Neurol. 372:27-36.

Maclaren RE, Taylor JS (1995) A critical period for axon regrowth through a lesion in the developing mammalian retina. Eur.J.Neurosci. 7:2111-2118.

Maclaren RE, Taylor JSH (1997) Regeneration in the developing optic nerve: Correlating observations in the opossum to other mammalian systems. Prog.Neurobiol. 53:381-398.

Margolis RK, Rauch U, Maurel P, Margolis RU (1996) Neurocan and phosphacan: two major nervous tissue-specific chondroitin sulfate proteoglycans. Perspect.Dev.Neurobiol. 3:273-290.

McKeon RJ, Höke A, Silver J (1995) Injury-induced proteoglycans inhibit the potential for laminin- mediated axon growth on astrocytic scars. Exp.Neurol. 136:32-43.

McKeon RJ, Schreiber RC, Rudge JS, Silver J (1991) Reduction of neurite outgrowth in a model of glial scarring following CNS injury is correlated with the expression of inhibitory molecules on reactive astrocytes. J.Neurosci. 11:3398-3411.

McKerracher L, David S, Jackson DL, Kottis V, Dunn RJ, Braun PE (1994) Identification of myelin-associated glycoprotein as a major myelin-derived inhibitor of neurite growth. Neuron 13:805-811.

Meiri KF, Saffell JL, Walsh FS, Doherty P (1998) Neurite outgrowth stimulated by neural cell adhesion molecules requires growth-associated protein-43 (GAP-43) function and is associated with GAP-43 phosphorylation in growth cones. Journal Of Neuroscience 18:10429-10437.

Meyer RL, Miotke J (1990) Rapid initiation of neurite outgrowth onto laminin from explants of adult mouse retina induced by optic nerve crush. Exp.Neurol. 107:214-221.

Miller FD, Tetzlaff W, Bisby MA, Fawcett JW, Milner RJ (1989) Rapid induction of the major embryonic alpha-tubulin mRNA, T alpha 1, during nerve regeneration in adult rats. J.Neurosci. 9:1452-1463.

Morrow DR, Campbell G, Lieberman AR, Anderson PN, (1993) Differential regenerative growth of CNS axons into tibial and peroneal nerve grafts in the thalamus of adult rats. Exper. Neurol. 120:60-69.

Muir E, Du J-S, Fok-Seang J, Smith-Thomas LC, Rogers JH, Fawcett JW (1998) Increased axon growth through astrocyte cell lines transfected with urokinase. Glia 23:24-34.

Ness R, David S (1997) Leptomeningeal cells modulate the neurite growth promoting properties of astrocytes in vitro. Glia 19:47-57.

Nothias F, Boyne L, Murray M, Tessler A, Fischer I (1995) The expression and distribution of tau proteins and messenger RNA in rat dorsal root ganglion neurons during development and regeneration. Neuroscience 66:707-719.

Pesheva P, Gennarini G, Goridis C, Schachner M (1993) The F3/11 cell adhesion molecule mediates the repulsion of neurons by the extracellular matrix glycoprotein J1-160/180. Neuron 10:69-82.

Plant GW, Dimitropolou A, BATES ML, Bunge MB (1998) The expression of inhibitory proteoglycans following transplantation of Schwann cell grafts into completely transected rat spinal cord. Soc.Neurosci.Abstr. 24:69

Rossi F, Jankovski A, Sotelo C (1995) Differential regenerative response of Purkinje cell and inferior olivary axons confronted with embryonic grafts: Environmental cues versus intrinsic neuronal determinants. J.Comp.Neurol. 359:663-677.

Sakurai T, Friedlander DR, Grumet M (1996) Expression of polypeptide variants of receptor-type protein- tyrosine- phosphatase-beta - the secreted form, phosphacan, increases dramatically during embryonic-development and modulates glial-cell behavior in-vitro. Journal Of Neuroscience Research 43:694-706.

Sakurai T, Friedlander DR, Grumet M (1996) Expression of polypeptide variants of receptor-type protein tyrosine phosphatase beta: the secreted form, phosphacan, increases dramatically during embryonic development and modulates glial cell behavior in vitro. J.Neurosci.Res. 43:694-706.

Sawai H, Clarke DB, Kittlerova P, Bray GM, Aguayo AJ (1996) Brain-derived neurotrophic factor and neurotrophin-4/5 stimulate growth of axonal branches from regenerating retinal ganglion cells. J.Neurosci. 16:3887-3894.

Schwab ME, Kapfhammer JP, Bandtlow CE (1993) Inhibitors of neurite growth. Annu.Rev.Neurosci. 16:565-595.

Shewan D, Berry M, Cohen J (1995) Extensive regeneration in-vitro by early embryonic neurons on immature and adult CNS tissue. Journal Of Neuroscience 15:2057-2062.

Sinclair SR, Torres ER, Fawcett JW, Dunnett SB (1999) Cell division in embryonic mesencephalic neurones before and after transplantation. Submitted.

Smith-Thomas L, Fok-Seang J, Stevens J, Du J-S, Muir E, Faissner A, Geller HM, Rogers JH, Fawcett JW (1994) An inhibitor of neurite outgrowth produced by astrocytes. J.Cell Sci. 107:1687-1695.

Smith-Thomas L, Stevens J, Fok-Seang J, Muir E, Faissner A, Rogers JH, Fawcett JW (1995) Increased axon regeneration in astrocytes grown in the presence of proteoglycan synthesis inhibitors. J.Cell Sci. 108:1307-1315.

Smith GM, Miller RH, Silver J (1986) Changing role of forebrain astrocytes during development, regenerative failure, and induced regeneration upon transplantation. J.Comp.Neurol. 251:23-43.

Snyder SE, Li J, Schauwecker PE, Mcneill TH, Salton SR (1996) Comparison of RPTP zeta/beta, phosphacan, and trkB mRNA expression in the developing and adult rat nervous system and induction of RPTP zeta/beta and phosphacan mRNA following brain injury. Brain Res.Mol.Brain Res. 40:79-96.

Snyder SE, Li J, Schauwecker PE, Mcneill TH, Salton SRJ (1996) Comparison of rptp-zeta/beta, phosphacan, and trkb messenger-rna expression in the developing and adult-rat nervous-system and induction of rptp-zeta/beta and phosphacan messenger-rna following brain injury. Molecular Brain Research 40:79-96.

Takahashi K, Schwartz E, Ljubetic C, Murray M, Tessler A, Saavedra RA (1999) A DNA plasmid that codes for humand BCL-2 gene preserves axotomized Clarke's nucleus neurons and reduces atrophy after spinal cord hemisection. J. Comp. Neurol.404:159-171.

Tang S, Woodhall RW, Shen YJ, deBellard ME, Saffell JL, Doherty P, Walsh FS, Filbin MT (1997) Soluble myelin-associated glycoprotein (MAG) found in vivo inhibits axonal regeneration. Mol.Cell Neurosci. 9:333-346.

Tetzlaff W, Kobayashi NR, Giehl KMG, Tsui BJ, Cassar SL, Bedard AM (1994) Response of rubrospinal and corticospinal neurons to injury and neurotrophins. Progress In Brain Research 103:271-286.

Varga ZM, Schwab ME, Nicholls JG (1995) Myelin-associated neurite growth-inhibitory proteins and suppression of regeneration of immature mammalian spinal cord in culture. Proc.Natl.Acad.Sci.USA 92:10959-10963.

Wang XM, Terman JR, Martin GF (1998) Regeneration of supraspinal axons after transection of the thoracic spinal cord in the developing opossum, Didelphis virginiana. J.Comp.Neurol. 398:83-97.

Wictorin K, Brundin P, Sauer H, Lindvall O, Björklund A (1992) Long distance directed axonal growth from human dopaminergic mesencephalic neuroblasts implanted along the nigrostriatal pathway in 6-hydroxydopamine lesioned adult rats. J.Comp.Neurol. 323:475-494.

Wiederkehr A, Staple J, Caroni P (1997) The motility-associated proteins GAP-43, MARCKS, and CAP-23 share unique targeting and surface activity-inducing properties. Exp.Cell Res. 236:103-116.

Wigley CB, Berry M (1988) Regeneration of adult rat retinal ganglion cell processes in monolayer culture: comparisons between cultures of adult and neonatal neurons. Brain.Res. 470:85-98.

Wizenmann A, Bähr M (1997) Growth characteristics of ganglion cell axons in the developing and regenerating retino-tectal projection of the rat. Cell Tissue Res. 290:395-403.

Woolhead CL, Zhang Y, Lieberman AR, Schachner M, Emson PC, Anderson PN (1998) Differential effects of autologous peripheral nerve grafts to the corpus striatum of adult rats on the regeneration of axons of striatal and nigral neurons and on the expression of GAP-43 and the cell adhesion molecules N-CAM and L1. J.Comp.Neurol. 391:259-273.

Yamada H, Fredette B, Shitara K, Hagihara K, Miura R, Ranscht B, Stallcup WB, Yamaguchi Y (1997) The brain chondroitin sulfate proteoglycan brevican associates with astrocytes ensheathing cerebellar glomeruli and inhibits neurite outgrowth from granule neurons. J.Neurosci. 17:7784-7795.

Zagrebelsky M, Buffo A, Skerra A, Schwab ME, Strata P, Rossi F (1998) Retrograde regulation of growth-associated gene expression in adult rat Purkinje cells by myelin-associated neurite growth inhibitory proteins. Journal Of Neuroscience 18:7912-7929.

Zuo J, Ferguson TA, Hernandez YJ, Stetler-Stevenson WG, Muir D (1998) Neuroanl matrix metalloproteinase-2 degraded and inactivates a neurite inhibitin chondroitin sulfate proteoglycan. J.Neurosci. 18:5203-5211.

7

Apoptotic Cell Death Following Axotomy

P. Chaudhary and S.C. Sharma
New York Medical College, Valhalla, New York

I. INTRODUCTION

Axotomy and/or removal of targets for developing neurons leads to widespread cell death (Hamburger 1934). The reason for this was unclear until Levi-Montalcini and Hamburger isolated a substance from mouse salivary glands that has the ability to keep sympathetic neurons alive even after axotomy. The discovery of this substance, nerve growth factor (NGF), led to the suggestion that cell death after axotomy may be due to the deprivation of substances (trophic factors) produced at the target sites (Cohen et al., 1954). Despite enormous advances in neuroscience over the ensuing decades, the signals initiating the changes in the cell body after axotomy are still not fully understood. In order to conceptualize the details of neuronal cell death that occurs in some neurons as a consequence of axotomy, we will first review what is known about cell death and then relate these events to the changes occurring following axotomy.

II. NEURONAL CELL DEATH

Every day millions of cells die as part of a dynamic, homeostatic, physiologic blueprint. The studies of Hamburger and Levi-Montalcini demonstrated that nearly 50% of sympathetic neurons die during embryogenesis in chicks (Hamburger and Levi-Montalcini 1949). Cell death occurring during development of neuronal populations (for earlier reviews see Oppenheim et al., 1989, Oppenheim, 1991) plays an important role in vertebrate embryogenesis (Glucksmann 1951). In developing neurons, cell death (usually termed programmed cell death) occurs due to the competition for limited amounts of trophic factors derived from the targets which the cells innervate (Johnson and Oppenheim 1994). Apoptosis is the term used to describe cell death taking place under a variety of conditions other than development. However, the term programmed cell death is also frequently used for any type of cell death that is dependent on a genetic program.

Different mechanisms control cell death under different conditions. Necrotic cell death usually occurs as a result of external damage which may be caused by a variety of agents or abrupt environment change and/or departure from physiological conditions. This has traditionally been visualized as disruption of structural and functional integrity, rapid influx of Ca^{2+} and water, swelling of mitochondria and a breakdown in membrane permeability which leads to death of the cell (Kerr 1969, Martin et al., 1998). The exact molecular mechanisms involved in necrosis are not well understood, but changes in cell volume homeostasis and mitochondrial dysfunction have been implicated in the process (Laiho et al., 1971). Plasma membranes undergo a process called ‘blebbing’ that may be the result of oxidative damage to the cytoskeleton (Mirabelli et al., 1988). Since necrosis is associated with release of intracellular debris, it is accompanied also by an inflammatory response.

While necrotic cell death does not follow a specific pathway of events, apoptosis is an orderly, active cell death characterized by condensation of the cytoplasm and nucleus,and breakdown of DNA (Kerr et al., 1972). Subsequently the cell shrinks while the plasma membrane remains intact. Condensation of the cytoplasm is also associated with formation of cytoplasmic vacuoles. Later, the nuclear and plasma membranes become convoluted and the cell undergoes budding. Internucleosomal cleavage of DNA (ladder pattern) appears to be a relatively late event in the apoptotic process. The dying cell fragments into membrane bound structures (apoptotic bodies) and is then phagocytosed without creating an inflammatory response. The cleavage of DNA occurring during apoptosis can be recognized as a DNA ladder on gel electrophoresis (Wyllie 1980), whereas in necrosis there is a random cleavage of DNA which is seen as a smear on the gel.

Apoptosis occurs in two parts: first, a commitment to the cell death pathway and second, the actual execution of the death. A variety of studies have shown that while there are many initiators of cell death, there are only a few executors and those executors act only if the cell reaches a ‘point of no return’ (Fig. 1). Apoptosis is accomplished by activation of specialized cellular machinery that is highly conserved among nematodes, insects and mammals. It is the path of cell death of neurons in early developmental stages and is also involved in pathological states following trauma, ischemia, stroke and in neurodegenerative disorders (Bredesen 1995; Thompson 1995).

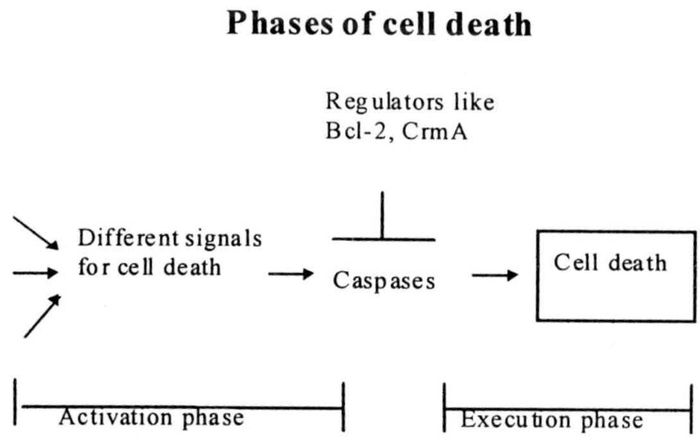

Figure 1 Phases of cell death. Multiple pathways are responsible for the activation of caspases which finally lead to execution of cell death. Caspase activation can in turn be blocked by various antiapoptotic proteins. Crm A – cytokine response modifier A, Bcl-2 – a protein which interferes with cell death.

The dependence of apoptotic cell death on new RNA and protein synthesis confirmed the active nature of this process *in vitro* (Martin et al., 1988 , Comella et al., 1994) and *in vivo* (Oppenheim 1990) systems (see also Ratan et al., 1994, 1995). Using fibroblast and oligodendrocyte cell lines, Jacobson et al., (1994) showed that apoptotic changes can occur in the absence of the nucleus, suggesting that the death machinery is constitutively expressed in all cells (Raff 1992). Apoptotic cell death is mediated by transduction mechanisms with subsequent changes either in gene expression or in the activation/inactivation of proteins already present in the cell (Merry and Korsmeyer 1997). It has been suggested that the signal for death of a cell may depend on the ratio of death suppressor and death effector proteins (Oltvai et al., 1993).

The execution phase of apoptosis requires the participation of ICE (interleukin-1ß-converting enzyme) like proteases, which are mammalian homologs of the *C. elegans* cell death protein ced-3 (Yuan 1997). ICE, a cysteine protease, that cleaves the 31kDa pro interleukin-1ß to its active 17 kDa mature form, was identified as the first mammalian homologue of ced-3 (Yuan et al., 1993). Additional members in this family such as Nedd2, CPP32, ICH-2, ICErelIII, ICE-LAP3 have also been identified (Cohen 1997).

One of the major differences between apoptosis and necrosis is that in apoptosis the cells are sequestered in phagocytes before they can cause an inflammatory reaction. Preventing the release of intracellular components of the cell is important in the nervous system, because the release of excitotoxic mediators such as glutamate can cause secondary injury to surrounding neurons and these injured neurons can then enter the apoptotic pathway (Leist and Nicotera 1998a). Sometimes cell death appears to be a hybrid between apoptosis and necrosis and intermediate forms of cell death may occur during neuronal degeneration where clear distinctions among the different forms of cell death is difficult. Apoptosis and necrosis have also been seen to coexist under various conditions; in some instances necrosis follows apoptosis while in others apoptosis follows necrosis. For example, when cerebellar granule cells were exposed to glutamate, some cells died by necrosis while the cells surviving necrosis died by delayed apoptosis (Ankarcrona et al., 1995). On the other hand, following glutamate induced excitotoxic injury of the rat striatum, internucleosomal DNA fragmentation (evidence of apoptosis) was seen at early time intervals and random DNA fragmentation (evidence of necrosis) at later time points (Portera-Cailliau et al., 1995). These studies indicate that the extent of the initial insult appears to determine whether death is necrotic or apoptotic (Beilharz et al., 1995), and that there is frequently primary death due to the triggering insult and secondary death due to release of excitotoxins or production of harmful oxygen radicals.

III. MEDIATORS OF CELL DEATH

A. EXCITOTOXICITY

Excitotoxicity, the excessive activation of excitatory amino acid (EAA) receptors, has been implicated in cell death in many neurological diseases as well as after axotomy. Glutamate has been reported to be a major cause of retinal ganglion cell death after axotomy (Yoles and Schwartz 1998; Fig. 2). Glutamate induced cell death may be prevented by the use of MK-801, an NMDA-glutamate receptor antagonist, further evidence that glutamate is involved in cell death after axotomy (Russelakis-Carneiro et al., 1996).

Loss of mitochondrial membrane potential ($\Delta\psi_M$) in the presence of Ca^{2+} overload also may be involved in excitotoxic conditions (Schinder et al., 1996, Montal, 1998). The breakdown of $\Delta\psi$ leads to the release of Ca^{2+} into the cytosol and the generation of reactive oxygen species (ROS). The alteration in intracellular calcium concentration leads to activation of caspases which results in cell death (Leist et al., 1997). Although NMDA receptor mediated Na^+ and Ca^+ influx have been thought to be the primary ions involved in excitotoxicity (Choi 1988), recently NMDA receptor-mediated K^+ efflux has been shown to promote neuronal apoptosis (Yu et al., 1999).

1997). NFκB has been shown to protect hippocampal neurons *in vitro* from oxidative stress induced apoptosis (Mattson et al., 1997).

4. Genetic regulators

Discovery of genes involved in cell death came from the studies on *Caenorhabditis elegans* (Hengartner and Horvitz 1994a). This nematode was ideal for study since about 1090 cells are born and 131 cells die in the making of the whole organism. This normal pattern can be disrupted by mutations in a number of genes e.g., CED-3, CED-4 and CED-9. Mutations inactivating CED-3 and 4 result in survival of cells which would normally die and mutations in CED-9 cause extensive cell death (Hengartner et al., 1992, Yuan and Horvitz 1990). Studies on double mutations indicated that CED-3 and 4 had killer activity and that CED-9 had protective effects. Bcl-2 was isolated as a mammalian homologue of CED-9, which is a negative regulator of CED-3 (Vaux et al., 1988, Hengartner and Horvitz HR 1994b). Bcl-2 was discovered in human follicular lymphomas where it plays a role in promoting cell survival. At present at least 15 members of the Bcl-2 gene family have been isolated (Adams and Cory 1998). The members are classified as to whether they are anti-apoptotic death suppressors (Bcl-2, Bclx$_L$, Bcl-w, Mcl-1) or pro-apoptotic death promoters (Bax, Bak, Bik, Bad, Bcl-x$_s$). They are known to have conserved domains called BH 1-4 (Bcl-2 homology). These family members differ in the presence or absence of homology domains. The interaction between these proteins is partly regulated by the BH-1 and BH-2 domains (Yin et al., 1994). The pro and anti- apoptotic proteins have interactions with each other and can heterodimerize. Depending upon the individual concentrations of anti or pro - apoptotic proteins the cell can survive or die. Bax, another member of the Bcl-2 family of proteins, if overexpressed antagonizes the effect of Bcl-2 (Oltvai et al., 1993). Bad, Bcl-xS, Bak and Bik are other members interacting with Bcl-2 (Yang et al., 1995, Chittenden et al., 1995, Boyd et al., 1995 and Farrow et al., 1995). Bcl-xL is also known to interact with Bcl-xS, Bak and Bik. The Bcl-xL protein distribution pattern is similar to Bcl-2 (Gonzalez-Garcia et al., 1994). Several Bcl family members, including Bcl-2, Bcl-xL and Bax, are expressed in the nervous system (Merry et al., 1994, Oltvai et al., 1993 and Gonzalez-Garcia et al., 1994).

Bcl-2, a 25 kDa protein, is attached to the mitochondrial, endoplasmic reticulum and nuclear membranes via a COOH-terminal hydrophobic stretch of amino acids (Hockenbery et al., 1990,1993). The three-dimensional structure of a Bcl-2 homologue, Bcl-xL, suggests striking similarity to the pore-forming domains of diphtheria toxin and the bacterial colicins (Schendel et al., 1997). It is now known that Bcl-2, Bcl-xL and Bax have pore-forming capacity. Cytoprotection by Bcl-2 requires the pore-forming alpha5 and alpha6 helices (Matsuyama et al., 1998). Moderate differences in ion selectivity are found in Bcl-2 and Bax. These channels also show unique characteristics of conductance, voltage dependence and rectification (Schlesinger et al., 1997) suggesting that they may regulate electrochemical gradients, osmotic balance and transport of critical substances

(Liu et al., 1996). Thus, apoptotic regulators share common features with the bacterial toxins suggesting their conserved nature from bacteria to mammals.

Bcl-2 has been shown to bind to Raf-1, protein phosphatase calcineurin, the GTPases R and H-Ras and p53 binding protein (Reed 1997). Bcl-2 associates with Raf-1 and calcineurin through the BH4 domain. The BH4 domain is specific for death suppressor proteins and its removal from Bcl-2 transforms it from an anti-apoptotic protein to a pro-apoptotic protein (Cheng et al., 1997). Phosphorylation plays an important role in regulating the activity of cell death proteins. Phosphorylation of Bcl-2 attenuates its anti-apoptotic activity. Bad, on being phosphorylated loses its pro-apoptotic activity. Bcl-2 can associate with Raf-1, a protein kinase, at the mitochondrial membrane and then Raf-1 can induce phosphorylation of Bad (Wang et al., 1996).

Bax can lead to cell death in a caspase independent manner. In the presence of caspase inhibitors Bax can kill cells, provoking DNA condensation and membrane alterations without DNA degradation (Xiang et al., 1996). Recently, it has been shown that Bax can directly induce the release of cytochrome c, without apparent requirement of caspases. Cytochrome c is a small heme protein localized in the inner mitochondrial membrane. Thus, these data cast doubts on previous models that envision Bax as an inhibitor of the Bcl-2 family of proteins that triggers the release of CED-4like proteins (Jurgensmeier et al., 1998). Bax and the constitutive mitochondrial protein ANT (adenine nucleotide translocator) cooperate within the permeability transition pore complex (PTPC) to increase mitochondrial membrane permeability and trigger cell death (Marzo et al., 1998 a,b).

5. Mitochondria

While the apoptotic cascade was initially thought to be independent of mitochondria (Jacobson et al., 1993), recent data suggest that under some conditions mitochondria play a role in signaling cell death (Green and Reed, 1998, Zamzami et al., 1997). The first evidence of mitochondria being involved in apoptosis came from studies in a Xenopus cell-free system (Newmeyer et al., 1994), a system that can reproduce some of the final intracellular events typically seen in apoptosis. Evidence now suggests that apoptosis involves a fall of mitochondrial membrane potential ($\Delta\psi_M$), opening of mitochondrial permeability transition pores (PTPs) and release of proteins called apoptosis inducing factors (Tatton and Chalmers-Redman 1998). Opening of PTPs causes free exchange of solutes and proteins between the mitochondria and cytosol, swelling and later bursting of the mitochondrial membrane (Hirsch et al., 1998). The mitochondrial PTP is a voltage dependent megachannel with a maximum conductance of $>$ 1nS and multiple subconductance stages (Simpson and Russell, 1998). The PTP is a complex structure made up of an adenine nucleotide translocator (ANT), porin and a benzodiazepine binding protein. PTP also interacts with a variety of proteins like hexokinases, Bcl-2, Bax, creatine kinase, phospholipid hydroperoxidase, and glutathione peroxidase (Ichas and Mazat 1998, Beutner et al., 1998).

Overexpression of the anti-apoptotic protein Bcl-2 could prevent the release of cytochrome c. Apoptosis activating factor (Apaf-1), a cytosolic partner of cytochrome c (Zou et al., 1997) has a nucleotide binding site where dATP, a cofactor binds during apoptosis. Apaf 1, cytochrome c, and dATP can lead to the activation of procaspase 9 which in turn leads to the activation of procaspase 3, a key enzyme involved in apoptosis (Fig. 3).

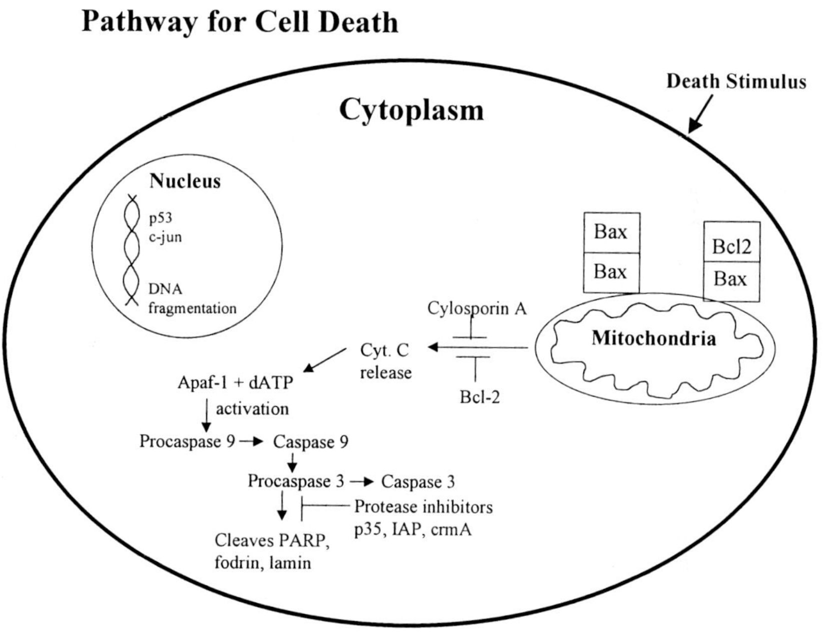

Figure 3 The pathway for cell death. The external stimulus operates through various transduction pathways to activate the cell death pathway in the nucleus.There are various points where the cell death pathway can be interrupted either by activation of anti-apoptotic proteins within the cell or by artificially introducing anti-apoptotic molecules.

Mitochondrial dysfunction may lead to impaired calcium buffering, generation of reactive oxygen species (ROS), and activation of the mitochondrial permeability transition pore (Beal 1998). Apoptosis inducing factor (AIF), an ICElike protease, is localized in the mitochondrial intermembrane space. When the PTPs are opened, AIF is released into the cytosol inducing apoptosis (Skulachev 1998). Factors which maintain closure of the PTP prevent apoptosis and those which effect opening of PTP promote apoptosis. Cyclosporin A, benzodiazepine receptor-binding agents and bongkrekic acid have been found to bind PTP and reduce apoptosis (Tatton and Chalmers-Redman 1998). Bcl-2 and Bcl-x_L are also responsible for maintaining the membrane potential of the mitochondrial membrane thus preventing apoptosis (Zamzami et al., 1998 and Marzo et al., 1998 a,b). The loss of a component of the mitochondrial electron transport chain (cyt c) also causes the generation of superoxide which can lead to oxidative stress, also a possible trigger for apoptotic cell death. Superoxide dismutase and glutathione, free radical scavengers that can prevent oxidative stress and cell death, may also play a role in preventing the PTP from opening (Chernyak 1997 and Vercesi et al., 1997).

6. Reactive oxygen species (ROS)

Cells generate ROS (hydroxyl and superoxide free radicals) as normal byproducts of aerobic metabolism. Hydroxyl radicals are harmful and responsible for most of the ROS damage. Under physiological conditions, there is a delicate balance between ROS and antioxidant protective mechanisms. Oxidative stress, an excess of free radicals that cannot be neutrallized by antioxidant defense mechanisms, causes cellular damage resulting in alteration of the redox state, lipid peroxidation and a loss of intracellular calcium homeostasis, all of which have been shown to occur during apoptosis. It is known that ROS can activate programmed cell death, but are not required for the execution of cell death (Jacobson 1996). Bcl-2 has been shown to have antioxidant properties and inhibits cell death either by suppressing the formation of ROS or by protecting the cell from the effects of ROS (Hockenbery et al., 1993). Bcl-2 is also known to prevent cell death in which ROS generation is not involved.

Many redox-regulated proteins are present in the cell. NFκB and AP-1 are involved in responding to the changes in the redox status within a cell and mediating apoptosis. ROS either directly mediate harmful effects or may affect the cell by acting as secondary mediators in signal transduction. Thus, ROS independent and dependent pathways for programmed cell death are known.

IV. NEURONAL CELL DEATH FOLLOWING AXOTOMY

A. Changes in the Nerve Cell Body After Axotomy

The responses of neurons to an insult may be diverse, involving enlargement of the cell body due to increased metabolic activity or shrinkage as a prelude to atrophy or cell death. Some of the typical responses to axotomy are vacuolation, enlargement of the nucleolus, displacement of the nucleus to eccentric or peripheral locations, swelling of the cell body and increased RNA metabolism and protein synthesis (discussed in detail elsewhere in this book).

After axotomy, mitochondria and lysosomes accumulate at the cut end of the axon as it retracts and begins to reseal (see this volume, chapter by Bittner and Fishman). Cell death that occurs in some neurons after axotomy may be due to interruption of trophic factors derived from target sources, excitotoxicity mediated by excess glutamate (see above) and/or a delay in the resealing of the severed axon. Recent experiments from our laboratory indicate that the latter may play a role in neuronal survival. These *in vivo* studies have shown that following axotomy, a CNS neuron (retinal ganglion cell) takes at least twice as long as a PNS neuron (DRG) to exclude a marker dye from entry into their cut ends (Ahmed et al., unpublished data). If CNS axons do, in fact, fail to reseal for an extensive period following injury, it may be a major reason for their death and inability to mount a regenerative response. The study of the events accompanying neuronal cell death following axotomy are important because it allows one to determine the stages where the axotomized cells can be rescued, so that they can be induced to grow axons and perhaps reinnervate their original target tissue (discussed in detail in this volume, chapter by Himes and Tessler).

B. Cell Death in Neonatal Animals After Axotomy

The extent of cell death after axotomy of neonatal CNS and PNS neurons is dependent on the developmental stage at which the lesion is performed and on whether the neuron has made appropriate connections with its target. The structural and morphological changes in the nucleus and the cytoplasm seen after axotomy are similar to those seen during naturally occurring programmed cell death.

1. PNS

In the immature nervous system axotomized neurons die rapidly whereas in the mature nervous system the neurons are likely to survive. Neonatal spinal motor neurons (Crews and Wigston 1990, Burls et al., 1990), cranial motor neurons (Snider and Thanedar 1989, Sendtner et al., 1990), dorsal root ganglion cells (Himes and Tessler 1989) and sympathetic ganglion cells (Hendry and Campbell 1976) respond with massive cell death after axotomy. Neonatal cell death appears to be due to deprivation of neurotrophic factors when contact between the neurons and their targets are severed (Hamburger et al., 1958). Facial neurons when axotomized in neonatal animals undergo cell death via the apoptotic pathway (Koliatsos and Price, 1996). Overexpression of Bcl-2 in transgenic mice protects motoneurons from apoptotic death following axotomy and during naturally occurring cell death (de Bilbao et al., 1996, Farlie et al., 1995, Dubois-Dauphin et al., 1994). Similarly, inactivation of Bcl-2 results in progressive degeneration of motoneurons, sympathetic and sensory neurons during early postnatal development (Michaelidis et al., 1996). Overexpression of Bcl-xL in transgenic mice prevented the death of nearly 65% of the motor neurons 7 days after axotomy, as opposed to only 15% in non-transgenic littermates (Parsadanian et al., 1998). Thus, Bcl-xL prevents neuronal death in postnatal animals and the levels of Bcl-xL may be a critical determinant to the susceptibility of a neuron to apoptosis. Bcl-2 has been known to rescue selectively neurotrophic factor dependent embryonic sensory neurons from apoptosis (Allsopp et. al., 1993). Hence Bcl-2 and Bcl-x protect PNS neonatal neurons from degeneration after axonal injury.

Growth factors such as BDNF and GDNF help in transient rescue of neonatal motoneurons after axotomy (Vejsada et al., 1998). Other neuronal growth factors, such as ciliary neurotrophic factor (CNTF), brain-derived neurotrophic factor (BDNF), leukemia inhibitory factor (LIF), basic fibroblast growth factor (bFGF) and platelet-derived growth factor (PDGF) are also involved in rescuing neurons after axotomy (reviewed by Snider et al., 1992). NT4/5 and BDNF are effective in preventing the death of neonatal motoneurons following axotomy (Koliatsos et al., 1994). Glutamate receptors and excitotoxicity are also known to participate in the cell death of axotomized motor neurons in newborns. Blockage of the NMDA and non NMDA glutamate receptors can also prevent neonatal neurons from cell death (Casanovas et al., 1996, Mentis et al., 1993).

2. CNS

Neurons with axons within the CNS, e.g., cortico-spinal neurons (Merline and Kalil 1990), retinal ganglion cells (Allcutt et al., 1984) and rubrospinal neurons (Prendergast and Stelzner 1976) also die when axotomized at an early developmental stage. Since axotomized neurons undergo apoptotic cell death, various studies have been performed in which axotomized neurons are protected by overexpression of anti-apoptotic protein Bcl-2. Protection of retinal ganglion cells from natural and axotomy induced cell death in neonatal transgenic mice overexpressing Bcl-2 has been demonstrated by Bonfanti et al., (1996) and Chierzi et. al., (1998). The majority of axotomized retinal ganglion cells survived and exhibited normal visual responses in mice overexpressing Bcl-2, whereas, in wild-type mice, the majority of axotomized retinal ganglion cells died and the physiological responses were abolished (Porciatti et al.,1996). An increase in Bcl-2 immunoreactivity was detected in the Muller cell processes after neonatal optic tract lesion or optic nerve transection in adult rats (Chen et al., 1994). Bcl-2-/- mutant mice are smaller but viable and about half of them die by 6 weeks of age. Surprisingly, eliminating Bcl-2 function in mice does not lead to a striking reduction of neuronal viability and produces viable mice (Nakayama et al., 1994). Other family members may compensate for the loss of Bcl-2 function. In fact, Bcl-x deficient mice die during embryogenesis and exhibit massive cell death in the nervous system (Motoyama et al., 1995).

C. Cell Death in Adults

1. PNS

Following axon damage, peripheral neurons undergo a series of changes including chromatolysis, alteration in protein synthesis patterns, changes in the distribution of cytoskeletal proteins, changes in the transport of proteins and in some cases, cell death. Spinal DRGs rarely die after peripheral nerve section in adult mammals

(Himes and Tessler, 1989). A large proportion of cranial motoneurons die after injury to the facial and hypoglossal nerves (Snider and Thanedar 1989), apparently because the cranial nerve lesions are closer to the soma than the nerve lesions in the spinal motoneurons. The extent of retrograde degeneration depends on the age, severity of lesion, location of the lesion in relation with the cell soma, the type of neurons and whether all the connections with the axon targets have been cut. Functional recovery from peripheral nerve injury and repair also depends on intrinsic and extrinsic factors. Neuronal survival after axotomy is a prerequisite for regeneration and is facilitated by trophic factors, neuropoietic cytokines, insulin-like growth factors (IGFs), and glial-cell-line-derived neurotrophic factors (GDNFs). Expression of the neuropoietic cytokines in injured neurons suggests an involvement in promoting the survival of the injured neurons.

Axotomized neurons switch to a growth mode and express growth-associated proteins, such as GAP-43, tubulin, and actin, as well as an array of novel neuropeptides and cytokines, while downregulating other genes (this volume, chapter by Fernandes and Tetzlaff). In addition to the axotomized neurons undergoing structural, metabolic and functional changes, Schwann cells also experience changes in order to make the environment favorable for regeneration. Schwann cells in the distal nerve stump appear to switch their function from myelination of axons to growth support for regenerating axons. Schwann cells increase the production of cell adhesion molecules (CAMs) such as N-CAM, N-cadherin and Ng-CAM (Nieke and Schachner, 1985; Martini and Schachner, 1988) and extracellular matrix proteins such as laminin and fibronectin (Bunge, 1993; Brodkey et al., 1993; Fu and Gordon, 1997) and downregulate genes that code for myelin associated proteins such as myelin basic protein (MBP) and MAG (Trapp et al., 1988, LeBlanc and Poduslo 1990; this volume, chapter by Grumet). L1 and N-CAM mediate cellular interactions by binding to the same molecules in a calcium dependent manner. N-CAM can also mediate cell adhesion by binding to integrins. Integrins are cell surface molecules which interact externally with extracellular matrix and internally with the cytoskeleton. Integrin-cytoskeletal assembly plays an important role in adhesion and growth. Expression of these molecules on the Schwann cells may also be a marker of survival promoting molecules for the injured neurons.

While the role of c-jun activation following axotomy is not well understood, it can regulate transcription of other genes affected by axotomy and it could be a key regulator of the neuronal axotomy response. Members of the *jun* family are expressed in axotomized motor and sensory neurons. One study indicates that c-jun is essential for regeneration to occur (Broude et al., 1997). But another study, where rat sympathetic neurons maintained *in vitro* were deprived of NGF, found that c-jun was involved in cell death (Estus et al., 1994). c-jun immunoreactivity has been detected after axotomy in facial motoneurons in neonatal rats (Garrah et al., 1998) and expression of c-jun was found in distal root-axotomized motoneurons. Since distal root axotomy does not cause motoneuron death, expression of c-jun is likely to be related to the regenerative process (Wu et al., 1994). Decreases in NFκB immediately after sciatic nerve crush and its recovery after one day suggest that its levels may play a role in controlling apoptosis in sensory neurons (Doyle and Hunt 1997).

Sciatic nerve transection in rats results in increases in nuclear c-jun and cytoplasmic Bax and decreases in Bcl-2 and Bcl-X immunoreactivity (Gillardon et al., 1996). The relative levels of Bcl-2 and Bax proteins are related to the threshold for cell death and appear to be modulated at the onset of neurodegeneration. (Gillardon et al., 1996).

There is compelling evidence that neuronal cell death after peripheral nerve axotomy is due, in large part, to deprivation of trophic factors. After axotomy, non-neuronal cells (primarily Schwann cells) in the distal nerve stump synthesize a variety of neurotrophins e.g., NT 4/5, BDNF, GDNF, IGFs (Richardson and Ebendal 1982, Raivich and Kreutzberg 1987, Meyer et al., 1992, Trupp et al., 1995). Nerve injury also induces a dramatic and rapid upregulation in bFGF mRNA levels, in 80% of all DRG neurons within 3 days after axotomy (Ji et al., 1995). Antisense p75NGFR oligonucleotides when applied at the proximal end of a transected peripheral nerve (sciatic, ulnar and median) significantly reduced the loss of axotomized sensory neurons suggesting a role for p75 in cell death (Cheema et al., 1996). Similarly, increases in BDNF and NT-4 in the distal part of an axotomized sciatic nerve were detected after 2 weeks and decreases in truncated Trk B and C appeared in the Schwann cell surrounding the peripheral nerve at the distal part of the nerve, indicating that the neurotrophins and their receptors may play a role in peripheral nerve regeneration (Funakoshi et al., 1993). Upregulation of the low affinity p75receptor in young adult rats and the high affinity Trk B receptor in aged rats after motoneuron axotomy has been reported (Johnson et al., 1999). In summary, evidence suggests that neurotrophic factors support the survival of neurons after axotomy and that they may provide useful as therapeutic agents (this volume, chapter by Thoenen).

2. CNS

Direct injury to grey matter leads to neuronal cell death. Injury to white matter also may result in cell death, but, in many cases neurons survive when their axons are severed. For example, when spinal cords in adult mammals are cut, both cortico-spinal and rubrospinal neurons survive (although they may atrophy and shrink), whereas optic nerve transection results in extensive death of retinal gang-

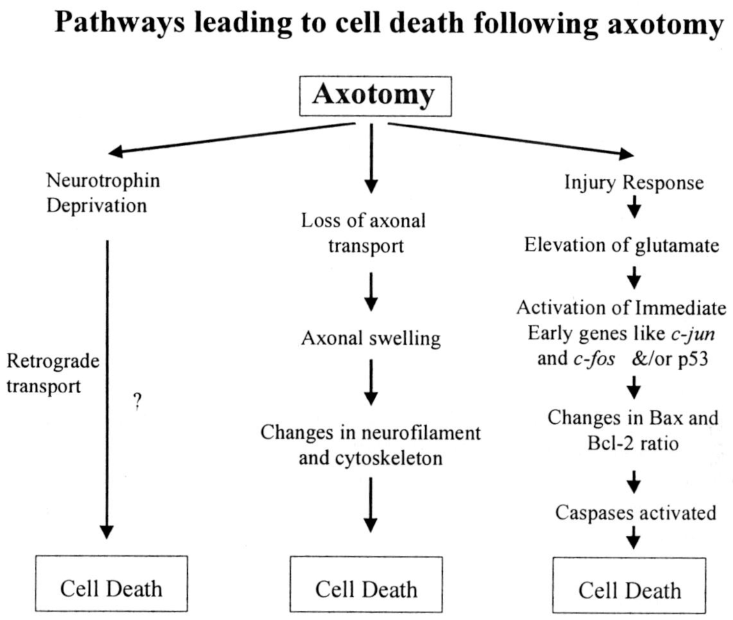

Figure 4 Potential mediators of cell death following axotomy. See text for details.

lion cells (see below). This variability in neuronal survival correlates with the distance between the lesion and the cell body and with the extent of axonal collateralization. One explanation for this phenomenon is that survival of distally axotomized neurons is due to their ability to procure target derived neurotrophic factors from intact collaterals proximal to the axotomy (Tetzlaff et al., 1994). While this topic deserves further experimental attention, in this chapter, we focus on the consequences of transecting the optic nerve on the viability of retinal ganglion cells.

Optic nerve axotomy provides a good model system to study the nature and mechanisms of cell death in the CNS. Apoptosis has been shown to be the mechanism of cell death of retinal ganglion cells (RGCs) after axotomy performed during development (Rabacchi et al., 1994) or in adult animals (Berkelaar et al., 1994, Garcia-Valenzuela et al., 1994). RGC cell death may be the result of lack of neurotrophins, excitotoxicity, alterations in anterograde or retrogradely transported signals and/or delayed resealing (Fig. 4). Following optic nerve axotomy RGCs progressively die and after two months a residual population of only about 5% survive (Mey and Thanos 1993). The ganglion cells die in two phases - initially there is massive loss of cells and later there is a gradual decline in their number. The number of retinal ganglion cells which die depends upon the distance between the site of transection and the optic nerve head (Villegas-Perez et al., 1993), the initial abrupt loss of ganglion cells in the first two weeks being more severe when the ON is cut close to the eye (Villegas-Perez et al., 1993). Only about 5% of RGCs survived by day 14 when the rat ON was cut about 0.5mm behind the eye, while 54% of RGCs survived when the ON was cut 8-9 mm from the eye. Growth associated protein, GAP-43, is upregulated when the optic nerve is cut about 3mm from the nerve head, but not following distal cuts (Lozano et. al., 1987). The relationship between axonal growth and the expression of GAP-43 after injury indicates that GAP-43 may be involved in the sequence of changes that modulate the responsiveness of a neuron after axotomy (Doster et al., 1991). c-jun immunoreactivity increased in retinal ganglion cells and was maximum 3 days after axotomy (Isenmann and Bahr 1997). NFκB was activated, in a time dependent manner, which may mediate apoptosis of retinal ganglion cells after optic nerve transection (Choi et al., 1998).

An important difference between axotomy in neonatal and adult animals is that in newborns the site of transection is less important whereas in adults cell death is dependent upon the distance between the site of transection and the soma. Another difference is that in young animals, axonal injury both in the PNS and CNS leads to massive degeneration, whereas neurons in the adult PNS generally survive and regenerate, while neurons in the CNS degenerate and die.

D. Phagocytic Response

Axon injury not only results in degeneration of distal nerve segments and in some cases the cell body, but also involves rapid activation of phagocytic cells. A prompt microglial reaction is characterized by a series of structural and phenotypic changes which in many ways are similar to an immune response, e.g., cell proliferation and upregulation of MHC antigens. The activated microglia express a number of inflammatory and immune mediators and when neuronal soma degeneration occurs, microglia act as phagocytes (Matsumoto and Fujiwara 1986). A similar reaction occurs following peripheral nerve injury but cell death after peripheral nerve injury is uncommon in the adult mammal. Thus, the functional implications of glial cell responses in this situation are unclear.

Phagocytic cells increase in numbers after axotomy either by direct proliferation or by recruitment from the circulating monocyte pool through an intact blood-brain barrier and subsequent differentiation into microglia (Perry et al., 1987; Lawson et al., 1992). Microglia transform into macrophages upon proper stimulation (Innocenti et al., 1983; Streit et al., 1988; Milligan et al., 1991). Experiments conducted in our lab have shown that the microglial cell number peaks at day 12 after optic nerve axotomy in adult rat retina and remains high for several months. The number of microglia present in the retina is proportional to the number of retinal ganglion cells that die. Intraocular administration of caspase inhibitors after axotomy rescues the ganglion cells, which correlates with a decrease in the number of microglial cells (Chaudhary et al., 1999). The complex interactions between microglial cells and neurons are not well understood. The hunt for new microglial genes responsible for the activation/action of microglial has recently resulted in the isolation of a new microglial gene, mrf-1 (microglial response factor-1) that appears to be one of the genes that responds to neuronal cell death and degeneration (Tanaka et al., 1998). Also, the increased expression of calcitonin gene related peptide (CGRP), in motoneurons following axotomy, suggests that it may play a role as a signaling molecule mediating the interactions between the damaged neurons and surrounding glial cells (Reddington et al., 1995).

V. PREVENTION OF CELL DEATH AFTER AXOTOMY IN RGCs

Experiments on attempts to intervene to prevent cell death are described in detail later in this volume, (chapter by Himes and Tessler). Here, we briefly describe specific efforts to save axotomized RGCs from entering the apoptotic cascade.

A. Cell Death Regulators After Axotomy

The entry of neurons, like most cells, into the apoptotic cascade involves the participation of Bcl-2 and Baxlike proteins. Over expression of Bcl-2 can block cell death (probably by inhibiting entry into the caspase cascade) whereas Bax stimulates the onset of the cascade (Korsmeyer et al., 1995). Our lab was one of the first to report that ganglion cells die via an apoptotic mechanism following axotomy (Garcia-Valenzuela 1994), a finding that was later supported by other studies (Quigley et al., 1995). The anti-death gene Bcl-xl is the predominant member of the Bcl-2 family in the adult rat retina and its levels decrease after optic nerve crush (Levin et al., 1997). Our recent studies and those of Isenmann et al., (1997), have shown differential expression of various apoptotic genes after adult rat optic nerve transection. Bcl-2 and Bcl-x decrease after axotomy whereas Bax expression increases. The ratio of Bcl-2/Bax appears to determine if the cell will undergo apoptosis (Korsmeyer et al., 1993). Approximately 65% of ganglion cells survived 3.5 months after axotomy in adult transgenic mice overexpressing Bcl-2 while in the wild type only about 10% of the ganglion cells survived two months after axotomy (Cenni et al., 1996). These studies support the role of Bcl-2 in rescuing axotomized RGCs.

B. Neurotrophic Factors

Target derived neurotrophic factors have been proposed to save RGCs from cell death after axotomy in a manner similar to the developing nervous system (Korsching 1993, Watanabe et al., 1997). Exogenous application of tropic factors such as BDNF, CNTF, GDNF, NT-4 – all have been reported to enhance survival of RGCs (Mey and Thanos 1993, Mansour Robaey et al., 1994, Klocker et al., 1997, Peinado-Ramon et al., 1996). BDNF can prevent lesion induced axonal dieback in young rat optic nerve (Weibel et al., 1995) and nerve growth factor (NGF) enhances survival and functional recovery of RGCs after ischemia (Siliprandi et al., 1993) and also after optic nerve section (Carmignoto et al., 1989). Fibroblast growth factor (FGF) implanted next to the proximal stump of a transected optic nerve of adult rats also promotes the survival of RGCs (Sievers et al., 1987).

Initially it was thought that the growth factors/neurotrophins for retinal ganglion cells are derived from targets in the optic tectum where axons of the RGCs project. Therefore, introducing growth factors into the eye was believed to be able to rescue the ganglion cells after axotomy. Although the neurotrophic factors were able to rescue some of the ganglion cells, these factors were not able to completely block cell death. It is now known that some growth factors are also derived locally in the retina (Mekada et al., 1998 and Xiao et al., 1999). While several studies have shown that ganglion cell death can be prevented by use of different growth factors, the mechanism of ganglion cell death is still not fully understood (Dreyfus et al., 1998 and Cui et al., 1998). In a recent study it was shown that neuroprotection by BDNF is limited because of excessive free radicals (Klocker et al., 1998). The free radical scavenger, N-tert-butyl-(2-sulfophenyl)-nitrone (S-PBN) alone did not have any survival effect on the ganglion cells. However, S-PBN potentiated the neuroprotective effects when administered along with BDNF (Klocker et al., 1998).

C. Peptide Inhibitors

The knowledge of cleavage sites of different substrates for caspases has helped to design peptides which could inhibit the action of caspases. Ac-DEVD-CHO and Ac-YVAD-CHO inhibit caspases 3 and 1 respectively. Recently, an irreversible tripeptide caspases inhibitor Z-VAD-FMK has helped to reveal the role of caspases in apoptosis (Gorman et al., 1999, Pronk et al., 1996). N-benzyloxycarbonyl-Val-Ala-Asp (OMe)-fluoromethylketone (z-VAD.FMK) is a cell permeable, nonselective inhibitor that blocks both ICElike and CPP32like activity. Acetyl-Tyr-Val-Ala-Asp-chloro-methylketone (YVAD-CMK) is more selective for ICE. N-benzyloxycarbonyl-Asp (OMe)-Glu (OMe)-Val-Asp (OMe)-fluoromethylketone (z-DEVD-FMK), inhibits CPP32like caspases more effectively due to an aspartate residue in the P4 position. Other irreversible, cell permeable inhibitors have now been designed which have been used to block apoptosis in a variety of systems.

Cell death in various systems (*in vitro* and *in vivo*) can be prevented by the administration of peptide inhibitors. Using retinal explants from postnatal rats at the age between 9 and 12 days Lucius and Sievers 1997 showed that YVAD protects retinal ganglion cells. This *in vitro* model could be compared to adult animals in their regenerative response. Caspase activation also contributes to death of RGCs after optic nerve axotomy (Kermer et al., 1998 and Chaudhary et al., 1999). Our lab has shown that intraocular application of caspase inhibitors e.g. DEVD-FMK and DEVD-CHO rescued up to 30-35% of RGCs that would otherwise have died (Chaudhary et al., 1999).

Calpains are non-lysosomal cysteine proteases that are activated by high Ca^{2+} levels. Calpain inhibitors blocked actin cleavage and DNA fragmentation (Villa et al., 1998). These inhibitors have also been used to block cell death in some systems.

D. Viral Proteins

The protein products of two viral anti-apoptotic genes, cytokine response modifier A (CrmA) and p35, have been found to be potent inhibitors of CED-3/ICE proteases. The cowpox serpin CrmA is a potent (Ki < 20 nM) and selective inhibitor of caspase-1, -4, and -5 and caspase-8, -9, and -10 (Garcia-Calvo et al., 1998). Microinjection of crmA, a specific inhibitor of ICE, inhibited neuronal cell death induced by trophic factor deprivation (Gagliardini et al., 1994). The baculovirus protein p35 inhibits programmed cell death in diverse animals such as insects, nematodes and mammals (Xue and Horvitz 1995). p35 inhibits the activity of caspases 1, 3, 6, 7, 8, and 10 (Zhou et al., 1998). Cell death in two Drosophila mutant strains exhibiting age-related retinal degeneration occurs by apoptosis. Studies by Davidson and Steller (1998) found that retinal cell death could be blocked by eye-specific expression of p35 and that the mutant flies expressing p35 showed significant retention of visual function. Although the viral proteins have not been used to prevent cell death after axotomy, they certainly have the potential to block cell death.

Another group of proteins known to block apoptosis are known as inhibitors of apoptosis (IAP). These proteins are conserved through evolution e.g., NAIP, XAIP, c-IAP-1, c-IAP-2. c-IAP-1 and c-IAP-2 function similarly to XIAP by inhibiting caspases-3 and -7, whereas NAIP presumably inhibits apoptosis via other targets. (Roy et al., 1997). IAPs have been identified as gene targets of NFκB transcriptional activity (Wang et al., 1998).

VI. FUTURE DIRECTIONS

Although there are different triggering mechanisms for cell death in different systems, all cells appear to have a final common pathway. Following axotomy, cells must be able to regain their integrity before any hope for regenerative repair is possible. One of the first and frequently overlooked steps, is for the neuron to reseal its cut process. Taking steps to find ways to assure that the severed axon reseals as quickly as possible after injury may be an important area for future studies. It is also important to understand the pathways of cell death in order to be able to block cell death before the cell gets committed to die. Overexpression of Bcl-2 provides protection to neurons in the central and peripheral nervous system after axotomy and its use in rescuing axotomized cells should be studied further. Changes in mitochondrial membrane potential play an important role in cell survival and developing specific inhibitors for the mitochondrial transition pore is another important avenue of investigation. Its use in combination with the caspase inhibitors may provide for better strategies in preventing cell death under different pathological conditions.

ACKNOWLEDGEMENT

The work from the authors laboratory, reported in this chapter was supported by N.I.H.N.E.I. 11295.

REFERENCES

Adams J.M and Cory S (1998) The Bcl2 protein family: arbiters of cell survival. Science 281:1322-1326.

Alcantara S, Frisen J, del Rio JA, Soriano E, Barbacid M, Silos-Santiago I (1997) TrkB signaling is required for postnatal survival of CNS neurons and protects hippocampal and motor neurons from axotomy-induced cell death. J Neurosci 17(10):3623-3633.

Allcutt D, Berry M, Sievers J (1984) A qualitative comparison of the reactions of retinal ganglion cell axons to optic nerve crush in neonatal and adult mice. Brain Res 318(2):231-240.

Allsopp TE, Wyatt S, Paterson HF, Davies AM (1993) The proto-oncogene bcl-2 can selectively rescue neurotrophic factor-dependent neurons from apoptosis. Cell 73(2):295-307.

Aloyz RS, Bamji SX, Pozniak CD, Toma JG, Atwal J, Kaplan DR, Miller FD (1998) p53 is essential for developmental neuron death as regulated by the TrkA and p75 neurotrophin receptors. J Cell Biol 143(6):1691-1703.

Ankarcrona M, Dypbukt JM, Bonfoco E, Zhivotovsky B, Orrenius S, Lipton SA, Nicotera P (1995) Glutamate-induced neuronal death: a succession of necrosis or apoptosis depending on mitochondrial function. Neuron 15(4):961-973.

Barbacid M (1994) The Trk family of neurotrophin receptors. J Neurobiol 25(11):1386-1403.

Beal MF (1998) Mitochondrial dysfunction in neurodegenerative diseases. Biochim Biophys Acta 1366(1-2):211-223.

Beilharz EJ, Williams CE, Dragunow M, Sirimanne ES, Gluckman PD (1995) Mechanisms of delayed cell death following hypoxic-ischemic injury in the immature rat: evidence for apoptosis during selective neuronal loss. Brain Res Mol Brain Res 29(1):1-14.

Berkelaar M, Clarke DB, Wang YC, Bray GM, and Aguayo AJ (1994) Axotomy results in delayed death and apoptosis of retinal ganglion cells in adult rats. J Neurosci 14(7): 4368-4374.

Beutner G, Ruck A, Riede B, Brdiczka D (1998) Complexes between porin, hexokinase, mitochondrial creatine kinase and adenylate translocator display properties of the permeability transition pore. Implication for regulation of permeability transition by the kinases. Biochim Biophys Acta 1368(1):7-18.

Bonfanti, L., Strettoi, E., Chierzi, S., Cenni, M.C., Liu, X.H., Martinou, J.C., Maffei, L. and Rabacchi, S.A. (1996) Protection of retinal ganglion cells from natural and axotomy-induced cell death in neonatal transgenic mice overexpressing bcl-2. J Neurosci 16(13): 4186-4194.

Bonfoco E, Leist M, Zhivotovsky B, Orrenius S, Lipton SA, Nicotera P (1996) Cytoskeletal breakdown and apoptosis elicited by NO donors in cerebellar granule cells require NMDA receptor activation. J Neurochem 67(6):2484-2493.

Bothwell M (1996) p75NTR: a receptor after all. Science 272(5261):506-507.

Boyd JM, Gallo GJ, Elangovan B, Houghton AB, Malstrom S, Avery BJ, Ebb RG, Subramanian T, Chittenden T, Lutz RJ (1995) Bik, a novel death-inducing protein shares a distinct sequence motif with Bcl-2 family proteins and interacts with viral and cellular survival-promoting proteins. Oncogene 11(9):1921-1928.

Bredesen, DE (1995) Neural apoptosis, Ann. Neurol., 38(6): 839-851.

Bredesen DE, Rabizadeh S (1997) p75NTR and apoptosis: Trk-dependent and Trk-independent effects. Trends Neurosci 20(7):287-290.

Brodkey JA, Gates MA, Laywell ED, Steindler DA (1993) The complex nature of interactive neuroregeneration-related molecules. Exp Neurol 123(2):251-270.

Broude E, McAtee M, Kelley MS, Bregman BS (1997) c-Jun expression in adult rat dorsal root ganglion neurons: differential response after central or peripheral axotomy. Exp Neurol 148(1):367-377.

Bunge RP (1993) Expanding roles for the Schwann cell: ensheathment, myelination, trophism and regeneration. Curr Opin Neurobiol 3(5):805-809.

Burls A., Subramaniam K, Lourie MB, and Vrbova G (1990) Absence of nerve-muscle interaction influences survival of developing motor neurons. Eur J Neurosci 3:216-221.

Caelles C, Helmberg A, Karin M (1994) p53-dependent apoptosis in the absence of transcriptional activation of p53-target genes. Nature 370(6486):220-223.

Cardone MH, Roy N, Stennicke HR, Salvesen GS, Franke TF, Stanbridge E, Frisch S, Reed JC (1998) Regulation of cell death protease caspase-9 by phosphorylation. Science 282(5392):1318-1321.

Carmignoto G, Maffei L, Candeo P, Canella R, Comelli C (1989) Effect of NGF on the survival of rat retinal ganglion cells following optic nerve section. J Neurosci 9(4):1263-1272.

Carter BD, Kaltschmidt C, Kaltschmidt B, Offenhauser N, Bohm-Matthaei R, Baeuerle PA, Barde YA (1996) Selective activation of NF-kappa B by nerve growth factor through the neurotrophin receptor p75. Science 272(5261):542-545.

Carter BD, Lewin GR (1997) Neurotrophins live or let die: does p75NTR decide? Neuron 18: 187-190.

Casanovas A, Ribera J, Hukkanen M, Riveros-Moreno V, Esquerda JE (1996) Prevention by lamotrigine, MK-801 and N-omega-nitro-L-arginine methyl ester of motoneuron cell death after neonatal axotomy. Neuroscience 71(2):313-325.

Casciola-Rosen LA, Miller DK, Anhalt GJ, Rosen A (1994) Specific cleavage of the 70-kDa protein component of the U1 small nuclear ribonucleoprotein is a characteristic biochemical feature of apoptotic cell death. J Biol Chem 269(49):30757-30760.

Cenni MC, Bonfanti L, Martinou JC, Ratto GM, Strettoi E and Maffei L (1996) Long-term survival of retinal ganglion cells following optic nerve section in adult bcl-2 transgenic mice. Eur J Neurosci 8(8):1735-1745.

Chaudhary P, Ahmed F, Quebada P and Sharma SC (1999) Caspase inhibitors block the retinal ganglion cell death following optic nerve transection. Brain Res Mol Brain Res 67(1):36-45.

Cheema SS, Barrett GL, Bartlett PF (1996) Reducing p75 nerve growth factor receptor levels using antisense oligonucleotides prevents the loss of axotomized sensory neurons in the dorsal root ganglia of newborn rats. J Neurosci Res 46(2):239-245.

Chen ST, Garey LJ, Jen LS (1994) Bcl-2 proto-oncogene protein immunoreactivity in normally developing and axotomised rat retinas. Neurosci Lett 172(1-2):11-14.
Cheng EH, Kirsch DG, Clem RJ, Ravi R, Kastan MB, Bedi A, Ueno K, Hardwick JM (1997) Conversion of Bcl-2 to a Bax-like death effector by caspases. Science 278(5345):1966-1968.
Chernyak BV (1997) Redox regulation of the mitochondrial permeability transition pore. Biosci Rep 17(3):293-302.
Chierzi S, Cenni MC, Maffei L, Pizzorusso T, Porciatti V, Ratto GM, Strettoi E (1998) Protection of retinal ganglion cells and preservation of function after optic nerve lesion in bcl-2 transgenic mice. Vision Res 38(10):1537-1543.
Chittenden T, Flemington C, Houghton AB, Ebb RG, Gallo GJ, Elangovan B, Chinnadurai G, Lutz RJ (1995) A conserved domain in Bak, distinct from BH1 and BH2, mediates cell death and protein binding functions. EMBO J 14(22):5589-5596.
Choi DW (1988) Calcium-mediated neurotoxicity: relationship to specific channel types and role in ischemic damage. Trends Neurosci 11(10):465-469.
Choi JS, Sungjoo KY, Joo CK (1998) NF-kappa B activation following optic nerve transection. Korean J Ophthalmol 12(1):19-24.
Cohen S, Levi-Montalcini R, Hamburger V (1954) A nerve growth factor isolated from sarcomas 37 and 180. Proc Natl Acad Sci USA 40: 1014-1018.
Cohen GM (1997) Caspases: the executioners of apoptosis. Biochem J 326: 1-16
Comella JX, Sanz-Rodriguez C, Aldea M, Esquerda JE (1994) Skeletal muscle-derived trophic factors prevent motoneurons from entering an active cell death program in vitro. J Neurosci 14(5 Pt 1):2674-2686.
Crews LL, Wigston DJ (1990) The dependence of motoneurons on their target muscle during postnatal development of the mouse. J Neurosci 10(5):1643-1653.
Cryns VL, Bergeron L, Zhu H, Li H, Yuan J (1996) Specific cleavage of alpha-fodrin during Fas- and tumor necrosis factor-induced apoptosis is mediated by an interleukin-1beta-converting enzyme/Ced-3 protease distinct from the poly(ADP-ribose) polymerase protease. J Biol Chem 271(49):31277-31282.
Cui Q, So KF, Yip HK (1998) Major biological effects of neurotrophic factors on retinal ganglion cells in mammals. Biol Signals Recept 7(4):220-226.
Davidson FF, Steller H (1998) Blocking apoptosis prevents blindness in Drosophila retinal degeneration mutants. Nature 391(6667):587-591.
de Bilbao F, Dubois-Dauphin M (1996) Time course of axotomy-induced apoptotic cell death in facial motoneurons of neonatal wild type and bcl-2 transgenic mice. Neuroscience 71(4):1111-1119.
Depraetere V, Golstein P (1997) Fas and other cell death signaling pathways. Semin Immunol 9(2):93-107.
Dobrowsky RT, Werner MH, Castellino AM, Chao MV, Hannun YA (1994) Activation of the sphingomyelin cycle through the low-affinity neurotrophin receptor. Science 265(5178):1596-1599.
Dobrowsky RT, Carter BD (1998). Coupling of the p75 neurotrophin receptor to sphingolipid signaling. Ann N Y Acad Sci 845:32-45.
Doster SK, Lozano AM, Aguayo AJ, Willard MB (1991) Expression of the growth-associated protein GAP-43 in adult rat retinal ganglion cells following axon injury. Neuron 6(4):635-647.
Doyle CA, Hunt SP (1997) Reduced nuclear factor kappaB (p65) expression in rat primary sensory neurons after peripheral nerve injury. Neuroreport 8(13):2937-2942.

Dreyfus H, Sahel J, Heidinger V, Mohand-Said S, Guerold B, Meuillet E, Fontaine V, Hicks D (1998) Gangliosides and neurotrophic growth factors in the retina. Molecular interactions and applications as neuroprotective agents. Ann N Y Acad Sci 845:240-252.

Dubois-Dauphin M, Frankowski H, Tsujimoto Y, Huarte J, Martinou JC (1994) Neonatal motoneurons overexpressing the bcl-2 protooncogene in transgenic mice are protected from axotomy-induced cell death. Proc Natl Acad Sci U S A 91(8):3309-3313.

Estus S, Zaks WJ, Freeman RS, Gruda M, Bravo R, Johnson EM Jr (1994) Altered gene expression in neurons during programmed cell death: identification of c-jun as necessary for neuronal apoptosis. J Cell Biol 127(6 Pt 1):1717-1727.

Frade JM, Rodriguez-Tebar A, Barde YA (1996) Induction of cell death by endogenous nerve growth factor through its p75 receptor. Nature 383(6596):166-168.

Farlie PG, Dringen R, Rees SM, Kannourakis G, Bernard O (1995) bcl-2 transgene expression can protect neurons against developmental and induced cell death. Proc Natl Acad Sci U S A 92(10):4397-4401.

Farrow SN, White JH, Martinou I, Raven T, Pun KT, Grinham CJ, Martinou JC, Brown R (1995) Cloning of a bcl-2 homologue by interaction with adenovirus E1B 19K. Nature 374(6524):731-733.

Fesus L, Thomazy V, Falus A (1987) Induction and activation of tissue transglutaminase during programmed cell death. FEBS Lett 224(1):104-108.

Folk JE (1980) Transglutaminases. Annu Rev Biochem 49:517-531.

Fu SY, Gordon T (1997) The cellular and molecular basis of peripheral nerve regeneration. Mol Neurobiol 14(1-2):67-116.

Funakoshi H, Frisen J, Barbany G, Timmusk T, Zachrisson O, Verge VM, Persson H (1993) Differential expression of mRNAs for neurotrophins and their receptors after axotomy of the sciatic nerve. J Cell Biol 123(2):455-465.

Gagliardini V, Fernandez PA, Lee RK, Drexler HC, Rotello RJ, Fishman MC, Yuan J (1994) Prevention of vertebrate neuronal death by the crmA gene. Science 263(5148):826-828.

Garcia-Calvo M, Peterson EP, Leiting B, Ruel R, Nicholson DW, Thornberry NA (1998) Inhibition of human caspases by peptide-based and macromolecular inhibitors. J Biol Chem 273(49):32608-32613.

Garcia-Valenzuela, E., Gorczyca, W., Darzynkiewicz,Z. and Sharma, S.C. (1994) Apoptosis in adult retinal ganglion cells after axotomy. J Neurobiol 25(4): 431-438.

Garrah JM, Bisby MA, Rossiter JP (1998) Immunolabelling of the cytoplasm and processes of apoptotic facial motoneurons following axotomy in the neonatal rat. Acta Neuropathol (Berl) 95(3):223-228.

Gillardon F, Klimaschewski L, Wickert H, Krajewski S, Reed JC, Zimmermann M (1996) Expression pattern of candidate cell death effector proteins Bax, Bcl-2, Bcl-X, and c-Jun in sensory and motor neurons following sciatic nerve transection in the rat. Brain Res 739(1-2):244-250.

Glucksmann, A (1951) Cell deaths in normal vertebrate development. Biol Rev 26: 59-86.

Gonzalez-Garcia M, Perez-Ballestero R, Ding L, Duan L, Boise LH, Thompson CB, Nunez G (1994) bcl-XL is the major bcl-x mRNA form expressed during murine development and its product localizes to mitochondria. Development 120(10):3033-3042.

Gorman AM, Bonfoco E, Zhivotovsky B, Orrenius S, Ceccatelli S (1999) Cytochrome c release and caspase-3 activation during colchicine-induced apoptosis of cerebellar granule cells. Eur J Neurosci 11(3):1067-1072.

Greene LA, Kaplan DR (1995) Early events in neurotrophin signalling via Trk and p75 receptors. Curr Opin Neurobiol 5(5):579-587.

Green, DR and Reed JC (1998) Mitochondria and Apoptosis. Science 281:1309-1312.

Hamburger V (1934) The effects of wing bud extirpation on the development of the central nervous system in chick embryos. J Exp Zool 68: 449-494.

Hamburger, V and Levi-Montalcini, R (1949) Proliferation, differentiation and degeneration in the spinal ganglia of the chick embryo under normal and experimental conditions. J Exp Zool 111:457-502.

Hamburger V (1958) Regression versus peripheral control of differentiation on motor hypoplasia. Am J Anat 102:365-409.

Haupt Y, Rowan S, Shaulian E, Kazaz A, Vousden K, Oren M (1997) p53 mediated apoptosis in HeLa cells: transcription dependent and independent mechanisms. Leukemia 11 Suppl 3:337-339.

Hendry IA, Campbell J (1976) Morphometric analysis of rat superior cervical ganglion after axotomy and nerve growth factor treatment. J Neurocytol 5(3):351-360.

Hengartner MO, Ellis RE, Horvitz HR (1992) Caenorhabditis elegans gene ced-9 protects cells from programmed cell death. Nature 356(6369):494-499.

Hengartner MO and Horvitz HR (1994a) Programmed cell death in *Caenorhabditis elegans.* Curr Opin Genet Dev 4(4): 581-586.

Hengartner MO and Horvitz HR (1994b) *C. elegans* cell survival gene ced-9 encodes a functional homolog of the mammalian proto-oncogene bcl-2. Cell 76(4) 665-676.

Herdegen T, Claret FX, Kallunki T, Martin-Villalba A, Winter C, Hunter T, Karin M (1998) Lasting N-terminal phosphorylation of c-Jun and activation of c-Jun N-terminal kinases after neuronal injury. J Neurosci 18(14):5124-5135.

Himes BT and Tessler A (1989) Death of some doral root ganglion neurons and plasticity of others following sciatic nerve section in adult and neonatal rats. J Comp Neurol 284: 215-230.

Hirsch DB, Steiner JP, Dawson TM, Mammen A, Hayek E and Snyder SH (1993) Neurotransmitter release regulated by nitric oxide in PC-12 cells and brain synaptosomes Curr Biol 3: 749-754.

Hirsch T, Susin SA, Marzo I, Marchetti P, Zamzami N, Kroemer G (1998) Mitochondrial permeability transition in apoptosis and necrosis. Cell Biol Toxicol 14(2):141-145.

Hockenbery D, Nunez G, Milliman C, Schreiber RD, Korsmeyer SJ (1990) Bcl-2 is an inner mitochondrial membrane protein that blocks programmed cell death. Nature 348(6299):334-336.

Hockenbery DM, Oltvai ZN, Yin XM, Milliman CL, Korsmeyer SJ (1993) Bcl-2 functions in an antioxidant pathway to prevent apoptosis. Cell 75(2):241-251.

Ichas F, Mazat JP (1998) From calcium signaling to cell death: two conformations for the mitochondrial permeability transition pore. Switching from low- to high-conductance state. Biochim Biophys Acta 1366(1-2):33-50.

Innocenti, G.M., Clarke, S., Koppel, H. (1983) Transitory macrophages in the white matter of the developing visual cortex. II. Development and relations with axonal pathways. Brain Res 313: 55-60.

Isenmann S, Wahl C, Krajewski S, Reed JC and Bahr M (1997) Up-regulation of Bax protein in degenerating retinal ganglion cells precedes apoptotic cell death after optic nerve lesion in rat. Eur J Neurosci 9: 1763-1772.

Isenmann S, Bahr M (1997) Expression of c-Jun protein in degenerating retinal ganglion cells after optic nerve lesion in the rat. Exp Neurol 147(1):28-36.

Jacobson MD, Burne JF, King MP, Miyashita T, Reed JC, Raff MC (1993) Bcl-2 blocks apoptosis in cells lacking mitochondrial DNA. Nature 361(6410):365-369.

Jacobson MD, Burne JF, Raff MC (1994) Programmed cell death and Bcl-2 protection in the absence of a nucleus. EMBO J 13(8):1899-1910.

Jacobson MD (1996) Reactive oxygen species and programmed cell death. Trends Biochem Sci 21(3):83-86.

Ji RR, Zhang Q, Zhang X, Piehl F, Reilly T, Pettersson RF, Hokfelt T (1995) Prominent expression of bFGF in dorsal root ganglia after axotomy. Eur J Neurosci 7(12):2458-2468.

Johnson J, Oppenheim R (1994) Neurotrophins. Keeping track of changing neurotrophic theory. Curr Biol 4(7):662-665.

Johnson H, Hokfelt T, Ulfhake B (1999) Expression of p75(NTR), trkB and trkC in non-manipulated and axotomized motoneurons of aged rats. Brain Res Mol Brain Res 69(1):21-34.

Jurgensmeier JM, Xie Z, Deveraux Q, Ellerby L, Bredesen D, Reed JC (1998) Bax directly induces release of cytochrome c from isolated mitochondria. Proc Natl Acad Sci U S A 95(9):4997-5002.

Kermer, P., Klocker N., Labes M. and Bahr M. (1998) Inhibition of CPP32 like proteases recsues axotomized retinal ganglion cells from secondary cell death *In Vivo.* J Neurosci 18(12) :4656-4662.

Kerr JF (1969) An electron-microscope study of liver cell necrosis due to heliotrine. J Pathol 97(3):557-562.

Kerr, JFR, Wyllie AH and CurrieAR (1972) Apoptosis: a basic biological phenomenon with wide-ranging implications in tissue kinetics. Br J Cancer 26: 239-257.

King LB, Ashwell JD (1993) Signaling for death of lymphoid cells. Curr Opin Immunol 5(3):368-373.

Klocker N, Braunling F, Isenmann S and Bahr M (1997) In vivo neurotrophic effects of GDNF on axotomized retinal ganglion cells. Neuroreport 8(16): 3439-3442.

Klocker N, Cellerino A, Bahr M (1998) Free radical scavenging and inhibition of nitric oxide synthase potentiates the neurotrophic effects of brain-derived neurotrophic factor on axotomized retinal ganglion cells In vivo. J Neurosci 18(3):1038-1046.

Koliatsos VE, Cayouette MH, Berkemeier LR, Clatterbuck RE, Price DL, Rosenthal A (1994) Neurotrophin 4/5 is a trophic factor for mammalian facial motor neurons. Proc Natl Acad Sci U S A 91(8):3304-3308.

Koliatsos VE, Price DL (1996) Axotomy as an experimental model of neuronal injury and cell death. Brain Pathol 6(4):447-465.

Korsching S (1993) The neurotrophic factor concept: a reexamination. J Neurosci 13(7):2739-2748.

Korsmeyer SJ, Shutter JR, Veis DJ, Merry DE, Oltvai ZN (1993) Bcl-2/Bax: a rheostat that regulates an anti-oxidant pathway and cell death. Semin Cancer Biol 4(6):327-332.

Korsmeyer SJ, Yin XM, Oltvai ZN, Veis-Novack DJ, Linette GP (1995) Reactive oxygen species and the regulation of cell death by the Bcl-2 gene family. Biochim Biophys Acta 1271(1):63-66.

Laiho KU, Shelburne JD, Trump BF (1971) Observations on cell volume, ultrastructure, mitochondrial conformation and vital-dye uptake in Ehrlich ascites tumor cells. Effects of inhibiting energy production and function of the plasma membrane. Am J Pathol 65(1):203-230.

Lawson, L.J., Perry, V.S., and Gordon, S. (1992) Turnover of resident microglia in the normal adult mouse brain. Neurosci 48: 405-410.

Lazebnik YA, Kaufmann SH, Desnoyers S, Poirier GG, Earnshaw WC (1994) Cleavage of poly(ADP-ribose) polymerase by a proteinase with properties like ICE. Nature 371(6495):346-347.

Lazebnik YA, Takahashi A, Moir RD, Goldman RD, Poirier GG, Kaufmann SH, Earnshaw WC (1995) Studies of the lamin proteinase reveal multiple parallel biochemical pathways during apoptotic execution. Proc Natl Acad Sci U S A 92(20):9042-9046.

LeBlanc AC, Poduslo JF (1990) Axonal modulation of myelin gene expression in the peripheral nerve. J Neurosci Res 26(3):317-326.

Leist M, Volbracht C, Kuhnle S, Fava E, Ferrando-May E, Nicotera P (1997) Caspase-mediated apoptosis in neuronal excitotoxicity triggered by nitric oxide. Mol Med 3(11):750-764.

Leist M, Nicotera P (1998a) Apoptosis, excitotoxicity, and neuropathology. Exp Cell Res 239(2):183-201.

Leist M, Nicotera P (1998b) Calcium and neuronal death. Rev Physiol Biochem Pharmacol 132:79-125.

Levin LA, Schlamp CL, Spieldoch RL, Geszvain KM and Nickells RW (1997) Identification of the bcl-2 family of genes in the rat retina. Invest Ophthalmol Vis Sci 38(12) 2545-2553.

Lewin GR, Barde YA (1996) Physiology of the neurotrophins. Annu Rev Neurosci 19:289-317.

Lipton SA (1997) Janus faces of NF-kappa B: neurodestruction versus neuroprotection. Nat Med 3(1):20-22.

Liu X, Kim CN, Yang J, Jemmerson R, Wang X (1996) Induction of apoptotic program in cell-free extracts: requirement for dATP and cytochrome c. Cell 86(1):147-157.

Lozano AM, Doster KS, Aguayo AJ, Willard MB (1987) Immunoreactivity to GAP-43 in axotomized and regenerating retinal ganglion cells of adult rat. Soc. Neurosci Abstr 13:1389.

Lucius R, and Sievers J (1997) YVAD protect post-natal retinal ganglion cells against axotomy-induced but not free radical-induced axonal degeneration in vitro. Brain Res Mol Brain Res 48(1): 181-184.

Mansour-Robaey S, Clarke DB, Wang YC, Bray GM and Aguayo AJ (1994) Effects of ocular injury and administration of brain-derived neurotrophic factor on survival and regrowth of axotomized retinal ganglion cells. Proc Natl Acad Sci USA 91(5) :1632-1636.

Martin DP, Schmidt RE, DiStefano PS, Lowry OH, Carter JG, Johnson EM Jr (1988) Inhibitors of protein synthesis and RNA synthesis prevent neuronal death caused by nerve growth factor deprivation. J Cell Biol 106(3):829-844.

Martin LJ, Al-Abdulla NA, Brambrink AM, Kirsch JR, Sieber FE, Portera-Cailliau C (1998) Neurodegeneration in excitotoxicity, global cerebral ischemia, and target deprivation: A perspective on the contributions of apoptosis and necrosis. Brain Res Bull 46(4): 281-309

Martini R, Schachner M (1988) Immunoelectron microscopic localization of neural cell adhesion molecules (L1, N-CAM, and myelin-associated glycoprotein) in regenerating adult mouse sciatic nerve. J Cell Biol 106(5):1735-1746.

Marzo I, Brenner C, Zamzami N, Susin SA, Beutner G, Brdiczka D, Remy R, Xie ZH, Reed JC, Kroemer G (1998a) The permeability transition pore complex: a target for apoptosis regulation by caspases and bcl-2-related proteins. J Exp Med Apr 20;187(8):1261-1271.

Marzo I, Brenner C, Zamzami N, Jurgensmeier JM, Susin SA, Vieira HL, Prevost MC, Xie Z, Matsuyama S, Reed JC, Kroemer G (1998b) Bax and adenine nucleotide translocator cooperate in the mitochondrial control of apoptosis. Science 281(5385):2027-2031.

Matsumoto Y, Fujiwara M (1986) *In situ* detection of class I and II major histocompatibility complex antigens in the rat central nervous system during experimental allergic encephalomyelitis. An immunohistochemical study. J Neuroimmunol 12(4):265-277.

Matsuyama S, Schendel SL, Xie Z, Reed JC (1998) Cytoprotection by bcl-2 requires the pore-forming alpha5 and alpha6 helices. J Biol Chem 273(47):30995-31001.

Mattson MP, Goodman Y, Luo H, Fu W, Furukawa K (1997) Activation of NF-kappaB protects hippocampal neurons against oxidative stress-induced apoptosis: evidence for induction of manganese superoxide dismutase and suppression of peroxynitrite production and protein tyrosine nitration. J Neurosci Res 49(6):681-697.

Meffert MK, Calakos NC, Scheller RH, Schulman H (1996) Nitric oxide modulates synaptic vesicle docking fusion reactions. Neuron 16(6):1229-1236.

Mekada A, Sasahara M, Yamada E, Kani K, Hazama F (1998) Platelet-derived growth factor B-chain expression in the rat retina and optic nerve: distribution and changes after transection of the optic nerve. Vision Res 38(20):3031-3039.

Melino G, Piacentini M (1998) Tissue transglutaminase in cell death: a downstream or a multifunctional upstream effector? FEBS Lett 430(1-2):59-63.

Mentis GZ, Greensmith L, Vrbova G (1993) Motoneurons destined to die are rescued by blocking N-methyl-D-aspartate receptors by MK-801. Neuroscience 54(2):283-285.

Merline M, Kalil K (1990) Cell death of corticospinal neurons is induced by axotomy before but not after innervation of spinal targets. Comp Neurol 296(3):506-516.

Merry DE, Veis DJ, Hickey WF, Korsmeyer SJ (1994) bcl-2 protein expression is widespread in the developing nervous system and retained in the adult PNS. Development 120(2):301-311.

Merry DE, Korsmeyer SJ (1997) Bcl-2 gene family in the nervous system. Annu Rev Neurosci 20:245-267.

Mey J and Thanos S (1993) Intravitreal injections of neurotrophic factors support the survival of axotomized retinal ganglion cells in adult rats in vivo. Brain Res 602(2): 304-317.

Meyer M, Matsuoka I, Wetmore C, Olson L, Thoenen H (1992) Enhanced synthesis of brain-derived neurotrophic factor in the lesioned peripheral nerve: different mechanisms are responsible for the regulation of BDNF and NGF mRNA. J Cell Biol 119(1):45-54.

Michaelidis TM, Sendtner M, Cooper JD, Airaksinen MS, Holtmann B, Meyer M, Thoenen H (1996) Inactivation of bcl-2 results in progressive degeneration of motoneurons, sympathetic and sensory neurons during early postnatal development. Neuron 17(1):75-89.

Milligan CE, Levitt P and Cunningham TJ (1991) Brain macrophages and microglia respond differently to lesions of the developing and adult visual system. J Comp Neurol 314: 136-146.

Mirabelli F, Salis A, Perotti M, Taddei F, Bellomo G, Orrenius S (1988) Alterations of surface morphology caused by the metabolism of menadione in mammalian cells are associated with the oxidation of critical sulfhydryl groups in cytoskeletal proteins. Biochem Pharmacol 37(18):3423-3427.

Montal M (1998) Mitochondria, glutamate neurotoxicity and the death cascade. Biochim Biophys Acta 1366(1-2):113-126.

Motoyama N, Wang F, Roth KA, Sawa H, Nakayama K, Nakayama K, Negishi I, Senju S, Zhang Q, Fujii S, et al (1995) Massive cell death of immature hematopoietic cells and neurons in Bcl-x-deficient mice. Science 267(5203):1506-1510.

Nakayama K, Nakayama K, Negishi I, Kuida K, Sawa H, Loh DY (1994) Targeted disruption of Bcl-2 alpha beta in mice: occurrence of gray hair, polycystic kidney disease, and lymphocytopenia. Proc Natl Acad Sci U S A 91(9):3700-3704.

Newmeyer DD, Farschon DM, Reed JC (1994) Cell-free apoptosis in Xenopus egg extracts: inhibition by Bcl-2 and requirement for an organelle fraction enriched in mitochondria. Cell 79(2):353-364.

Nicholson DW, Ali A, Thornberry NA, Vaillancourt JP, Ding CK, Gallant M, Gareau Y, Griffin PR, Labelle M, Lazebnik YA, et al (1995) Identification and inhibition of the ICE/CED-3 protease necessary for mammalian apoptosis. Nature 376(6535):37-43.

Nicholson DW and Thornberry NA (1997) Caspases: killer proteases. Trends Biochem Sci 22: 299-306.

Nieke J, Schachner M (1985) Expression of the neural cell adhesion molecules L1 and N-CAM and their common carbohydrate epitope L2/HNK-1 during development and after transection of the mouse sciatic nerve. Differentiation 30(2):141-151.

Oltvai ZN, Milliman CL and Korsmeyer SJ (1993) Bcl-2 heterodimerizes in vivo with a conserved homolog, Bax, that accelerates programmed cell death. Cell 74(4) 609-619.

Oppenheim RW (1989) The neurotrophic theory and naturally occurring motoneuron death. Trends Neurosci 12(7):252-255.

Oppenheim RW, Prevette D, Tytell M, Homma S (1990) Naturally occurring and induced neuronal death in the chick embryo in vivo requires protein and RNA synthesis: evidence for the role of cell death genes. Dev Biol 138(1):104-113.

Oppenheim RW (1991) Cell death during development of the nervous system. Annu Rev Neurosci 14:453-501.

Parsadanian AS, Cheng Y, Keller-Peck CR, Holtzman DM, Snider WD (1998) Bcl-xL is an antiapoptotic regulator for postnatal CNS neurons. J Neurosci 18(3):1009-1019.

Peinado-Ramon, P., Salvador, M., Villegas-Perez, M.P. and Vidal-Sanz, M. (1996) Effects of axotomy and intraocular administration of NT-4, NT-3, and brain-derived neurotrophic factor on the survival of adult rat retinal ganglion cells. A quantitative in vivo study. Invest Ophthalmol Vis Sci 37(4): 489-500.

Perry VH, Brown MC and Gordon S (1987) The macrophage response to central and peripheral nerve injury. A possible role for macrophages in regeneration. J Exp Med 165: 1218-1223.

Polyak K, Xia Y, Zweier JL, Kinzler KW, Vogelstein B (1997) A model for p53-induced apoptosis. Nature 389(6648):300-305.

Porciatti V, Pizzorusso T, Cenni MC, Maffei L (1996) The visual response of retinal ganglion cells is not altered by optic nerve transection in transgenic mice overexpressing Bcl-2. Proc Natl Acad Sci U S A 93(25):14955-14959.

Portera-Cailliau C, Hedreen JC, Price DL, Koliatsos VE (1995) Evidence for apoptotic cell death in Huntington disease and excitotoxic animal models. J Neurosci 15(5 Pt 2):3775-3787.

Prendergast J, Stelzner DJ (1976) Changes in the magnocellular portion of the red nucleus following thoracic hemisection in the neonatal and adult rat. J Comp Neurol 166(2):163-171.

Pronk GJ, Ramer K, Amiri P, Williams (1996) LT Requirement of an ICE-like protease for induction of apoptosis and ceramide generation by REAPER. Science 271(5250):808-810.

Quigley HA, Nickells RW, Kerrigan LA, Pease ME, Thibault DJ and Zack DJ (1995) Retinal ganglion cell death in experimental glaucoma and after axotomy occurs by apoptosis. Invest Ophthalmol Vis Sci 36(5): 774-786.

Rabacchi SA, Bonfanti L, Liu XH and Maffei L (1994) Apoptotic cell death induced by optic nerve lesion in the neonatal rat. J Neurosci 14(9): 5292-5301.

Raff MC (1992) Social controls on cell survival and cell death. Nature 356(6368):397-400.

Raivich G, Kreutzberg GW (1987) Expression of growth factor receptors in injured nervous tissue. I. Axotomy leads to a shift in the cellular distribution of specific beta-nerve growth factor binding in the injured and regenerating PNS. J Neurocytol 6(5):689-700.

Ratan RR, Murphy TH, Baraban JM (1994) Oxidative stress induces apoptosis in embryonic cortical neurons. J Neurochem 62(1):376-379.

Ratan RR, Baraban JM (1995) Apoptotic death in an in vitro model of neuronal oxidative stress. Clin Exp Pharmacol Physiol 22(4):309-310.

Reddington M, Priller J, Treichel J, Haas C, Kreutzberg GW (1995) Astrocytes and microglia as potential targets for calcitonin gene related peptide in the central nervous system. Can J Physiol Pharmacol 73(7):1047-1049.

Reed JC (1997) Double identity for proteins of the Bcl-2 family. Nature 387(6635):773-776.

Richardson PM, Ebendal T (1982) Nerve growth activities in rat peripheral nerve. Brain Res 246(1):57-64.

Rodriguez-Tebar A, Dechant G, Barde YA (1990) Binding of brain-derived neurotrophic factor to the nerve growth factor receptor. Neuron 4(4):487-492.

Roy N, Deveraux QL, Takahashi R, Salvesen GS, Reed JC (1997) The c-IAP-1 and c-IAP-2 proteins are direct inhibitors of specific caspases. EMBO J 16(23):6914-6925.

Rudin CM, Van Dongen J, Thompson CB (1996) Apoptotic signaling in lymphocytes. Curr Opin Hematol 3(1):35-40.

Russelakis-Carneiro M, Silveira LC, PerryVH (1996) Factors affecting the survival of cat retinal ganglion cells after optic nerve injury. J Neurocytol 25(6): 393-402.

Sakhi S, Bruce A, Sun N, Tocco G, Baudry M, Schreiber SS (1994) p53 induction is associated with neuronal damage in the central nervous system. Proc Natl Acad Sci U S A 91(16):7525-7529.

Schendel SL, Xie Z, Montal MO, Matsuyama S, Montal M, Reed JC (1997) Channel formation by antiapoptotic protein Bcl-2. Proc Natl Acad Sci U S A 94(10):5113-5118.

Schinder AF, Olson EC, Spitzer NC, Montal M (1996) Mitochondrial dysfunction is a primary event in glutamate neurotoxicity. J Neurosci 16(19):6125-6133.

Schlesinger PH, Gross A, Yin XM, Yamamoto K, Saito M, Waksman G, Korsmeyer SJ (1997) Comparison of the ion channel characteristics of proapoptotic BAX and antiapoptotic BCL-2. Proc Natl Acad Sci U S A 94(21):11357-11362.

Schwartz LM and Milligan CE (1996) Cold thoughts of death : the role of ICE proteases in neuronal cell death. Trends Neurosci 19 :555-562.

Sendtner M, Kreutzberg GW, Thoenen H (1990) Ciliary neurotrophic factor prevents the degeneration of motor neurons after axotomy. Nature 345(6274):440-441.

Sievers J, Hausmann B, Unsicker K, Berry M (1987) Fibroblast growth factors promote the survival of adult rat retinal ganglion cells after transection of the optic nerve. Neurosci Lett 76(2):157-162.

Siliprandi R, Canella R, Carmignoto G (1993) Nerve growth factor promotes functional recovery of retinal ganglion cells after ischemia. Invest Ophthalmol Vis Sci 34(12):3232-3245.

Simpson PB, Russell JT (1998) Role of mitochondrial Ca2+ regulation in neuronal and glial cell signalling. Brain Res Rev 26(1):72-81.

Skulachev VP (1998) Cytochrome c in the apoptotic and antioxidant cascades. FEBS Lett 423(3):275-280.

Snider WD and Thanedar S (1989) Target dependence of hypoglossal motor neurons during development and in maturity. J Comp Neurol 279: 489-497.

Snider WD, Elliott JL, Yan Q (1992) Axotomy-induced neuronal death during development. J Neurobiol 23(9):1231-1246.

Streit WJ, Graeber MB and Kreutzberg GW (1988) Functional plasticity of microglia: a review. Glia 1: 301-315.

Tanabe H, Eguchi Y, Shimizu S, Martinou JC, Tsujimoto Y (1998) Death-signalling cascade in mouse cerebellar granule neurons. Eur J Neurosci 10(4):1403-1411.

Tanaka S, Suzuki K, Watanabe M, Matsuda A, Tone S, Koike T (1998) Upregulation of a new microglial gene, mrf-1, in response to programmed neuronal cell death and degeneration. J Neurosci 18(16):6358-6369.

Tatton WG, Chalmers-Redman RM (1998) Mitochondria in neurodegenerative apoptosis: an opportunity for therapy? Ann Neurol 44(3 Suppl 1):S134-141.

Tetzlaff, W, NR Kobayashi, KMG Giebl, BJ Tusi, SL Cassar, AM Bedard (1994). Response of rubrospinal and cortico spinal neurons to injury and neurotrophins. Prog. Brain Res. 103: 271-286.

Thompson CB (1995) Apoptosis in the pathogenesis and treatment of disease Science 267(5203):1456-1462.

Thornberry NA and Lazebnik Y (1998) Caspases: Enemies within. Science 281:1317-1322.

Trapp BD, Hauer P, Lemke G (1988) Axonal regulation of myelin protein mRNA levels in actively myelinating Schwann cells. J Neurosci 8(9):3515-3521.

Troy CM, Stefanis L, Greene LA, Shelanski ML (1997) Mechanisms of neuronal degeneration: a final common pathway? Adv Neurol 72:103-111.

Trupp M, Ryden M, Jornvall H, Funakoshi H, Timmusk T, Arenas E, Ibanez CF (1995) Peripheral expression and biological activities of GDNF, a new neurotrophic factor for avian and mammalian peripheral neurons. J Cell Biol 130(1):137-148.

Ucker DS, Obermiller PS, Eckhart W, Apgar JR, Berger NA, Meyers J (1992) Genome digestion is a dispensable consequence of physiological cell death mediated by cytotoxic T lymphocytes. Mol Cell Biol 12(7):3060-3069.

Vanags DM, Porn-Ares MI, Coppola S, Burgess DH, Orrenius S (1996) Protease involvement in fodrin cleavage and phosphatidylserine exposure in apoptosis. J Biol Chem 271(49):31075-31085.

Vaux DL, Cory S, Adams JM (1988) Bcl-2 gene promotes haemopoietic cell survival and cooperates with c-myc to immortalize pre-B cells. Nature 335(6189):440-442.

Vejsada R, Tseng JL, Lindsay RM, Acheson A, Aebischer P, Kato AC (1998) Synergistic but transient rescue effects of BDNF and GDNF on axotomized neonatal motoneurons. Neuroscience 84(1):129-139.

Vercesi AE, Kowaltowski AJ, Grijalba MT, Meinicke AR, Castilho RF (1997) The role of reactive oxygen species in mitochondrial permeability transition. Biosci Rep 17(1):43-52.

Villa PG, Henzel WJ, Sensenbrenner M, Henderson CE, Pettmann B (1998) Calpain inhibitors, but not caspase inhibitors, prevent actin proteolysis and DNA fragmentation during apoptosis. J Cell Sci 111 (Pt 6):713-722.

Villegas-Perez, M.P., Vidal-Sanz, M., Rasminsky, M., Bray, G.M. and Aguayo, A.J. (1993) Rapid and protracted phases of retinal ganglion cell loss follow axotomy in the optic nerve of adult rats. J Neurobiol 24(1) : 23-36.

Wang CY, Mayo MW, Korneluk RG, Goeddel DV, Baldwin AS Jr (1998) NF-kappaB antiapoptosis: induction of TRAF1 and TRAF2 and c-IAP1 and c-IAP2 to suppress caspase-8 activation. Science 281(5383):1680-1683.

Wang HG, Rapp UR, Reed JC (1996) Bcl-2 targets the protein kinase Raf-1 to mitochondria. Cell 87(4):629-638.

Ware CF, VanArsdale S, VanArsdale TL (1996) Apoptosis mediated by the TNF-related cytokine and receptor families. J Cell Biochem 60(1):47-55.

Watanabe M, Sawai H, Fukuda Y (1997) Survival of axotomized retinal ganglion cells in adult mammals. Clin Neurosci 4(5):233-239.

Weibel D, Kreutzberg GW and Schwab ME (1995) Brain-derived neurotrophic factor (BDNF) prevents lesion-induced axonal die-back in young rat optic nerve. Brain Res 679 (2): 249-254.

Wu W, Li Y, Schinco FP (1994) Expression of c-jun and neuronal nitric oxide synthase in rat spinal motoneurons following axonal injury. Neurosci Lett 179(1-2): 157-161.

Wyllie AH (1980) Glucocorticoid-induced thymocyte apoptosis is associated with endogenous endonuclease activation. Nature 284(5756):555-556.

Xiao M, McLeod D, Cranley J, Williams G, Boulton M (1999) Growth factor staining patterns in the pig retina following retinal laser photocoagulation. Br J Ophthalmol 83(6):728-736.

Xiang J, Chao DT and Korsmeyer SJ (1996) BAX-induced cell death may not require interleukin 1 beta-converting enzyme-like proteases. Proc Natl Acad Sci USA 93(25): 14559-14563.

Xiang H, Kinoshita Y, Knudson CM, Korsmeyer SJ, Schwartzkroin PA, Morrison RS (1998) Bax involvement in p53-mediated neuronal cell death. J Neurosci 18(4):1363-1373.

Xue D, Horvitz HR (1995) Inhibition of the *Caenorhabditis elegans* cell-death protease CED-3 by a CED-3 cleavage site in baculovirus p35 protein. Nature 377(6546):248-251.

Yang E, Zha J, Jockel J, Boise LH, Thompson CB, Korsmeyer SJ (1995) Bad, a heterodimeric partner for Bcl-XL and Bcl-2, displaces Bax and promotes cell death. Cell 80(2):285-291.

Yin XM, Oltvai ZN, Korsmeyer SJ (1994) BH1 and BH2 domains of Bcl-2 are required for inhibition of apoptosis and heterodimerization with Bax. Nature 369(6478):321-323.

Yoles E, Schwartz M (1998) Elevation of intraocular glutamate levels in rats with partial lesion of the optic nerve. Arch Ophthalmol 116(7): 906-910.

Yu SP, Yeh C, Strasser U, Tian M, Choi DW (1999) NMDA receptor-mediated K+ efflux and neuronal apoptosis. Science 284(5412):336-339.

Yuan JY, Horvitz HR (1990) The Caenorhabditis elegans genes ced-3 and ced-4 act cell autonomously to cause programmed cell death. Dev Biol 138(1):33-41.

Yuan J, Shaham S, Ledoux S, Ellis HM and Horvitz HR (1993) The *C. elegans* cell death gene ced-3 encodes a protein similar to mammalian interleukin-1 beta-converting enzyme. Cell 75(4): 641-652.

Yuan J (1997) Transducing signals of life and death. Curr Opin Cell Biol 9(2):247-251.

Zamzami N, Hirsch T, Dallaporta B, Petit PX, Kroemer G (1997) Mitochondrial implication in accidental and programmed cell death: apoptosis and necrosis. J Bioenerg Biomembr 29(2):185-193.

Zamzami N, Brenner C, Marzo I, Susin SA, Kroemer G (1998) Subcellular and submitochondrial mode of action of Bcl-2-like oncoproteins. Oncogene 16(17):2265-2282.

Zhou Q, Krebs JF, Snipas SJ, Price A, Alnemri ES, Tomaselli KJ, Salvesen GS (1998) Interaction of the baculovirus anti-apoptotic protein p35 with caspases. Specificity, kinetics, and characterization of the caspase/p35 complex. Biochemistry 37(30):10757-10765.

Zou H, Henzel WJ, Liu X, Lutschg A, Wang X (1997) Apaf-1, a human protein homologous to *C. elegans* CED-4, participates in cytochrome c-dependent activation of caspase-3. Cell 90(3):405-413.

8

Gene Expression in Axotomized Neurons: Identifying the Intrinsic Determinants of Axonal Growth

Karl J. L. Fernandes and Wolfram G. Tetzlaff
University of British Columbia, Vancouver, Canada

I. INTRODUCTION

One of the most striking features of neurons in the mature peripheral nervous system (PNS) is their ability to survive and to regenerate their axons following axonal injury (i.e. axotomy) (reviewed in Fu and Gordon, 1997). In contrast, those neurons confined to the CNS of higher vertebrates fail to regenerate their axons, an outcome that has been attributed to an inhibitory CNS environment (Fitch and Silver, 1997; Keirstead and Steeves, 1998; Schwab, 1996). It has become increasingly evident that the success of axonal regeneration is also dependent on the intrinsic growth properties of the axotomized neuron. This notion was most elegantly demonstrated in a landmark experiment by Richardson and Issa (1984), in which they showed that a preceding axotomy of the peripheral axon of DRG neurons elicits an enhanced growth response from the central axon. In comparison to PNS neurons, CNS neurons generally display weak intrinsic survival and growth responses, and are highly susceptible to the numerous growth-inhibitory molecules found within the CNS microenvironment (Fawcett, 1997; this volume, chapters by Schwab and David &McKerracher).

It has long been noted that the capacity for axonal growth varies according to the injured neuron's age, type/localization in the nervous system, and axotomy to cell body distance (Lieberman, 1974; Ramon y Cajal, 1991). Cross-age transplantation experiments, using co-cultures of retinal ganglion cells with tectum explants (Chen *et al.*, 1995) or entorhinal cortex neurons with dentate gyrus explants (Li *et al.*, 1995), have provided support for the concept that immature neurons generally have a greater propensity than adult neurons to regenerate within the adult mammalian CNS (Chen *et al.*, 1995; Davies *et al.*, 1994; Dusart *et al.*, 1997; Li *et al.*, 1995; Wictorin *et al.*, 1990). Within the mature mammalian nervous system, different neuron types also have varying growth capacities; for instance, while many CNS neuron types readily extend axons into peripheral nerve or embryonic tissue transplants, cerebellar Purkinje cells are notorious for their reluctance to regenerate in these paradigms (Dusart and Sotelo, 1994; Rossi *et al.*, 1997; Rossi *et al.*, 1995). The complexity is further compounded by the demonstration that individual CNS neurons exhibit different capacities for growth depending on whether they are axotomized relatively close or distant from their cell bodies (Figure 1) (Richardson *et al.*, 1984; Tetzlaff *et al.*, 1994). This growth is tightly correlated with the expression of regeneration-associated genes following a close but not distant axotomy (Doster *et al.*, 1991; Tetzlaff *et al.*, 1991; Fernandes et al., 1999).

Studies such as those above have laid the foundation for the concept that the intrinsic growth state of the axotomized neuron is a fundamental determinant of its potential for regenerative success. Consequently, a weak intrinsic growth state may limit the possibility for axonal regeneration even in situations where a permissive growth environment is offered. Conversely, a strong intrinsic growth state may allow axotomized neurons to override the growth-inhibitory influences associated with the CNS microenvironment (Berry *et al.*, 1996; Davies *et al.*, 1994; Davies *et al.*, 1997). For example, embryonic hippocampal or adult peripheral neurons implanted into the CNS can undergo extensive axonal elongation within myelinated tracts of the CNS (Davies *et al.*, 1994; Davies *et al.*, 1997). Similarly, activation of the growth program in adult DRG neurons by axotomy of the peripheral axon stimulates some of the central axons to overcome the site of injury and grow a few millimeters within the spinal cord (Neumann and Woolf, 1999).

First steps towards enhancing the intrinsic capacity for growth have been taken, as treatments of the neuronal cell body have been shown to enhance axonal regeneration of rubrospinal neurons into peripheral nerve transplants (Kobayashi *et al.*, 1997) and of retinal ganglion cells within the inhibitory environment of the optic nerve (Berry *et al.*, 1996). Thus, the current challenge is to identify the essential molecular determinants of axonal regeneration and to delineate the mechanisms involved in their regulation.

Axotomized neurons undergo a wide spectrum of changes in gene expression, which affect levels of transcription factors (Section IV.C), cytoskeletal proteins (Section III.B), growth cone proteins (Section III.C), cell adhesion and guidance proteins (Section III.D), secreted proteins (Section III.E), ion channels, signaling molecules, and a variety of other stress response/homeostatic/housekeeping proteins (Table 1). Recent transgenic studies have begun to evaluate the functional importance of specific gene products for axonal elongation (Aigner *et al.*, 1995; Caroni, 1997a; Caroni et al., 1997a; Chen et al., 1997; Hilton et al., 1997).

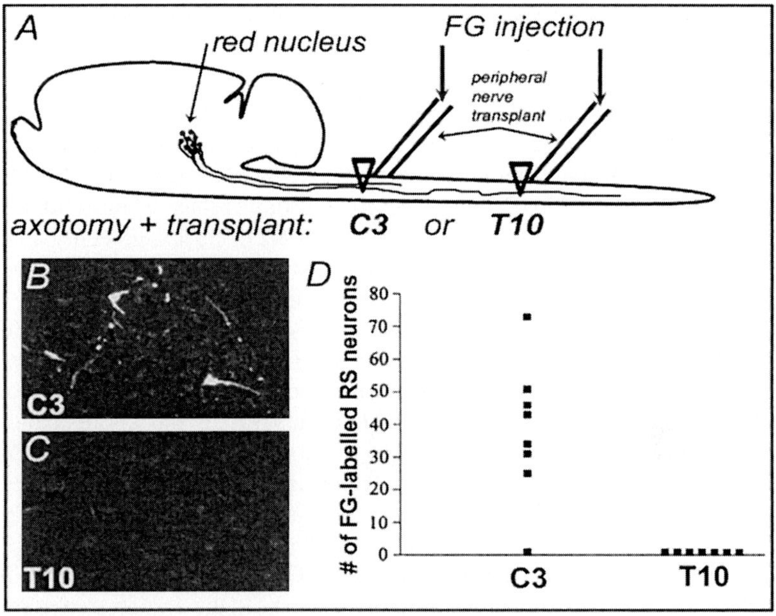

Figure 1 Rubrospinal neurons regenerate into peripheral nerve transplants after cervical (proximal) but not thoracic (distal) axotomy. (A) The rubrospinal tract was severed at either the C3 or T10 level of the rat spinal cord, and an autologous sciatic nerve graft was implanted into the lesion site. 2 months later the free end of the graft was exposed to 5% FluoroGold, and 14d later the animals were sacrificed. (B) Numerous retrogradely labelled rubrospinal neurons were found in the axotomized red nucleus of cervically axotomized rats. (C) No FluoroGold-positive neurons were identified in the red nucleus after thoracic axotomy. (D) Numbers of regenerating rubrospinal neurons after C3 or T10 procedures. (Modified from Fernandes et al., 1999)

However, as many changes are outside the scope of this review, they are only listed in Table 1. Furthermore, as the precise significance of many of these changes is uncertain, in this review we have focused on the changes in neuronal gene expression having demonstrated roles in axonal growth, and that appear to be mitigated in CNS neurons having impaired survival/growth responses. Given the very large number of studies examining the responses of axotomized neurons, it is inevitable that some work will inadvertently be omitted from this review, and we apologize to our colleagues in advance for such oversights.

II. SURVIVAL FACTORS FOR AXOTOMIZED NEURONS

Axotomized PNS neurons in the adult nervous system are exposed to an abundant supply of non-target-derived neurotrophic factors (NTFs) (Korsching, 1993; Oppenheim, 1996). The sources of these NTFs include the Schwann cells and invading macrophages of the distal nerve segment (BDNF, NT-3, NT-4/5, CNTF, LIF, GDNF, IGFs, interleukins), the axotomized motoneurons themselves (BDNF, FGF-2, IL-6) and their perineuronal cells (LIF,CNTF, IL-6, and TGF-β), as well as afferents which terminate on the cell bodies of the axotomized neurons (BDNF). This situation contrasts to that of the developing nervous system, where PNS neurons are critically dependent on target-derived NTFs (reviewed in: Davies, 1994; Lewin and Barde, 1996; Snider *et al.*, 1992). This also contrasts with the situation of CNS neurons in the mature nervous system, which are exposed to insufficient quantities of NTFs to maintain survival of the entire axotomized population. For example, only about 50% of subcortically axotomized corticospinal neurons are detectable after 7 days, and this is reduced to 30 % in the presence of function blocking BDNF antibodies, indicating that BDNF is an endogenous survival factor for the surviving neurons (Giehl *et al.*, 1998). Infusion of BDNF into the cortex rescues the entire population (Giehl and Tetzlaff, 1996), further indicating insufficient endogenous trophic support for the axotomized corticospinal neurons. Similarly, cervically axotomized rubrospinal neurons undergo considerable atrophy, which can be prevented by infusion of BDNF into the vicinity of the red nucleus (Kobayashi *et al.*, 1997). One reason for the inadequate level of NTFs for axotomized CNS neurons may be lack of autocrine/paracrine support, as comparatively little trophic factor expression has been detected in CNS neurons after injury. For example, although both motoneurons and rubrospinal neurons express the trkB and FGFR-1 receptors, axotomized motoneurons upregulate these receptors and their ligands BDNF and FGF-2, while axotomized rubrospinal neurons decrease their expression of these receptors and ligands (Kobayashi *et al.*, 1996b; Stilwell et al., 1997).

Which NTFs have been implicated in the survival of axotomized PNS neurons? At present, three families of NTFs (neurotrophins, the gp130-dependent family of cytokines, and insulin-like growth factors) have clearly been shown to contribute to PNS neuron survival. Adenoviral-mediated over-expression of these NTFs is sufficient to prolong the survival of axotomized neonatal motoneurons for as long as five weeks (Gravel *et al.*, 1997). The evidence for their involvement in the survival of axotomized adult PNS neurons is discussed below.

Firstly, the trkB high affinity receptor for the neurotrophins BDNF and NT-4/5 is up-regulated in axotomized adult sensory and motoneurons (Ernfors *et al.*, 1993; Kobayashi *et al.*, 1996a; Piehl *et al.*, 1994; Tonra *et al.*, 1998). Since these PNS neurons are exposed to BDNF both in peripheral nerve (Funakoshi *et al.*, 1993) and at the level of their cell bodies (Altar *et al.*, 1997; Fawcett *et al.*, 1998; Kobayashi *et al.*, 1996a; Tonra *et al.*, 1998), trkB up-regulation may be an important factor contributing to survival after axotomy. In accord with this idea, in trkB knockout mice there is a 50% decrease in the apparent number of surviving facial motoneurons five days after transection of the facial nerve on postnatal day 5 (Alcantara *et al.*, 1997).

Secondly, axotomized motoneurons up-regulate gp130 (Yao *et al.*, 1997), the common signal transducing component for the receptor complexes of the CNTF/LIF/IL-6/cardiotrophin family of cytokines (Heinrich *et al.*, 1998; Murphy *et al.*, 1997). CNTF is synthesized by myelinating Schwann cells and perineuronal astrocytes (Friedman *et al.*, 1992; Richardson, 1994; Sendtner *et al.*, 1994; Sendtner *et al.*, 1992). Although it is not known to be actively secreted, CNTF appears to be released from injured Schwann cells (Sendtner *et al.*, 1992), and its retrograde transport is enhanced following axotomy (Curtis *et al.*, 1993). Studies of CNTF knockout mice have demonstrated that it is an endogenous survival factor for both normal (Masu *et al.*, 1993) and axotomized (Sendtner *et al.*, 1997) motoneurons. Unlike CNTF, whose expression in the distal stump decreases after axotomy (Sendtner *et al.*, 1992), LIF production increases in the injured nerve (Curtis *et al.*, 1994), and LIF/CNTF double knockout mice have nearly 35% fewer countable facial motoneurons 14 days after facial nerve axotomy of 4 week old mice (Sendtner *et al.*, 1996). Recent studies have also demonstrated a role for a third gp130-dependent member of this cytokine family. IL-6 is normally up-regulated in axotomized sensory and motoneurons (Klein *et al.*, 1997; Murphy *et al.*, 1999; Murphy *et al.*, 1995). It may act in an autocrine/paracrine fashion, but it also appears to be involved in the activation of perineuronal glial cells (Klein *et al.*, 1997). IL-6 knockout mice have a 20% reduction in survival of axotomized adult sensory neurons after two weeks, as well as impaired regeneration of the sensory axons (Murphy *et al.*, 1999; Zhong *et al.*, 1999).

Thirdly, insulin-like growth factors (IGFs) have been implicated in partially mediating the survival and regeneration of axotomized PNS neurons (Glazner *et al.*, 1993; Pu *et al.*, 1999). Following axotomy, IGFs are up-regulated within the distal nerve segment (Glazner *et al.*, 1994). Sequestering IGFs by infusion of IGF binding proteins or IGF antibodies onto the axotomized neonatal sciatic nerve reduced survival of sciatic motoneurons by 20% five days after axotomy on P2 (Pu *et al.*, 1999).

Taken together, the above studies indicate that there is a rich enough quantity of trophic support in and around axotomized adult rodent PNS neurons to support survival of the majority of the population. This is correlated with increased retrograde transport of CNTF, LIF, and neurotrophins after axotomy (Curtis *et al.*, 1993; Curtis *et al.*, 1994; Curtis *et al.*, 1998). Although these neurotrophic factor signalling pathways converge, their actions can be synergistic (Mitsumoto *et al.*, 1994; Rajan *et al.*, 1998; Wu and Bradshaw, 1996), and in some cases, they may have differential effects on health of the neuronal cell body or axon (Haase *et al.*, 1997; Sagot *et al.*, 1998).

Recent studies have begun to unravel the underlying mechanisms by which neurotrophic factors regulate neuronal survival. The majority of the neurotrophic factor receptors described above possess an intracellular tyrosine kinase domain that, when in a phosphorylated state, binds adaptor proteins that initiate several downstream signalling pathways (Kaplan and Miller, 1997; Kaplan and Stephens, 1994). The essential pathway involved in maintaining neuronal survival appears to be the PI-3-kinase induced activation of the serine/threonine kinase Akt (Dudek *et al.*, 1997; (Klesse *et al.*, 1999; Nunez and Delpeso, 1998). Studies of neurotrophin-dependent primary cultures of sympathetic neurons indicate that inhibition of an endogenous Akt/PKB/RAC pathway, by transfection with dominant negative Akt, inhibits neurotrophin-mediated survival of these neurons (Crowder and Freeman, 1998); conversely, stimulation of this pathway using constitutively active constructs is sufficient to enable these neurons to survive in the absence of neurotrophins (Crowder and Freeman, 1998; Philpott *et al.*, 1997). Activation of the PI-3-kinase/Akt kinase pathway has been shown to elicit a number of downstream effects, including phosphorylation-induced inactivation of proteins involved in apoptotic cell death processes (i.e. BAD, caspase 9, and a forkhead transcription factor) (Brunet *et al.*, 1999; Cardone *et al.*, 1998; Datta *et al.*, 1997; Delpeso *et al.*, 1997; Nunez and Delpeso, 1998), potentiation of Ca^{2+} currents through L-type calcium channels (Blair *et al.*, 1999), suppression of jun N-terminal kinase (JNK)–associated apoptosis (Cerezo *et al.*, 1998; Okubo *et al.*, 1998; Shimoke *et al.*, 1999), activation of the transcription factor CREB (Du and Montminy, 1998), and posttranscriptional regulation of gene expression for the cell cycle regulator cyclin D (Muisehelmericks *et al.*, 1998), perhaps by regulating activity of mRNA binding proteins (Gingras *et al.*, 1998). The PI-3-kinase/Akt kinase pathway appears to be negatively regulated within cells by phosphatases such as SHIP (Liu *et al.*, 1999), the PTEN tumor suppressor (Ramaswamy *et al.*, 1999; Stambolic *et al.*, 1998), and perhaps calcineurin (Wang *et al.*, 1999). Moderate increases in intracellular calcium through ligand or voltage gated Ca^{2+} channels, which can increase survival of many cultured neurons, can also activate Akt directly via phosphorylation by the Ca^{2+}/calmodulin-dependent protein kinase kinase (CaM-KK) (Bhave *et al.*, 1999; Foulstone *et al.*, 1999; Yano *et al.*, 1998). Future work will determine how these insights can be utilized to prevent the axotomy-induced degeneration of CNS neurons.

III. GROWTH OF THE INJURED AXON

A. Role of the cell body in different axonal growth modes

1. Axonal regeneration and axonal sprouting are mechanistically distinct.

The terms *axonal regeneration* and *axonal sprouting* have been variously defined on anatomical, functional or molecular criteria. Here we assign these terms to the two extreme modes of axonal growth, based respectively on the participation and lack of participation of the cell body. The distinction on the basis of cell body involvement is supported by recent *in vitro* experiments by Smith & Skene (1997), who observed that DRG neurons grow long extended axons if axotomized prior to explantation ("regeneration"), but only short and highly branched axons if explanted without a prior axotomy ("sprouting"). The ability of the pre-axotomized neurons to "regenerate" was dependent on the transcription of new gene products, as the "regeneration" growth mode was lost in the presence of RNA synthesis inhibitors. The gene expression associated with axonal regeneration (regeneration-associated genes, or "RAGs") is the subject of Sections III.B–E. Importantly, however, it has become apparent that intermediate phenotypes of axonal growth exist between the extremes of local sprouting and rapid long distance regeneration. Thus, as discussed below, while axonal growth *per se* does not require RAG expression, the axonal growth ultimately achieved depends on both the level/types of RAGs expressed and the growth permissiveness of the axonal environment.

2. Limited axonal growth can occur without up-regulation of RAGs

In the growth permissive environment of the PNS, motoneurons expressing only low levels of RAGs can terminally sprout into adjacent denervated muscle fibers without up-regulating markers of RAG expression such as GAP-43 (Bisby *et al.*, 1996). However, low levels of RAG expression allows only slow axonal elongation, even in a growth permissive environment. This is illustrated following central axotomy of DRG neurons, which have a heterogeneous baseline expression of RAGs. After axonal injury of their central axons, DRG neurons show little change in RAG expression - most notably no increase in GAP-43 (Schreyer and Skene, 1993). While the subpopulation of DRG neurons expressing high baseline levels of GAP-43 can still regrow at several mm/d within the permissive dorsal roots, the majority of DRG neurons have only a low baseline expression of GAP-43 and these regrow with a markedly reduced rate of axonal elongation (Andersen and Schreyer, 1999). Thus, in the absence of a cell body response, differences in the baseline levels of RAGs result in different growth abilities.

3. Rapid long distance axonal regeneration is associated with pronounced changes in RAG expression

Rapid axonal growth (3-4 mm/d in the rodent) in the presence of pronounced changes in RAG expression reliably occurs in axotomized PNS neurons. The strong up-regulation of RAGs observed in PNS neurons is contrasted by the incomplete induction of, and failure to sustain, RAG expression in axotomized CNS neurons. For example, different populations of brainstem-spinal cord neurons of the fish show different regenerative propensities after spinal cord injury. Those neurons which express a fuller complement of regeneration-associated genes, i.e. GAP-43 + L1, show greater axonal regeneration than those which increase only GAP-43, which is greater than those that show no changes at all (Becker *et al.*, 1998). Similarly, neurons over-expressing multiple growth-associated proteins, i.e.

GAP-43 and CAP-23, have greater axonal growth than those expressing either protein individually (Caroni, 1997a).

In most cases of axonal growth elicited through experimental manipulations of the CNS environment, it remains to be determined whether these manipulations have stimulated (i) rapid axonal growth via enhanced expression of RAGs (peripheral-type "regeneration"), or (ii) intermediate forms of slower/limited axonal growth driven only by the pre-existing baseline levels of RAG expression. Stimulating RAG expression in axotomized CNS neurons is presumably a prerequisite to enabling them to undergo rapid axonal regeneration, and should ultimately result in more vigorous and effective regeneration within the CNS.

B. Cytoskeletal proteins involved in axonal extension and growth cone function

The roles of cytoskeletal proteins in regenerating neurons have been reviewed elsewhere (Bisby and Tetzlaff, 1992; Tetzlaff *et al.*, 1991; Tetzlaff *et al.*, 1988). Axotomized PNS neurons strongly up-regulate tubulins and actin, and down-regulate the intermediate filaments with the exception of peripherin. In the following section, we briefly summarize recent data on actin and intermediate filaments in regenerating neurons, and focus on the roles of tubulins and microtubule-associated proteins.

Actin plays an important role in cytoskeletal motility (Mitchison and Cramer, 1996) and is the major cytoskeletal element of filopodia and lammellipodia of the growth cone. In growing neurons, the mRNA and protein for the β-actin isotype is particularly up-regulated, and is enriched within the growth cone and axon (Bassell *et al.*, 1998; Micheva *et al.*, 1998). While the vast majority of actin in synthesized in the cell body, recent *in vitro* data on sympathetic neurons suggest that a small portion (<1%) may be produced in the axon itself (Eng *et al.*, 1999). The biological significance of this fraction is at present not understood. Actin is known to interact with myosins and present models favor a myosin V and myosin II-powered retrograde f-actin flow in the leading edge of the growth cone (Lin *et al.*, 1996; Suter and Forscher, 1998). The forward advancement of the growth cone seems to involve the assembly of actin at the distal plus end and the anchoring of the filament to the cell membrane (Suter and Forscher, 1998). Myosin II immunoreactivity has been reported at the leading edge of the axonal growth cone, and the inhibition of the myosin IIB isoform expression with antisense oligonucleotides attenuated filopodial extension *in vitro* (Wylie *et al.*, 1998). It remains to be shown whether myosin expression changes after axotomy. Actin-myosin II interactions are regulated by myosin light-chain kinase which shows increased expression in axotomized retinal ganglion cells (Jian *et al.*, 1996). The crucial involvement of this molecular machinery in axonal regeneration *in vivo* can only be inferred since most data are based on *in vitro* studies. It may be of interest to learn that the increased expression of actin is only transient and normalizes in facial motoneurons between 3-4 weeks after axotomy even in the absence of target contact. The increased expression in rubrospinal neurons lasted for one week only (Tetzlaff *et al.*, 1991).

The intermediate filaments include the type IV neurofilaments, α-internexin and nestin, and the type III peripherin (Lee and Cleveland, 1996). The type IV intermediate filaments are down-regulated by axotomy, and are therefore likely not critical to axonal regeneration *per se*. For example, mice lacking neurofilaments are capable of motoneuron axonal regeneration, but have hampered axonal maturation (Zhu *et al.*, 1997). Down-regulation of the neurofilament network may in fact facilitate the axonal transport of actin and tubulins (Tetzlaff *et al.*, 1996; Zhu *et al.*, 1998), as neurofilaments interact with both tubulin and actin and are as much as 10 fold more abundant within the axon than microtubules (Hirokawa *et al.*, 1988). Supporting this idea, the rate of tubulin transport is dramatically increased in mice lacking the neurofilament light chain, and reduced in mice over-expressing the neurofilament heavy chain (Collard *et al.*, 1995). Interestingly, in some nonmammalian vertebrates whose CNS neurons do regenerate, high levels of neurofilaments are observed (Asch *et al.*, 1998; Jacobs *et al.*, 1997; Zhao and Szaro, 1995). This may be due to differences in the chemical properties of neurofilaments between mammals and various other vertebrates (Pleasure *et al.*, 1989). Although neurofilaments are down-regulated in axotomized mammalian neurons, the self-assembly competent type III intermediate filament, peripherin, is up-regulated in axotomized sensory and motoneurons, suggesting that it may be involved in the outgrowth process (Chadan *et al.*, 1994a; Chadan *et al.*, 1994b; Oblinger *et al.*, 1989; Troy *et al.*, 1990). Similarly, the type III intermediate filament, plasticin, is up-regulated in regenerating goldfish optic nerves (Canger *et al.*, 1998; Fuchs *et al.*, 1994; Glasgow *et al.*, 1992).

Microtubules are of central importance for cell motility and are critically involved in the process of axonal transport and elongation of the axonal shaft (comprehensively reviewed in Kobayashi and Mundel, 1998; Laferriere *et al.*, 1997). Several isotypes (in mouse, 7 α and 6 β isotypes) are known to exist, and the high neuronal expression of tubulins during developmental and regenerative axonal elongation is due to the selective up-regulation of the Tα1 α-tubulin isotype and the βII and βIII β-tubulin isotypes. The exact chemical significance of these specific isotypes is unclear; as in many studies the various α or β isotypes appear to be functionally redundant. However, the strong up-regulation of tubulins is most likely required as substrate for elongation of the microtubule-based cytoskeleton. Axotomized PNS neurons maintain their high expression of tubulins throughout the process of axonal regeneration, and indefinitely if target reconnection is prevented (Jiang *et al.*, 1994).

In comparison to the PNS, tubulin expression is significantly less robust in nonregenerating axotomized CNS neurons, such as corticospinal neurons (Kost and Oblinger, 1993), transcollosal cortical neurons (Elliott *et al.*, 1999), retinal ganglion cells (Fournier and McKerracher, 1997), or rubrospinal neurons (Tetzlaff *et al.*, 1991). However, if provided with a growth-permissive peripheral nerve environment, those CNS neurons regenerating into the transplants do exhibit high expression of growth-associated tubulin isotypes (Fournier and McKerracher, 1997; Fernandes et al., 1999). This observation may indicate the presence of trophic molecules within the peripheral nerve transplants capable of enhancing tubulin gene expression (for further discussion see Sections 4.4 and 5.1).

Microtubule associated proteins (MAPs) are critical stabilizers of tubulin polymerization and microtubule dynamics (Chau *et al.*, 1998; Drewes *et al.*, 1998; Tokuraku *et al.*, 1999). The members of the families of MAPs found in neurons are the high molecular weight MAP1A, MAP1B, and MAP2, and the low molecular weight MAP2c, MAP2d, and tau isoforms. Axonal elongation during development is associated with expression of MAP1B, MAP2c and juvenile isoforms of tau. The expression of all of these decline with neuronal maturation, and is replaced with MAP1A, MAP2, and mature tau isoforms. Interestingly, following axotomy the expression of MAPs does not recapitulate the pattern observed during development, demonstrating that developmental and regenerative axon growth are not identical (Chambers and Muma, 1997; Fawcett *et al.*, 1994). However, in the particular case of the axon-specific MAP1B, homozygous knockout mutant mice fail to develop, and heterozygotes exhibit delayed brain development and structural abnormalities of the nervous system (Takei *et al.*, 1997), confirming a critical role in neuronal development. Furthermore, MAP1B inhibition *in vitro* inhibits axonal elaboration on laminin (DiTella *et al.*, 1996). Tau appears to facilitate axonal regeneration, as high levels correlate with fast regeneration (Fawcett *et al.*, 1994). The binding of MAPs to microtubules, in turn, is critically regulated by phosphorylation by the recently discovered microtubule-affinity-regulating kinases (Drewes *et al.*, 1998), however at present there is little information available on changes in their activity during regeneration.

C. Cytoplasmic growth cone proteins mediating plasticity of the terminal axon

The major functions of the axonal growth cone are to sense the axonal environment and direct the growth of the axon in response to appropriate cues. Classical axonal transport studies by Skene identified substantial increases in the levels of specific proteins within the fast axonal transport fraction of injured peripheral nerves, but which are virtually undetectable in normal nerves (reviewed in Skene, 1989). Of these Growth Associated Proteins (GAPs), the most intensely studied has been the 27.6 kD protein GAP-43 (F1, B-50, neuromodulin).

GAP-43 protein has been demonstrated to interact with several other growth cone proteins, including cytoskeletal proteins (actin, spectrin, fodrin), calmodulin, and the α subunits of the G proteins (reviewed in Benowitz and Routtenberg, 1997). GAP-43 is involved in the transduction of extracellular signals to the actin based submembrane cytoskeleton. In support of this, gene deletion shows that GAP-43 is necessary for FGF receptor-mediated increases in growth cone motility in response to cell adhesion molecules N-CAM and L1 (Meiri *et al.*, 1998). In the context of CNS regeneration, it is interesting to note that GAP-43 over-expression *in vitro* renders DRG growth cones more resistant to myelin-associated growth cone inhibitors (Aigner and Caroni, 1995). It is possible that this overriding effect of GAP-43 is mediated by cAMP dependent mechanisms, as cAMP and pertussis toxin-sensitive pathways appear to underlie neurotrophin-induced resistance to myelin-associated growth inhibitors *in vitro* (Cai *et al.*, 1999).

Other functionally-related proteins, such as CAP-23, MARKS and paralemmin have many similar properties to GAP-43 (Kutzleb *et al.*, 1998; Wiederkehr *et al.*, 1997) and unpublished data from our laboratory show that the expression of at least CAP-23 (others not studied) is increased after axonal injury.

Expression of GAP-43 has been a useful and reliable marker of an enhanced intrinsic neuronal growth state. Ample evidence correlates the induction of GAP-43 expression in axotomized neurons with their subsequent growth propensity. For example, the expression of GAP-43 is virtually undetectable in most parts of the mature nervous system, but it is highly expressed in developing and regenerating PNS neurons (Fernandes *et al.*, 1999; Schreyer and Skene, 1993; Skene, 1989; Tetzlaff *et al.*, 1991). Within the mature CNS, basal levels of GAP-43 expression are typically very low in most areas, though it remains highly expressed in some regions such as the neocortex. Induction of GAP-43 following axotomy in the CNS is generally extremely limited, and highly dependent on the axotomy-to-cell body distance (discussed in Section 4.4). As in the PNS, rapid axonal regeneration only occurs in those situations where CNS neurons express GAP-43, i.e. axonal regeneration into peripheral nerve transplants only occurs with more proximal (GAP-43-inducing) injuries (Doster *et al.*, 1991; Fernandes *et al.*, 1999; Richardson *et al.*, 1984). It is important to note that GAP-43 expression is not, by itself, sufficient for axonal regeneration. Specific transgenic over-expression of GAP-43 did not stimulate axonal regeneration of CNS neurons, but did, however, increase axonal sprouting (Buffo *et al.*, 1997). Neither is GAP-43 absolutely necessary for axonal growth *per se*. GAP-43 knockout mice appear to have a grossly normal nervous system, but exhibit defects in axonal pathfinding (Kruger *et al.*, 1998; Sretavan and Kruger, 1998; Strittmatter *et al.*, 1995; Zhu and Julien, 1999). However, GAP-43 is presumably regulated in a similar fashion as a full complement of genes involved in axonal growth, which when expressed together, enhance the intrinsic ability of axons to grow. For example, neurons over-expressing GAP-43 and a closely related growth-associated protein, CAP-23, have greater growth properties than those over-expressing either protein alone (Caroni, 1997a; Caroni, 1997b). Taken together, these results suggest that the expression of certain growth cone proteins reduces the threshold (as proposed by Caroni) or enhances the sensitivity of axons to respond to local environmental cues.

D. Membrane-associated cell adhesion/guidance molecules and their receptors

Cell adhesion molecules and axonal guidance molecules play an important role in the development of the PNS and CNS (Walsh and Doherty, 1997). The expression of CAMs changes considerably in regenerating peripheral nerves (Martini, 1994; Schachner *et al.*, 1995). L1, a member of the immunoglobulin superfamily, has been observed to increase in regenerating peripheral nerves (Bernhardt *et al.*, 1996; Kamiguchi and Lemmon, 1997; Martini *et al.*, 1994). L1 has a specific sequence that directly targets its transport to the neuronal growth cone (Kamiguchi and Lemmon, 1998). More than one binding mechanism may account for the broad range of functions of L1: homophilic binding, binding to integrin or axogenin-1, as well as FGF-receptor dimerization and activation (Brummendorf *et al.*, 1998). Antibodies to FGF receptors or dominant negative FGF receptors inhibit the L1 stimulation of neurite outgrowth (Viollet and Doherty, 1997; Walsh and Doherty, 1997). Consistent with this idea, transgenic L1 over-expression in astrocytes enhanced axonal sprouting characteristics (Mohajeri *et al.*, 1996). *In vivo*, L1 knock out mice show hypoplasia of the corticospinal tract which also fails to decussate properly at the pyramid (Cohen *et al.*, 1998; Dahme *et al.*, 1997). While the development of peripheral nerves in these mice shows only minor impairment in the ensheathment of axons by Schwann cells (Dahme *et al.*, 1997), it remains to be shown whether regeneration after peripheral nerve injury is hampered or whether other CAMs compensate for a deficit in L1 expression. In spinal cord projection neurons of lower vertebrates, the expression of L1 and N-CAM corresponds well with their regenerative propensity (Becker *et al.*, 1998). Similarly, L1 is expressed in retinal ganglion cells successfully regenerating into peripheral nerve transplants (Jung *et al.*, 1997). Thus, the expression of cell adhesion molecules correlates with better regenerative success.

Expression of FGFRs, which are receptors for FGFs as well as for cell adhesion molecules like L1 and NCAM, is probably critical for axonal growth (Saffell *et al.*, 1997). Dominant negative FGFR receptors perturb the formation of the retino-tectal projection (McFarlane *et al.*, 1996) and changes of FGFR expression after axotomy suggest a role in regeneration. Motoneurons and sensory neurons express high levels of FGFR-1 which are maintained or even increase after axotomy (Huber *et al.*, 1997; Klimaschewski *et al.*, 1999; Stilwell *et al.*, 1997). This most likely enhances their responsiveness to the ligands mentioned above. Interestingly, the expression of FGFR-1 decreases in rubrospinal neurons after axotomy which may contribute to their failure to regenerate (Stilwell *et al.*, 1997).

The functional distinction between the above mentioned cell adhesion molecules (CAMs) and the currently identified families of axonal guidance molecules (Semaphorins, Netrins and Ephrins) may be somewhat artificial. Both play roles in axonal guidance during neural development. Since semaphorins, netrins and ephrins can have axonal growth inhibiting as well as growth promoting effects it is conceivable that they are re-expressed after axotomy and that they may also contribute to the failure of axonal regeneration in the CNS of higher vertebrates. While there are no published studies on the involvement of netrins in axonal regeneration thus far, recent work by Pasterkamp and colleagues (Pasterkamp *et al.*, 1998b) demonstrated co-expression of Semaphorin III/D and its neuropilin-1 receptor component in peripheral motoneurons. After axotomy, the expression of

Sema III/D was down-regulated while neuropilin-1 expression remained unchanged. A possible involvement in CNS regeneration failure was recently suggested by demonstrating the expression of Sema III and its neuropilin receptor after olfactory bulb lesions (Pasterkamp *et al.*, 1998a; Pasterkamp *et al.*, 1999).

The Eph receptor family, named after the first member discovered in an erythropoietin-producing hepatocellular carcinoma cell line, is the largest known receptor tyrosine kinase family with over a dozen members (Flanagan and Vanderhaeghen, 1998). This family has been implicated in a variety of patterning events during embryonic development, particularly in the nervous system. Ephrins play a role in axonal guidance and topographic map formation of neural projections (Gale and Yancopoulos, 1997; Orioli and Klein, 1997). After denervation of the optic tectum some guidance properties are re-expressed, suggesting a role for this "family" in the reformation of the retino-tectal map (Drescher *et al.*, 1997; Wizenmann *et al.*, 1993). The gene deletion of Eph4 demonstrated an involvement of the Eph/ephrin-family in the formation of the corticospinal tract. Hence, it is conceivable that these factors also play a role in neural regeneration (Aubert *et al.*, 1995; Miranda *et al.*, 1999).

E. Secreted neuronal proteins modifying the axonal environment

A general pattern observed in axotomized PNS neurons is a shift in the cellular targets of proteins secreted from the axon. There is (i) a down-regulation of proteins involved in modifying the post-synaptic cell, and (ii) an up-regulation of proteins involved in remodelling the extracellular matrix (ECM) and Schwann cell micro-environment. In the case of (i), among the down-regulated proteins are agrins and neuregulins (Bermingham-McDonogh *et al.*, 1997; Thomas *et al.*, 1995), which are involved in assembling and maintaining the post-synaptic structure, and neurotransmitter enzymes, such as the cholinergic enzymes choline acetyltransferase and acetylcholinesterase in motoneurons (Fernandes *et al.*, 1998). These reductions in features of the differentiated phenotype of neurons are likely passive in nature, resulting from interruption of target contact, and may contribute to axonal regeneration only by reducing nonessential metabolic costs. In the case of (ii), however, given the importance of the Schwann cell and ECM microenvironment for axonal growth, it is reasonable to postulate that such changes contribute significantly to the successful outcome of peripheral nerve regeneration. Some of these changes are described below.

Regenerating axons appear to actively condition the environment through which they are growing, a function largely performed by secretion of proteases such as the serine protease Plasminogen Activator (PA) (reviewed in Seeds *et al.*, 1997), and matrix metalloproteinases (MMPs). MMPs are a family of calcium-dependent zinc-containing proteases critically involved in the remodelling of the extracellular matrix. They are expressed in the developing CNS and PNS (Nordstrom *et al.*, 1995), as well as by regenerating PNS neurons. Their endopeptidase activity cleaves a variety of extracellular matrix molecules, including collagen, chondroitin sulfate proteoglycans, laminin and fibronectin, which can be potent growth-inhibitory influences for axons in the CNS and PNS. In the periphery, MMPs are secreted by Schwann cells in the distal nerve segment (Kherif *et al*., 1998) as well as from the growth cone of the growing axons (Zuo *et al*., 1998). *In vitro* studies have demonstrated that neuronal MMP expression and activity is stimulated by neurite outgrowth-promoting trophic factors, such as NGF, FGF-1 and FGF-2 (Fillmore *et al*., 1992; Machida *et al*., 1991; Nordstrom *et al*., 1995). Furthermore, inhibition of this MMP activity prevents trophic-factor promoted growth into gels of ECM or collagen (Muir, 1994; Pittman and Williams, 1989). Interestingly, MMP activity is also required for process outgrowth of oligodendrocytes (Uhm *et al*., 1998) and for migration of glioblastomas (Belien *et al*., 1999; Hensel *et al*., 1998). Similar to MMPs, PAs are also secreted from the growth cone (Pittman, 1985) and are associated with enhanced migratory and growth abilities of neurons (Pittman and DiBenedetto, 1995; Yuguchi *et al*., 1997), including during activity-dependent plasticity (Seeds *et al*., 1995).

Neuronal production of Schwann cell mitogens also appears to be an important mechanism by which growing peripheral axons influence their environment. The protein REG-2 has recently been identified as a powerful proliferative agent for Schwann cells, and is expressed by growing peripheral neurons during axonal development and regeneration (Livesey *et al*., 1997). Inhibition of Reg-2 actions compromised the regenerative ability of peripheral motoneurons (Livesey *et al*., 1997). Whether axonally-derived mitogenic factors, such as Reg-2, play a role in CNS regeneration remains to be shown.

IV. REGULATION OF AXOTOMY-INDUCED GENE EXPRESSION

A. Signals of axotomy

Some thirty years ago, Cragg published a seminal review on the possible signals of axonal injury (Cragg, 1970). He summarized over 10 conceivable scenarios by which the neuronal cell body might be informed about an axonal injury to trigger those changes important for axonal regeneration Despite this early conceptualization of the possible signals of axotomy, our understanding of their molecular nature is still incomplete. Since unveiling the signals of axotomy may help in the development of strategies for optimizing the growth state of the axotomized neuron, a brief summary on recent progress in this area is provided below.

The temporal sequence of events following axotomy suggests that more than one type of signal is responsible for the multitude of changes observed. Both rapid and slower retrograde signals appear to be involved. For instance, an unmasking of a connexin-43 epitope is seen in glial cells surrounding axotomized rat facial motoneurons within 45 minutes of axonal injury (Rohlmann *et al*., 1994), lending support to the notion that some injury signals are electrically propagated (Ambron and Walters, 1996) and might act via Ca++ and cAMP to regulate gene expression. This first phase may be followed by a wave of rapid molecular signals, e.g. the loss of "NF-kB binding" which somehow spreads from the site of axonal injury as fast as 2.5 cm within 15min (Povelones *et al.*, 1997). This reflects a velocity of 2400 mm/day and would by far exceed the reported speed of retrograde transport at 50-200 mm/day.

These first two rapid phases of changes are believed to be followed by signals travelling at the velocity of retrograde transport. A retrogradely transported signal appears to be involved in the increase in c-Jun-kinase and is seen within 30 min after axonal injury close to the cell body, yet it takes 3 hours when the axon is injured further distally (Kenney and Kocsis, 1997b). Retrogradely transported signals may include *intrinsic* neuronal molecules modified/activated at the site of injury (Bisby, 1982; Cragg, 1970), e.g. MAP-kinases (Ambron and Walters, 1996), as well as *extrinsic* molecules obtained from the injury site or axonal targets. *Extrinsic* retrogradely transported signals can be classified as "positive" or "negative" in nature. Positive signals include factors originating at the injury site while negative signals are due to the interruption of axonally transported factors normally reaching the cell body from the target or the axonal environment (Skene, 1989; Woolf *et al.*, 1990). The transcription of growth-associated genes such as GAP-43 and Tα1-tubulin appears to be the result of negative signals, as their expression can be stimulated by blockade of axonal transport without axotomy (Skene, 1989; Wu *et al.*, 1993). The GAP-43 repressor is likely derived from the terminal or target cells rather than the sheath cells of the nerve, as no difference in GAP-43 expression was observed after proximal versus distal axotomies in spinal motoneurons and DRG neurons (Fernandes *et al.*, 1999; Liabotis and Schreyer, 1995). Although the identity of the presumed target-derived repressor(s) for GAP-43 and Tα1-tubulin in PNS neurons is not known, there is general agreement that negative signals resulting from interruption of target-derived trophic factors trigger a large number of changes after axonal injury. This concept is based on the identification of target-derived trophic factors that, when applied exogenously, normalize axotomy-induced changes. For example, application of BDNF to axotomized motoneurons normalizes the decrease in ChAT and AChE (Fernandes *et al.*, 1998). However, since such results are often achieved with high non-physiological concentrations of factors, the inverse approach of inhibiting endogenous trophic factors should help clarify the functions of the endogenous factors.

The concept of a lesion site derived positive signal is exemplified by the actions of Leukemia Inhibitory Factor (LIF). LIF is produced within hours after injury by non-neuronal cells, most likely Schwann cells and satellite cells (Matsuoka *et al.*, 1997). A variety of axotomy-induced neuropeptide changes, most prominently galanin, are not observed in mice with gene deletions for LIF (Sun and Zigmond, 1996; Zigmond *et al.*, 1996). LIF application to intact neurons has only a partial effect on the induction of galanin and the induction seen after axotomy is due to a concomittant depletion of target-derived NGF (Zigmond and Sun, 1997; Shadiack *et al.*, 1998) (Corness *et al.*, 1998). Thus, positive and negative signals operate in concert. In addition to deficiencies in neuropeptide expression, peripheral neurons of LIF knockout mice also fail to up-regulate the Schwann cell mitogen Reg-2 (Livesey *et al.*, 1997). The effects of LIF are likely to be mediated via gp130-JAK-STAT signalling, as LIF knockout mice also fail to activate STAT signalling after injury (Rajan *et al.*, 1995). LIF mRNA expression can be induced by a variety of cytokines and growth factors and it appears that activation of cAMP, diacylglycerol, Ca++ signalling as well as the ERK-pathways are involved (Nagamoto-Combs *et al.*, 1999).

Positive signals are also likely to contribute to the survival of axotomized PNS neurons, as an apparent signal from mast cells is responsible for the up-regulation of IL-6 in axotomized PNS neurons, and IL-6 knockout mice have elevated axotomy-induced motoneuron death (Murphy *et al.*, 1999).

In addition to these lesion site derived "positive signals," other positive signals seem to come from the denervated distal nerve and are taken up as the regenerating axons grow through it. In hypoglossal motoneurons, the re-expression of the low affinity p75-neurotrophin receptor was only observed if the crushed axons were allowed to regenerate; nerve ligation or blockade of axonal transport inhibited p75 up-regulation (Bussmann and Sofroniew, 1999).

B. Transcriptional/post-transcriptional regulation of gene expression

As a tool for investigating the transcriptional regulation of growth-associated gene expression, transgenic mice have been generated expressing the bacterial lacZ gene from either a 1.1 kb promoter region of the Tα1 α-tubulin gene (Gloster *et al.*, 1994) or promoter plus intronic regions of the GAP-43 gene (Vanselow *et al.*, 1994). Although GAP-43 transcription is known to be repressed by specific DNA-binding proteins (Chiaramello *et al.*, 1996), mouse lines from both transgenic models show a transcriptional up-regulation of these genes during development and axonal regeneration. It remains to be determined, however, whether this transcriptional up-regulation accounts for most or only some of the axotomy-induced up-regulation of their respective mRNAs. In the case of tubulin, for example, the 168-fold reduction in β-II tubulin mRNA expression between postnatal day 5 and adult rats has been shown to be accompanied by only a 3.6-fold reduction in the rate of transcription, suggesting that decreased mRNA stability is the predominant regulatory process involved (Bhattacharya *et al.*, 1991; Moskowitz and Oblinger, 1995b). Furthermore, an autoregulatory feedback mechanism by which soluble tubulin monomers reduce the stability of tubulin mRNAs has been demonstrated for β-tubulins (Yen *et al.*, 1988a; Yen *et al.*, 1988b). Similarly, in the case of GAP-43, elements within the 3' untranslated region bind to mRNA-binding proteins that regulate the mRNA stability (Neve *et al.*, 1999). Since *in vitro* studies suggest that GAP-43 mRNA is stabilized by neurotrophic factors, (Nishizawa, 1994; Perrone-Bizzozero *et al.*, 1993; Tsai *et al.*, 1997) *in vivo* observations of increases in GAP-43 expression in response to trophic or inflammatory factors may be mediated via alterations in GAP-43 mRNA stability rather than transcription (discussed further in Section D.). Interestingly, one recent study has shown that the protein kinase Akt/PKB, which is activated downstream of many growth factor tyrosine kinase receptors, phosphorylates and inactivates 4E-BP1, a translational repressor (Gingras *et al.*, 1998). However, the relative importance of transcriptional and posttranscriptional mechanisms in the regulation of injury- and trophic factor-induced gene expression has yet to be evaluated.

C. Transcription factors mediating neuronal gene expression

DNA-binding proteins are important transcriptional regulators of gene expression. In light of the vast array of changes in gene expression following axotomy, which are mediated at least in part via altered transcription rates (Section IV.B), it has been of interest to determine whether specific transcription factors may act upstream as global switches for an axonal growth/regeneration "program." The independent expression of subsets of RAGs indicates that there is most likely not one simple program. Extensive research has investigated axotomy-induced changes in the activation state of constitutive transcription factors (i.e. CREB, CREM, ICER, ATF-1, ATF-2, SRF, NFkB) or the expression level of inducible transcription factors (i.e. c-jun, junB, junD, c-fos, fra-1, fra-2, krox-20, krox-24), However, their downstream targets and functional role in regeneration has for the most part remained elusive and we therefore refer the reader to Table 1 and more comprehensive reviews (Herdegen and Leah, 1998). Of these transcription factors, c-jun is the most highly correlated with axotomy.

Despite extensive investigation, the role of c-jun after axotomy has nevertheless remained enigmatic, as its expression is paradoxically associated with both neuronal survival/regeneration, and neuronal degeneration (Herdegen *et al.*, 1997b). In support of a function in survival/regeneration, for example, c-jun is induced and maintained in DRG neurons after peripheral axotomy but is only transiently up-regulated in a small proportion of them after dorsal rhizotomy (Broude *et al.*, 1997; Kenney and Kocsis, 1997a); allowing access of the injured dorsal roots to fetal transplant tissue promotes their growth and up-regulates c-jun expression (Broude *et al.*, 1997). Similarly, when axotomized CNS neurons are given access to peripheral nerve transplants, c-jun expression is selectively maintained in those neurons that regenerate into the transplants (Anderson *et al.*, 1998; Broude *et al.*, 1999; Hull and Bahr, 1994; Robinson, 1995). Contrasting these findings are studies implicating c-jun in neuronal death. For instance, direct overexpression of c-jun in cultured sympathetic neurons provokes their death, while inhibiting c-jun prevents their death following NGF-deprivation (Estus *et al.*, 1994; Ham *et al.*, 1995). Similarly, JNK inhibitors rescue neurons from apoptosis in several models of injury (Glicksman *et al.*, 1998).

Elucidating the precise effects mediated by c-jun has been complicated by its widespread expression following a variety of stimuli, including axotomy, trophic factor withdrawal, ischemia, irradiation, and metabolic stress (reviewed in Herdegen *et al.*, 1997b). Since formation of AP-1 transcription factors requires c-jun to dimerize with either other jun or fos family members or with non-AP-1-

binding transcription factors, such as ATF-2, the complexity of its apparent functions may be due to variable affinities of different AP-1 complexes for (i) AP-1 consensus binding sites, (ii) other regulatory nuclear factors (Wasylyk *et al.*, 1998) , or (iii) regulation by kinases such as JNKs (Herdegen *et al.*, 1998).

Inhibition of c-jun expression is likely to provide some indication of its functions. Although c-jun knockout mice die developmentally, RGC in c-jun -/- retinae extended axons normally when transplanted into wildtype mice, demonstrating that c-jun is dispensable for developmental axonal growth (Herzog *et al.*, 1999). However, an involvement of c-jun in the expression of neuropeptides by axotomized sensory neurons has been demonstrated using anti-sense knockdown of c-jun expression: inhibition of c-jun expression in cultures of sensory neurons specifically inhibited their expression of VIP and neuropeptide Y (Mulderry and Dobson, 1996).

D. Influence of the axotomy-to-cell body distance on neuronal gene expression

Direct comparison of the influence of the axotomy-to-cell body distance on growth-associated gene expression in PNS motoneurons and CNS rubrospinal neurons has revealed important differences (Figure 2) (Fernandes *et al.*, 1999). While successfully regenerating sciatic motoneurons up-regulated GAP-43 mRNA expression to comparable levels (5-20 fold) regardless of the axotomy-to-cell body distance, rubrospinal neurons showed a 5-fold increase after cervical axotomy and no increase after thoracic axotomy. GAP-43 expression in axotomized RGCs is also sensitive to the axotomy-to-cell body distance, as injuries must be closer than 3 mm to stimulate an up-regulation (Doster *et al.*, 1991). In corticospinal neurons, the threshold distance is as little as 200 microns (K.M. Giehl and W. Tetzlaff, unpublished observations).

Tubulin expression also shows differences between axotomized rubrospinal and sciatic motoneurons. In both systems, tubulin mRNA increases to a greater extent with proximal than distant axotomy. However, in the case of sciatic motoneurons the tubulin up-regulation was sustained for at least 3 weeks, while the up-regulation was aborted after only 7 days in rubrospinal neurons (Fernandes *et al.*, 1999; Tetzlaff *et al.*, 1991).

There is currently no simple explanation for the stronger up-regulation of regeneration-associated genes following axotomy proximal than distal from the cell body of CNS neurons. As discussed in Sections 4A and 4.B, the GAP-43 gene is believed to be transcriptionally repressed by retrogradely transported target-derived factors in PNS neurons; thus, regardless of lesion site, PNS neurons up-regulate it to similar levels. One possible explanation for the distance-dependent expression in the CNS is continued transcriptional repression supplied from axonal collaterals located more proximal to an injury site. However, this simple model does not fit in the optic system, where there are no collaterals. It has also been proposed that CNS myelin along the proximal axon is an additional source of transcriptional GAP-43 repression (Kapfhammer and Schwab, 1994; Skene, 1992), so that shorter proximal axons exert less inhibition of GAP-43 expression than longer axons. However, myelin fractions do not repress GAP-43 expression in developing cortical neurons (Karimi-Abdolrezaee and Schreyer, 1998), and treatment of Purkinje cell axons with antibodies to the NI-35/250 components of myelin fail to induce expression of GAP-43 (Zagrebelsky *et al.*, 1998).

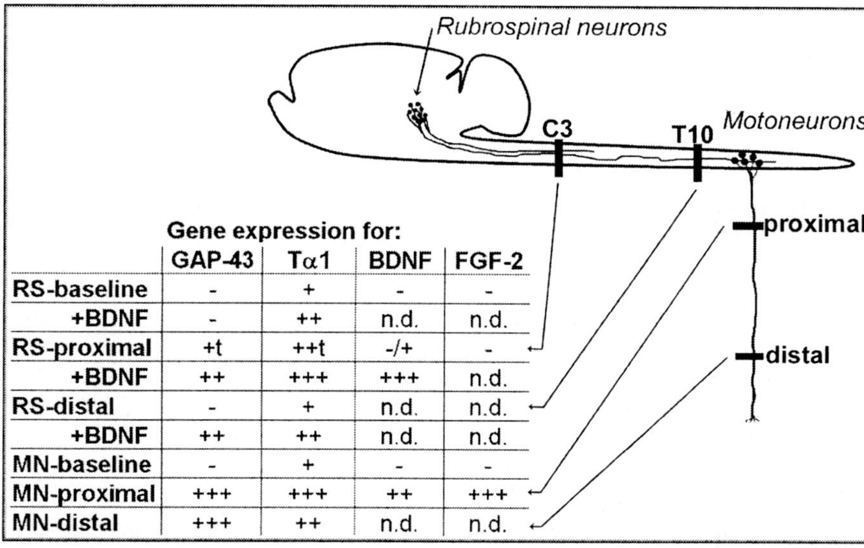

	Gene expression for: GAP-43	Tα1	BDNF	FGF-2
RS-baseline	-	+	-	-
+BDNF	-	++	n.d.	n.d.
RS-proximal	+t	++t	-/+	-
+BDNF	++	+++	+++	n.d.
RS-distal	-	+	n.d.	n.d.
+BDNF	++	++	n.d.	n.d.
MN-baseline	-	+	-	-
MN-proximal	+++	+++	++	+++
MN-distal	+++	++	n.d.	n.d.

Figure 2 Changes in regeneration-associated gene expression after proximal and distal axotomy of rubrospinal neurons and motoneurons, and effects of BDNF.(Expression is not detectable (-), low (+), medium (++), high (+++), or not determined (n.d.). "t" = transient).

We propose an alternative explanation, that prolonged injury-induced expression of GAP-43 involves two processes: (i) increased transcription of mRNAs via release from target-derived transcriptional repression, and (ii) additional positive signals to maintain the elevated mRNA expression. Such positive signals may occur in the form of neurotrophic factors (Kobayashi *et al.*, 1997) or inflammatory factors (Section 5A) (Lu and Richardson, 1991; Lu and Richardson, 1995; Richardson and Lu, 1994). Since NGF has been shown to increase GAP-43 expression *in vitro* via posttranscriptional mechanisms (Nishizawa, 1994; Perrone-Bizzozero *et al.*, 1993; Tsai *et al.*, 1997) , we further suggest that the positive signals of neurotrophic or inflammatory factors on GAP-43 expression are mediated via mRNA binding proteins that increase its mRNA stability (Neve *et al.*, 1999) and/or rate of translation into protein. Using this model, we would interpret the above observations in the following fashion: (i) Axotomy of PNS neurons derepresses GAP-43 transcription, and the variety of neurotrophic factors and cytokines to which they are exposed (Section II) stabilize the GAP-43 mRNAs; (ii) Cervically axotomized rubrospinal neurons show an initial up-regulation of growth-associated genes due to loss of target-derived repression, but this is attenuated and transient due to the lack of trophic/inflammatory factors to stabilize the growth-associated mRNAs; (iii) Thoracically axotomized rubrospinal neurons neither atrophy nor up-regulate GAP-43 because sustaining collaterals continue to supply both target-derived GAP-43 repressors *and* adequate trophic support to prevent the massive atrophy seen following cervical axotomy; (iv) Retinal ganglion cells increase GAP-43 expression after lesions that are within 3 mm from the retina but not farther (Doster *et al.*, 1991) because injury-related cytokines and trophic factors reach the neuronal cell bodies from the intra-orbital lesion sites but not from the more distant intracranial lesion sites; (v) Furthermore, positive signals arising from peripheral nerve transplants may explain why only those neurons regenerating into them maintain high expression of axotomy-induced genes such as GAP-43, tubulins, and c-jun. Conceptually, this model provides an attractive mechanism (i.e. enhancement/stabilization of the pre-existing transcriptional state of the neuron) with which to explain the diverse effects of neurotrophic factors over the course of neurodevelopment (proliferation, growth, terminal differentiation). However, at present this model is speculative.

V. PROSPECTS FOR AXONAL GROWTH OF CNS NEURONS

The success of axonal growth in the CNS appears to be determined by the relative levels of environmental growth inhibition and intrinsic neuronal growth capability, subjects described in detail in other chapters in this volume. Shifting the balance in favor of axonal growth has been mainly attempted by modifying the axonal environment, via removal of CNS myelin (Dyer *et al.*, 1998; Keirstead *et al.*, 1995), antibody-mediated masking of inhibitory myelin epitopes (Raineteau *et al.*, 1999; Thallmair *et al.*, 1998; von Meyenburg *et al.*, 1998), transplants of peripheral nerve or embryonic tissue (Bregman *et al.*, 1998; Bregman *et al.*, 1997; Bregman and Reier, 1986; Cheng *et al.*, 1996), or the use of Schwann cells (Xu *et al.*, 1997; Xu *et al.*, 1999), olfactory ensheathing glia (Li *et al.*, 1997; Li *et al.*, 1998; Ramon-Cueto *et al.*, 1998), cells genetically modified to over-express growth factors (Grill *et al.*, 1997; Menei *et al.*, 1998) or sensitized macrophages (Lazarov-Spiegler *et al.*, 1996; Schwartz *et al.*, 1999a; Schwartz *et al.*, 1999b).

An alternative strategy is to enhance the intrinsic growth capacity of the axotomized neurons in an effort to overcome the growth inhibitory molecules within the CNS. This strategy may be subdivided into two approaches: (1) enhancing the vigor of the neuronal growth response, and (2) enhancing the resistance of the axon to growth inhibitors. Both approaches are only in their beginnings and the first promising results are described below.

A. Improving neuronal cell body responses to axotomy with neurotrophic factors

Experiments from the laboratory of Martin Berry (Berry *et al.*, 1996) have shown that placement of a peripheral nerve segment into the vitreous of the eye stimulates the regeneration of crushed retinal ganglion cell (RGC) axons within the growth inhibitory environment of the optic nerve. In these experiments, it is most likely

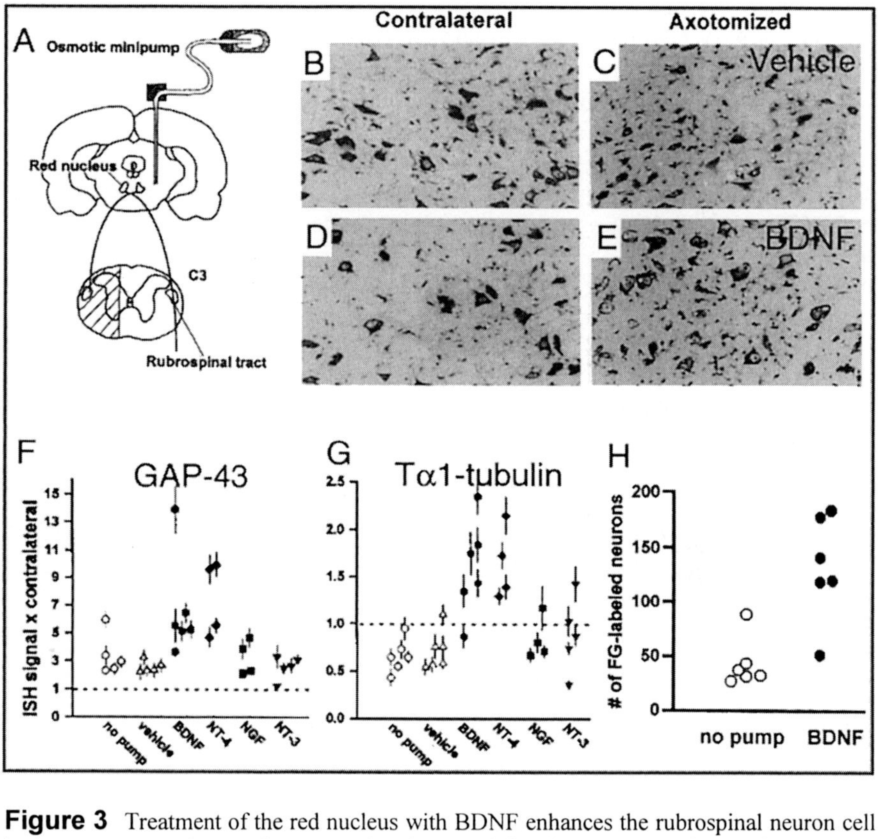

Figure 3 Treatment of the red nucleus with BDNF enhances the rubrospinal neuron cell body response and axonal regeneration into peripheral nerve transplants after cervical axotomy. (A) The rubrospinal tract was transected at the C3 level of the rat spinal cord, and neurotrophin or vehicle solution was infused into the red nucleus for 7-14d using an osmotic pump. (B-E) Axotomized rubrospinal neurons are highly atrophied in control or vehicle (C) treated animals, but the atrophy is prevented with BDNF (E) or NT-4/5 application. The BDNF or NT-4/5-treated rubrospinal neurons also have enhanced expression of regeneration-associated genes such as GAP-43 (F) and Tα1-tubulin (G). Implantation of peripheral nerve transplants into the C3 injury site together with distal application of FluoroGold (as in figure 1) demonstrated that BDNF treatment at the cell bodies stimulated more rubrospinal neurons to regenerate their axons (I). (Modified from Kobayshi et al., 1997).

that Schwann cells of the degenerating peripheral nerve segment served as a source of neurotrophic factors (NTFs) for the cell bodies of the axotomized RGCs. The specific NTFs mediating this response have not been deter-mined, but Schwann cells in degenerating peripheral nerve are known to release a variety of factors, including various members of neurotrophin and cytokine families (Section II.). We have recently shown that direct infusion of neurotrophins into the cortex maintains the survival of subcortically axotomized corticospinal neurons and simultaneously enhances their expression of the regeneration-associated genes GAP-43 and Tα1 α-tubulin (Giehl and Tetzlaff, 1996). Similarly, neurotrophin infusion into the midbrain prevents rubrospinal neuron atrophy and also stimulates GAP-43 and Tα1 α-tubulin expression (Kobayashi *et al.*, 1997). Furthermore, the BDNF treatment increases the number of rubrospinal axons regenerating into peripheral nerve transplants at cervical (Figure 3) (Kobayashi *et al.*, 1997) and, for the first time, at thoracic spinal cord levels (Kobayashi et al., in preparation). The expression of GAP-43 may be particularly relevant to CNS axonal regeneration, as overexpression of GAP-43 *in vitro* prevents growth cone collapse in response to myelin (Aigner and Caroni, 1995), apparently rendering the actin cytoskeleton of the growth cone less susceptible to collapse in response to environmental growth inhibitors.

In addition to neurotrophins, inflammation can also stimulate GAP-43 expression. Lu and Richardson (Lu and Richardson, 1991; Lu and Richardson, 1995) have shown that an inflammatory reaction created by injection of *Corynebacterium parvum* into rat dorsal root ganglia stimulates the expression of GAP-43 in a similar manner as peripheral axotomy, and also accelerates the regeneration of the crushed dorsal root. More recently, an intracellular purine sensitive mechanism has been found to play a role in axonal outgrowth of goldfish retinal ganglion cells, giving rise to strategies of neuronal treatment with inosine-derivates (Benowitz *et al.*, 1998).

B. Enhancing growth cone resistance to growth inhibitors

The intracellular mechanisms of growth cone collapse appear to converge onto members of the Rho family of small GTPases (Gallo and Letourneau, 1998). Promising recent efforts have focused on rendering growth cones at the site of a CNS lesion resistant to growth inhibitors by "short-circuiting" their intracellular growth cone collapse pathways. McKerracher and coworkers showed that crushed optic nerves treated with a bacterial inhibitor of RhoA, the C3 subunit of botulinum toxin, allowed profuse sprouting of the injured axons beyond the lesion site (Lehmann et al., 1999).

Intriguing recent developments indicate that neurotrophic factors at the level of the injury site may also be able to inhibit growth cone collapse. Cerebellar or DRG neurons treated with BDNF *in vitro* had increased intracellular levels of cAMP and acquired the ability to subsequently extend neurites over growth-inhibitory myelin substrates (Cai *et al.*, 1999). Furthermore, inhibition of the cAMP-dependent protein kinase (PKA) during neurotrophic factor "priming" blocked this resistance to myelin growth inhibitors. Since PKA has been shown to inactivate Rho (Lang *et al.*, 1996), these experiments offer a novel rationale for treating the CNS injury site with neurotrophic factors or Rho inhibitors.

C. Conclusions

Although recent experimental approaches for increasing the intrinsic neuronal growth capacity have shown promising results (Berry *et al.*, 1996; Cai *et al.*, 1999; Kobayashi *et al.*, 1997; Neumann and Woolf, 1999) , it remains unclear whether large-scale axonal regeneration within the CNS can be achieved solely by this approach. For example, even if neurons with a high intrinsic growth capacity can overcome or avoid myelin-associated growth inhibition, the physical and chemical barrier presented by the lesion site scar and cavitation may still require additional treatments (Davies *et al.*, 1997; Fitch and Silver, 1997; Silver, 1994). Furthermore, proper functioning of restored circuits will necessitate remyelination of the regenerated axons and appropriate sensori-motor retraining (Muir and Steeves, 1997). Thus, it is likely that therapeutic strategies for spinal cord injury will require combinatorial approaches to address both intrinsic neuronal and extrinsic glial aspects of the problem.

Table 1 Survey of axotomy-induced changes in neuronal gene expression.

Molecule	M	S	A	CNS	Ref
Transcription factors					
c-jun	⇑	⇑	⇑	regenerating into PN grafts	1
Oct-2		⇑			1
CREB, CREM, ICER, ATF-1, ATF-2, SRF, NFkB, junB, junD, c-fos, fra-1, fra-2, krox-20, krox-24 – various changes					1
NTF receptors, ligands and signalling components					
Neurotrophins:					
TrkA		⇑⇓			2
NGF		⇑			2
TrkB	⇑	⇑			3
BDNF	⇑	⇑		⇑ RGCs, ⇔ rubrospinal	3
TrkC	⇓				4
>>ERK (MAP kinase)	⇑				5
>>MEK (ERK kinase)	⇑				5
>>ShcA (Shc)	⇑				6
>>ShcB (SCK)	⇔				6
>>ShcC (N-Shc)	⇓				6
>>Grb2	⇔				6
gp130 cytokines:					
gp130	⇑				7
IL-6	⇑	⇑			7
CNTFRα				⇑ septal	7
>>JAK2,3	⇑				7
Others:					
FRFR-1	⇑			⇓ rubrospinal	8
FGF-2	⇑	⇑		⇔ rubrospinal (very low)	8
ret	⇑	⇑			9
GDNFRα	⇑	⇑			9
TGF-β2	⇑				10
PDGF	⇑				11
IFN-γ	⇑				12

Table 1 (cont'd)

Molecule	M	S	A	CNS	Ref
Death/survival genes					
Death:					
bax	⇑	⇔		⇑RGCs, neonate sc. MNs	13
caspase-3	⇑				13
bcl-x_S	⇑			(neonate motoneurons)	13
Survival:					
bcl-2	⇓	⇓		⇓RGCs	13
bcl-x_L	⇑	⇓			13
Cytoskeletal proteins					
actin	⇑	⇑	⇑	⇑rubrospinal (transient)	14
α1-tubulin	⇑	⇑	⇑	⇑regenerating into PN grafts; ⇑rubrospinal (transient)	15
T26 α-tubulin	⇔				15
βII tubulin	⇑	⇑		⇑RGCs regenerating into PN grafts	15
βIII tubulin	⇑	⇑		⇑RGCs regenerating into PN grafts	15
neurofilaments	⇓	⇓	⇓	⇓RGCs, ⇓rubrospinal	16
peripherin	⇑	⇑			17
kinesins and dynein	⇑				18
Growth-associated proteins (GAPs), guidance and adhesion molecules					
GAP-43	⇑	⇑	⇑	regenerating into PN grafts	19
CAP-23/NAP-23	⇑				20
sema III/collapsin-1	⇓				21
neuropilin-1	⇔				21
ninjurin		⇑			22
L1/L1-like	⇑			⇑ in regenerating hippocampal and RGCs	23
NCAM	⇑	⇑			24
c-src	⇑	⇑			25
thrombospondin	⇑				26
plasminogen activators (tPA, uPA)	⇑				27

Table 1 (cont'd)

Molecule	M	S	A	CNS	Ref
Neurotransmission & other inter-cellular signalling-related molecules					
Transmitter systems:					
ChAT	⇓				28
VAChT	⇓				28
AChE	⇓				28
VAMP-1	⇓				29
VAMP-2	⇑				29
SNAP-25	⇓				29
mGluR2,3	⇓				30
mGluR1,4	⇔				30
NMDA receptors					
NR1, NR2B, NR2D	⇓				31
NR1B				⇑ RGCs	31
GABA(A)		⇑			32
Neuropeptides:					
galanin	⇑	⇑	⇑		33
NPY		⇑	⇓		33
VIP	⇑	⇑	⇑		33
SP		⇓			33
PACAP		⇑	⇑		34
CGRP	⇑	⇓		⇑ rubrospinal	35
Others:					
neuregulins	⇓	⇓			36
agrin			⇓		37
Reg-2	⇑	⇑			38

Table 1 (cont'd)

Molecule	M	S	A	CNS	Ref
Housekeeping/metabolic/intra-cellular signalling proteins					
cyclin G	⇑				39
CaMKIIα	⇑				40
CaMKIIβ	⇓				40
PKA	⇓				41
PKC type II			⇑		42
calbindin	⇑				43
calmodulin	⇔				43
14-3-3 family	⇑				44
NOS	⇑	⇑	⇑	⇑hypothalamic, ⇓during regeneration into PN grafts	45
Mn-SOD	⇑	⇑			46
Cu/Zn-SOD	⇔	⇔			46
hsc70		⇔			47
hsp68		⇑			47
hsp27		⇑	⇑		47
cytochrome oxidase	⇓				48
tra2beta	⇑				49
ubiquitin			⇑		50
glucose-regulated p78	⇑				51
receptor tyrosine phosphatases:					
PTPsigma		⇑			52
LAR, PTPalpha		⇓			52
Ion channels					
Na^+ channel III		⇑			53
Na^+ SNS		⇓			53
Na^+ NaN		⇓			53
K^+ 1.2, 2.1		⇓			54
K^+ 1.1, 1.3		⇓			54
K^+ 1.4, 1.6		⇔			54

(1) (Begbie *et al.*, 1996; Herdegen *et al.*, 1997a; Herdegen and Leah, 1998; Herdegen *et al.*, 1997b; Herdegen and Zimmermann, 1994). (2) (Kashiba *et al.*, 1998; Shen *et al.*, 1999). (3) (Ernfors *et al.*, 1993; Gao *et al.*, 1997; Kobayashi *et al.*, 1996a; Piehl *et al.*, 1994; Shen *et al.*, 1999; Tonra *et al.*, 1998; Kobayashi *et al.*, 1996b). (4) (Fernandes *et al.*, 1998). (5) (Kiryu *et al.*, 1995). (6) (Tanabe *et al.*, 1998). (7) (Klein *et al.*, 1997; Lee *et al.*, 1997; Murphy *et al.*, 1999; Murphy *et al.*, 1995; Yao *et al.*, 1997). (8) (Huber *et al.*, 1997; Ji *et al.*, 1995; Stilwell *et al.*, 1997).(9) (Burazin and Gundlach, 1998; Colucci-D'Amato *et al.*, 1996; Kashiba *et al.*, 1998; Naveilhan *et al.*, 1997). (10) (Hermanson *et al.*, 1995). (11) (Colosetti *et al.*, 1995). (12) (Kristensson *et al.*, 1994). (13) (de Bilbao *et al.*, 1999;

Gillardon *et al.*, 1996; Gillardon *et al.*, 1994; Guarin *et al.*, 1999; Isenmann *et al.*, 1997; Vanderluit et al., 1999; Vanderluit et al., 1997). (14) (Bisby and Tetzlaff, 1992; Koo *et al.*, 1988; Lund and McQuarrie, 1996; Tetzlaff *et al.*, 1991). (15) (Bisby and Tetzlaff, 1992; Fernandes *et al.*, 1999; Fournier and McKerracher, 1997; Gloster *et al.*, 1994; Laferriere *et al.*, 1997; Miller *et al.*, 1987; Miller *et al.*, 1989; Moskowitz and Oblinger, 1995a). (16) (Bisby and Tetzlaff, 1992; Tetzlaff *et al.*, 1991; Tetzlaff *et al.*, 1996) (17) (Chadan *et al.*, 1994a; Chadan *et al.*, 1994b; Oblinger *et al.*, 1989; Troy *et al.*, 1990). (18) (Su *et al.*, 1997). (19) (Benowitz and Routtenberg, 1997; Fernandes *et al.*, 1999; Schaden *et al.*, 1994). (20) (Caroni, 1997a) . W. Tetzlaff, unpublished observations. (21) (Pasterkamp *et al.*, 1998a; Pasterkamp *et al.*, 1998b). (22) (Araki and Milbrandt, 1996). (23) (Anderson *et al.*, 1998; Aubert *et al.*, 1998; Bahr *et al.*, 1988; Chaisuksunt et al., 1998; Jung *et al.*, 1997). (24) (Daniloff *et al.*, 1986). (25) (Isozumi *et al.*, 1997; Le Beau *et al.*, 1991). (26) (Moller *et al.*, 1996). (27) (Yuguchi *et al.*, 1997). (28) (Fernandes *et al.*, 1998 and references therein; Gilmor *et al.*, 1998; Matsuura *et al.*, 1997). (29) (Jacobsson *et al.*, 1998). (30) (Kennis and Holstege, 1997; Tang and Sim, 1997). (31) (Kreutz *et al.*, 1998; Piehl *et al.*, 1995). (32) (Oyelese *et al.*, 1995). (33) (Corness *et al.*, 1996; Corness *et al.*, 1998; Zigmond *et al.*, 1996; Zigmond and Sun, 1997). (34) (Klimaschewski *et al.*, 1996a; Larsen *et al.*, 1997; Moller *et al.*, 1997; Zhang *et al.*, 1995; Zhang *et al.*, 1996). (35) (Blake-Bruzzini *et al.*, 1997; Fukuoka *et al.*, 1997; Fukuoka *et al.*, 1999; Mulder *et al.*, 1997; Piehl *et al.*, 1998). (36) (Bermingham-McDonogh *et al.*, 1997). (37) (Thomas *et al.*, 1995). (38) (Livesey *et al.*, 1997). (39) (Morita *et al.*, 1996). (40) (Lund and McQuarrie, 1997). (41) (Kiryu *et al.*, 1995; Ohno *et al.*, 1994). (42) (Yamada *et al.*, 1994). (43) (Dassesse *et al.*, 1998; Krebs *et al.*, 1997). (44) (Namikawa *et al.*, 1998) . (45) (Jia *et al.*, 1994; Klimaschewski *et al.*, 1996b; Lumme *et al.*, 1997; Vizzard *et al.*, 1995; Wu *et al.*, 1994a; Wu *et al.*, 1994b). (46) (Rosenfeld *et al.*, 1997). (47) (Costigan *et al.*, 1998; Hopkins *et al.*, 1998; Tedeschi and Ciavarra, 1997). (48) (Iannuzzelli *et al.*, 1994). (49) (Kiryu-Seo *et al.*, 1998). (50) (De Stefano *et al.*, 1998). (51) (Moreno-Flores *et al.*, 1997). (52) (Haworth *et al.*, 1998). (53) (Dib-Hajj *et al.*, 1998; Okuse *et al.*, 1997; Waxman *et al.*, 1994). (54) (Ishikawa *et al.*, 1999) .

M = motor, S = sensory, A = autonomic

REFERENCES

Aigner L, Arber S, Kapfhammer JP, Laux T, Schneider C, Botteri F *et al.* (1995) Overexpression of the neural growth-associated protein GAP-43 induces nerve sprouting in the adult nervous system of transgenic mice. Cell 83: 269-278.

Aigner L, Caroni P (1995) Absence of persistent spreading, branching, and adhesion in GAP-43-depleted growth cones. J Cell Biol 128: 647-660.

Alcantara S, Frisen J, del Rio JA, Soriano E, Barbacid M, Silos-Santiago I (1997) TrkB signaling is required for postnatal survival of CNS neurons and protects hippocampal and motor neurons from axotomy-induced cell death. J Neurosci 17: 3623-3633.

Altar CA, Cai N, Bliven T, Juhasz M, Conner JM, Acheson AL *et al.* (1997) Anterograde transport of brain-derived neurotrophic factor and its role in the brain. Nature 389: 856-860.

Ambron RT, Walters ET (1996) Priming events and retrograde injury signals. A new perspective on the cellular and molecular biology of nerve regeneration. Mol Neurobiol 13: 61-79.

Andersen LB, Schreyer DJ (1999) Constitutive expression of GAP-43 correlates with rapid, but not slow regrowth of injured dorsal root axons in the adult rat. Exp Neurol 155: 157-164.

Anderson PN, Campbell G, Zhang Y, Lieberman AR (1998) Cellular and molecular correlates of the regeneration of adult mammalian CNS axons into peripheral nerve grafts. Prog Br Res 117: 211-32.

Araki T, Milbrandt J (1996) Ninjurin, a novel adhesion molecule, is induced by nerve injury and promotes axonal growth. Neuron 17: 353-61.

Asch WS, Leake D, Canger AK, Passini MA, Argenton F, Schechter N (1998) Cloning of zebrafish neurofilament cDNAs for plasticin and gefiltin: increased mRNA expression in ganglion cells after optic nerve injury. J Neurochem 71: 20-32.

Aubert I, Ridet JL, Gage FH (1995) Regeneration in the adult mammalian CNS: guided by development. Curr Opin Neurobiol 5: 625-35.

Aubert I, Ridet JL, Schachner M, Rougon G, Gage FH (1998) Expression of L1 and PSA during sprouting and regeneration in the adult hippocampal formation. J Comp Neurol 399: 1-19.

Bahr M, Vanselow J, Thanos S (1988) In vitro regeneration of adult rat ganglion cell axons from retinal explants. Exp Brain Res 73: 393-401.

Bassell GJ, Zhang H, Byrd AL, Femino AM, Singer RH, Taneja KL *et al.* (1998) Sorting of beta-actin mRNA and protein to neurites and growth cones in culture. J Neurosci 18: 251-65.

Becker T, Bernhardt RR, Reinhard E, Wullimann MF, Tongiorgi E, Schachner M (1998) Readiness of zebrafish brain neurons to regenerate a spinal axon correlates with differential expression of specific cell recognition molecules. J Neurosci 18: 5789-5803.

Begbie JL, Wood JN, Anderson PN, Latchman DS (1996) Specific up-regulation of the POU domain transcription factor Oct-2 following axotomy. Neurosci Lett 207: 183-186.

Belien ATJ, Paganetti PA, Schwab ME (1999) Membrane-type 1 matrix metalloprotease (MT1-MMP) enables invasive migration of glioma cells in central nervous system white matter. J Cell Biol 144: 373-384.

Benowitz LI, Jing Y, Tabibiazar R, Jo SA, Petrausch B, Stuermer CAO *et al.* (1998) Axon Outgrowth Is Regulated By an Intracellular Purine-Sensitive Mechanism in Retinal Ganglion Cells. J Biol Chem 273: 29626-29634.

Benowitz LI, Routtenberg A (1997) GAP-43: an intrinsic determinant of neuronal development and plasticity. Trends Neurosci 20: 84-91.

Bermingham-McDonogh O, Xu YT, Marchionni MA, Scherer SS (1997) Neuregulin espression in PNS neurons: isoforms and regulation by target interactions. Mol Cell Neurosci 10: 184-195.

Bernhardt RR, Tongiorgi E, Anzini P, Schachner M (1996) Increased expression of specific recognition molecules by retinal ganglion cells and by optic pathway glia accompanies the successful regeneration of retinal axons in adult zebrafish. J Comp Neurol 376: 253-264.

Berry M, Carlile J, Hunter A (1996) Peripheral nerve explants grafted into the vitreous body of the eye promote the regeneration of retinal ganglion cell axons severed in the optic nerve. J Neurocyt 25: 147-170.

Bhattacharya B, Saha S, Sarkar PK (1991) Post-transcriptional regulation of tubulin mRNA in developing rat brain. Brain Res Mol Brain Res 10: 347-350.

Bhave SV, Ghoda L, Hoffman PL (1999) Brain-derived neurotrophic factor mediates the anti-apoptotic effect of NMDA in cerebellar granule neurons: Signal transduction cascades and site of ethanol action. J Neurosci 19: 3277-3286.

Bisby MA (1982) Functions of retrograde axonal transport. Federation Proceedings 41: 2307-2311.

Bisby MA, Tetzlaff W (1992) Changes in cytoskeletal protein synthesis following axon injury and during axon regeneration. Mol Neurobiol 6: 107-123.

Bisby MA, Tetzlaff W, Brown MC (1996) GAP-43 mRNA in mouse motoneurons undergoing axonal sprouting in response to muscle paralysis of partial denervation. J Neurosci 8: 1240-1248.

Blair LAC, Bence-Hanulec KK, Mehta S, Franke T, Kaplan D, Marshall J (1999) Akt-dependent potentiation of L channels by insulin-like growth factor-1 is required for neuronal survival. J Neurosci 19: 1940-1951.

Blake-Bruzzini KM, Borke RC, Anders JJ, Potts JD (1997) Calcitonin gene-related peptide and alpha-CGRP mRNA expression in cranial motoneurons after hypoglossal nerve injury during postnatal development. J Neurocyt 26: 163-179.

Bregman BS, Broude E, McAtee M, Kelley MS (1998) Transplants and neurotrophic factors prevent atrophy of mature CNS neurons after spinal cord injury. Exp Neurol 149: 13-27.

Bregman BS, McAtee M, Dai HN, Kuhn PL (1997) Neurotrophic factors increase axonal growth after spinal cord injury and transplantation in the adult rat. Exp Neurol 148: 475-494.

Bregman BS, Reier PJ (1986) Neural tissue transplants rescue axotomized rubrospinal cells from retrograde death. J Comp Neurol 244: 86-95.

Broude E, McAtee M, Kelley MS, Bregman BS (1997) c-Jun expression in adult rat dorsal root ganglion neurons: differential response after central or peripheral axotomy. Exp Neurol 148: 367-377.

Broude E, McAtee M, Kelley MS, Bregman BS (1999) Fetal spinal cord transplants and exogenous neurotrophic support enhance c-Jun expression in mature axotomized neurons after spinal cord injury. Exp Neurol 155: 65-78.

Brummendorf T, Kenwrick S, Rathjen FG (1998) Neural cell recognition molecule L1: from cell biology to human hereditary brain malformations. Curr Opin Neurobiol 8: 87-97.

Brunet A, Bonni A, Zigmond MJ, Lin MZ, Juo P, Hu LS *et al.* (1999) Akt promotes cell survival by phosphorylating and inhibiting a forkhead transcription factor. Cell 96: 857-868.

Buffo A, Holtmaat AJ, Savio T, Verbeek JS, Oberdick J, Oestreicher AB *et al.* (1997) Targeted overexpression of the neurite growth-associated protein B-50/GAP-43 in cerebellar Purkinje cells induces sprouting after axotomy but not axon regeneration into growth-permissive transplants. J Neurosci 17: 8778-91.

Burazin TCD, Gundlach AL (1998) Up-regulation of GDNFR-α and C-Ret mRNA in facial motor neurons following facial nerve injury in the rat. Mol Brain Res 55: 331-336.

Bussmann KAV, Sofroniew MV (1999) Re-expression of p75(NTR) by adult motor neurons after axotomy is triggered by retrograde transport of a positive signal from axons regrowing through damaged or denervated peripheral nerve tissue. Neurosci 91: 273-281.

Cai DM, Shen YJ, De Bellard M, Tang S, Filbin MT (1999) Prior exposure to neurotrophins blocks inhibition of axonal regeneration by MAG and myelin via a cAMP-dependent mechanism. Neuron 22: 89-101.

Canger AK, Passini MA, Asch WS, Leake D, Zafonte BT, Glasgow E *et al.* (1998) Restricted expression of the neuronal intermediate filament protein plasticin during zebrafish development. J Comp Neurol 399: 561-72.

Cardone MH, Roy N, Stennicke HR, Salvesen GS, Franke TF, Stanbridge E *et al.* (1998) Regulation of cell death protease caspase-9 by phosphorylation. Science 282: 1318-1321.

Caroni P (1997a) Intrinsic neuronal determinants that promote axonal sprouting and elongation. Bioessays 19: 767-75.

Caroni P (1997b) Overexpression of growth-associated proteins in the neurons of adult transgenic mice. J Neurosci Methods 71: 3-9.

Caroni P, Aigner L, Schneider C (1997) Intrinsic neuronal determinants locally regulate extrasynaptic and synaptic growth at the adult neuromuscular junction. J Cell Biol 136: 679-92.

Cerezo A, Martinez C, Lanzarot D, Fischer S, Franke TF, Rebollo A (1998) Role of Akt and c-Jun N-terminal kinase 2 in apoptosis induced by interleukin-4 deprivation. Mol Biol Cell 9: 3107-3118.

Chadan S, Le Gall JY, Di Giamberardino L, Filliatreau G (1994a) Axonal transport of type III intermediate filament protein peripherin in intact and regenerating motor axons of the rat sciatic nerve. J Neurosci Res 39: 127-39.

Chadan S, Moya KL, Portier MM, Filliatreau G (1994b) Identification of a peripherin dimer: changes during axonal development and regeneration of the rat sciatic nerve. J Neurochem 62: 1894-905.

Chaisuksunt V, Zhang Y, Schachner M, Anderson PN, Lieberman AR (1998) Expression of the cell recognition molecule CHL1 (close homologue of L1), in adult rat brain following peripheral nerve graft implantation. Soc Neurosci Abstr 24(2):2009.

Chambers CB, Muma NA (1997) Tau mRNA isoforms following sciatic nerve axotomy with and without regeneration. Brain Res Mol Brain Res 48: 115-24.

Chau MF, Radeke MJ, de Ines C, Barasoain I, Kohlstaedt LA, Feinstein SC (1998) The microtubule-associated protein tau cross-links to two distinct sites on each alpha and beta tubulin monomer via separate domains. Biochem 37: 17692-17703.

Chen DF, Jhaveri S, Schneider GE (1995) Intrinsic changes in developing retinal neurons result in regenerative failure of their axons. Proc Natl Acad Sciences USA 92: 7287-91.

Chen DF, Schneider GE, Martinou JC, Tonegawa S (1997) Bcl-2 promotes regeneration of severed axons in mammalian CNS. Nature 385: 434-9.

Cheng H, Cao Y, Olson L (1996) Spinal cord repair in adult paraplegic rats: partial restoration of hind limb function. Science 273: 510-3.

Chiaramello A, Neuman T, Peavy DR, Zuber MX (1996) The GAP-43 gene is a direct downstream target of the basic helix-loop-helix transcription factors. J Biol Chem 271: 22035-43.

Cohen NR, Taylor JSH, Scott LB, Guillery RW, Soriano P, Furley AJW (1998) Errors in corticospinal axon guidance in mice lacking the neural cell adhesion molecule L1. Curr Biol 8: 26-33.

Collard JF, Cote F, Julien JP (1995) Defective axonal transport in a transgenic mouse model of amyotrophic lateral sclerosis. Nature 375: 61-4.

Colosetti P, Olsson T, Miyazono K, Funa K (1995) Axotomy of rat facial nerve induces TGF-beta and latent TGF-beta binding protein. Brain Res Bull 37: 561-7.

Colucci-D'Amato GL, D'Alessio A, Filliatreau G, Florio T, Di Giamberardino L, Chiappetta G *et al.* (1996) Presence of physiologically stimulated RET in adult rat brain: induction of RET expression during nerve regeneration. Cell Growth Diff 7: 1081-6.

Corness J, Shi TJ, Xu ZQ, Brulet P, Hokfelt T (1996) Influence of leukemia inhibitory factor on galanin/GMAP and neuropeptide Y expression in mouse primary sensory neurons after axotomy. Exp Brain Res 112: 79-88.

Corness J, Stevens B, Fields RD, Hokfelt T (1998) NGF and LIF both regulate galanin gene expression in primary DRG cultures. Neuroreport 9: 1533-6.

Costigan M, Mannion RJ, Kendall G, Lewis SE, Campagna JA, Coggeshall RE *et al.* (1998) Heat shock protein 27: developmental regulation and expression after peripheral nerve injury. J Neurosci 18: 5891-900.

Cragg BG (1970) What is the signal for chromatolysis? Brain Res 23: 1-21.

Crowder RJ, Freeman RS (1998) Phosphatidylinositol 3-kinase and Akt protein kinase are necessary and sufficient for the survival of nerve growth factor-dependent sympathetic neurons. J Neurosci 18: 2933-2943.

Curtis R, Adryan KM, Zhu Y, Harkness PJ, Lindsay RM, DiStefano PS (1993) Retrograde axonal transport of ciliary neurotrophic factor is increased by peripheral nerve injury. Nature 365: 253-5.

Curtis R, Scherer SS, Somogyi R, Adryan KM, Ip NY, Zhu Y *et al.* (1994) Retrograde axonal transport of LIF is increased by peripheral nerve injury: correlation with increased LIF expression in distal nerve. Neuron 12: 191-204.

Curtis R, Tonra JR, Stark JL, Adryan KM, Park JS, Cliffer KD *et al.* (1998) Neuronal injury increases retrograde axonal transport of the neurotrophins to spinal sensory neurons and motor neurons via multiple receptor mechanisms. Mol Cell Neurosci 12: 105-18.

Dahme M, Bartsch U, Martini R, Anliker B, Schachner M, Mantei N (1997) Disruption of the mouse L1 gene leads to malformations of the nervous system. Nature Genetics 17: 346-9.

Daniloff JK, Levi G, Grumet M, Rieger F, Edelman GM (1986) Altered expression of neuronal cell adhesion molecules induced by nerve injury and repair. J Cell Biol 103: 929-45.

Dassesse D, Cuvelier L, Krebs C, Streppel M, Guntinas-Lichius O, Neiss WF *et al.* (1998) Differential expression of calbindin and calmodulin in motoneurons after hypoglossal axotomy. Brain Res 786: 181-8.

Datta SR, Dudek H, Tao X, Masters S, Fu H, Gotoh Y *et al.* (1997) Akt phosphorylation of BAD couples survival signals to the cell-intrinsic death machinery. Cell 91: 231-41.

Davies AM (1994) The role of neurotrophins in the developing nervous system. J Neurobiol 25: 1334-1348.

Davies SJ, Field PM, Raisman G (1994) Long interfascicular axon growth from embryonic neurons transplanted into adult myelinated tracts. J Neurosci 14: 1596-612.

Davies SJ, Fitch MT, Memberg SP, Hall AK, Raisman G, Silver J (1997) Regeneration of adult axons in white matter tracts of the central nervous system. Nature 390: 680-3.

de Bilbao F, Guarin E, Nef P, Dubois-Dauphin M (1999) The mouse cpp32 mRNA transcript is early up-regulated in axotomized motoneurons following facial nerve transection. Neurosci Lett 266: 65-68.

De Stefano ME, Squitti R, Toschi G (1998) The rise in cytoplasmic ubiquitin levels is an early step in the response of parasympathetic ganglionic neurons to axonal injury followed by regeneration. J Neuropathol Exp Neurol 57: 1000-1012.

Delpeso L, Gonzalezgarcia M, Page C, Herrera R, Nunez G (1997) Interleukin-3-induced phosphorylation of Bad through the protein kinase Akt. Science 278: 687-689.

Dib-Hajj SD, Tyrrell L, Black JA, Waxman SG (1998) NaN, a novel voltage-gated Na channel, is expressed preferentially in peripheral sensory neurons and down-regulated after axotomy. Proc Natl Acad Sci U S A 95: 8963-8968.

DiTella MC, Feiguin F, Carri N, Kosik KS, Caceres A (1996) MAP-1B/TAU functional redundancy during laminin-enhanced axonal growth. J Cell Sci 109: 467-77.

Doster SK, Lozano AM, Aguayo AJ, Willard MB (1991) Expression of the growth-associated protein GAP-43 in adult rat retinal ganglion cells following axon injury. Neuron 6: 635-47.

Drescher U, Bonhoeffer F, Muller BK (1997) The Eph family in retinal axon guidance. Curr Opin Neurobiol 7: 75-80.

Drewes G, Ebneth A, Mandelkow EM (1998) MAPS, MARKS and microtubule dynamics. Trends Biochem Sci 23: 307-311.

Du KY, Montminy M (1998) CREB is a regulatory target for the protein kinase Akt/PKB. J Biol Chem 273: 32377-32379.

Dudek H, Datta SR, Franke TF, Birnbaum MJ, Yao R, Cooper GM *et al.* (1997) Regulation of neuronal survival by the serine-threonine protein kinase Akt. Science 275: 661-5.

Dusart I, Airaksinen MS, Sotelo C (1997) Purkinje cell survival and axonal regeneration are age dependent: an in vitro study. J Neurosci 17: 3710-26.

Dusart I, Sotelo C (1994) Lack of Purkinje cell loss in adult rat cerebellum following protracted axotomy: degenerative changes and regenerative attempts of the severed axons. J Comp Neurol 347: 211-32.

Dyer JK, Bourque JA, Steeves JD (1998) Regeneration of brainstem-spinal axons after lesion and immunological disruption of myelin in adult rat. Exp Neurol 154: 12-22.

Elliott EJ, Parks DA, Fishman PS (1999) alpha(1)-tubulin expression in proximally axotomized mouse cortical neurons. J Neurotrauma 16: 333-339.

Eng H, Lund K, Campenot RB (1999) Synthesis of beta-tubulin, actin, and other proteins in axons of sympathetic neurons in compartmented cultures. J Neurosci 19: 1-9.

Ernfors P, Rosario CM, Merlio JP, Grant G, Aldskogius H, Persson H (1993) Expression of mRNAs for neurotrophin receptors in the dorsal root ganglion and spinal cord during development and following peripheral or central axotomy. Brain Res Mol Brain Res 17: 217-26.

Estus S, Zaks WJ, Freeman RS, Gruda M, Bravo R, Johnson EM, Jr. (1994) Altered gene expression in neurons during programmed cell death: identification of c-jun as necessary for neuronal apoptosis. J Cell Biol 127: 1717-27.

Fawcett JP, Bamji SX, Causing CG, Aloyz R, Ase AR, Reader TA *et al.* (1998) Functional evidence that BDNF is an anterograde neuronal trophic factor in the CNS. J Neurosci 18: 2808-21.

Fawcett JW (1997) Astrocytic and neuronal factors affecting axon regeneration in the damaged central nervous system. Cell Tissue Res 290: 371-377.

Fawcett JW, Mathews G, Housden E, Goedert M, Matus A (1994) Regenerating sciatic nerve axons contain the adult rather than the embryonic pattern of microtubule associated proteins. Neurosci 61: 789-804.

Fernandes KJL, Kobayashi NR, Jasmin BJ, Tetzlaff W (1998) Acetylcholinesterase gene expression in axotomized rat facial motoneurons is differentially regulated by neurotrophins: correlation with trkB and trkC mRNA levels and isoforms. J Neurosci 18: 9936-47.

Fernandes KJL, Fan D-P, Tsui BJ, Cassar SL, Tetzlaff W (1999) Influence of the axotomy to cell body distance in rat rubrospinal and spinal motoneurons: differential regulation of GAP-43, tubulins, and neurofilament-M. J. Comp Neurol 414 (4): 495-510.

Fillmore HL, Mainardi CL, Hasty KA (1992) Differentiation of PC12 cells with nerve growth factor is associated with induction of transin synthesis and relase. J Neurosci. 31: 662-669.

Fitch MT, Silver J (1997) Glial cell extracellular matrix: boundaries for axon growth in development and regeneration. Cell Tissue Res 290: 379-84.

Flanagan JG, Vanderhaeghen P (1998) The ephrins and Eph receptors in neural development. Ann Rev Neurosci 21: 309-45.

Foulstone EJ, Tavare JM, Gunn-Moore FJ (1999) Sustained phosphorylation and activation of protein kinase B correlates with brain-derived neurotrophic factor and insulin stimulated survival of cerebellar granule cells. Neurosci Lett 264: 125-128.

Fournier AE, Beer J, Arregui CO, Essagian C, Aguayo AJ, McKerracher L (1997) Brain-derived neurotrophic factor modulates GAP-43 but not Tα1 expression in injured retinal ganglion cells of adult rats. J Neurosci Research 47: 561-72.

Fournier AE, McKerracher L (1997) Expression of specific tubulin isotypes increases during regeneration of injured CNS neurons, but not after the application of brain-derived neurotrophic factor (BDNF). J Neurosci 17: 4623-32.

Friedman B, Scherer SS, Rudge JS, Helgren M, Morrisey D, McClain J *et al.* (1992) Regulation of ciliary neurotrophic factor expression in myelin-related Schwann cells in vivo. Neuron 9: 295-305.

Fu SY, Gordon T (1997) The cellular and molecular basis of peripheral nerve regeneration. Mol Neurobiol 14: 67-116.

Fuchs C, Glasgow E, Hitchcock PF, Schechter N (1994) Plasticin, a newly identified neurofilament protein, is preferentially expressed in young retinal ganglion cells of adult goldfish. J Comp Neurol 350: 452-62.

Fukuoka T, Miki K, Yoshiya I, Noguchi K (1997) Expression of beta-calcitonin gene-related peptide in axotomized rubrospinal neurons and the effect of brain derived neurotrophic factor. Brain Res 767: 250-8.

Fukuoka T, Tokunaga A, Kondo E, Miki K, Tachibana T, Noguchi K (1999) Differential regulation of alpha- and beta-CGRP mRNAs within oculomotor, trochlear, abducens, and trigeminal motoneurons in response to axotomy. Brain Res Mol Brain Res 63: 304-315.

Funakoshi H, Frisen J, Barbany G, Timmusk T, Zachrisson O, Verge VM *et al.* (1993) Differential expression of mRNAs for neurotrophins and their receptors after axotomy of the sciatic nerve. J Cell Biol 123: 455-65.

Gale NW, Yancopoulos GD (1997) Ephrins and their receptors: a repulsive topic? Cell Tissue Res 290: 227-41.

Gallo G, Letourneau PC (1998) Axon guidance: GTPases help axons reach their targets. Current Biol 8: R80-2.

Gao H, Qiao XX, Hefti F, Hollyfield JG, Knusel B (1997) Elevated mRNA expression of brain-derived neurotrophic factor in retinal ganglion cell layer after optic nerve injury. Investigative Ophthalmology & Visual Science 38: 1840-1847.

Giehl KM, Schutte A, Mestres P, Yan Q (1998) The survival-promoting effect of glial cell line-derived neurotrophic factor on axotomized corticospinal neurons in vivo is mediated by an endogenous brain-derived neurotrophic factor mechanism. J Neurosci 18: 7351-60.

Giehl KM, Tetzlaff W (1996) BDNF and NT-3, but not NGF, prevent axotomy-induced death of rat corticospinal neurons in vivo. Eur J Neurosci 8: 1167-75.

Gillardon F, Klimaschewski L, Wickert H, Krajewski S, Reed JC, Zimmermann M (1996) Expression pattern of candidate cell death effector proteins Bax, Bcl-2, Bcl-X, and c-Jun in sensory and motor neurons following sciatic nerve transection in the rat. Brain Res 739: 244-50.

Gillardon F, Wickert H, Zimmermann M (1994) Differential expression of bcl-2 and bax mRNA in axotomized dorsal root ganglia of young and adult rats. J Neurosci 6: 1641-4.

Gilmor ML, Counts SE, Wiley RG, Levey AI (1998) Coordinate expression of the vesicular acetylcholine transporter and choline acetyltransferase following septohippocampal pathway lesions. J Neurochem 71: 2411-2420.

Gingras AC, Kennedy SG, Oleary MA, Sonenberg N, Hay N (1998) 4e-Bp1, a repressor of mRNA translation, is phosphorylated and inactivated by the Akt(Pkb) signaling pathway. Genes & Development 12: 502-513.

Glasgow E, Druger RK, Levine EM, Fuchs C, Schechter N (1992) Plasticin, a novel type III neurofilament protein from goldfish retina: increased expression during optic nerve regeneration. Neuron 9: 373-81.

Glazner GW, Lupien S, Miller JA, Ishii DN (1993) Insulin-like growth factor-II increases the rate of sciatic nerve regeneration in rats. Neurosci 54: 791-797.

Glazner GW, Morrison AE, Ishii DN (1994) Elevated insulin-like growth factor (IGF) gene expression in sciatic nerves during IGF-supported nerve regeneration. Mol Brain Res 25: 265-272.

Glicksman MA, Chiu AY, Dionne CA, Harty M, Kaneko M, Murakata C *et al.* (1998) CEP-1347/KT7515 prevents motor neuronal programmed cell death and injury-induced dedifferentiation in vivo. J Neurobiol 35: 361-70.

Gloster A, Wu W, Speelman A, Weiss S, Causing C, Pozniak C *et al.* (1994) The T alpha 1 alpha-tubulin promoter specifies gene expression as a function of neuronal growth and regeneration in transgenic mice. J Neurosci 14: 7319-30.

Gravel C, Gotz R, Lorrain A, Sendtner M (1997) Adenoviral gene transfer of ciliary neurotrophic factor and brain-derived neurotrophic factor leads to long-term survival of axotomized motor neurons. Nature Medicine 3: 765-70.

Grill R, Murai K, Blesch A, Gage FH, Tuszynski MH (1997) Cellular delivery of neurotrophin-3 promotes corticospinal axonal growth and partial functional recovery after spinal cord injury. J Neurosci 17: 5560-72.

Guarin E, Seuret P, Nef S, de Bilbao F, Nef P, Dubois-Dauphin M (1999) cpp32 messenger RNA neosynthesis is induced by fatal axotomy and is not regulated by athanatal Bcl-2 over-expression. Neurosci 90: 653-664.

Haase G, Kennel P, Pettmann B, Vigne E, Akli S, Revah F *et al.* (1997) Gene therapy of murine motor neuron disease using adenoviral vectors for neurotrophic factors. Nature Medicine 3: 429-436.

Ham J, Babij C, Whitfield J, Pfarr CM, Lallemand D, Yaniv M *et al.* (1995) A c-Jun dominant negative mutant protects sympathetic neurons against programmed cell death. Neuron 14: 927-39.

Haworth K, Shu KK, Stokes A, Morris R, Stoker A (1998) The expression of receptor tyrosine phosphatases Is responsive to sciatic nerve crush. Mol Cell Neurosci 12: 93-104.

Heinrich PC, Behrmann I, Muller-Newen G, Schaper F, Graeve L (1998) Interleukin-6-type cytokine signalling through the gp130/Jak/STAT pathway. Biochem J 334 (Pt 2): 297-314.

Hensel T, Amberger VR, Schwab ME (1998) A metalloprotease activity from C6 glioma cells inactivates the myelin-associated neurite growth inhibitors and can be neutralized by antibodies. British Journal of Cancer 78: 1564-1572.

Herdegen T, Blume A, Buschmann T, Georgakopoulos E, Winter C, Schmid W *et al.* (1997a) Expression of activating transcription factor-2, serum response factor and cAMP/Ca response element binding protein in the adult rat brain following generalized seizures, nerve fibre lesion and ultraviolet irradiation. Neurosci 81: 199-212.

Herdegen T, Claret FX, Kallunki T, Martin-Villalba A, Winter C, Hunter T *et al.* (1998) Lasting N-terminal phosphorylation of c-Jun and activation of c-Jun N-terminal kinases after neuronal injury. J Neurosci 18: 5124-35.

Herdegen T, Leah JD (1998) Inducible and constitutive transcription factors in the mammalian nervous system: control of gene expression by Jun, Fos and Krox, and CREB/ATF proteins. Brain Res - Brain Res Rev 28: 370-490.

Herdegen T, Skene P, Bahr M (1997b) The c-Jun transcription factor--bipotential mediator of neuronal death, survival and regeneration. Trends Neurosci 20: 227-31.

Herdegen T, Zimmermann M (1994) Expression of c-Jun and JunD transcription factors represent specific changes in neuronal gene expression following axotomy. Prog Br Res 103: 153-71.

Hermanson M, Olsson T, Westermark B, Funa K (1995) PDGF and its receptors following facial nerve axotomy in rats: expression in neurons and surrounding glia. Exp Br Res 102: 415-22.

Herzog KH, Chen S-C, Morgan JI (1999) c-jun is dispenable for developmental cell death and axogenesis in the retina. J Neurosci 19: 4349-4359.

Hilton M, Middleton G, Davies AM (1997) Bcl-2 influences axonal growth rate in embryonic sensory neurons. Curr Biol 7: 798-800.

Hirokawa N, Hisanaga S, Shiomura Y (1988) MAP2 is a component of crossbridges between microtubules and neurofilaments in the neuronal cytoskeleton: quick-freeze, deep-etch immunoelectron microscopy and reconstitution studies. J Neurosci 8: 2769-79.

Hopkins DA, Plumier JC, Currie RW (1998) Induction of the 27-kDa heat shock protein (Hsp27) in the rat medulla oblongata after vagus nerve injury. Exp Neurol 153: 173-183.

Huber K, Meisinger C, Grothe C (1997) Expression of fibroblast growth factor-2 in hypoglossal motoneurons is stimulated by peripheral nerve injury. J Comp Neurol 382: 189-98.

Hull M, Bahr M (1994) Differential regulation of c-JUN expression in rat retinal ganglion cells after proximal and distal optic nerve transection. Neurosci Lett 178: 39-42.

Iannuzzelli PG, Wang XH, Wang Y, Murphy EH (1994) Axotomy-induced changes in cytochrome oxidase activity in the cat trochlear nucleus. Brain Res 637: 267-272.

Isenmann S, Wahl C, Krajewski S, Reed JC, Bahr M (1997) Up-regulation of bax protein in degenerating retinal ganglion cells precedes apoptotic cell death after optic nerve lesion in the rat. J Neurosci 9: 1763-1772.

Ishikawa K, Tanaka M, Black JA, Waxman SG (1999) Changes in expression of voltage-gated potassium channels in dorsal root ganglion neurons following axotomy. Muscle & Nerve 22: 502-507.

Isozumi T, Yamada E, Hazama F, Handa J (1997) Altered expression of src tyrosine kinase after axotomy. Acta Neuropathol (Berl) 93: 438-442.

Jacobs AJ, Swain GP, Snedeker JA, Pijak DS, Gladstone LJ, Selzer ME (1997) Recovery of neurofilament expression selectively in regenerating reticulospinal neurons. J Neurosci 17: 5206-20.

Jacobsson G, Piehl F, Meister B (1998) VAMP-1 and VAMP-2 gene expression in rat spinal motoneurones: differential regulation after neuronal injury. J Neurosci 10: 301-16.

Ji RR, Zhang Q, Zhang X, Piehl F, Reilly T, Pettersson RF *et al.* (1995) Prominent expression of bFGF in dorsal root ganglia after axotomy. J Neurosci 7: 2458-68.

Jia YS, Wang XA, Ju G (1994) Nitric oxide synthase expression in vagal complex following vagotomy in the rat. Neuroreport 5: 793-6.

Jian X, Szaro BG, Schmidt JT (1996) Myosin light chain kinase: expression in neurons and upregulation during axon regeneration. J Neurobiol 31: 379-91.

Jiang YQ, Pickett J, Oblinger MM (1994) Long-term effects of axotomy on beta-tubulin and NF gene expression in rat DRG neurons. Journal of Neural Transplantation & Plasticity 5: 103-14.

Jung M, Petrausch B, Stuermer CA (1997) Axon-regenerating retinal ganglion cells in adult rats synthesize the cell adhesion molecule L1 but not TAG-1 or SC-1. Mol Cell Neurosci 9: 116-31.

Kamiguchi H, Lemmon V (1997) Neural cell adhesion molecule L1: signaling pathways and growth cone motility. J Neurosci Res 49: 1-8.

Kamiguchi H, Lemmon V (1998) A neuronal form of the cell adhesion molecule L1 contains a tyrosine-based signal required for sorting to the axonal growth cone. J Neurosci 18: 3749-56.

Kapfhammer JP, Schwab ME (1994) Increased expression of the growth-associated protein GAP-43 in the myelin-free rat spinal cord. J Neurosci 6: 403-11.

Kaplan DR, Miller FD (1997) Signal transduction by the neurotrophin receptors. Curr Opin Cell Biol 9: 213-21.

Kaplan DR, Stephens RM (1994) Neurotrophin signal transduction by the Trk receptor. J Neurobiol 25: 1404-17.

Karimi-Abdolrezaee S, Schreyer DJ (1998) CNS myelin fails to inhibit GAP-43 expression in developing cortical neurons in vivo and in vitro. Soc Neurosci Abstr 24: 29.

Kashiba H, Hyon B, Senba E (1998) Glial cell line-derived neurotrophic factor and nerve growth factor receptor mRNAs are expressed in distinct subgroups of dorsal root ganglion neurons and are differentially regulated by peripheral axotomy in the rat. Neurosci Lett 252: 107-110.

Keirstead HS, Dyer JK, Sholomenko GN, McGraw J, Delaney KR, Steeves JD (1995) Axonal regeneration and physiological activity following transection and immunological disruption of myelin within the hatchling chick spinal cord. J Neurosci 15: 6963-74.

Keirstead HS, Steeves JD (1998) CNS myelin: Does a stabilizing role in neurodevelopment result in inhibition of neuronal repair after injury. The Neuroscientist 4: 273-284.

Kenney AM, Kocsis JD (1997a) Temporal variability of jun family transcription factor levels in peripherally or centrally transected adult rat dorsal root ganglia. Brain Res Mol Brain Res 52: 53-61.

Kenney AM, Kocsis JD (1997b) Timing of c-jun protein induction in lumbar dorsal root ganglia after sciatic nerve transection varies with lesion distance. Brain Res 751: 90-5.

glutamate receptor subunits in spinal motoneurons after sciatic nerve injury. Exp Neurol 147: 18-27.

Kherif S, Dehaupas M, Lafuma C, Fardeau M, Alameddine HS (1998) Matrix metalloproteinases MMP-2 and MMP-9 in denervated muscle and injured nerve. Neuropathology and Applied Neurobiology 24: 309-319.

Kiryu S, Morita N, Ohno K, Maeno H, Kiyama H (1995) Regulation of mRNA expression involved in Ras and PKA signal pathways during rat hypoglossal nerve regeneration. Brain Res Mol Brain Res 29: 147-56.

Kiryu-Seo S, Matsuo N, Wanaka A, Ogawa S, Tohyama M, Kiyama H (1998) A sequence-specific splicing activator, tra2beta, is up-regulated in response to nerve injury. Brain Res Mol Brain Res 62: 220-223.

Klein MA, Moller JC, Jones LL, Bluethmann H, Kreutzberg GW, Raivich G (1997) Impaired neuroglial activation in interleukin-6 deficient mice. Glia 19: 227-33.

Klesse LJ, Meyers KA, Marshall CJ, Parada LF (1999) Nerve growth factor induces survival and differentiation through two distinct signaling cascades in PC12 cells. Oncogene 18: 2055-2068.

Klimaschewski L, Hauser C, Heym C (1996a) PACAP immunoreactivity in the rat superior cervical ganglion in comparison to VIP. Neuroreport 7: 2797-801.

Klimaschewski L, Meisinger C, Grothe C (1999) Localization and regulation of basic fibroblast growth factor (FGF-2) and FGF receptor-1 in rat superior cervical ganglion after axotomy. J Neurobiol 38: 499-506.

Klimaschewski L, Obermuller N, Majewski M, Bachmann S, Heym C (1996b) Increased expression of nitric oxide synthase in a subpopulation of rat sympathetic neurons after axotomy - correlation with vasoactive intestinal peptide. Cell Tissue Res 285: 419-25.

Kobayashi N, Mundel P (1998) A role of microtubules during the formation of cell processes in neuronal and non-neuronal cells. Cell Tissue Res 291: 163-174.

Kobayashi NR, Bedard AM, Hincke MT, Tetzlaff W (1996a) Increased expression of BDNF and trkB mRNA in rat facial motoneurons after axotomy. Eur J Neurosci 8: 1018-29.

Kobayashi NR, Fan DP, Giehl KM, Bedard AM, Wiegand SJ, Tetzlaff W (1997) BDNF and NT-4/5 prevent atrophy of rat rubrospinal neurons after cervical axotomy, stimulate GAP-43 and Talpha1-tubulin mRNA expression, and promote axonal regeneration. J Neurosci 17: 9583-95.

Kobayashi NR, Harrington KC, Tetzlaff W (1996b) Further evidence for autocrine trophic support of rat facial motoneurons but not rubrospinal neurons after axotomy. Soc Neurosci Abstr 22: 547.

Koo EH, Hoffman PN, Price DL (1988) Levels of neurotransmitter and cytoskeletal protein mRNAs during nerve regeneration in sympathetic ganglia. Brain Res 449: 361-3.

Korsching S (1993) The neurotrophic factor concept: a reexamination. J Neurosci 13: 2739-48.

Kost SA, Oblinger MM (1993) Immature corticospinal neurons respond to axotomy with changes in tubulin gene expression. Brain Res Bull 30: 469-75.

Krebs C, Neiss WF, Streppel M, Guntinas-Lichius O, Dassesse D, Stennert E *et al.* (1997) Axotomy induces transient calbindin D28K immunoreactivity in hypoglossal motoneurons in vivo. Cell Calcium 22: 367-72.

Kreutz MR, Bockers TM, Bockman J, Seidenbecher CI, Kracht B, Vorwerk CK *et al.* (1998) Axonal injury alters alternative splicing of the retinal NR1 receptor: the preferential expression of the NR1b isoforms is crucial for retinal ganglion cell survival. J Neurosci 18: 8278-8291.

Kristensson K, Aldskogius M, Peng ZC, Olsson T, Aldskogius H, Bentivoglio M (1994) Co-induction of neuronal interferon-gamma and nitric oxide synthase in rat motor neurons after axotomy: a role in nerve repair or death? J Neurocyt 23: 453-9.

Kruger K, Tam AS, Lu C, Sretavan DW (1998) Retinal ganglion cell axon progression from the optic chiasm to initiate optic tract development requires cell autonomous function of GAP-43. J Neurosci 18: 5692-5705.

Kutzleb C, Sanders G, Yamamoto R, Wang XL, Lichte B, Petraschparwez E *et al.* (1998) Paralemmin, a prenyl-palmitoyl-anchored phosphoprotein abundant in neurons and implicated in plasma membrane dynamics and cell process formation. J Cell Biol 143: 795-813.

Laferriere B, MacRae TH, Brown DL (1997) Tubulin synthesis and assembly in differentiating neurons. Biochem Cell Biol 75: 103-117.

Lang P, Gesbert F, Delespine-Carmagnat M, Stancou R, Pouchelet M, Bertoglio J (1996) Protein kinase A phosphorylation of RhoA mediates the morphological and functional effects of cyclic AMP in cytotoxic lymphocytes. EMBO Journal 15: 510-9.

Larsen JO, Hannibal J, Knudsen SM, Fahrenkrug J (1997) Expression of pituitary adenylate cyclase-activating polypeptide (PACAP) in the mesencephalic trigeminal nucleus of the rat after transsection of the masseteric nerve. Brain Res Mol Brain Res 46: 109-17.

Lazarov-Spiegler O, Solomon AS, Zeev-Brann AB, Hirschberg DL, Lavie V, Schwartz M (1996) Transplantation of activated macrophages overcomes central nervous system regrowth failure. FASEB Journal 10: 1296-302.

Le Beau JM, Tedeschi B, Walter G (1991) Increased expression of pp60c-src protein-tyrosine kinase during peripheral nerve regeneration. J Neurosci Res28: 299-309.

Lee MK, Cleveland DW (1996) Neuronal intermediate filaments. Ann Rev Neurosci 19: 187-217.

Lee MY, Naumann T, Kirsch M, Frotscher M, Hofmann HD (1997) Transient up-regulation of ciliary neurotrophic factor receptor-alpha mRNA in axotomized rat septal neurons. J Neurosci 9: 622-6.

Lehman M, Fournier A, Selles-Navarro (1999) Inactivation of Rho signalling pathway promotes CNS axon regeneration. J. Neurosci 19 (17): 7537-7547.

Lewin GR, Barde YA (1996) Physiology of the neurotrophins. Ann Rev Neurosci 19: 289-317.

Li D, Field PM, Raisman G (1995) Failure of axon regeneration in postnatal rat entorhino-hippocampal slice coculture is due to maturation of the axon, not that of the pathway or target. Eur J Neurosci 7: 1164-71.

Li Y, Field PM, Raisman G (1997) Repair of adult rat corticospinal tract by transplants of olfactory ensheathing cells. Science 277: 2000-2002.

Li Y, Field PM, Raisman G (1998) Regeneration of adult rat corticospinal axons induced by transplanted olfactory ensheathing cells. J Neurosci 18: 10514-10524.

Liabotis S, Schreyer DJ (1995) Magnitude of GAP-43 induction following peripheral axotomy of adult rat dorsal root ganglion neurons is independent of lesion distance. Exp Neurol 135: 28-35.

Lieberman AR (1974) Some factors affecting retrograde neuronal responses to axonal lesions. in: Essays on the Nervous System: a festschrift for Professor J.Z.Young. Edited by R. Bellairs and E.G. Gray. Clarendon Press, Oxford.

Lin CH, Espreafico EM, Mooseker MS, Forscher P (1996) Myosin drives retrograde F-actin flow in neuronal growth cones. Neuron 16: 769-82.

Liu QR, Sasaki T, Kozieradzki I, Wakeham A, Itie A, Dumont DJ *et al.* (1999) SHIP is a negative regulator of growth factor receptor-mediated PKB/Akt activation and myeloid cell survival. Genes & Development 13: 786-791.

Livesey FJ, O'Brien JA, Li M, Smith AG, Murphy LJ, Hunt SP (1997) A Schwann cell mitogen accompanying regeneration of motor neurons. Nature 390: 614-8.

Lu X, Richardson PM (1991) Inflammation near the nerve cell body enhances axonal regeneration. J Neurosci 11: 972-8.

Lu X, Richardson PM (1995) Changes in neuronal mRNAs induced by a local inflammatory reaction. J Neurosci Res 41: 8-14.

Lumme A, Vanhatalo S, Sadeniemi M, Soinila S (1997) Expression of nitric oxide synthase in hypothalamic nuclei following axonal injury or colchicine treatment. Exp Neurol 144: 248-57.

Lund LM, McQuarrie IG (1996) Axonal regrowth upregulates beta-actin and Jun D mRNA expression. J Neurobiol 31: 476-86.

Lund LM, McQuarrie IG (1997) Calcium/calmodulin-dependent protein kinase II expression in motor neurons - effect of axotomy. J Neurobiol 33: 796-810.

Machida CM, Scott JD, Ciment G (1991) NGF-induction of the metalloproteinase-trasin/stromelysin in PC12 cells: involvement of multiple protein kinases. J Cell Biol 114: 1037-1048.

Martini R (1994) Expression and functional roles of neural cell surface molecules and extracellular matrix components during development and regeneration of peripheral nerves. J Neurocyt 23: 1-28.

Martini R, Xin Y, Schachner M (1994) Restricted localization of L1 and N-CAM at sites of contact between Schwann cells and neurites in culture. Glia 10: 70-4.

Masu Y, Wolf E, Holtmann B, Sendtner M, Brem G, Thoenen H (1993) Disruption of the CNTF gene results in motor neuron degeneration. Nature 365: 27-32.

Mathew TC, Miller FD (1993) Induction of T alpha 1 alpha-tubulin mRNA during neuronal regeneration is a function of the amount of axon lost. Dev Biol 158: 467-74.

Matsuoka I, Nakane A, Kurihara K (1997) Induction of LIF-mRNA by TGF-beta 1 in Schwann cells. Brain Res 776: 170-80.

Matsuura J, Ajiki K, Ichikawa T, Misawa H (1997) Changes of expression levels of choline acetyltransferase and vesicular acetylcholine transporter mRNAs after transection of the hypoglossal nerve in adult rats. Neurosci Lett 236: 95-98.

McFarlane S, Cornel E, Amaya E, Holt CE (1996) Inhibition of FGF receptor activity in retinal ganglion cell axons causes errors in target recognition. Neuron 17: 245-54.

Meiri KF, Saffell JL, Walsh FS, Doherty P (1998) Neurite outgrowth stimulated by neural cell adhesion molecules requires growth-associated protein-43 (GAP-43) function and is associated with GAP-43 phosphorylation in growth cones. J Neurosci 18: 10429-37.

Menei P, Montero-Menei C, Whittemore SR, Bunge RP, Bunge MB (1998) Schwann cells genetically modified to secrete human BDNF promote enhanced axonal regrowth across transected adult rat spinal cord. Eur J Neurosci 10: 607-21.

Micheva KD, Vallee A, Beaulieu C, Herman IM, Leclerc N (1998) beta-actin is confined to structures having high capacity of remodelling in developing and adult rat cerebellum. Eur J Neurosci 10: 3785-3798.

Miller FD, Naus CC, Durand M, Bloom FE, Milner RJ (1987) Isotypes of alpha-tubulin are differentially regulated during neuronal maturation. J Cell Biol 105: 3065-73.
Miller FD, Tetzlaff W, Bisby MA, Fawcett JW, Milner RJ (1989) Rapid induction of the major embryonic alpha-tubulin mRNA, T alpha 1, during nerve regeneration in adult rats. J Neurosci 9: 1452-63.
Miranda JD, White LA, Marcillo AE, Willson CA, Jagid J, Whittemore SR (1999) Induction of Eph B3 after spinal cord injury. Exp Neurol 156: 218-222.
Mitchison TJ, Cramer LP (1996) Actin-based cell motility and cell locomotion. Cell 84: 371-379.
Mitsumoto H, Ikeda K, Klinkosz B, Cedarbaum JM, Wong V, Lindsay RM (1994) Arrest of motor neuron disease in wobbler mice cotreated with CNTF and BDNF. Science 265: 1107-10.
Mohajeri MH, Bartsch U, van der Putten H, Sansig G, Mucke L, Schachner M (1996) Neurite outgrowth on non-permissive substrates in vitro is enhanced by ectopic expression of the neural adhesion molecule L1 by mouse astrocytes. Eur J Neurosci 8: 1085-97.
Moller JC, Klein MA, Haas S, Jones LL, Kreutzberg GW, Raivich G (1996) Regulation of thrombospondin in the regenerating mouse facial motor nucleus. Glia 17: 121-132.
Moller K, Reimer M, Ekblad E, Hannibal J, Fahrenkrug J, Kanje M *et al.* (1997) The effects of axotomy and preganglionic denervation on the expression of pituitary adenylate cyclase activating peptide (PACAP), galanin and PACAP type 1 receptors in the rat superior cervical ganglion. Brain Res 775: 166-82.
Moreno-Flores MT, Olazabal UE, Kreutzberg GW (1997) Axotomy increases the expression of glucose-regulated protein 78 kDa in rat facial nucleus. Exp Neurol 146: 10-16.
Morita N, Kiryu S, Kiyama H (1996) p53-independent cyclin G expression in a group of mature neurons and its enhanced expression during nerve regeneration. J Neurosci 16: 5961-5966.
Moskowitz PF, Oblinger MM (1995a) Sensory neurons selectively upregulate synthesis and transport of the beta III-tubulin protein during axonal regeneration. J Neurosci 15: 1545-55.
Moskowitz PF, Oblinger MM (1995b) Transcriptional and post-transcriptional mechanisms regulating neurofilament and tubulin gene expression during normal development of the rat brain. Brain Res Mol Brain Res 30: 211-22.
Muir D (1994) Metalloproteinase-dependent neurite outgrowth within a synthetic extracellular matrix is induced by nerve growth factor. Exp Cell Res 210: 243-252.
Muir GD, Steeves JD (1997) Sensorimotor stimulation to improve locomotor recovery after spinal cord injury. Trends Neurosci 20: 72-7.
Muisehelmericks RC, Grimes HL, Bellacosa A, Malstrom SE, Tsichlis PN, Rosen N (1998) Cyclin D expression is controlled post-transcriptionally via a phosphatidylinositol 3-kinase Akt-dependent pathway. J Biol Chem 273: 29864-29872.
Mulder H, Zhang Y, Danielsen N, Sundler F (1997) Islet amyloid polypeptide and calcitonin gene-related peptide expression are down-regulated in dorsal root ganglia upon sciatic nerve transection. Brain Res Mol Brain Res 47: 322-30.
Mulderry PK, Dobson SP (1996) Regulation of VIP and other neuropeptides by c-Jun in sensory neurons: implications for the neuropeptide response to axotomy. Eur J Neurosci 8: 2479-91.
Murphy M, Dutton R, Koblar S, Cheema S, Bartlett P (1997) Cytokines which signal through the LIF receptor and their actions in the nervous system. Prog Neurobiol 52: 355-78.

Murphy PG, Borthwick LS, Johnston RS, Kuchel G, Richardson PM (1999) Nature of the retrograde signal from injured nerves that induces interleukin-6 mRNA in neurons. J Neurosci 19: 3791-3800.
Murphy PG, Grondin J, Altares M, Richardson PM (1995) Induction of interleukin-6 in axotomized sensory neurons. J Neurosci 15: 5130-8.
Nagamoto-Combs K, Vaccariello SA, Zigmond RE (1999) The levels of leukemia inhibitory factor mRNA in a Schwann cell line are regulated by multiple second messenger pathways. J Neurochem. 72: 1871-1881.
Namikawa K, Su QN, Kiryuseo S, Kiyama H (1998) Enhanced expression of 14-3-3 family members in injured motoneurons. Mol Brain Res 55: 315-320.
Naveilhan P, ElShamy WM, Ernfors P (1997) Differential regulation of mRNAs for GDNF and its receptors Ret and GDNFR alpha after sciatic nerve lesion in the mouse. J Neurosci 9: 1450-60.
Neumann S, Woolf CJ (1999) Regeneration of dorsal column fibers into and beyond the lesion site following adult spinal cord injury. Neuron 23: 83-91.
Neve RL, Ivins KJ, Tsai KC, Rogers SL, Perrone-Bizzozero NI (1999) cis-acting regulatory elements in the GAP-43 mRNA 3'-untranslated region can function in trans to suppress endogenous GAP-43 gene expression. Brain Res Mol Brain Res 65: 52-60.
Nishizawa K (1994) NGF-induced stabilization of GAP-43 mRNA is mediated by both 3' untranslated region and a segment encoding the carboxy-terminus peptide. Biochem Biophys Res Comm 200: 789-96.
Nordstrom LA, Lochner J, Yeung W, Ciment G (1995) The metalloproteinase stromelysin-1 (transin) mediates PC12 cell growth cone invasiveness through basal laminae. Mol Cell Neurosci 6: 56-68.
Nunez G, Delpeso L (1998) Linking extracellular survival signals and the apoptotic machinery. Curr Opin Neurobiol 8: 613-618.
Oblinger MM, Wong J, Parysek LM (1989) Axotomy-induced changes in the expression of a type III neuronal intermediate filament gene. J Neurosci 9: 3766-75.
Ohno K, Kitahara T, Takeda N, Kubo T, Kiyama H (1994) Gene regulation of cyclic AMP-dependent protein kinase subunits (C alpha, beta; RI alpha, beta and RII alpha, beta) in rat facial motoneurons after nerve transection. Neurosci 63: 1101-9.
Okubo Y, Blakesley VA, Stannard B, Gutkind S, Leroith D (1998) Insulin-like growth factor-I inhibits the stress-activated protein kinase/C-Jun N-terminal Kinase. J Biol Chem 273: 25961-25966.
Okuse K, Chaplan SR, McMahon SB, Luo ZD, Calcutt NA, Scott BP *et al.* (1997) Regulation of expression of the sensory neuron-specific sodium channel SNS in inflammatory and neuropathic pain. Mol Cell Neurosci 10: 196-207.
Oppenheim RW (1996) Neurotrophic survival molecules for motoneurons: an embarrassment of riches. Neuron 17: 195-7.
Orioli D, Klein R (1997) The Eph receptor family: axonal guidance by contact repulsion. Trends Genetics 13: 354-9.
Oyelese AA, Eng DL, Richerson GB, Kocsis JD (1995) Enhancement of GABAA receptor-mediated conductances induced by nerve injury in a subclass of sensory neurons. J Neurophys 74: 673-83.
Pasterkamp RJ, Dewinter F, Holtmaat A, Verhaagen J (1998a) Evidence for a role of the chemorepellent semaphorin III and its receptor, neuropilin-1 in the regeneration of primary olfactory axons. J Neurosci 18: 9962-9976.
Pasterkamp RJ, Giger RJ, Ruitenberg MJ, Holtmaat A, De Wit J, De Winter F *et al.* (1999) Expression of the gene encoding the chemorepellent semaphorin III is induced in the fi-

broblast component of neural scar tissue formed following injuries of adult but not neonatal CNS. Mol Cell Neurosci 13: 143-166.
Pasterkamp RJ, Giger RJ, Verhaagen J (1998b) Regulation of semaphorin III collapsin-1 gene expression during peripheral nerve regeneration. Exp Neurol 153: 313-327.
Perrone-Bizzozero NI, Cansino VV, Kohn DT (1993) Posttranscriptional regulation of GAP-43 gene expression in PC12 cells through protein kinase C-dependent stabilization of the mRNA. J Cell Biol 120: 1263-70.
Philpott KL, McCarthy MJ, Klippel A, Rubin LL (1997) Activated phosphatidylinositol 3-kinase and Akt kinase promote survival of superior cervical neurons. J Cell Biol 139: 809-815.
Piehl F, Frisen J, Risling M, Hokfelt T, Cullheim S (1994) Increased trkB mRNA expression by axotomized motoneurones. Neuroreport 5: 697-700.
Piehl F, Hammarberg H, Tabar G, Hokfelt T, Cullheim S (1998) Changes in the mRNA expression pattern, with special reference to calcitonin gene-related peptide, after axonal injuries in rat motoneurons depends on age and type of injury. Exp Br Res 119: 191-204.
Piehl F, Tabar G, Cullheim S (1995) Expression of NMDA receptor mRNAs in rat motoneurons is down-regulated after axotomy. J Neurosci 7: 2101-10.
Pittman RN (1985) Release of plasminogen activator and calcium-dependent metalloprotease from cultured sympathetic and sensory neurons. Dev Biol 110: 91-101.
Pittman RN, DiBenedetto AJ (1995) PC12 cells overexpressing tissue plasminogen activator regenerate neurites to a greater extent and migrate faster than control cells in complex extracellular matrix. J Neurochem 64: 566-75.
Pittman RN, Williams AG (1989) Neurite penetration into collagen gels requires a Ca2+-dependent metalloproteinase activity. Dev Neurosci 11: 41-51.
Pleasure SJ, Selzer ME, Lee VM (1989) Lamprey neurofilaments combine in one subunit the features of each mammalian NF triplet protein but are highly phosphorylated only in large axons. J Neurosci 9: 698-709.
Povelones M, Tran K, Thanos D, Ambron RT (1997) An NF-kappaB-like transcription factor in axoplasm is rapidly inactivated after nerve injury in Aplysia. J Neurosci 17: 4915-20.
Pu S-F, Zhuang H-X, Marsh DJ, Ishii DN (1999) Insulin-like growth factor II increases and IGF is required for postnatal rat spinal motoneurons survival following sciatic nerve axotomy. J Neurosci Res 55: 9-16.
Raineteau O, Z'Graggen WJ, Thallmair M, Schwab ME (1999) Sprouting and regeneration after pyramidotomy and blockade of the myelin-associated neurite growth inhibitors NI 35/250 in adult rats. J Neurosci 11: 1486-1490.
Rajan P, Gearan T, Fink JS (1998) Leukemia Inhibitory Factor and NGF regulate Signal Transducers and Activators of Transcription activation in sympathetic ganglia - convergence of cytokine- and neurotrophin-signaling pathways. Brain Res 802: 198-204.
Rajan P, Stewart CL, Fink JS (1995) Lif-mediated activation of stat proteins after neuronal injury in vivo. Neuroreport 6: 2240-2244.
Ramaswamy S, Nakamura N, Vazquez F, Batt DB, Perera S, Roberts TM *et al.* (1999) Regulation of G(1) progression by the PTEN tumor suppressor protein is linked to inhibition of the phosphatidylinositol 3-kinase/Akt pathway. Proc Natl Acad Sci USA 96: 2110-2115.
Ramon-Cueto A, Plant GW, Avila J, Bunge MB (1998) Long-distance axonal regeneration in the transected adult rat spinal cord is promoted by olfactory ensheathing glia transplants. J Neurosci 18: 3803-15.

Ramon y Cajal S (1991) Cajal's degeneration and regeneration of the nervous system . Translated by RM May. Editors: DeFelipe J and Jones EG.. New York : Oxford University Press.
Richardson PM (1994) Ciliary neurotrophic factor: a review. Pharmacology and Therapeutics 63(2):187-198.
Richardson PM, Issa VM, Aguayo AJ (1984) Regeneration of long spinal axons in the rat. J Neurocyt 13: 165-82.
Richardson PM, Lu X (1994) Inflammation and axonal regeneration. J Neurol 242: S57-60.
Robinson GA (1995) Axotomy-induced regulation of c-Jun expression in regenerating rat retinal ganglion cells. Brain Res Mol Brain Res 30: 61-9.
Rohlmann A, Laskawi R, Hofer A, Dermietzel R, Wolff JR (1994) Astrocytes as rapid sensors of peripheral axotomy in the facial nucleus of rats. Neuroreport 5: 409-12.
Rosenfeld J, Cook S, James R (1997) Expression of superoxide dismutase following axotomy. Exp Neurol 147: 37-47.
Rossi F, Bravin M, Buffo A, Fronte M, Savio T, Strata P (1997) Intrinsic properties and environmental factors in the regeneration of adult cerebellar axons. Prog Br Res 114: 283-96.
Rossi F, Jankovski A, Sotelo C (1995) Differential regenerative response of Purkinje cell and inferior olivary axons confronted with embryonic grafts: environmental cues versus intrinsic neuronal determinants. J Comp Neurol 359: 663-77.
Saffell JL, Williams EJ, Mason IJ, Walsh FS, Doherty P (1997) Expression of a dominant negative FGF receptor inhibits axonal growth and FGF receptor phosphorylation stimulated by CAMs. Neuron 18: 231-42.
Sagot Y, Rosse T, Vejsada R, Perrelet D, Kato AC (1998) Differential effects of neurotrophic factors on motoneuron retrograde labeling in a murine model of motoneuron disease. J Neurosci 18: 1132-41.
Schachner M, Martini R, Hall H, Orberger G (1995) Functions of the L2/HNK-1 carbohydrate in the nervous system. Prog Br Res 105: 183-8.
Schaden H, Stuermer CA, Bahr M (1994) GAP-43 immunoreactivity and axon regeneration in retinal ganglion cells of the rat. J Neurobiol 25: 1570-8.
Schreyer DJ, Skene JH (1993) Injury-associated induction of GAP-43 expression displays axon branch specificity in rat dorsal root ganglion neurons. J Neurobiol 24: 959-70.
Schwab ME (1996) Molecules inhibiting neurite growth: a minireview. Neurochem Res 21: 755-61.
Schwartz M, Lazarov-Spiegler O, Rapalino O, Agranov I, Velan G, Hadani M (1999a) Potential repair of rat spinal cord injuries using stimulated homologous macrophages. Neurosurgery 44: 1041-1045.
Schwartz M, Moalem G, Leibowitz-Amit R, Cohen IR (1999b) Innate and adaptive immune responses can be beneficial for CNS repair. Trends Neurosci 22: 295-299.
Seeds NW, Siconolfi LB, Haffke SP (1997) Neuronal extracellular proteases facilitate cell migration, axonal growth, and pathfinding. Cell Tissue Res 290: 367-370.
Seeds NW, Williams BL, Bickford PC (1995) Tissue plasminogen activator induction in Purkinje neurons after cerebellar motor learning. Science 270: 1992-4.
Sendtner M, Carroll P, Holtmann B, Hughes RA, Thoenen H (1994) Ciliary neurotrophic factor. J Neurobiol 25: 1436-53.
Sendtner M, Gotz R, Holtmann B, Escary JL, Masu Y, Carroll P *et al.* (1996) Cryptic physiological trophic support of motoneurons by LIF revealed by double gene targeting of CNTF and LIF. Curr Biol 6: 686-94.

Sendtner M, Gotz R, Holtmann B, Thoenen H (1997) Endogenous ciliary neurotrophic factor is a lesion factor for axotomized motoneurons in adult mice. J Neurosci 17: 6999-7006.

Sendtner M, Stockli KA, Thoenen H (1992) Synthesis and localization of ciliary neurotrophic factor in the sciatic nerve of the adult rat after lesion and during regeneration. J Cell Biol 118: 139-48.

Shen H, Chung JM, Chung K (1999) Expression of neurotrophin mRNAs in the dorsal root ganglion after spinal nerve injury. Brain Res Mol Brain Res 64: 186-192.

Shimoke K, Yamagishi S, Yamada M, Ikeuchi T, Hatanaka H (1999) Inhibition of phosphatidylinositol 3-kinase activity elevates c-Jun N-terminal kinase activity in apoptosis of cultured cerebellar granule neurons. Brain Research. Dev Brain Res 112: 245-253.

Skene JH (1989) Axonal growth-associated proteins. Ann Rev Neurosci 12: 127-56.

Skene JHP (1992) Retrograde pathways controlling expression of a major growth cone component in the adult CNS. In: P.C. Letourneau, S.B. Kater and E.R. Macagno, (Eds.), *The Nerve Growth Cone*, Raven Press, New York, pp.463-375.

Smith DS, Skene JH (1997) A transcription-dependent switch controls competence of adult neurons for distinct modes of axon growth. J Neurosci 17(2):646-658.

Snider WD, Elliott JL, Yan Q (1992) Axotomy-induced neuronal death during development. J Neurobiol 23: 1231-1246.

Sretavan DW, Kruger K (1998) Randomized retinal ganglion cell axon routing at the optic chiasm of GAP-43-deficient mice: Association with midline recrossing and lack of normal ipsilateral axon turning. J Neurosci 18: 10502-10513.

Stambolic V, Suzuki A, Delapompa JL, Brothers GM, Mirtsos C, Sasaki T *et al.* (1998) Negative regulation of PKB/Akt-dependent cell survival by the tumor suppressor PTEN. Cell 95: 29-39.

Stilwell K, Kobayashi NR, Steeves JD, Tetzlaff W (1997) Changes in FGF-2, FGFR-1 and FGFR-2 in the axotomized facial nucleus and red nucleus of the adult rat. Soc Neurosci Abstr 23: 2247.

Strittmatter SM, Fankhauser C, Huang PL, Mashimo H, Fishman MC (1995) Neuronal pathfinding is abnormal in mice lacking the neuronal growth cone protein GAP-43. Cell 80(3):455-452.

Su QN, Namikawa K, Toki H, Kiyama H (1997) Differential display reveals transcriptional up-regulation of the motor molecules for both anterograde and retrograde axonal transport during nerve regeneration. J Neurosci 9: 1542-1547.

Sun Y, Zigmond RE (1996) Involvement of leukemia inhibitory factor in the increases in galanin and vasoactive intestinal peptide mRNA and the decreases in neuropeptide Y and tyrosine hydroxylase mRNA in sympathetic neurons after axotomy. J Neurochem 67: 1751-1760.

Suter DM, Forscher P (1998) An emerging link between cytoskeletal dynamics and cell adhesion molecules in growth cone guidance. Curr Opin Neurobiol 8: 106-16.

Takei Y, Kondo S, Harada A, Inomata S, Noda T, Hirokawa N (1997) Delayed development of nervous system in mice homozygous for disrupted microtubule-associated protein 1B (MAP1B) gene. J Cell Biol 137: 1615-26.

Tanabe K, Kiryu-Seo S, Nakamura T, Mori N, Tsujino H, Ochi T *et al.* (1998) Alternative expression of Shc family members in nerve-injured motoneurons. Brain Res Mol Brain Res 53: 291-296.

Tang FR, Sim MK (1997) Expression of glutamate receptor sunits 2/3 and 4 in the hypoglossal nucleus of the rat after neurectomy. Exp Brain Res 117: 453-456.

Tedeschi B, Ciavarra RP (1997) Differential effects of axotomy on the in vivo synthesis of the stress-inducible and constitutive 70-kDa heat-shock proteins in rat dorsal root ganglia. Brain Res Mol Brain Res 45: 199-206.

Tetzlaff W, Alexander SW, Miller FD, Bisby MA (1991) Response of facial and rubrospinal neurons to axotomy: changes in mRNA expression for cytoskeletal proteins and GAP-43. J Neurosci 11: 2528-44.

Tetzlaff W, Bisby MA, Kreutzberg GW (1988) Changes in cytoskeletal proteins in the rat facial nucleus following axotomy. J Neurosci 8: 3181-9.

Tetzlaff W, Kobayashi NR, Giehl KM, Tsui BJ, Cassar SL, Bedard AM (1994) Response of rubrospinal and corticospinal neurons to injury and neurotrophins. Prog Br Res 103: 271-86.

Tetzlaff W, Leonard C, Krekoski CA, Parhad IM, Bisby MA (1996) Reductions in motoneuronal neurofilament synthesis by successive axotomies: a possible explanation for the conditioning lesion effect on axon regeneration. Exp Neurol 139: 95-106.

Thallmair M, Metz GAS, Zgraggen WJ, Raineteau O, Kartje GL, Schwab ME (1998) Neurite Growth Inhibitors Restrict Plasticity and Functional Recovery Following Corticospinal Tract Lesions. Nature Neuroscience 1: 124-131.

Thomas WS, Jacob MH, O'Dowd DK, Smith MA (1995) Agrin gene expression in ciliary ganglion neurons following preganglionic denervation and postganglionic axotomy. Dev Biol (Orlando) 168: 662-669.

Tokuraku K, Katsuki M, Nakagawa H, Kotani S (1999) A new model for microtubule-associated protein (MAP)-induced microtubule assembly - The Pro-rich region of MAP4 promotes nucleation of microtubule assembly in vitro. Eur J Biochem 259: 158-166.

Tonra JR, Curtis R, Wong V, Cliffer KD, Park JS, Timmes A *et al.* (1998) Axotomy upregulates the anterograde transport and expression of brain-derived neurotrophic factor by sensory neurons. J Neurosci 18: 4374-83.

Troy CM, Muma NA, Greene LA, Price DL, Shelanski ML (1990) Regulation of peripherin and neurofilament expression in regenerating rat motor neurons. Brain Res 529: 232-8.

Tsai KC, Cansino VV, Kohn DT, Neve RL, Perrone-Bizzozero NI (1997) Post-transcriptional regulation of the GAP-43 gene by specific sequences in the 3' untranslated region of the mRNA. J Neurosci 17: 1950-8.

Uhm JH, Dooley NP, Oh LY, Yong VW (1998) Oligodendrocytes utilize a matrix metalloproteinase, MMP-9, to extend processes along an astrocyte extracellular matrix. Glia 22: 53-63.

Vanderluit JL, McPhail LT, Fernandes KJL, McBride CB, Huguenot C, Roy S, Robertson GS, Nicholson DW, Tetzlaff W (1999) Caspase 3 is developmentally regulated in facial motoneurons and activated following axotomy in neonatal rodents but is ultimately not required for cell death. Submitted.

Vanderluit JL, McPhail LT, Harrington KC, Barclay S, Anderson LL, Rossiter JR, Tetzlaff W (1997) Expression of cell death and survival genes in axotomized facial motoneurons in the adult versus newborn rat. Soc Neurosci Abstr 23(2):1157.

Vanselow J, Grabczyk E, Ping J, Baetscher M, Teng S, Fishman MC (1994) GAP-43 transgenic mice: dispersed genomic sequences confer a GAP-43-like expression pattern during development and regeneration. J Neurosci 14: 499-510.

Viollet C, Doherty P (1997) CAMS and the FGF receptor - an interacting role in axonal growth. Cell Tissue Res 290: 451-455.

Vizzard MA, Erdman SL, de Groat WC (1995) Increased expression of neuronal nitric oxide synthase (NOS) in visceral neurons after nerve injury. J Neurosci 15: 4033-45.

von Meyenburg J, Brosamle C, Metz GAS, Schwab ME (1998) Regeneration and sprouting of chronically injured corticospinal tract fibers in adult rats promoted by NT-3 and the mAb IN-1, which neutralizes myelin-associated neurite growth inhibitors. Exp Neurol 154: 583-594.

Walsh FS, Doherty P (1997) Neural cell adhesion molecules of the immunoglobulin superfamily: role in axon growth and guidance. Ann Rev Cell Dev Biol 13: 425-56.

Wang HG, Pathan N, Ethell IM, Krajewski S, Yamaguchi Y, Shibasaki F *et al.* (1999) Ca2+-induced apoptosis through calcineurin dephosphorylation of BAD. Science 284: 339-343.

Wasylyk B, Hagman J, Gutierrez-Hartmann A (1998) Ets transcription factors: nuclear effectors of the Ras-MAP-kinase signaling pathway. Trends Biochem Sci 23: 213-216.

Waxman SG, Kocsis JD, Black JA (1994) Type III sodium channel mRNA is expressed in embryonic but not adult spinal sensory neurons, and is reexpressed following axotomy. J Neurophys 72: 466-70.

Wictorin K, Brundin P, Gustavii B, Lindvall O, Bjorklund A (1990) Reformation of long axon pathways in adult rat central nervous system by human forebrain neuroblasts. Nature 347: 556-8.

Wiederkehr A, Staple J, Caroni P (1997) The motility-associated proteins GAP-43, MARCKS, and CAP-23 share unique targeting and surface activity-inducing properties. Exp Cell Res 236: 103-16.

Wizenmann A, Thies E, Klostermann S, Bonhoeffer F, Bahr M (1993) Appearance of target-specific guidance information for regenerating axons after CNS lesions. Neuron 11: 975-83.

Woolf CJ, Reynolds ML, Molander C, O'Brien C, Lindsay RM, Benowitz LI (1990) The growth-associated protein GAP-43 appears in dorsal root ganglion cells and in the dorsal horn of the rat spinal cord following peripheral nerve injury. Neurosci 34: 465-78.

Wu W, Han K, Li L, Schinco FP (1994a) Implantation of PNS graft inhibits the induction of neuronal nitric oxide synthase and enhances the survival of spinal motoneurons following root avulsion. Exp Neurol 129: 335-9.

Wu W, Liuzzi FJ, Schinco FP, Depto AS, Li Y, Mong JA *et al.* (1994b) Neuronal nitric oxide synthase is induced in spinal neurons by traumatic injury. Neurosci 61: 719-26.

Wu W, Mathew TC, Miller FD (1993) Evidence that the loss of homeostatic signals induces regeneration-associated alterations in neuronal gene expression. Dev Biol 158: 456-66.

Wu YY, Bradshaw RA (1996) Synergistic induction of neurite outgrowth by nerve growth factor or epidermal growth factor and interleukin-6 in PC12 cells. J Biol Chem 271: 13033-9.

Wylie SR, Wu PJ, Patel H, Chantler PD (1998) A conventional myosin motor drives neurite outgrowth. Proc Natl Acad Sci USA 95: 12967-12972.

Xu XM, Chen A, Guenard V, Kleitman N, Bunge MB (1997) Bridging Schwann cell transplants promote axonal regeneration from both the rostral and caudal stumps of transected adult rat spinal cord. J Neurocyt 26: 1-16.

Xu XM, Zhang SX, Li HY, Aebischer P, Bunge MB (1999) Regrowth of axons into the distal spinal cord through a Schwann-cell-seeded mini-channel implanted into hemisected adult rat spinal cord. J Neurosci 11: 1723-1740.

Yamada E, Kataoka H, Hazama F (1994) Specific expression of type II protein kinase c after axotomy in the dorsal motor nucleus of the vagus nerve and the hypoglossal nucleus. Brain Res 639: 341-6.

Yano S, Tokumitsu H, Sodeling TR (1998) Calcium promotes cell survival through CaM-K kinase activation of the protein-kinase-B pathway. Nature 396: 584-587.

Yao GL, Kato H, Khalil M, Kiryu S, Kiyama H (1997) Selective upregulation of cytokine receptor subchain and their intracellular signalling molecules after peripheral nerve injury. Eur J Neurosci 9: 1047-1054.

Yen TJ, Gay DA, Pachter JS, Cleveland DW (1988a) Autoregulated changes in stability of polyribosome-bound beta-tubulin mRNAs are specified by the first 13 translated nucleotides. Mol Cell Biol 8: 1224-35.

Yen TJ, Machlin PS, Cleveland DW (1988b) Autoregulated instability of beta-tubulin mRNAs by recognition of the nascent amino terminus of beta-tubulin. Nature 334: 580-5.

Yuguchi T, Kohmura E, Yamada K, Otsuki H, Sakaki T, Yamashita T *et al.* (1997) Expression of tPA mRNA in the facial nucleus following facial nerve transection in the rat. Neuroreport 8: 419-22.

Zagrebelsky M, Buffo A, Skerra A, Schwab ME, Strata P, Rossi F (1998) Retrograde regulation of growth-associated gene expression in adult rat Purkinje cells by myelin-associated neurite growth inhibitory proteins. J Neurosci 18: 7912-29.

Zhang Q, Shi TJ, Ji RR, Zhang YZ, Sundler F, Hannibal J *et al.* (1995) Expression of pituitary adenylate cyclase-activating polypeptide in dorsal root ganglia following axotomy: time course and coexistence. Brain Res 705: 149-158.

Zhang YZ, Hannibal J, Zhao Q, Moller K, Danielsen N, Fahrenkrug J *et al.* (1996) Pituitary adenylate cyclase activating peptide expression in the rat dorsal root ganglia: up-regulation after peripheral nerve injury. Neurosci 74: 1099-1110.

Zhao Y, Szaro BG (1995) The optic tract and tectal ablation influence the composition of neurofilaments in regenerating optic axons of Xenopus laevis. J Neurosci 15: 4629-40.

Zhong J, Dietzel ID, Wahle P, Kopf M, Heumann R (1999) Sensory impairments and delayed regeneration of sensory axons in interleukin-6-deficient mice. J Neurosci 19: 4305-4313.

Zhu Q, Couillard-Despres S, Julien JP (1997) Delayed maturation of regenerating myelinated axons in mice lacking neurofilaments. Exp Neurol 148: 299-316.

Zhu QZ, Julien JP (1999) A key role for GAP-43 in the retinotectal topographic organization. Exp Neurol 155: 228-242.

Zhu QZ, Lindenbaum M, Levavasseur F, Jacomy H, Julien JP (1998) Disruption of the NF-H gene increases axonal microtubule content and velocity of neurofilament transport - relief of axonopathy resulting from the toxin beta,beta'-iminodipropionitrile. J Cell Biol 143: 183-193.

Zigmond RE, Hyatt-Sachs H, Mohney RP, Schreiber RC, Shadiack AM, Sun Y *et al.* (1996) Changes in neuropeptide phenotype after axotomy of adult peripheral neurons and the role of leukemia inhibitory factor. Persp Dev Neurobiol 4: 75-90.

Zigmond RE, Sun Y (1997) Regulation of neuropeptide expression in sympathetic neurons. Paracrine and retrograde influences. Annals NY Acad Sci 814: 181-97.

Zuo J, Ferguson TA, Hernandez YJ, Stetler-Stevenson WG, Muir D (1998) Neuronal matrix metalloproteinase-2 degrades and inactivates a neurite-inhibiting chondroitin sulfate proteoglycan. J Neurosci 18: 5203-5211.

9

A-fiber Central Sprouting After Peripheral Nerve Injury – New Pathways for Pain?

Richard J. Mannion and Clifford J. Woolf
Massachusetts General Hospital & Harvard Medical School, Boston, Massachusetts

Can primary sensory neurons grow within the spinal cord during adulthood? After traumatic injury to the dorsal column pathways, almost no growth is observed under normal circumstances (Richardson & Issa, 1984). However, A-fiber primary afferent central terminals can sprout in the spinal cord. Remarkably, this occurs after peripheral nerve injury, where central terminals of A-fibers sprout into regions of the dorsal horn that normally only receive C-fiber input. The aim of this chapter is to highlight the structural reorganization of primary afferent central terminals that occurs following peripheral nerve injury, and explain how this mechanism may contribute to the neuropathic pain that often accompanies nerve injury in humans.

I. INTRODUCTION

Primary sensory neurons are the interface between the periphery and the central nervous system, informing the brain about the outside world. To cope with the vast range of sensory stimuli that they encounter, they are a morphologically and functionally heterogeneous population, classified as either A- or C-fibers, the 'large light' and 'small dark' neurons respectively (Lawson, 1979). Approximately two thirds of somatic sensory afferents are the small unmyelinated C-fiber neurons, many of which are nociceptors (Willis & Coggeshall, 1991). The other third of primary sensory neurons are the A-fiber population, which are generally larger neurons with myelinated axons (Lawson et al. 1984). A-fibers are classified into three groups; the thinly myelinated Aδ-fibers, which are predominantly nociceptive, the myelinated Aβ-fibers, many of which are cutaneous mechanoreceptors that can be slowly or rapidly adapting, and the large myelinated Aα-fibers that innervate muscle spindles and golgi-tendon organs and are involved in proprioceptive function.

II. PRIMARY AFFERENTS PROJECT TO THE DORSAL HORN

The central projections of dorsal root ganglion (DRG) neurons are highly ordered in three dimensions. Rostrocaudally and mediolaterally, projections are arranged somatotopically, that is, specific nerves project centrally to respect the same boundaries as they do in the periphery, forming a two dimensional body map with little or no overlap among nerves (Molander and Grant, 1985; Molander and Grant, 1986; Swett and Woolf, 1985). Dorsoventrally, specific types of neuron project to cytoarchitectonically distinct laminae of the dorsal horn. Aδ-fibers project to laminae I and V, Aβ-fibers to the deeper dorsal horn laminae (III-V, with some input to lamina II inner, II_i), while C-fibers project to lamina II (Figure 1). Lamina II outer (II_o), therefore, receives C-fiber input exclusively (Light & Perl, 1979; Rivero-Melian & Grant, 1990; Willis & Coggeshall, 1991).

III. IS CENTRAL DENERVATION SUFFICIENT TO INDUCE PRIMARY AFFERENT SPROUTING?

Primary sensory neurons are classified as pseudounipolar, having a stem axon that leaves the cell body in the DRG and divides into two axons, one projecting peripherally to targets in the skin, muscle, joints and viscera, and another that projects centrally into the spinal cord. This population of neurons therefore offers an opportunity to study the ability of axons belonging to the same neuron to grow in the peripheral and central nervous system (P/CNS). Some of the original studies into the effects of cutaneous nerve injury on sensibility were done by Henry Head early in this century. He and others documented the sensory disturbances that accompanied the crush of their own cutaneous nerves in the arm, describing sensory deficits across modalities that eventually returned after denervated targets were reinnervated by regenerating axons (Head & Sherren, 1905). It is now fully accepted that both sensory and motor axons in peripheral nerves have the capacity to regenerate efficiently, particular if the perineurium remains intact so that individual Schwann cell tubes can act as physical guidance cues to the periphery (Madison et al. 1996). This ability to regenerate, however, has long been known not to be the case within the mammalian CNS. When Liu and Chambers (1958) first presented evidence for sprouting within the spinal cord of *uninjured* primary affer-

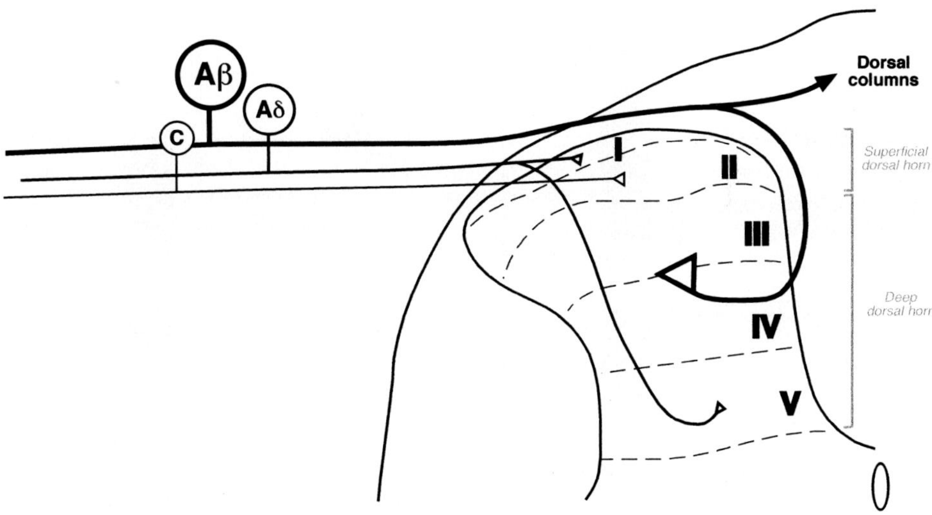

Figure 1 Primary afferent terminations within the dorsal horn. The sensory neurons have cell bodies that sit in the DRG and central axons that project into the dorsal horn to terminate within specific cytoarchitectonically distinct laminae. Large, myelinated Aβ-fibers terminate in the deep dorsal horn (laminae IIi-V), Aδ-fibers in I and V, and C-fibers in lamina II. Aα-fibers have been omitted for clarity.

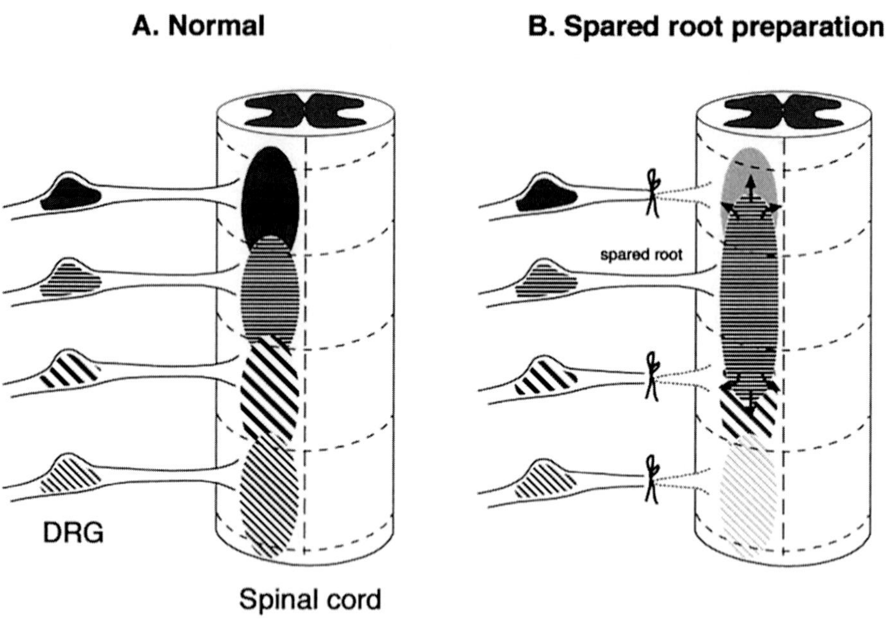

Figure 2 **Spared root preparation.** Denervation within the spinal cord dorsal horn is created by ligating and cutting a number of dorsal roots ipsilaterally except one that is left intact (the spared root). The central projections of the DRG with intact dorsal roots are mapped before and after denervation to assess whether these axons can sprout into the deafferented regions (shaded regions). Conclusions from different studies have been controversial.

ent central axons into dorsal horn territories that had been denervated by dorsal root section (the 'spared root preparation'; Figure 2), this was greeted with great interest and excitement. Indeed, these studies suggested that under some circumstances, uninjured axons could demonstrate significant growth within the CNS, as well as proposing a possible central mechanism to account for some of the long term sensory disturbances that occur following nerve injury. Since then, many investigators have attempted to repeat and extend the findings of Liu & Chambers, using a number of different techniques (e.g., Polistena et al., 1990). Whether this phenomenon is real, however, remains controversial.

Many of the studies that have used transganglionic tracers to assess primary afferent central terminal sprouting have concluded that very little growth of uninjured axons occurs into regions denervated either from dorsal rhizotomy (McMahon & Kett-White, 1991) or transganglionic degeneration after nerve injury (Molander et al. 1988). However, some growth is observed in the dorsal horn if the neurons are 'primed' into an increased growth status. Priming is achieved by injuring the peripheral axons of sensory neurons, e.g., with a nerve crush. This results in the dissociation of sensory neurons from their innervation targets so that neurons no longer receive retrograde signals from the periphery. Subsequently, alterations in neuronal phenotype are observed, including the upregulation of structural and growth related molecules (Skene, 1989), cell adhesion molecules involved in homo- and heterophilic binding (Araki & Milbrandt, 1996) and Schwann cell mitogens (Livesey et al., 1997), all of which act to increase the rate of regenerative growth of these cells. The consequences of nerve injury on neuronal phenotype are discussed elsewhere in this book. However, it is interesting to note that many of the injury-regulated molecules, synthesized in cell bodies within the DRG, are transported centrally to the spinal cord as well as peripherally to the injured axon tip (Bisby, 1981). Growth Associated Protein (GAP)-43 is one such molecule, dramatically upregulated within the DRG after peripheral nerve injury and transported bidirectionally, that is, peripherally into the growth cones of regenerating axons and centrally to the superficial laminae of the dorsal horn of the spinal cord (Chong et al., 1992). These observations offer a possible explanation as to why primary afferent sprouting occurs into denervated dorsal horn territory following injury to peripheral axons, but not in its absence (Molander et al., 1988; McMahon & Kett-White, 1991); i.e., the central terminal of a sensory neuron with an injured peripheral axon may acquire the molecular machinery necessary for axonal growth.

The studies initiated by Liu and Chambers were concerned with the ability of primary afferent central terminals to sprout outside their normal projection fields in a rostrocaudal direction. However, it turns out that it is in the dorsoventral plane that significant sprouting occurs after peripheral nerve injury. Axotomy or crush induces the sprouting of A-fibers into lamina II_o, a region that normally only receives noxious C-fiber input (Woolf et al. 1992), that lasts for over 9 months regardless of whether the peripheral nerve is allowed to regenerate to its peripheral targets (Woolf et al. 1995). This was first shown using the transganglionic tracer horseradish peroxidase conjugated to the B subunit of cholera toxin (B-HRP), a modificaton that allows the tracer to be taken up only by myelinated fibers, that is the A- but not the C-population. B-HRP can be bulk injected into the peripheral nerve in order to label transganglionically the central terminals in the dorsal horn. This technique identifies the central termination sites of A-fibers, which are in all laminae of the dorsal horn apart from II_o. After nerve injury, however, all laminae of the dorsal horn are densely labeled, including lamina II_o (Figure 3; Woolf et al., 1992).

A criticism of this technique has been that bulk B-HRP labeling throughout lamina II after nerve injury may simply reflect a post-injury ability of C-fibers to uptake and transport B-HRP, rather than the result of central sprouting of A-fiber terminals into this region (Tong et al., 1999). The following data suggest that this is not the case. First, if this were the case, the number of small C-fiber cell bodies and the number of unmyelinated axons in the dorsal root that were positive for B-HRP labeling after nerve injury should increase dramatically. Neither of these phenomena appear to occur (Woolf et al. 1995; Bennett et al. 1996 but see Tong et al. 1999). Second, using intra-axonal tracer injections, single A-fiber collateral axons have been filled (Woolf et al. 1992; Shortland et al. 1993; Koerber et al. 1994). After nerve injury, these axons extend past their normal boundary in lamina II_i and begin to innervate novel dorsal horn territory within lamina II_o and lamina I. Third, it has been shown using electron microscopy that after nerve injury, lamina II contains many synapses with B-HRP-filled pre-synaptic terminals with a synaptic structure different from C-fibers (Woolf et al., 1995). Consistent with these anatomical observations are data from whole cell patch-clamp recordings within lamina II neurons in adult spinal cord slices. These studies have revealed that in normal animals, no monosynaptic A-fiber input can be elicited. Two weeks after peripheral nerve injury, however, monosynaptic as well as polysynaptic A-fiber inputs to these neurons increase dramatically (Okamoto et al. 1996; Kohama et al. 1998).

Peripheral nerve injury also induces a transganglionic degeneration of primary afferent terminals, particularly within the superficial dorsal horn layers innervated predominantly by C-fiber terminals (Knyihar-Csillik et al. 1987; Castro-Lopes et al. 1990). The exact reasons for this are unknown, although it is known that many C-fibers have a phenotype that is maintained by peripherally derived Nerve Growth Factor (NGF) and Glial cell-derived Growth Factor (GDNF), with two distinct subpopulations of C-fiber neurons expressing, almost mutually exclusively, the cognate receptors for these molecules (Molliver et al. 1997; Bennett et al. 1998). It is highly likely that the transganglionic degenerative atrophy occurring after nerve injury results from the decreased availability of factors that are retrogradely transported from the periphery (Csillik & Knyihar-Csillik, 1982). The application of exogenous NGF to the proximal stump of the injured sciatic nerve dramatically reduces the extent of transganglionic degenerative atrophy observed within the superficial dorsal horn (Csillik et al. 1985).

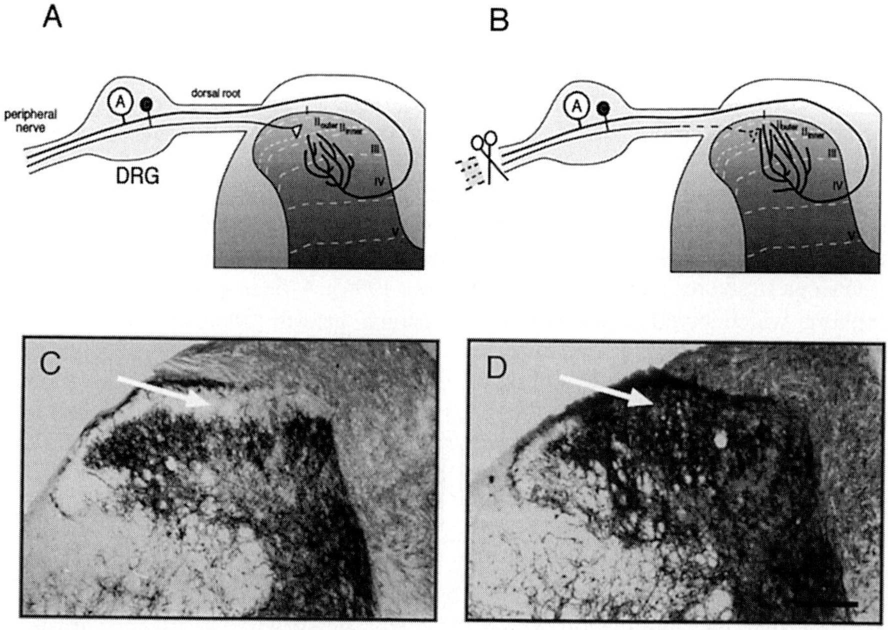

Figure 3 **A-fibers sprout into lamina II following peripheral nerve injury**. (A) Normally, A-fiber central terminals innervate all laminae other than IIo. (C) This is observed using B-HRP to preferentially label A-fibers. Note the absence of staining within lamina II (arrow). (B, D) Two weeks after nerve injury, and lasting for over nine months, A-fibers sprout into lamina II and make functional connections. Nerve injury, therefore, induces a rewiring of spinal circuitry in the dorsal horn. Scale bars = 20 um. Adapted from Mannion et al. (1998).

A-fiber sprouting into lamina II after nerve injury was, therefore, initially thought to occur through a combination of two main factors; first, that injured A-fiber neurons increase their propensity for growth as a consequence of peripheral axonal injury, and second, that transganglionic degeneration within the superficial dorsal horn creates synaptic space for the primed A-fiber central terminals to grow into. A-fiber sprouting was termed *regenerative-collateral* sprouting, because it exhibits features of both types of growth (Woolf et al. 1995).

Collateral sprouting, defined as the growth of uninjured axons into a denervated region, has been studied in detail within the skin. Following a denervation produced by injuring dorsal cutaneous nerves, intact C- and Aδ-fibers innervating adjacent regions sprout into denervated territory in an NGF dependent manner (Diamond et al. 1987; Mearow et al. 1993). This type of growth is increased if the intact nerves are electrically stimulated (Doucette & Diamond, 1987), and the sprouting neurons upregulate growth related molecules such as GAP-43 (Mearow et al. 1994). Low threshold Aβ-fiber collateral sprouting has also been observed in cutaneous structures (Doubleday & Robinson, 1994). A-fiber sprouting in the dorsal horn, which includes Aβ-fiber central terminal growth (Shortland et al. 1993), occurs after a peripheral nerve injury, which injures both C- and A-fiber peripheral axons. The central A-fiber sprouting could be the effect of damage to the peripheral branch of the A-fibers with the injury induced upregulation of growth related molecules in these fibers leading to central terminal growth. Alternatively, if the C-fiber injury alone was the key factor for initiating the A-fiber central terminal growth, then this would be an example of true collateral sprouting, occurring independently of any peripheral axon 'priming' injury to the neurons that grow.

To address this possibility, we have used two different approaches. The first, using the C-fiber specific neurotoxin capsaicin, aimed to injure selectively the unmyelinated fiber population within the sciatic nerve without affecting myelinated A-fibers. Capsaicin, applied topically to the sciatic nerve, causes transganglionic degeneration within the superficial dorsal horn in a fashion similar to that observed following nerve injury (Jancso, 1992). It also causes a depletion in C-fiber neuron peptide content, in particular substance P and CGRP (Ainsworth et al. 1981; Fitzgerald, 1983) as well as a significant reduction in thiamine monophosphatase (TMP) staining within the superficial dorsal horn (Gamse et al. 1982; Mannion et al. 1996). In contrast, no changes in the phenotype of post-ganglionic sympathetic neurons are observed following topical capsaicin treatment to the sciatic nerve (Gamse et al. 1982), an observation that suggests a specific action of this toxic compound on C-fibers and not unmyelinated axons *per se*. These findings are supported by recent studies that have characterized the expression of the capsaicin receptor, VR1, on DRG neurons. Only small neurons are found to express this molecule, where it colocalizes with both the TrkA-expressing and IB4-binding populations of C-fibers (Tominaga et al. 1998). Following capsaicin treatment to the sciatic nerve, B-HRP transganglionic labeling reveals that A-fibers, in contrast to the normal pattern of staining now innervate all laminae of the dorsal horn including lamina II_o (Mannion et al., 1996). This labeling is indistinguishable from that observed two weeks after a sciatic nerve injury. Thus, selective C-fiber injury to the sciatic nerve is sufficient to induce the sprouting of *uninjured* sciatic A-fibers.

The second approach depended on the particular arrangement of the somatotopic innervation of the dorsal horn by primary afferents (Swett & Woolf, 1985). The saphenous and sciatic nerves innervate adjacent territories with almost no overlap between the two nerves, reflecting the innervation patterns in the skin. An interesting feature of primary termination patterns in the dorsal horn, though, is that hindlimb nerve A-fiber neurons innervate a larger area rostrocaudally and mediolaterally than C-fibers within the same nerve, and this is particularly evident for the sciatic nerve. The mediolateral extent of B-HRP labeling within lamina III of the L5 spinal segment occupies approximately 80% of the medial dorsal horn. Sciatic C-fiber central terminals, however, only occupy approximately 60-70% of the medial dorsal horn in lamina II (Doubell et al., 1997). Therefore, a region of dorsal horn neuropil exists within lateral lamina II that contains C-fiber central terminals of another hindlimb nerve, while sciatic A-fibers innervate lamina III directly below, in the same dorsoventral plane. This lateral region is occupied by C-fiber neurons of the posterior cutaneous nerve (Figure 4; Swett & Woolf, 1985).

Selective axotomy of the posterior cutaneous nerve offers an opportunity to study the effects of transganglionic degeneration in lateral lamina II on A-fiber central terminals of the sciatic nerve that has experienced no manipulation whatsoever and is, therefore, indisputably uninjured. Two weeks after posterior cutaneous nerve axotomy, sciatic B-HRP labeling in the spinal cord reveals that no A-fiber label is observed in sciatic regions of lamina II, but laterally, the region that under normal circumstances is innervated by posterior cutaneous C-fibers, now contains dense staining, suggestive of A-fiber sprouting into this territory (Figure 5). Once again, this result is consistent with the hypothesis that uninjured A-fibers can sprout into lamina II, suggesting that nerve-injury induced A-fiber central terminal growth is a genuine example of collateral sprouting. Such sprouting may be the consequence of peripheral nerve injury acting on C-fibers to either induce the creation of vacant synaptic space in lamina II due to withdrawal of C-fiber terminals, or the production of a chemoattractive ‘factor’ by C-fiber terminal that attracts A-fiber terminals to grow in this region and make synapses.

These possibilities can be addressed by experimentally creating true denervation within the superficial dorsal horn using a dorsal rhizotomy. Sectioning the dorsal roots induces Wallerian degeneration of the distal axon segments and significant deafferentation within the dorsal horn (Murray & Goldberger, 1986). The lumbar dorsal root ganglion neurons project to the spinal cord and innervate a region that is larger, at the lamina III level, than the relevant spinal segment (Rivero-Melian & Grant, 1990). Therefore, the lumbar DRGs have central projection fields that overlap rostrocaudally, even though individual peripheral nerves, such as the sciatic and saphenous, which for example both have sensory cell bodies in the L4 ganglion (Puigdellivol-Sanchez, 1998), have very little overlap centrally (Swett & Woolf, 1985). This means that an L5 rhizotomy will remove all L5 DRG input to

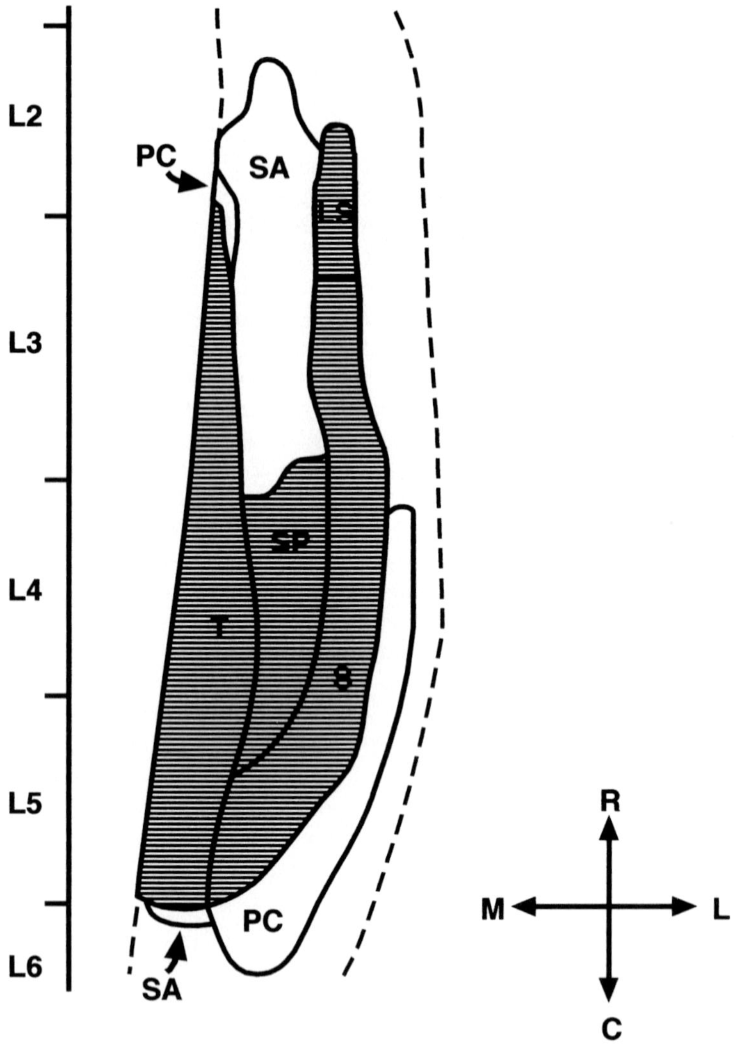

Figure 4 Somatotopic map of hindlimb nerve C-fiber projections to lamina II of the dorsal horn. A dorsal view of the spinal cord at the lamina II level. Each nerve projects to a region of lamina II that has almost no overlap with other hindlimb nerves. Note that the posterior cutaneous nerve (PC) starts more caudally then lies laterally to those that constitute the sciatic nerve (shaded region; T = tibial, SP = superficial peroneal, S = sural). SA = saphenous. The dotted lines represent boundaries of dorsal horn grey matter. Adapted from Swett & Woolf (1985).

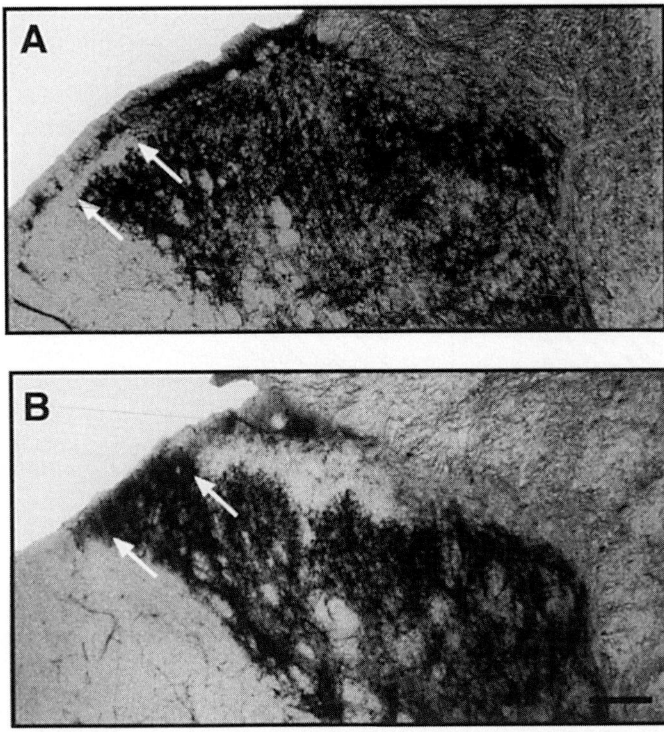

Figure 5 Photomicrographs showing sciatic nerve B-HRP labeling in the superficial dorsal horn 2 weeks after (A) sciatic nerve injury and (B) posterior cutaneous nerve injury. Note that sciatic A-fibers sprout into territory normally occupied by C-fiber terminals of the injured nerve (arrows). Scale bar = 100 μm. Adapted from Doubell et al. (1977).

the dorsal horn of the L5 spinal segment, but it will still be partially innervated by sensory neurons located within the L4 DRG that have central collaterals extending outside the L4 spinal segment. Remarkably, these axon collaterals can extend for many segments within the spinal cord and make functional connections (Wilson & Kitchener, 1996).

Using an L5 dorsal rhizotomy, we studied whether deafferentation to the dorsal horn, particularly lamina II, was sufficient to induce the sprouting of intact A-fiber terminals innervating territory outside their respective spinal segment. After L5 rhizotomy, bulk B-HRP labeling revealed that lamina III in the rostral L5 segment was still partially innervated (Figure 6), yet two weeks later, staining was never observed within lamina II (Mannion et al. 1998). This suggests that A-fiber sprouting into the superficial dorsal horn is not a true example of collateral sprouting, and that the mechanism responsible for this type of structural reorganization is different from that causing sprouting of cutaneous primary afferent peripheral terminals into denervated regions.

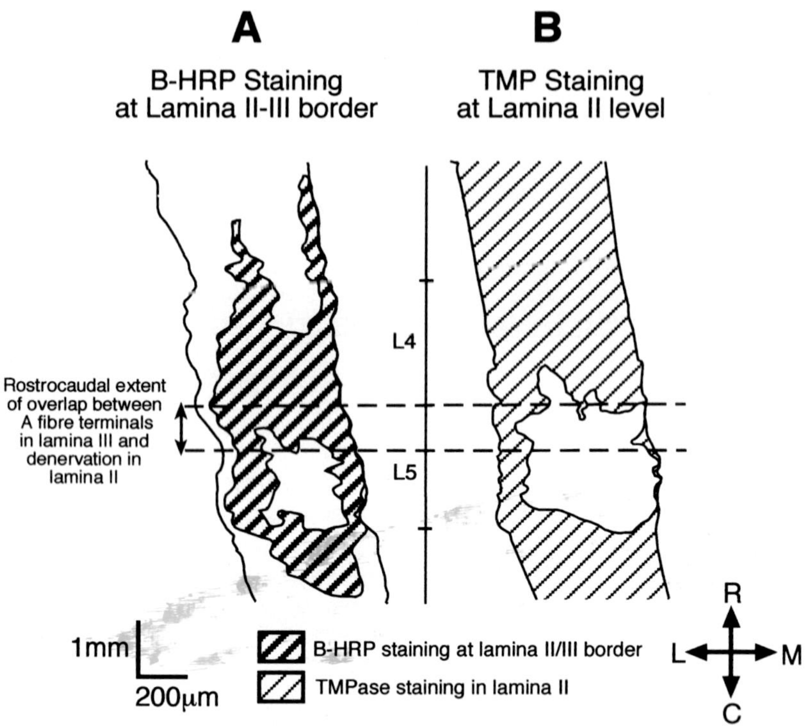

Figure 6 Somatotopic maps comparing the extent of territories in lamina III (A) and lamina II (B) that are denervated after L5 rhizotomy. The area in (A) is measured using B-HRP labeling in the dorsal horn, while the area in (B) is measured from regions that are depleted of TMP staining after rhizotomy. Note that the extent of the region that contains A-fiber terminals in lamina III but no C-fiber terminals in lamina II stretches for a few hundred microns within the rostral L5 spinal segment (arrows). Adapted from Mannion et al. (1998).

IV. WHAT CAUSES A-FIBER SPROUTING IN THE DORSAL HORN?

Following the initial observation of a reorganization of the distribution of A fiber central terminals after nerve injury, it was thought that growth related molecules transported centrally may be involved in sprouting into lamina II (Woolf et al. 1995), for example, GAP-43, where immunoreactivity increases significantly within this region over a time course consistent with A-fiber sprouting (Chong et al. 1992). If this were the case, it would follow that B-HRP, which labels the sprouting A-fibers, would colocalize with GAP-43. However, despite finding thousands of B-HRP labeled terminals in this region after nerve injury (Woolf et al. 1995), GAP-43 never colocalized with B-HRP in primary afferent central terminals within lamina II (Doubell & Woolf, 1997). It seems that GAP-43 immunoreactivity within the dorsal horn is located in C-fiber terminals, many of which undergo terminal atrophy during this time. This is consistent with GAP-43 immunoreactivity in the peripheral nerve after nerve injury, when it is only observed in unmyelinated axons (Verkade et al. 1995).

While it is not yet known whether peripheral injury to A-fibers will induce sprouting in the absence of C-fiber injury, the studies outlined above suggest that A-fiber injury is not necessary for sprouting. Only two factors are common to all the different manipulations that have been shown to produce sprouting in the dorsal horn: first, peripheral C-fiber injury, either physical or chemical, and second, that the injured C-fibers and the sprouting A-fibers are located within the same DRG. In trying to identify a mechanism for A-fiber growth, these features offer a useful starting point.

It is possible that C-fiber injury causes a switch in phenotype that leads to the production of a tropic/trophic factor for A-fibers. This molecule could potentially be released in the DRG, as has been shown for substance P from sensory neuron cell bodies (Huang & Neher, 1996), or it could be transported centrally and released in the dorsal horn. While the first suggestion is a possibility, two factors make it less likely to be a predominant mediator of sprouting. The areas into which A-fibers sprout are extremely specific within lamina II; sprouting does not occur radially, but only within the dorsoventral plane and boundaries are extremely distinct. Therefore, for this to be controlled entirely within the DRG through a factor that increase A-fiber growth propensity is difficult to imagine without at least some local guidance cues in the superficial dorsal horn. An alternative hypothesis is that injured C-fibers upregulate a factor that is transported centrally and released within lamina II. A good candidate for this molecule is the neurotrophin, Brain Derived Neurotrophic Factor (BDNF). BDNF is expressed in the DRG by small neurons, upregulated after nerve injury and transported centrally to the dorsal horn. Many myelinated A-fiber neurons express the high affinity receptor for BDNF, TrkB, so that any BDNF released from C-fiber central terminals after nerve injury could potentially act on A-fiber terminals to induce sprouting. Unfortunately, many attempts in our laboratory to induce A-fiber sprouting with acute or chronic BDNF infusion intrathecally with or without dorsal rhizotomy have failed. Likewise, the intrathecal infusion of TrkB-IgG fusion proteins to sequester BDNF in the dorsal horn has failed to prevent sprouting after nerve injury (unpublished observations).

Sprouting has, however, been shown to be prevented by NGF, supplied either chronically into the intrathecal space (Bennett et al., 1996), or as a bolus to the proximal stump of the transected sciatic nerve (Eriksson et al., 1997). TrkA, the high affinity NGF receptor, is expressed by approximately 40% of lumbar DRG neurons that also express CGRP (Averill et al., 1995) and project to lamina I and II_o (Alvarez et al., 1991). These are predominantly Aδ- and C-fiber neurons, of which many are thought to exhibit transganglionic degenerative changes after nerve injury. It is thought that exogenous NGF acts as a therapeutic agent to C-fibers and prevents any subsequent changes responsible for A-fiber sprouting (Bennett et al., 1996), such as the reduction in perikaryon size and many of the phenotypic changes of nerve injury (Fitzgerald et al., 1985). Transganglionic degenerative atrophy is preceded by an astroglial cell reaction in the superficial laminae, observed by an increase in Glial Fibrillary Acidic Protein (GFAP) (Svensson et al., 1993) as well as microglial reactivity (Eriksson et al., 1993), both of which have been implicated in the proceeding transganglionic changes (Eriksson et al. 1993) as well as A-fiber sprouting (Svensson et al. 1993). However, supplying exogenous NGF to the injured nerve does not prevent the astroglial or microglial response in the dorsal horn (Erikkson et al. 1997).

That NGF can totally prevent growth into lamina II is somewhat surprising, considering that only 50% of C-fibers express TrkA (Averill et al. 1995; Molliver et al. 1995). This means either that it is this subpopulation of C-fibers and not those that do not express TrkA that after injury are involved in A-fiber sprouting, or that a certain threshold of C-fiber injury is required in order for sprouting to occur. Certainly, non-TrkA expressing C-fibers are affected by capsaicin treatment – around 60% of IB4-binding neurons express VR1 (Tominaga et al. 1998), and TMP, a marker for this population of fibers, is massively depleted from the superficial dorsal horn (Mannion et al. 1996; Doubell et al. 1997). An indication that these findings with exogenous NGF are likely to represent a 'threshold' phenomenon comes from the recent observation that TMP-expressing C-fiber neurons also express the receptor complex for GDNF (Molliver et al. 1998; Bennett et al. 1998), and that intrathecal GDNF at the same dose as NGF, can prevent nerve injury induced central sprouting of myelinated fiber collaterals (Bennett et al.1998).

V. STRUCTURAL REORGANIZATION IN THE SPINAL CORD AND NEUROPATHIC PAIN

Nerve injury is a condition that is commonly seen in humans as a consequence of trauma, infection, malignancy, metabolic disturbances, drug toxicities and other conditions. A recognized complication of nerve injury is the generation of neuropathic pain, which manifests in many different ways but is extremely distressing and commonly unresponsive to current modes of analgesia such as the opiates and non-steroidal anti-inflammatory agents (Jensen, 1996). Over the last two decades, important inroads have been made, such as the recognition that the neuropathic symptoms can be caused not only by nociceptive Aδ- and C-fibers but also by the low threshold Aβ-fibers that normally do not signal pain (Treede et al. 1992; Gracely et al. 1992). For example, nerve injury is thought to result in an increase in primary nociceptive transmission to the dorsal horn, a state that is associated with the induction of hyperexcitability in dorsal horn neurons. This hyperexcitability, commonly termed central sensitization (Woolf et al. 1983), manifests in a number of different ways, one of which being that dorsal horn neurons can respond in an exaggerated fashion to low intensity Aβ-fiber input. In this way, a non-painful stimulus can elicit the sensation of pain, the phenomenon of mechanical allodynia. In the absence of ongoing nociceptor drive, it is thought that central sensitization is diminished and Aβ-mediated pain reduced (Gracely et al. 1992; Treede et al. 1992; Koltzenburg et al. 1994). However, many patients experience mechanical allodynia in the absence of ongoing nociceptor drive, and a potential underlying mechanism for their pain in primary afferents has not been identified. A-fiber sprouting creates a situation where a region of spinal cord that normally only receives nociceptive information, lamina II_o, begins to receive innocuous information. If the neurons that receive information from lamina II_o misinterpret novel A-fiber input as noxious, it is possible that sprouting represents an anatomical substrate for mechanical allodynia (Woolf et al. 1992). Furthermore, during the first three weeks of postnatal life, A-fiber central terminals exist in lamina II (Fitzgerald et al. 1994) where they make synapses (Coggeshall et al. 1996). During this time, lamina II neurons are far more excitable by Aβ-fiber inputs than in adult animals (Park et al. 1998) and repetitive A-fiber input is able to elicit a form of central sensitization (Jennings & Fitzgerald, 1998), a situation never normally seen in adult animals (Neumann et al. 1996).

In addition, A-fiber input may cause further structural changes in lamina II neurons. Many of these cells are inhibitory interneurons, and varying levels of trans-synaptic cell death have been described in this region following peripheral nerve injury (Sugimoto et al. 1990; Oliveira et al. 1997). Under normal conditions, cells within this region are excited by C-fiber inputs, characterized by longer lasting EPSCs than those elicited by A-fiber inputs. Repetitive A-fiber inputs to these neurons causes the accumulation of intracellular calcium, a key feature in the induction of central sensitization (Woolf, 1996). In addition, increased levels of calcium are associated with the induction of excitotoxicity, and it is possible that A-fiber input to this region may induce excitotoxic cell death within lamina II (Lekan et al. 1998). A reduction in the number of inhibitory neurons within the dorsal horn would produce a *disinhibition*, leading to an increase in excitability and in the amount of information that is relayed to higher centers. In this way, accompanying the downregulation of opioid receptors by primary afferents after nerve injury as well as the reduction in GABA content within superficial dorsal horn layers (Ibuki et al. 1997), A-fiber sprouting may contribute to neuropathic pain.

VI. SUMMARY AND FUTURE DIRECTIONS

Nerve injury induced A-fiber sprouting into the superficial dorsal horn is a long lasting, robust example of axonal growth in the adult mammalian central nervous system. The mechanism by which this anatomical plasticity occurs is not yet understood, but C-fiber injury seems to be a key feature. It is possible that A-fiber central sprouting is a modified form of collateral growth, where injured C-fibers release a factor centrally that acts to guide A-fiber terminals into regions denervated by transganglionic degeneration. These changes in primary afferent central terminal connectivity within the dorsal horn may underlie some of the features of neuropathic pain, and approaches aimed at preventing or reversing A-fiber sprouting after nerve injury may offer new strategies in the treatment of this condition.

REFERENCES

Ainsworth A, Hall P, Wall PD, Allt G, Lynn Mackenzie M, Gibson S, Polak JM (1981) Effects of capsaicin applied locally to adult peripheral nerve II: Anatomy and enzyme and peptide chemistry of peripheral nerve and spinal cord. Pain 11:379-388.

Alvarez FJ, Morris HR, Priestley JV (1991) Sub-populations of smaller diameter trigeminal primary afferent neurons defined by expression of calcitonin gene-related peptide and the cell surface oligosaccharide recognized by monoclonal antibody LA4. J Neurocytol 20:716-731.

Araki T, Milbrandt J (1996) Ninjurin, a novel adhesion molecule, is induced by nerve injury and promotes axonal growth. Neuron 17 (2):353-361.

Averill, S., S.B. McMahon, S.B. Clary, L.F. Reichardt, and J.V. Priestley (1995) Immunocytochemical localization of trkA receptors in chemically identified subgroups of adult rat sensory neurons. Eur.J.Neurosci. 7:1484-1494.

Baba H, Doubell TP, Woolf CJ (1999) Peripheral inflammation facilitates Aβ fiber-mediated synaptic input to the substantia gelatinosa of the adult rat spinal cord. J.Neurosci. In Press.

Bennett, D.L.H., J. French, J.V. Priestley, and S.B. McMahon (1996) NGF but not NT-3 or BDNF prevents the A fiber sprouting into lamina II of the spinal cord that occurs following axotomy. Mol.Cell.Neurosci. 8:211-220.

Bennett DL, Averill S, Clary DO, Priestley JV, McMahon SB (1996) Postnatal changes in the expression of the trkA high-affinity NGF receptor in primary sensory neurons.Eur. J. Neurosci 8(10):2204-2208.

Bisby MA (1981) Axonal transport in the central axon of sensory neurons during regeneration of their peripheral axon. Neurosci. Lett 21(1):7-11.

Castro-Lopes JM, Coimbra A, Grant G, Arvidsson J (1990) Ultrastructural changes of the central scalloped (C1) primary afferent endings of synaptic glomeruli in the substantia gelatinosa Rolandi of the rat after peripheral neurotomy. J Neurocytol 19:329-337.

Chong M-S, Fitzgerald M, Winter J, Hu-Tsai M, Emson PC, Weise U, Woolf CJ (1992) GAP-43 mRNA in rat spinal cord and dorsal root ganglia neurons: developmental changes and re-expression following peripheral nerve injury. Eur J Neurosci 4:883-895.

Coggeshall RE, Jennings E, Fitzgerald M (1996) Evidence that large myelinated primary afferent fibers make synaptic contacts in lamina II of neonatal rats. Dev. Brain Res. 92:81-90.

Csillik B, Knyihar-Csillik E (1982) Reversibility of microtubule inhibitor-induced transganglionic degenerative atrophy of central terminals of primary nociceptive neurons. Neuroscience 7:1149-1154.

Csillik B, Schwab ME, Thoenen H (1985) Transganglionic regulation of central terminals of dorsal root ganglion cells by nerve growth factor (NGF). Brain Res 331:11-15.

Diamond, J., M.D. Coughlin, L. MacIntyre, M. Holmes, and B. Visheau (1987) Evidence that endogenous NGF is responsible for the collateral sprouting, but not the regeneration, of nociceptive axons in adult rats. Proc.Natl.Acad.Sci 84:6596-6600.

Doubell TP, Mannion RJ, Woolf CJ (1997) Intact sciatic myelinated primary afferent terminals collaterally sprout in the adult rat dorsal horn following section of a neighbouring peripheral nerve. J Comp Neurol 380(1):95-104.

Doubell TP, Woolf CJ (1997) Growth-associated protein 43 immunoreactivity in the superficial dorsal horn of the rat spinal cord is localized in atrophic C-fiber, and not in sprouted A-fiber, central terminals after peripheral nerve injury. J. Comp. Neurol. 386(1):111-118.

Doubleday B, Robinson PP (1994) NGF depletion reduces collateral sprouting of cutaneous mechanoreceptive and tooth-pulp axons in ferrets. J Physiol (Lond) 481(3):709-718.

Doucette R, Diamond J (1987) Normal and precocious sprouting of heat nociceptors in the skin of adult rats.J. Comp. Neurol 261(4):592-603.

Eriksson NP, Persson JK, Svensson M, Arvidsson J, Molander C, Aldskogius H (1993) A quantitative analysis of the microglial cell reaction in central primary sensory projection territories following peripheral nerve injury in the adult rat. Exp. Brain Res. 96(1):19-27.

Eriksson, N.P., Aldskogius, H. Grant, G. Lindsay, R.M. Rivero-Melian, C. (1997) Effects of NGF, BDNF and NT-3 on the laminar distribution of transganglionically transported choleragenoid in the spinal cord dorsal horn following transection of the sciatic nerve in the adult rat. Neuroscience Jun 78(3): 863-872.

Fitzgerald M (1983) Capsaicin and sensory neurones - a review. Pain 15:109-130

Fitzgerald, M., T. Butcher, and P. Shortland (1994) Developmental changes in the laminar termination of A fibre cutaneous sensory afferents in the rat spinal cord dorsal horn. J.Comp.Neurol. 348:225-233.

Fitzgerald, M., P.D. Wall, M. Goedert, and P.C. Emson (1985) Nerve growth factor counteracts the neurophysiological and neurochemical effects of chronic sciatic nerve section. Brain Res. 332:131-141.

Gamse R, Petsche U, Lembeck F, Jancso G (1982) Capsaicin applied to peripheral nerve inhibits axoplasmic transport of substance P and somatostatin. Brain Res 239:447-462.

Gracely RH, Lynch SA, Bennett GJ (1992) Painful neuropathy: altered central processing maintained dynamically by peripheral input. Pain 51(2):175-194.

Head H, Sherren J (1905) The consequences of injury to peripheral nerves in man. Brain, 28, 116.

Huang LY, Neher E (1996) Ca(2+)-dependent exocytosis in the somata of dorsal root ganglion neurons. Neuron 17(1): 135-145.

Ibuki T, Hama AT, Wang XT, Pappas GD, Sagen J (1997) Loss of GABA-immunoreactivity in the spinal dorsal horn of rats with peripheral nerve injury and promotion of recovery by adrenal medullary grafts. Neuroscience 76:845-858.

Jancso G (1992) Pathobiological reactions of C-fibre primary sensory neurones to peripheral nerve injury. Exp Physiol 77:405-431.

Jennings E, Fitzgerald M (1998) Postnatal changes in responses of rat dorsal horn cells to afferent stimulation; a fibre-induced senstitization. J Physiol 509.3:859-868.

Jensen TS (1996) Mechanisms of Neuropathic pain. IASP Press, Seattle

Knyihar-Csillik E, Rakic P, Csillik B (1987) Transganglionic degenerative atrophy in the substantia gelatinosa of the spinal cord after peripheral nerve transection in rhesus monkeys. Cell & Tis Res 247:599-604.

Koerber HR, Mirnics K, Brown PB, Mendell LM (1994) Central sprouting and functional plasticity of regenerated primary afferents. J Neurosci 14(6):3655-3671.

Kohama I, Agulian S, Kocsis JD (1998) Changes in synaptic transmission of rat spinal dorsal horn neurons after sciatic nerve transection. Soc. Neurosci. Abstr. 154.8.

Koltzenburg M, Torebjork HE, Wahren LK (1994) Nociceptor modulated central sensitisation causes mechanical hyperalgesia in acute chemogenic and chronic neuropathic pain. Brain 117(Pt 3):579-591.

Lawson SN (1979) The postnatal development of large light and small dark neurons in mouse dorsal root ganglia: a statistical analysis of cell numbers and size. J. Neurocytol. 8(3):275-294.

Lawson SN, Harper AA, Harper EI, Garson JA, Anderton BH (1984) A monoclonal antibody against neurofilament protein specifically labels a subpopulation of rat sensory neurones. J. Comp Neurol 228(2):263-272.

Lekan HA, Woolf CJ, Coggeshall RE (1998) Loss of dorsal horn neurons following Aβ stimulation of the transected sciatic nerve. Soc. Neurosci. Abstr. 154.9.

Light AR, Perl ER (1979) Reexamination of the dorsal root projection to the spinal dorsal horn including observations on the differential termination of coarse and fine fibers. J. Comp Neurol 186(2):117-131.

Liu CN, Chambers WW (1958) Intraspinal sprouting of dorsal root axons. Arch Neurol 79:46-61.

Livesey F, O'Brien J, Li M, Smith A, Murphy L, Hunt S (1997) A Schwann cell mitogen accompanying regeneration of motor neurons. Nature; 390:614-618.

McMahon SB, Kett-White R (1991) Sprouting of peripherally regenerating primary sensory neurones in the adult central nervous system. J Comp Neurol 304:307-315.

Madison RD, Archibald SJ, Brushart TM (1996) Reinnervation accuracy of the rat femoral nerve by motor and sensory neurons. J. Neurosci 16:5698-5703.

Mannion RJ, Doubell TP, Coggeshall RE, Woolf CJ (1996) Collateral sprouting of uninjured primary afferent A-fibers into the superficial dorsal horn of the adult rat spinal cord after topical capsaicin treatment to the sciatic nerve. J Neurosci 16(16):5189-5195.

Mannion RJ, Doubell TP, Gill H, Woolf CJ (1998) Deafferentation is insufficient to induce sprouting of A-fibre central terminals in the rat dorsal horn. J Comp Neurol 393(2):135-144.

Mearow KM, Kril Y, Diamond J (1993) Increased NGF mRNA expression in denervated rat skin. Neuroreport 4(4):351-354.

Mearow KM, Kril Y, Gloster A, Diamond J (1994) Expression of NGF receptor and GAP-43 mRNA in DRG neurons during collateral sprouting and regeneration of dorsal cutaneous nerves. J. Neurobiol 25(2):127-142.

Molander, C., and G. Grant (1985) Cutaneous projections from the rat hindlimb foot to the substantia gelatinosa of the spinal cord studied by transganglionic transport of WGA-HRP conjugate. J.Comp.Neurol. 237:476-484.

Molander, C., and G. Grant (1986) Laminar distribution and somatotopic organization of primary afferent fibers from hindlimb nerves in the dorsal horn. A study by transganglionic transport of horseradish peroxidase in the rat. Neuroscience 19:297-312.

Molander C, Kinnman E, Aldskogius H (1988) Expansion of spinal cord primary sensory afferent projection following combined sciatic nerve resection and saphenous nerve crush: A horseradish peroxidase study in the adult rat. J Comp Neurol 276:436-441.

Molliver DC, Radeke MJ, Feinstein SC, Snider WD (1995) Presence or absence of TrkA protein distinguishes subsets of small sensory neurons with unique cytochemical characteristics and dorsal horn projections.J. Comp Neurol 361(3):404-416.

Molliver DC, Wright DE, Leitner ML, Parsadanian AS, Doster K, Wen D, Yan Q, Snider WD (1997) IB4-binding DRG neurons switch from NGF to GDNF dependence in early postnatal life. Neuron 19(4):849-861.

Murray M, Goldberger ME (1986) Replacement of synaptic terminals in lamina II and Clarke's nucleus after unilateral lumbosacral dorsal rhizotomy in adult cats. J Neurosci 6(11):3205-3217.

Neumann S, Doubell TP, Leslie TA, Woolf CJ (1996) Inflammatory pain hypersensitivity mediated by a phenotypic switch in myelinated primary sensory neurons. Nature 384:360-364.

Okamoto M, Yoshimura M, Baba H, Higashi H, Shimoji K (1996) Synaptic plasticity of substantia gelatinosa neurons in the chronic pain model rat. Jpn J Physiol 46:S136.

Oliveira AL, Risling M, Deckner M, Lindholm T, Langone F, Cullheim S (1997) Neonatal sciatic nerve transection induces TUNEL labeling of neurons in the rat spinal cord and DRG. Neuroreport 8(13):2837-2840

Park JS, Higashi H, Yoshimura M (1998) Plastic changes in primary afferent inputs to substantia gelatinosa during post-natal development: patch clamp study. Soc. Neurosci. Abstr. 152.4.

Polistina DC, Murray M, Goldberger ME (1990) Plasticity of dorsal root and descending serotinergic projections after partial deafferentation of the adult rat spinal cord. J. Comp. Neurol. 299(3):349-363.

Puigdellivol-Sanchez A, Prats-Galino A, Ruano-Gil D, Molander C (1998) Sciatic and femoral nerve sensory neurones occupy different regions of the L4 dorsal root ganglion in the adult rat. Nneurosci Lett 251(3):169-172.

Richardson PM, Issa VMK (1984) Peripheral injury enhances central regeneration of primary sensory neurones. Nature 309:791-793.

Rivero-Melian C, Grant G (1990) Distribution of lumbar dorsal root fibres in the lower thoracic and lumbosacral spinal cord of the rat studied with choleragenoid horseradish peroxidase conjugate. J Comp Neurol 299:470-481.

Shortland P, Woolf CJ (1993) Chronic peripheral nerve section results in a rearrangement of the central axonal arborizations of axotomized A beta primary afferent neurons in the rat spinal cord. J Comp Neurol 330:65-82.

Skene JHP (1989) Axonal growth associated proteins. Ann Rev Neurosci 12:127-156.

Sugimoto T, Bennett GJ, Kajander KC (1990) Transsynaptic degeneration in the superficial dorsal horn after sciatic nerve injury: effects of a chronic constriction injury, transection, and strychnine. Pain 42(2):205-213.

Svensson M, Eriksson P, Pesson JKE, Molander C, Avvidsson Aldskogius H (1993) The response of central glial to peripheral nerve injury. Brain Res Bull 30:499-506.

Swett JE, Woolf CJ (1985) Somatotopic organization of primary afferent terminals in the superficial dorsal horn of the rat spinal cord. J Comp Neurol 231:66-71.

Tominaga M, Caterina MJ, Malmberg AB, Rosen TA, Gilbert H, Skinner K, Raumann BE, Basbaum AI, Julius D (1998) The cloned capsaicin receptor integrates multiple pain-producing stimuli. Neuron 21(3):531-543.

Tong YG, Wang HF, Ju G, Grant G, Hokfelt T, Zhang X (1999) Increased uptake and transport of cholera toxin B-subunit in dorsal root ganglion neurons after peripheral axotomy: possible implications for sensory sprouting. J Comp Neurol 404:143-158.

Treede RD, Davis KD, Campbell JN, Raja SN (1992) The plasticity of cutaneous hyperalgesia during sympathetic ganglion blockade in patients with neuropathic pain. Brain 115(Pt 2):607-621.

Verkade P, Oestreicher AB, Verkleij AJ, Gispen WH (1995) The increase in B-50/GAP-43 in regenerating rat sciatic nerve occurs predominantly in unmyelinated axon shafts: a quantitative ultrastructural study. J. Comp Neurol 356(3):433-443.

Willis WD, Coggeshall RE (1991) Sensory Mechanisms of the Spinal Cord. Plenum press, New York

Wilson P, Kitchener PD (1996) Plasticity of cutaneous primary afferent projections to the spinal dorsal horn.Prog Neurobiol 48(2):105-129.

Woolf CJ (1983) Evidence for a central component of post-injury pain hypersensitivity. Nature 306:686-688.

Woolf CJ (1996) Windup and central sensitization are not equivalent. Pain 66:105-108.

Woolf CJ, Shortland P, Coggeshall RE (1992) Peripheral nerve injury triggers central sprouting of myelinated afferents. Nature 355:75-77.

Woolf CJ, Shortland P, Reynolds ML, Ridings J, Doubell TP, Coggeshall RE (1995) Central regenerative sprouting: the reorganization of the central terminals of myelinated primary afferents in the rat dorsal horn following peripheral nerve section or crush. J Comp Neurol 360:121-134.

10

Inflammatory Response Following Nerve Injury

Gennadij Raivich and Georg W. Kreutzberg
Max-Planck Institute for Neurobiology, Martinsried, Germany

I. INTRODUCTION

Inflammation in the brain, spinal cord and peripheral nerves is a unique and finely-tuned response different from most other tissues. In non-neural tissues, inflammation is normally defined by the classical triad of heat, redness and pain, combined with a reduction or loss of normal function. At the cellular level, it is characterized by an influx of different white blood cells, activation of the phagocytotic system, edema, and at later stages by a proliferation of mesenchyme leading to fibrosis. Inflammatory changes in the nervous system differ in many respects. Brain and spinal cord lack intrinsic pain receptors and thus a perception of pain in response to central damage. The vascular system is regulated autonomously and committed to the maintenance of constant conditions, dampening the increase in blood flow and heat production. The influx of leukocytes is restricted, and occurs in massive form only after severe neural injury. Despite all this, there are important core similarities - the ability to regenerate, to phagocytose and to form scars - which reflect a deeply engraved program involved in tissue repair and defense against infection. The aim of this chapter is to summarize these inflammatory changes in the injured central and peripheral nervous system, describe our current knowledge of the molecules involved and then discuss the functional role of these changes in the process of nerve regeneration.

II. LOCAL INFLAMMATION

A. Peripheral Nerve - Early changes

The most rapid changes are observed at the site of injury. Rupture of the blood vessels leads to immediate bleeding at the injury site, local blood clotting, platelet degranulation, and release of signaling molecules such as platelet-derived growth factor (PDGF), histamine or serotonin, with secondary effects on surrounding blood vessels, axons and endoneurial tissue.

Of particular interest is the reaction of endoneurial mast cells, which degranulate within minutes after local injury (MacDonald et al., 1981) and play an important role in shaping the cellular response to trauma. Thus, chemical induction of mast cell degranulation in normal nerves with compound 48/80 causes an opening of the blood-nerve barrier to soluble molecules (Harvey et al., 1994, Olsson, 1966), increased endoneurial tissue pressure, granulocyte influx (Powell et al., 1980), and a strong induction of interleukin-6 (IL6) synthesis by sensory neurons projecting through the treated peripheral nerve (Murphy et al., 1999). Inhibition of mast cell degranulation reduces or abolishes the induction of IL6 by the axotomized neurons (Murphy et al., 1999) and a rapid treatment of human patients with Bell's palsy with the mast cell blocking agent chromolyn sodium has been shown to prevent nerve degeneration and accelerate neurological recovery (McGovern and Estevez, 1980).

1. Molecular Signals

Within hours, the initial activation after injury is followed by a local synthesis of molecules involved in cell signaling. Immediate early genes, such as c-fos, c-jun and KROX-20, show a rapid increase and serve as important transcription regulatory factors (Pyykonen and Koistinaho, 1991; Herdegen et al., 1993; Stewart, 1995; Liu et al., 1995, Shy et al., 1996). Induced molecules also include cytokines (IL1, IL6, FGF), neurotrophic factors (NGF, LIF), mitogen receptors (TfR, PDGF-Ra) and chemokines including KC, MIF and MCP1 (Nishio et al., 1999; Carroll and Frohnert, 1998; Toews et al., 1998; Bourde et al., 1996; Bolin et al., 1995; Lindholm et al., 1987; Raivich et al., 1987b). These rapidly induced cytokines create an inflammatory network that appears to play a pivotal role in the further regulation of cellular changes in the damaged neural tissue.

2. Infiltration of White Blood Cells

Activation of local endoneurial cells is accompanied by a recruitment of leukocytes, beginning within hours after trauma. Neutrophil granulocytes and macrophages predominate, but show different temporal and spatial patterns. The increase in neutrophils is transient, with a maximum 2-3 days after injury and a diffuse distribution up to 10 mm away from the site of trauma.

The macrophages peak at day 4 and attain a very high density in and around the injury site (Fig. 1, 2). They express a number of typical monocyte antigens e.g., the ED1-3 series (Monaco et al., 1992), aMb2 and aLb2 integrins (Vougioukas et al., 1997; Dailey et al., 1998) and activation markers such as the transferrin receptor (Raivich et al., 1991a). These macrophages invade the basal membranes of endoneurial tubes, producing a typical appearance of strands of up to 10 macrophages squeezed one after the other inside an endoneurial tube (Fig. 2C). Surprisingly, these endoneurial macrophages are concentrated in a narrow, 1 mm cuff around the initial site of injury between day 1 and day 4 (Fig. 1), suggesting the presence of a highly localized chemotactic factor at the site of the initial vascular disruption. Peritraumatic macrophages aggregating around this site express high levels of activation markers such as functional transferrin receptors and the associated uptake of iron (Raivich et al., 1991). They are also avid and effective phagocytes, leading to a rapid breakdown and disappearance of myelin at the lesion site 6 days after injury, with myelin 2-5 mm further distally still largely intact.

3. Local Scarring

In addition to the phagocytosis of myelin, activated macrophages are a rich source of cytokines and mitogens such as IL1, IL6, TNFa, TGFb1 or PDGF (Lindholm et al., 1987; Wagner and Myers, 1996; Kiefer et al., 1995). Although some of the cytokines act on Schwann cells, fibroblasts are particularly good responders for the mitogenic action of most of these molecules (for a review see Raivich et al., 1993). Cell proliferation, including the proliferation of fibroblasts, begins particularly early at the site of injury, after 1-2 days, and it is considerably stronger than further distally. Importantly, this action on fibroblasts also leads to a sizable increase in endoneural mesenchyme and extensive deposition of extracellular matrix. Thus, as in many other tissues, local trauma and the resulting inflammation will lead to a gradual build-up of connective tissue and the formation of a scar in the peripheral nerve. This is not a big clinical problem in experimental animals like mice and rats, where axons regenerate robustly across the cellular bridge forming between the proximal and distal nerve end and where proliferation of mesenchyme is held in check. However, it is a frequent problem in human patients with nerve injury, with proliferating connective tissue leading to a progressive squeezing of the regenerating peripheral nerve.

III. CELLULAR CHANGES AFTER DAMAGE TO CENTRAL WHITE MATTER TRACTS

As in peripheral nerves, a similar set of early changes is also observed following central damage at the site of trauma. Axonal injury leads to the destruction of the distal, disconnected neurites. Vascular damage leads to local bleeding and then to hypoxia. There is recruitment of leukocytes, again with predominance of granulocytes and macrophages. Proliferating astrocytes, and to a lesser extent, meningeal

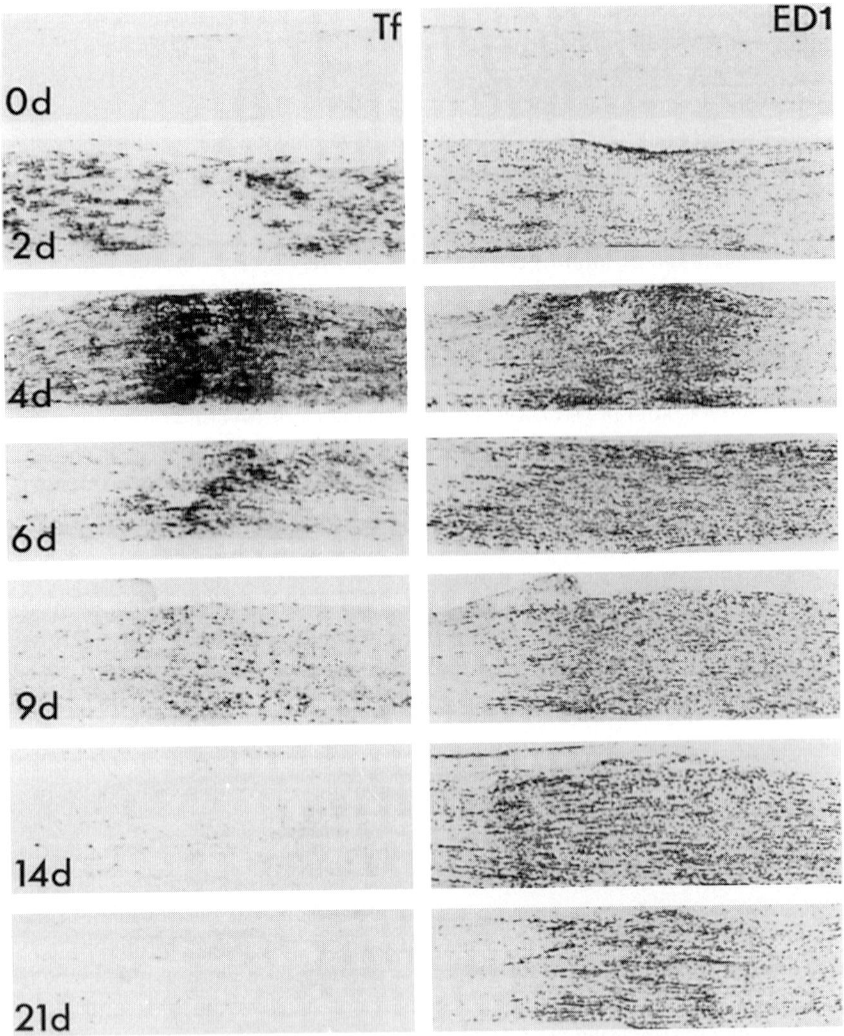

Figure 1 Macrophage influx to the injured rat sciatic nerve. The activated macrophages were detected using autoradiography for [^{125}I]-transferrin binding (left) and ED1-immunoreactivity (right) of adjacent longitudinal tissue sections of normal (0 days) and crushed (2 - 21 days) sciatic nerves. The crush site is in the middle of each micrograph, the proximal part of the nerve is to the left. There are 2 phases of macrophage influx. In the first, 0-4 days after crush, macrophages are restricted to a 1 mm wide peritrauma cuff distal and proximal to the crush. In the second phase, day 6-14, high numbers of macrophages are present throughout the distal nerve. All magnifications 18x. Reproduced from Raivich et al. 1991b, Fig 3.

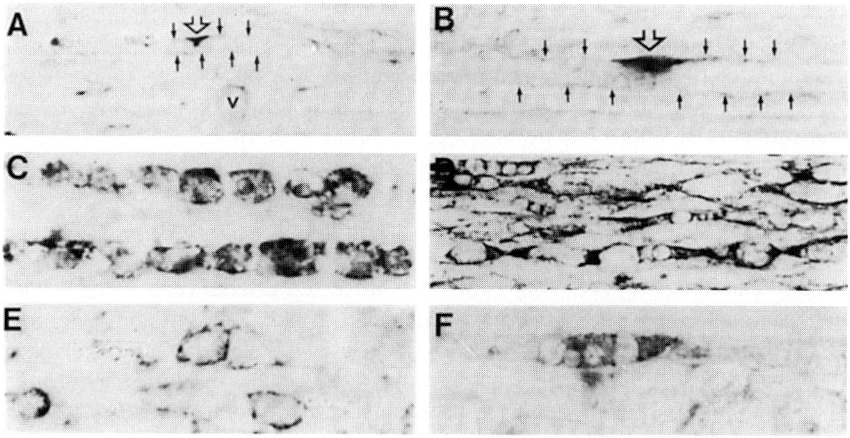

Figure 2 Cellular activation in the injured peripheral nerve using transferrin receptor (TfR) as a marker of Schwann cell and macrophage activation. A, B: In the normal sciatic nerve, TfR immunoreactivity is largely restricted to the perinuclear Schwann cell cytoplasm (big arrow) of myelinated nerve fibers. Weak labeling on axonal membranes (small arrows) endoneurial vcessels (v). C, D: Four days after crush, there is strong immunostaining on strings of large macrophages at the site of injury (C) and on Schwann cell tubes (Büngner bands) in the distal part of the crushed sciatic nerve (D). E, F: Six days after crush, there is a clear reduction in TfR immunoreactivity. Heavy staining is observed only on single macrophages (E, injury site) and single Schwann cells (F, distal nerve). A: 410x, B: 590x. C: 510x, D: 350x. E: 660x, F: 860x. Reproduced from Raivich et al. 1991b, Fig 1.

cells, are the main contributors of the central scar formation, leading to a deposition of the extracellular matrix, and later to a novel glia limitans.

There are, however, functional differences. Central axons degenerate more slowly (Pesini et al., 1999; Stoll et al., 1989). The overall macrophage recruitment is also slower, and takes more time, approximately twice as long, to reach a maximum (Stoll et al., 1989; Raivich et al., 1991, Raivich et al., 1994; Avellino et al., 1995; Lawson et al., 1994; Hirschberg and Schwartz, 1995). Most importantly, unlike the peripheral fibroblasts and Schwann cells, reactive astrocytes form scars that are an effective barrier to axonal regeneration (Davies et al., 1997). This ability to impede neurite outgrowth is a specific property of this central glial cell type. Implantation of peripheral nerves into the CNS restores the ability of central axons to cross the trauma site and grow into the peripheral implant (see this volume, chapter by So). At the cellular level, posttraumatic influx of Schwann cells after spinal cord trauma also permits effective axonal regeneration in the vicinity of the lesion site (Brook et al., 1998). This ability to support axonal outgrowth in the adult mammal CNS is not limited to peripheral cells. Successful axonal regeneration in the olfactory bulb appears to be due to the presence of olfactory ensheathing cells (OEC) that have an intermediate phenotype between astrocytes, oligodendroglia and Schwann cells (Raisman, 1985, Ramon-Cueto, 1998; this volume, see chapter by Plant et al.,). Transplantation of the olfactory ensheathing cells into damaged spinal cord white matter also allows regeneration of descending projections and inhibits astrocyte scar formation (Li et al., 1998). Moreover, neurite outgrowth is also successful in ventromedial hypothalamus, where tanycytes, a cell similar to the ensheathing cells of the olfactory bulb, are the predominant scar-forming cell (Alonso and Privat, 1993).

Why do astrocytes react in a way that is different from tanycytes or olfactory ensheathing cells? One reason could be an evolutionary adaptation to a physiological function. Olfactory bulb and, to lesser extent, ventrobasal hypothalamus are exposed to a continuous replacement of old axons with newly generated sprouts. This function, supported by local glial cells, apparently is also recruited during regeneration after trauma. Interestingly, the ability of scar-forming astrocytes to block growing axons, is itself amenable to proinflammatory signals. Implantation of activated macrophages into the optic nerve or spinal cord has been shown to reverse the inhibition (Lazarov-Spiegler et al., 1996; Franzen et al., 1998). Similar effects are observed after injection of cultured, brain-derived microglia transformed into phagocytes (Rabchevsky and Streit 1997; Prewitt et al., 1997). Matrix metalloproteinases produced by activated macrophages (La Fleur et al., 1996) degrade chondroitin sulfate proteoglycans synthesized in glial scars, and eliminate the inhibitory effects of these molecules on axonal regeneration *in vitro* (Ferguson et al., 1997). In spite of this, there is a decisive difference from the normal situation. Under normal conditions, monocytes are recruited to the site of central trauma and local debris also causes a transformation of resident microglia into phagocytotic cells (Lawson et. al., 1994; Stoll et al., 1989). However, these cells are incapable of reprogramming astrocytes under physiological conditions. This appears due to the presence of intrinsic inhibitory factors in most parts of the mammalian brain (Hirschberg and Schwartz, 1995), an inhibition that can be circumvented by the injection of activated macrophages.

IV. INFLAMMATORY CHANGES IN THE DISTAL PART OF THE NERVE

A. Axonal degeneration and myelin removal

Compared to the site of injury, cellular changes more distally are delayed. This applies to peripheral nerves as well as to central white matter tracts in the brain and spinal cord. At both sites, cellular changes begin with the degeneration of axons, in peripheral nerves as early as 24 hours after injury, in the central projections after approximately 3 days (Pesini et al., 1999). This axonal degeneration is crucial for the inflammatory and noninflammatory changes in the distal part. Thus, the prolonged survival of transected nerve fibers in mice with inherited slow Wallerian degeneration (WLDs), will cause a similar retardation in Schwann cell activation, influx of macrophages and axonal regeneration (Lunn et al., 1989; Brown et al., 1991; Chen and Bisby, 1993). The molecular defect in WLDs is apparently due to selective resistance of axonal neurofilaments to Ca-activated proteases (Bernier et al., 1999).

In the peripheral nerve, axonal degeneration is typically followed by the activation of associated Schwann cells, summarized schematically in Fig. 3. There is rapid detachment of myelin, opening of the vascular tight junctions and an influx of plasma proteins and monocytes (Williams and Hall, 1971; Ohara and Ikuta, 1985; Clemence et al., 1989; Stoll et al., 1989). Schwann cells initiate myelin breakdown in the absence of macrophages but these professional phagocytes are apparently needed to complete the process (Stoll et al., 1989; Reichert et al., 1994; Fernandez-Valle et al., 1995; Dailey et al., 1998). In the central white matter tracts, oligodendrocytes show little activation and the detachment of myelin is slow. Except at the site of injury, there is no recruitment of hematogenous macrophages (Berner et al., 1973; Skoff, 1975; Ling, 1979; Zammit et al., 1993; Blight, 1994; Hirschberg and Schwartz, 1995). Myelin debris is taken up by local microglia, and to a lesser extent, by astrocytes. Although microglia are functionally related to macrophages, they are not efficient removers of myelin. Thus, phagocytosis and degradation of myelin is a rather slow process, with debris-laden microglia in the pyramidal tract still present years after the original cerebral insult (Kösel et al., 1998). Overall, peripheral injury leads to activation of myelin-forming cells and efficient removal of myelin in the distal part of the nerve while central injury leads to little activation and tardy myelin breakdown. Both central and peripheral myelin contain substances that inhibit axonal outgrowth (Fruchtiger et al., 1996; Schwab, 1990), pointing to the functional significance of myelin removal.

B. Origin and function of cells involved in myelin degradation

It is now well accepted that macrophages are recruited into degenerating peripheral nerves to digest myelin debris. However, it was unclear for a long time if they are needed to start myelin degradation (Ramon y Cajal, 1928; Crang and Blakemore, 1986; Brown et al., 1991) or whether they play a more passive role as additional scavengers of myelin already detached and processed by the Schwann cells (Nathaniel and Pease, 1963, Stoll et al., 1989; Fernandez-Valle et al., 1995). The most striking evidence for the first possibility were experiments by the group of R.L. Friede in peripheral nerves explanted in Millipore chambers into the peritoneal cavity (Beuche and Friede, 1986). This study showed successful degradation of myelin if the chambers contained pores large enough to allow the entry of activated, peritoneal macrophages. This function relies on the presence of receptors for complement, complement itself and the macrophage scavenger receptors (Bruck and Friede, 1990; 1991; da Costa, 1997). Myelin removal did not occur when recruitment of macrophages was prevented by Millipore chamber pores smaller than 5 mm (Beuche and Friede, 1984). Recent *in vivo* studies suggest a more complex role, i.e., as late phase scavengers. The effects of whole body irrad-

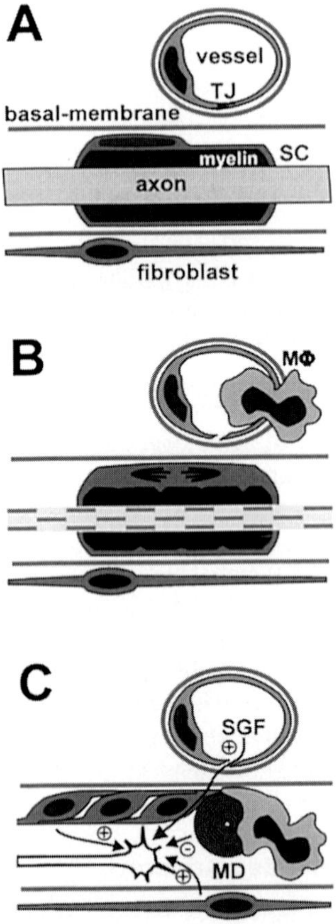

Figure 3 Schematic summary of cellular changes in the injured and regenerating peripheral nerve. A: A longitudinal section through a normal neural tube with myelinated motor axons and associated Schwann cells (SC) surrounded by basal lamina. The tight junctions (TJ) of the adjacent endoneurial vessels form the structural basis of the blood-nerve barrier in the normal, uninjured peripheral nerve. B: Axonal injury causes a rapid degeneration of the distal, diconnected axon, followed by a destabilization of the associated myelin and Schwann cell proliferation. Axonal degeneration also leads to a breakdown of the blood-nerve barrier and adhesion of circulating monocytes, which transform into tissue macrophages (Mf) and later invade the endoneurial tubes. C: Proliferating Schwann cells form endoneural Büngner bands that strongly support axonal regeneration. They are assisted by adjacent fibroblasts which provide neurotrophic factors and nutritional material for axonal growth. The absence of the blood-nerve barrier also provides access for serum growth factors (SGF) like transferrin, that aid ongoing axonal regeneration. In contrast, the myelin debris (MD) contains a number of inhibitory molecules that block neurite outgrowth. The removal of the myelin by macrophages plays a central role in promoting nerve regeneration. Reproduced from Kreutzberg and Raivich, 1999, Figure 4-12.

idiation are particularly informative. This treatment leads to an almost complete, >90% inhibition of macrophage recruitment but does not affect the disappearance of compact myelin during the first 5 days after axotomy (Perry et al., 1995). However, this treatment blocks myelin degradation between day 5 and day 10, stressing the role of macrophages as late scavengers. Similar effects on late myelin degradation by macrophages were also observed in complement-depleted animals (Dailey et al., 1998). To summarize these findings, the detachment of myelin and the initial breakdown is a function normally performed by the denervated Schwann cells. In cell cultures, denervated Schwann cells are efficent removers of myelin in the absence of cocultured macrophages (Fernandez-Valle et al., 1995). *In vivo*, these denervated Schwann cells also express a large set of phagocyte-associated molecules such as CD68, Ki-M1P and MAC-2, which may be important for myelin breakdown (Kaiserling et al., 1993; Reichert et al., 1994).

Myelin degradation by Schwann cells is surprisingly poor, however, in peripheral nerve explants. This applies both *in vivo*, in the classical Millipore chamber experiment (Beuche and Friede, 1984), but also *in vitro*, with desheathed sciatic nerves (Crang and Blakemore, 1986). This is probably due to insufficient oxygenation and nutrient supply, compared with the situation *in situ* (Raivich et al., 1987b; Dahlin LB, 1995). Studies using receptors for NGF and PDGF showed an extensive delay in the activation of Schwann cells and fibroblasts in peripheral nerve explants, which coincides with revascularization (Raivich and Kreutzberg, 1987b). Activated endoneural fibroblasts are also the primary source of GMCSF, a cytokine needed for the induction of MAC-2, that shifts the Schwann cells from the myelinating to the phagocytotic phenotype (Saada et al., 1996). Thus, the inability of Schwann cells to degrade myelin in explants may be due to the insufficient supply of nutrients. Apparently, the macrophage function is not impeded under these suboptimal conditions, stressing the importance of macrophage recruitment as a default mechanism to ensure the removal of debris (Fig. 4).

Vascular adhesion molecules, chemotactic peptides and their receptors all play an important role in this process of phagocyte influx into the damaged nerve (Archelos et al., 1999, Toews et al., 1998). Transgenic deletion of ICAM1, the endothelial ligand for the macrophage receptors aMb2 and aLb2-integrin, leads to a 40-50% reduction in the number of recruited macrophages (Vougioukas et al., 1998). A similar reduction is also observed in animals lacking CCR2 (Siebert and Bruck, 1999; Gschwendtner and Raivich, unpublished observations), the principal receptor for the monocyte chemotactic protein-1/MCP1. The decrease is more moderate in the CCR5-deficient animals. Neutralization of the aMb2-integrin had no effect (Brown et al., 1998). Overall, the regulation of macrophage recruitment into the damaged nerve is a multifactorial process, with a lot of inherent redundancy. In spite of the striking inability to recruit macrophages to the distal part of damaged central white matter tracts, it is unclear if this is the reason for the failure of axonal regeneration in the mammalian CNS. For example, axonal regeneration is successful in the axolotl spinal cord, despite the absence of macrophage recruitment (Zammit et al., 1993).

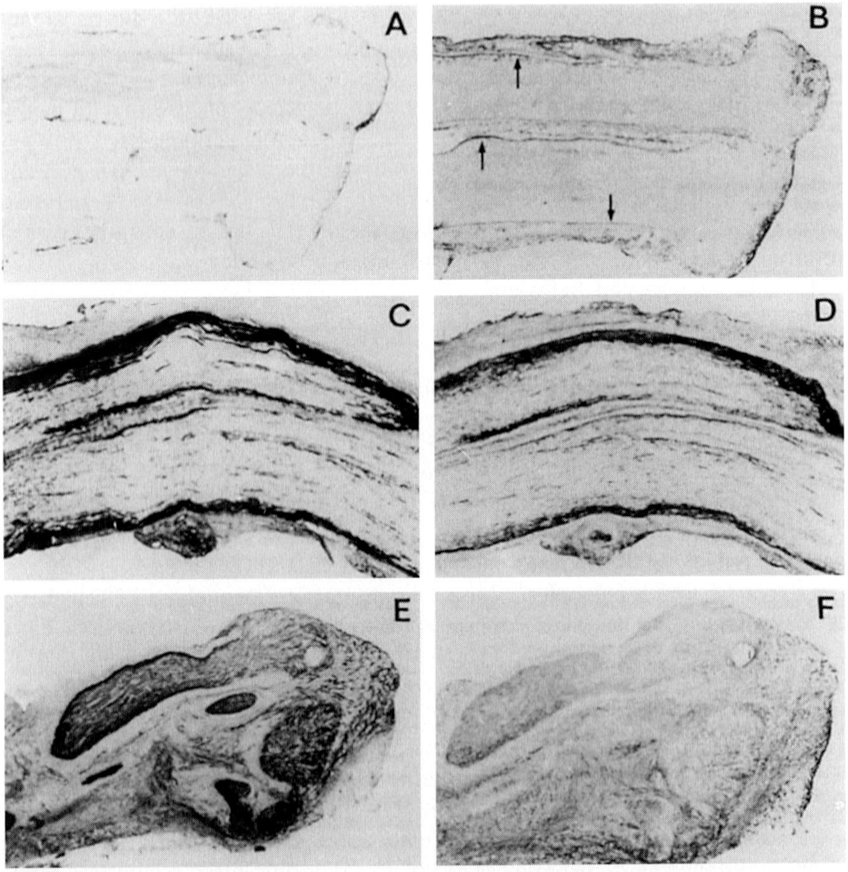

Figure 4 Receptor expression in peripheral nerve explants is delayed and follows the pattern of nerve revascularization. The autoradiographs show specific binding for [^{125}I]-bNGF on denervated Schwann cells (A,C,E) and [^{125}I]-PDGF binding on endoneurial fibroblasts (B,D,F). Longitudinal rat sciatic nerve sections 2, 6 and 14 days after explantation. A, B: At day 2, there is no specific bNGF binding; the PDGF binding is limited to a thin layer of subperineural mesenchyme (arrows). C, D: At day 6, binding to both receptors is restricted to the external part of the endoneurium in the explanted nerve. E, F: The 14 day nerve explants show specific binding for NGF and PDGF throughout the endoneurium of the explanted nerve and on the growing neuromatous tissue surrounding the explants. A, B: 16x ; C, D: 18x; E. 11x. F. 13x. Reproduced from Raivich et al. 1987b, Figure 4.

Macrophage depletion and the ensuing reduction in myelin breakdown do affect axonal regeneration in the peripheral nerve, but the effects are moderate, in the range of 20-30% (Tanaka et al., 1992; Calcutt et al., 1994; Dahlin, 1995; Dailey et al., 1998). However, successful regeneration in the peripheral nerve is a multifactorial process. Peripheral nerves contain laminin-coated basal membrane scaffolds that support moderate axonal regeneration even in acellular grafts (Wang et al., 1992; Agius and Cochard, 1998). The presence of activated Schwann cells clearly enhances the speed of axonal outgrowth (Wang et al., 1992; Dahlin, 1995). Finally, macrophages contribute to the success of the process, by removing inhibitory myelin molecules like MAG (Fruchtiger et al., 1996).

The situation in the CNS is very different. Central projections lack the numerous endoneurial basal membrane scaffolds and there is no recruitment of macrophages. Thus, success in the CNS only depends on one factor, the intrinsic glial cell function. Interestingly, these glial cells are rapidly activated after injury and support central axonal regeneration in fish and amphibia (see this volume, Part I), but this support is apparently lost in the higher vertebrates (Bernhardt, 1999).

V. THE RETROGRADE REACTION

In addition to molecular and morphological changes in the affected neuronal cell bodies, axotomy will cause the activation of the surrounding non-neuronal cells. In the peripheral ganglia, this leads to inflammatory changes in satellite cells and local macrophages (Mathews and Nelson, 1975; Lu and Richardson, 1991, 1993; Gehrmann et al., 1991a, Schreiber et al., 1995; Stephenson and Byers, 1995) and in the brain, there is a similar activation of astrocytes and of microglia, the brain-resident, macrophage-related cell type (Kreutzberg and Graeber, 1998; Raivich et al., 1999). This is accompanied by a rapid recruitment of leukocytes, primarily T-lymphocytes and NK-cells, to the sites of the neuronal reaction, both in the peripheral and central nervous system (Schmidt et al., 1990; Raivich et al., 1998; Kurkowska-Jastrzebska et al., 1999). Similar neuroglial activation is also a consistent feature in almost all forms of central and peripheral pathology. It appears to reflect an evolutionarily-conserved program which plays an important role in the repair of the injured nervous system. This program is particularly well characterized in a model of central retrograde reaction, the axotomized facial motor nucleus and involves microglia, astrocytes and T-cells.

A. Microglial response

The rapid transformation of ramified microglial from a resting to an activated state has been recognized for over a century. Morphologically, the microglia show a gradual increase in cell body size, thickening of proximal processes, increase in cell number and reduction in ramification. However, studies using quantitative immunofluorescence showed that this activation proceeds through several discrete and very different stages (fig. 5).

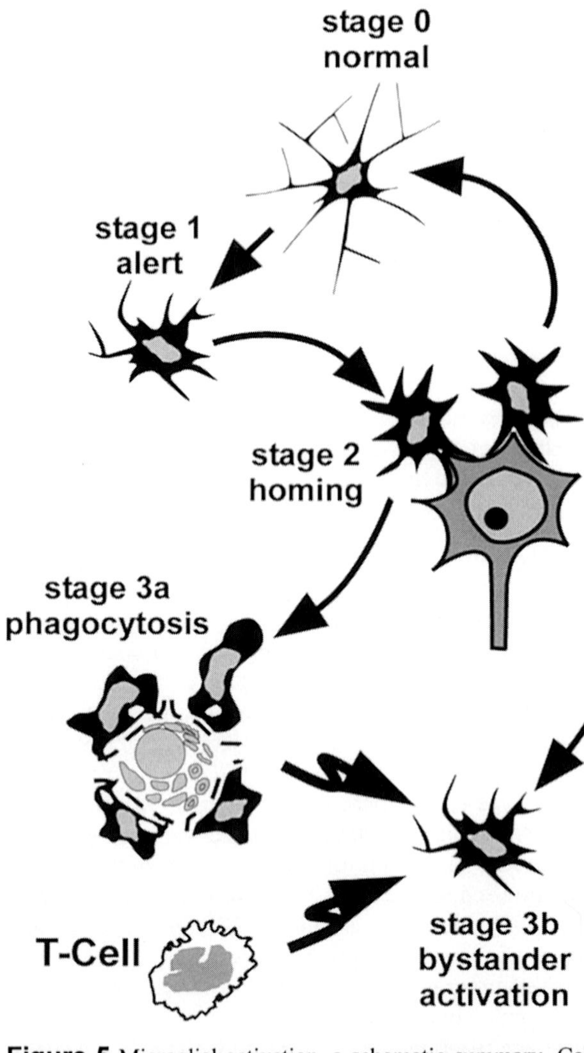

Figure 5 Microglial activation, a schematic summary. Cellular changes in activated microglia proceed through a series of steps which differ in their morphology and molecular profile. Neural injury leads to a rapid transformation of the highly ramified resting microglia (stage 0) to more stout and deramified form (stage 1: state of alert), which home on damaged structures like injured neurons (stage 2: homing), but without additional damage, gradually return to the normal, resting state (stage 0). Cell death leads to a further transformation of microglia into phagocytotic cells (stage 3a: phagocytosis). Interestingly, these foci of phagocytosis also lead to an activation of the surrounding, non-phagocytotic microglia (stage 3b: bystander activation). Microglial activation is also observed during immune response or infection in the presence of antigen-reactive lymphocytes. Reproduced from Raivich et al., 1999; Figure 2.

Early microglial activation, the state of alert, is characterized by a rapid increase in molecules involved in immune recognition. There is an increase in receptors for complement (aMb2-integrin, complement receptor type 3), leukocyte adhesion molecules like ICAM1, receptors for IgG (FcgR) and the associated IgG-immunoreactivity reaching a maximum within the first 24 hours (Raivich et al. 1998a, Werner et al., 1998). Amyloid precursor protein (APP) is also upregulated and may contribute to neurodegenerative changes (Banati et al., 1993a).

The second step, beginning 2-3 days after injury, is characterized by homing and adhesion to damaged structures such as degenerating terminals or injured neurons. Microglia adhere to the surface of neuronal cell bodies and remove the synaptic boutons, a phenomenon known as synaptic stripping. The molecular basis of this behavior is a subject of intense investigation, with a particular interest in chemokines and their receptors (Harrison et al., 1998; Schreiber et al., 1998). Homing and adhesion is accompanied by induction of several integrins, a5b1 and a6b1 in mice, a4b1 and aLb2 in rats, cytoskeletal proteins like vimentin, and further reduction in ramification (Graeber et al., 1998; Moneta et al., 1993, Hailer et al., 1998; Kloss et al., 1999). Early activation markers aMb2 and ICAM1 decrease, documenting the transition to the second stage (Raivich et al., 1998a; Werner et al., 1998). These homing microglia increase their receptors for monocytic mitogens such as MCSF and GMCSF (Raivich et al., 1991b; 1998a) and proliferate, a behavior controlled by the presence of MCSF. Homozygous mice with a loss of function mutation for MCSF show an almost complete absence in microglial proliferation after injury (Raivich et al., 1994).

Neuronal cell death causes a further transformation of microglia into phagocytotic cells that remove neuronal debris. Phagocytotic behavior is also observed in the removal of degenerating terminals or myelin. Removal of such large structures as degenerating pyramidal cells or motoneurons leads to the formation of microglial nodules, consisting of 3-20 phagocytes. This state of phagocytosis leads to the induction of most activation markers already present during stage 1 and stage 2, particularly the adhesion molecules, which could participate in the binding and internalization of the cellular debris (Fig. 5). Phagocytosis is also associated with the induction of molecules needed for antigen presentation. There is an increase in Major Histocompatibility Complex (MHC) molecules, proteases and proinflammatory cytokines e.g., IL1b and TNFa (Banati et al., 1993; Bohatschek et al., 1998; Raivich et al., 1998b). There is also an induction of many costimulatory molecules e.g., ICAM1, B7 and aXb2-integrin (Werner et al., 1998; Bohatschek et al., 1998; Kloss et al., 1999). Because of the lymphocyte influx to brain areas showing retrograde response and adhesion to microglial nodules (Raivich et al., 1998b), the microglial expression of these costimulatory molecules could cause successful antigen presentation, orchestrating an immune response in the damaged nervous system.

The process of phagocytosis also leads to the activation of neighboring, non-phagocytotic microglia, a process called bystander activation. This activation is absent in mice deficient in the p55 TNF receptor, pointing to the involvement of the TNFa in this process (Deckert-Schluter et al., 1998; Bohatschek et al., 1998). Bystander-activated microglia show an increase in MHC molecules, a4b1 and aMb2-integrins, and ICAM1. However, they appear to lack two decisive costimulatory factors, B7 and aXb2-integrin (Bohatschek et al., 1998, Kloss et al., 1999). Absence of costimulatory factors can lead to inactivation (anergy) in lymphocytes interacting with antigen-presenting cells (Bretscher and Cohn, 1970; Robey and Allison, 1995). Although hypothetical, such a mechanism could be used in the CNS to differentiate between microglia with constitutively expressed peptides, and microglia with antigens recovered from the phagocytosed debris, directing the lymphocyte response against the latter (Raivich et al., 1999). The microglial effects on the neighboring injured neurons are still a matter of debate. *In vitro*, activated microglia produce a series of neurotoxic molecules including excitotoxins, free oxygen radicals, proinflammatory cytokines and tissue destroying proteases (Banati et al., 1993; Giulian et al., 1996). However, they are also a source of trophic molecules, that promote neuronal survival (Elkabes et al., 1996; Mallat et al., 1989). *In vivo*, the overall results are egually equivocal. Reduction of microglial activation in MCSF or TNF receptor deficient mice is detrimental to neuronal survival in cerebral ischemia (Berezovskaya et al., 1995; Bruce et al., 1996). On the other hand, inhibition of microglia reduces cell death in axotomized retinal ganglion cells (Thanos et al., 1993). Activated microglia are also the main source of IL1 in the ischemic cerebral cortex (Zhang et al, 1998), and neutralization of this activity strongly inhibits the postischemic tissue damage (Relton and Rothwell, 1992). It is possible that microglial function is not directed primarily at killing or protecting neighboring cells. Such effects do occur, but they may be secondary, and their direction can differ depending on location and the tested cytokine. It is unlikely that this is their main role, considering the highly consistent nature of microglial activation in different brain regions and different forms of pathology. Instead, microglial activation leads to the appearance of a competent cell capable of antigen presentation, a basic function that is needed for the immune surveillance of the damaged, and potentially infected brain.

B. Leukocyte recruitment

Enhanced entry of leukocytes occurs rapidly after injury. As in the activation of microglia, this response differs according to the severity of the injury. Major trauma, infection or autoimmune disease will lead to a profuse recruitment of many different cell types, including neutrophil granulocytes, macrophages, and different B and T lymphocyte subclasses, which show clear regional preferences (Fig. 6). However, following the mild or indirect trauma, the response is limited to a small number of T and NK cells (for a review see Raivich et al., 1999). This entry is selective for the affected brain region and is already apparent one day after injury. In the mouse facial axotomy model, it is restricted to the retrogradely reacting neurons (Raivich et al., 1998b). This site-specific entry of lymphocytes appears to be a crucial factor in the development of precocious inflammation in

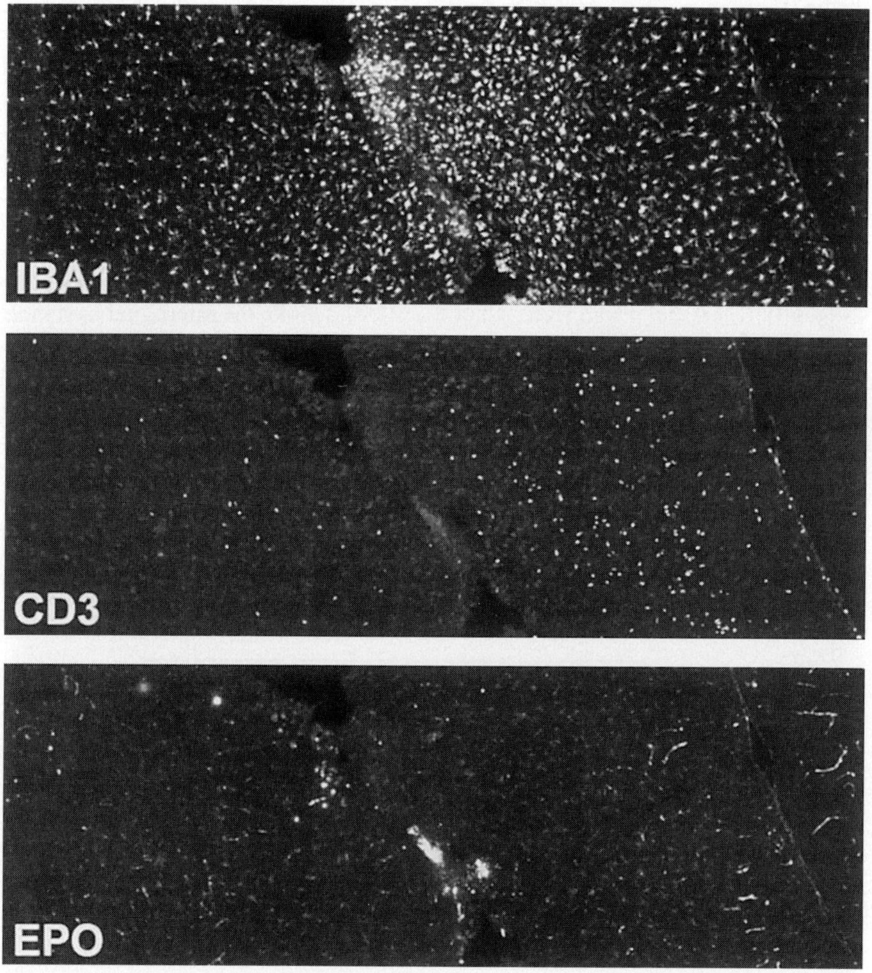

Figure 6 Leukocyte recruitment in direct cerebral trauma. 4 days after a parasagital cortical hemisection. A-C: Triple fluorescence labeling for macrophages/microglia uisng immunoreactivity for IBA1 (A), for T-lymphocytes using immunoreactivity for CD3 (B) and for neutrophil granulocytes and inflamed vessels using endogenous peroxidase (C). Note the conflagration of peroxidase activity at the site of the wound. Infiltration of IBA1+ macrophages is particularly strong at the wound site and decreases with further distance. The CD3+ lymphocytes are more numerous farther out into the parenchyma and avoid the wound site. 60x. Reproduced from Raivich et al., 1999; Figure 6E.

the cryoinjured cerebral cortex or the deafferented superior colliculus in experimental allergic encephalomyelitis (Molleston et al., 1993, Phillips et al., 1997).

Posttraumatic neural cell death leads to a further potentiation of this lymphocyte extravasation. In the mouse facial model, neuronal cell death peaks at day 14 after injury, and coincides with an approximately 100-fold increase in the number of CD3-positive cells, compared with the unoperated, contralateral side (Fig. 7). Both the CD4-positive T helper and the CD8-positive T suppressor/cytotoxic cells contribute to this increase and aggregate around the phagocytotic, MHC, B7 and aXb2-positive microglial nodules (Bohatschek et al., 1998). Studies in transgenic animals show an important role for several proinflammatory cytokines, including IL1, IL6 and TNFa (Raivich et al., 1999). Unlike the microglial bystander activation, the TNF effects on lymphocyte recruitment are apparently mediated by the p75 TNF receptor (Lucas et al., 1997, Raivich et al., 1999). Similar recruitment of lymphocytes to phagocytotic microglia was also observed in the substantia nigra, following MPTP-mediated destruction of the nigrostriatal pathway (Kurkowska-Jastrzebska et al., 1999). Lymphocyte infiltration also occurs in human neurodegenerative diseases such as Alzheimer's dementia (McGeer et al., 1993) or amyotrophic lateral sclerosis (Troost et al., 1989; Engelhardt et al., 1993), stressing the importance of immune surveillance in degenerating neural tissue.

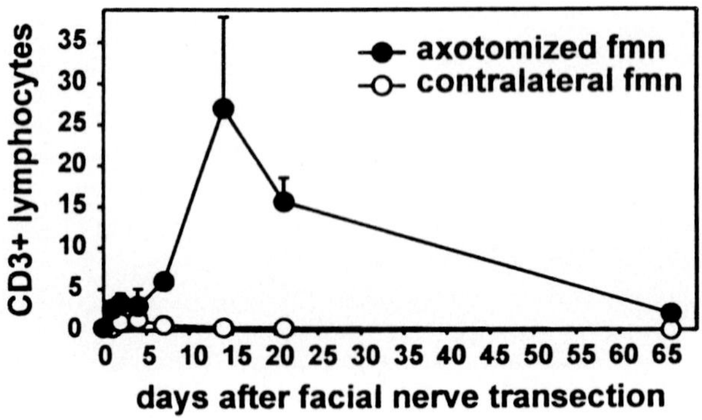

Figure 7 Time course of lymphocyte influx into the axotomized facial motor nucleus using immunohistochemistry for CD3 as a T-lymphocyte cell marker. Note the early plateau of 2-3 labeled cells per section 1-4 days after axotomy, and a further 10-fold increase at day 14. No statistically significant increase on the contralateral side (mean + standard error of the mean/SEM, n = 3 animals per time point). Reproduced from Raivich et al., 1998b; Figure 1F.

C. Astrocyte reaction

As with microglia and leukocytes, the astrocyte response to injury proceeds through several stages and depends on the extent of trauma and astrocyte type. The fibrillary astrocytes, with long slender processes contacting glia limitans, blood vessels and axonal nodes of Ranvier (Butt et al.1994), are normally located in the white matter and become activated in response to direct injury and Wallerian degeneration. They play an important role in the formation of inhibitory glial scars described in detail in other chapters of this volume.

The protoplasmatic astrocytes are located in the grey matter and exhibit numerous short and flappy processes contacting neuronal cell bodies, synapses and blood vessels, and play a crucial role in the transport of nutrients from the perivascular space to sites of high metabolism (Tsacopoulos and Magistretti, 1996; Kettenmann et al., 1999). Even mild, indirect forms of injury, such as neuronal axotomy rapidly activate this cell type. Within 24 h after injury, there is an increase in the synthesis of GFAP. At first, immunoreactivity for this cytoskeletal protein is distributed throughout the cytoplasm of the reactive astrocyte, causing a frequently blobby appearance (Fig. 8). This protein is redistributed 2-3 days after injury, becomes concentrated in the cell body and the main astrocyte branches, leading to the familiar appearance of the GFAP-immunoreactive, stellar astrocytes. Cytoskeletal proteins increase the stability of cells in the presence of tensile forces and the redistribution of GFAP to the cell body and main processes may thus add rigidity to the damaged neural parenchyma. This increased tissue rigidity may help to prevent damage around strained or lacerated blood vessels (Pekny et al., 1999).

Astrocyte transformation is tightly controlled by cytokines in the neural parenchyma, which regulate different steps in this activation process. IL6 plays a stimulatory and TGFb1 an inhibitory role. Thus, transgenic absence of IL6 does not inhibit the induction of GFAP immunoreactivity, but the cytokine is needed for the process of stellarization (Klein et al., 1997; Raivich et al., 1999). Endogenous IL6 stimulates the astrocyte expression of the microglial mitogen GMCSF (Penkowa et al., 1998) and has indirect effects on microglial proliferation (Klein et al., 1997). On the other hand, the absence of TGFb1 induces the expression of GFAP and the appearance of stellar astrocytes even in the normal, undamaged brain.

Absence of TGFb1 also promotes the astrocyte response after injury (Jones et al., 1998), suggesting that the function of this cytokine is to counteract the proinflammatory stimuli, like that of IL6, in the normal and damaged parenchyma. A main function of reactive astrocytes is to separate damaged and healthy cells, or on a macroscopical scale, between damaged and healthy tissue. Although the extent of scarring depends on the severity of brain damage, a rudimentary response around affected neurons is readily observed even after indirect trauma. Two to four weeks after axotomy, reactive astrocytes displace microglia from the neuronal surface and surround injured neurons with flat cytoplasmic processes (Graeber and

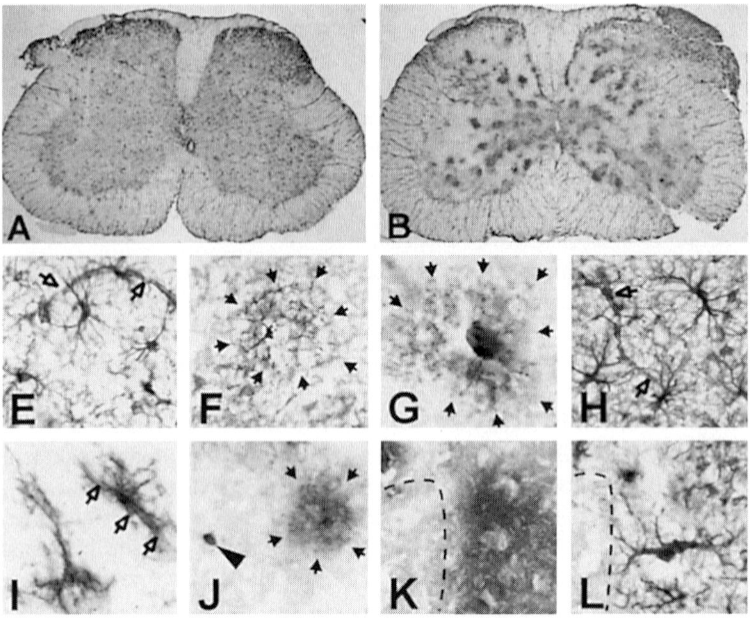

Figure 8 CNS injury leads to changes in astrocyte morphology and molecular markers. A, B: Effects of transgenic IL6-deficiency on the immunoreactivity for GFAP, a typical astrocyte cytoskelettal protein. Mouse lumbar spinal cord in wildtype (A) and IL6-deficient animals (B), 3 days after transection of the right sciatic nerve. A: Normal animals show a strong increase in the number of GFAP-positive, stellar astrocytes throughout the spinal cord gray matter on the operated side. There is also a moderate increase on the contralateral side. B: IL6-deficient animals show 60 mm large blobs of GFAP-immunoreactivity throughout the affected gray matter. The constitutive GFAP immunoreactivity on the slender, fibrillar astrocytes in the spinal cord white matter (fiber tracts) is not affected by IL6-deficiency. E-L: Astrocyte morphology at high light microscopic magnification using staining for GFAP (E-H, L) and CD44 (I-K), an astrocyte cell membrane glycoprotein. E, I: Stellar, fibrillary astrocytes in the white matter of normal mouse corpus callosum. The open arrows point to the adjacent vessels covered with GFAP (E) or CD44 (I) immunostaining. F, G, J: Early reactive astrocytes in the cerebral cortex gray matter following cerebral ischemia (F: 6 hour, J: 24 hour reperfusion) or infection with pneumococci (G: 36 hours after inocculation). The GFAP-immunoreactivity (F, G) reveals a diffuse staining of 30-50 μm large plaques (arrows), with a more intense staining of the cell body and fragments of the main astrocyte branches. Similar diffuse staining is also observed with CD44 (J). The large arrow points to a CD44-positive leukocyte. H, L: Late astrocyte response 6 days after ischemia. Astrocytes hypertrophy and reorient their GFAP-immunoreactive proximal processes at the margin between necrotic and surviving tissue (L, strippled line). Many astrocytes are also reactive outside the directly postischemic region, but these appear slender and multipolar (H). K: CD44 Immunoreactivity in the issue section adjacent to L. Note the diffuse distribution of this astrocyte membrane antigen around the necrotic zone (fig. 8K). A,B: 50x;D: 60x; E-L: 465x. Reproduced from Raivich et al., 1999; Figure 5.

Kreutzberg, 1988). These processes adhere to each other, creating stacks of astrocyte lamellae, which could act as a small glial scar. Interestingly, the production of thin astrocyte processes appears to depend on the presence of another cytoskeletal protein, vimentin (Colucci-Guyon et al., 1999), a common component of astroglial scars. Successful regeneration leads to a retraction of these astrocyte processes and a gradual repopulation of neuronal surface with some synaptic terminals. Thus, synaptic stripping and the astrocyte response to this event is, at least in part, a reversible process.

V. NEURAL INFLAMMATION: CUES TO PHYSIOLOGICAL FUNCTION

In the preceding sections, we described in detail the cellular changes in the damaged nervous system, at the site of injury, in the distal projections and around the injured neuronal cell bodies. One common denominator was their inflammatory nature, particularly the activation of a phagocytotic system and the induction of cells responsible for scar formation. Studies using transgenic and knockout models have started to provide information on the proinflammatory cytokines, chemokines and cell adhesion molecules that orchestrate these cellular changes. Specifically, this work now sheds light on the molecular targets for possible pharmacological manipulation. However, the crucial question is the specific biological function subserved by a more or less common set of inflammatory changes during neural repair.

In most tissues, the posttraumatic cellular response is considered to serve two different functions: (1) to allow repair, regeneration and resumption of normal function and (2) to protect against infectious pathogens. This dual role does not fully apply in the nervous system. In fact, as has been pointed out throughout this volume, there is a striking difference in the mammalian nervous system's ability to repair itself; i.e., peripheral nerves regenerate following injury while central nerves do not. This inability to regenerate has been interpreted as a protective mechanism that arose during vertebrate evolution, to ensure the maintenance of an increasingly complex CNS, where the intricate circuitry could be disturbed by a massive invasion of misdirected axons. However, the specific features of the inflammatory reaction in the injured brain: the recruitment of immune cells, antigen presentation and the effective insulation of the damaged tissue by astrocytes, all point to an alternative explanation, i.e., to prevent the spread of infectious disease. Moreover, the differences in the ability to regenerate after central or peripheral trauma, may reflect an adaptation to the predominant form of neural injury. The peripheral axons innervate many tissues, and are frequently injured by physical damage. The situation is very different for the CNS. The vertebrate brain and spinal cord are shielded by the skull and vertrebral column. The CNS is also suspended in the isodense cerebrospinal fluid to minimize indirect damage following blows to the head or body. Because of this physical protection, we recently suggested that the cellular response in the injured brain may represent a selective adaptation against the other major source of neural injury: the infectious pathogens (Raivich et al., 1999).

This interpretation of the cellular response to injury in the CNS is supported by several lines of evidence: Lymphocytes are rapidly recruited into the damaged brain, screening neural parenchyma for possible pathogens. This suveillance function is assisted by the transformation of microglia into antigen presenting cells that express MHC and a large set of costimulatory molecules. These microglia adhere to damaged cells, particularly neurons, placing the microglia in a strategic position to take up, process and present any infectious material leaking out from these cells, before they begin to die. The ability of astrocytes to produce dense glial scars and wall off the damaged brain region may stop or retard the spread of infection. Dense astrocyte lamellae around individual lesioned neurons may play a similar role, by preventing the transsynaptic propagation of viral particles from one infected neuron to the next. The inability to regenerate may also reflect such a device to limit the spread of infection by affected axons.

Apparently, all three central glial cell types, astrocytes, oligodendrocytes and microglia, contribute to this inability to regenerate. Thus, prevention of astrocyte scar formation by microsurgery, neutralization of collagen 4 or X-ray inhibition, elicits axonal regeneration in central white matter tracts. Neutralization of the oligodendrocyte inhibitory molecule NI-35, removal of myelin or ablation of the myelin-forming cells has a similar, regeneration-stimulatory effect. Microglial phagocytosis and degradation of myelin is an extremely slow process, with debris-laden microglia in the pyramidal tract still present years after the original cerebral insult (Kösel et al., 1998). Since activated microglia are effective removers of neuronal debris (Möller et al., 1996; Raivich et al., 1998b), this points to a specific problem with the degradation of myelin, which could be functionally desirable. The presence of several converging mechanisms to block axonal regeneration underlines the importance attached to this phenomenon. Glial scars and myelin also inhibit migration of astrocytes, fibroblasts and oligodendroglia, causing a successful insulation of the damaged brain. From an evolutionary point of view, this end result is probably highly desirable in combating infection, at least for the time before the advent of antibiotic and antiviral agents. However, the CNS appears ill equipped in dealing with noninfectious pathology, particularly with trauma to the central axonal projections.

VII. FUTURE DIRECTIONS

As shown in the preceding paragraphs, there is considerable functional plasticity in the inflammatory response in the damaged nervous system. In the peripheral nerve, the inflammatory response supports axonal regeneration, although the overall effect is probably moderate. In the CNS, the local inflammatory response is apparently modified and contributes to the overall lack of success in axonal elongation. Recent studies on inflammatory cytokines, chemokines and cell adhesion molecules have just begun to uncover the mechanisms involved in this plastic reponse, following central or peripheral damage. Of particular interest are the molecule, or the set of molecules, that are responsible for the unfavorable course in the CNS. Here, we are just at the beginning, with many discoveries still ahead. The presence of several converging mechanisms to block regeneration, does suggest considerable redundancy. Clearly, a better knowledge of these molecules could provide us with targets for intervention and thus improve our ability to help neural repair in the lesioned central or peripheral part of the nervous system.

REFERENCES

Agius E, Cochard P (1998) Comparison of neurite outgrowth induced by intact and injured sciatic nerves: a confocal and functional analysis. J Neurosci 18:328-338.

Alonso G, Privat A (1993) Reactive astrocytes involved in the formation of lesional scars differ in the mediobasal hypothalamus and in other forebrain regions. J Neurosci Res 34:523-538.

Archelos JJ, Previtali SC, Hartung HP (1999) The role of integrins in immune-mediated diseases of the nervous system Trends Neurosci 22:30-38.

Avellino AM, Hart D, Dailey AT, MacKinnon M, Ellegala D, Kliot M (1995) Differential macrophage responses in the peripheral and central nervous system during Wallerian degeneration of axons. Exp Neurol 136:83-98.

Banati RB, Gehrmann J, Czech C, Monning U, Jones LL, Konig G, Beyreuther K, Kreutzberg GW (1993a) Early and rapid de novo synthesis of Alzheimer beta A4-amyloid precursor protein (APP) in activated microglia. Glia 9:199-210.

Banati RB, Gehrmann J, Schubert P, Kreutzberg GW (1993b) Cytotoxicity of microglia. Glia 7:111-118.

Berezovskaya O, Maysinger D, Fedoroff S (1995) The hematopoietic cytokine, colony-stimulating factor 1, is also a growth factor in the CNS: congenital absence of CSF-1 in mice results in abnormal microglial response and increased neuron vulnerability to injury. Int J Dev Neurosci 13 285-299.

Berner A, Torvik A, Stenwig AE (1973) Origin of macrophages in traumatic lesions and Wallerian degeneration in peripheral nerves. Acta Neuropathol 25:228-236.

Bernhardt RR (1999) Cellular and molecular bases of axonal regeneration in the fish central nervous system. Exp Neurol 157:223-240.

Bernier B, Castejon S, Culver DG, Glass JD (1999) Axonal neurofilaments are rsistant to calpain-mediated degraddation in the WLDs mouse. NeuroReport 10:1423-1426.

Beuche W, Friede RL (1984) The role of non-resident cells in Wallerian degeneration. J Neurocytol 13:767-796.

Beuche W, Friede RL (1986) Myelin phagocytosis in Wallerian degeneration of peripheral nerves depends on silica-sensitive, bg/bg-negative and Fc-positive monocytes. Brain Res 378:97-106.

Bignami A, Eng LF, Dahl D, Uyeda CT (1972) Localization of the glial fibrillary acidic protein in astrocytes by immunofluorescence. Brain Res 43 429-435.

Blight AR (1994) Effects of silica on the outcome from experimental spinal cord injury: implication of macrophages in secondary tissue damage. Neurosci 60:263-273.

Bohatschek M, Galiano M, Bluethmann H, Labow M, Kreutzberg GW, Raivich G (1999) Cytokine-mediated regulation of antigen presenting molecules MHC1, MHC2 and B7-2 in the axotomized facial motor nucleus of the mouse. Ann Anat 181 S57-S58.

Bohatschek M., Jones L.L., Kreutzberg G.W., Raivich G (1998) Expression of immunoregulatory molecules MHC1, MHC2 and B7-2 in the axotomized mouse facial motor nucleus. Clin.Neuropathol. 17:286.

Bolin LM, Verity AN, Silver JE, Shooter EM, Abrams JS (1995) Interleukin-6 production by Schwann cells and induction in sciatic nerve injury. J Neurochem 64:850-858.

Bourde O, Kiefer R, Toyka KV, Hartung HP (1996) Quantification of interleukin-6 mRNA in wallerian degeneration by competitive reverse transcription polymerase chain reaction. J Neuroimmunol 69:135-140.

Bretscher P, Cohn M (1970) A theory of self-nonself discrimination. Science 169 1042-1049.

Brook GA, Plate D, Franzen R, Martin D, Moonen G, Schoenen J, Schmitt AB, Noth J, Nacimiento W (1998) Spontaneous longitudinally orientated axonal regeneration is associated with the Schwann cell framework within the lesion site following spinal cord compression injury of the rat. J Neurosci Res 53:51-65.

Brown HC, Castano A, Fearn S, Townsend M, Edwards G, Streuli C, Perry VH (1997) Adhesion molecules involved in macrophage responses to Wallerian degeneration in the murine peripheral nervous system. Eur J Neurosci 9:2057-2063.

Brown MC, Perry VH, Lunn ER, Gordon S, Heumann R (1991) Macrophage dependence of peripheral sensory nerve regeneration: possible involvement of nerve growth factor. Neuron 6:359-370.

Bruce AJ, Boling W, Kindy MS, Peschon J, Kraemer PJ, Carpenter MK, Holtsberg FW, Mattson MP (1996) Altered neuronal and microglial responses to excitotoxic and ischemic brain injury in mice lacking TNF receptors. Nature Med 2 788-794.

Bruck W, Friede RL (1990) Anti-macrophage CR3 antibody blocks myelin phagocytosis by macrophages in vitro. Acta Neuropathol 80:415-418.

Bruck W, Friede RL (1991) The role of complement in myelin phagocytosis during PNS Wallerian degeneration. J Neurol Sci 103:182-187.

Butt AM, Duncan A, Berry M (1994) Astrocyte associations with nodes of Ranvier: ultrastructural analysis of HRP-filled astrocytes in the mouse optic nerve. J Neurocytol 23:486-499.

Calcutt NA, McMurray HF, Moorhouse DF, Bache M, Parthasarathy S, Powell HC, Mizisin AP (1994) Inhibition of macrophage chemotaxis and peripheral nerve regeneration in normal and hyperglycemic rats by the aldose reductase inhibitor Tolrestat. Exp Neurol 128:226-232.

Carroll SL, Frohnert PW (1998) Expression of JE (monocyte chemoattractant protein-1) is induced by sciatic axotomy in wild type rodents but not in C57BL/Wld(s) mice. J Neuropathol Exp Neurol 57:915-930.

Chen S, Bisby MA (1993) Long-term consequences of impaired regeneration on facial motoneurons in the C57BL/Ola mouse. J Comp Neurol 335:576-585.

Clemence A, Mirsky R, Jessen KR (1989) Non-myelin-forming Schwann cells proliferate rapidly during Wallerian degeneration in the rat sciatic nerve. J Neurocytol 18:185-192.

Colucci-Guyon E, Gimenez y Ribotta M, Maurice T, Babinet C, Privat A (1999), Cerebellar defect and impaired motor coordination in mice lacking vimentin. Glia 25:33-43.

Crang AJ, Blakemore WF (1986) Observations on Wallerian degeneration in explant cultures of cat sciatic nerve. J Neurocytol 15:471-482.

da Costa CC, van der Laan LJ, Dijkstra CD, Bruck W (1997) The role of the mouse macrophage scavenger receptor in myelin phagocytosis. Eur J Neurosci 9:2650-2657.

Dahlin LB (1995) Prevention of macrophage invasion impairs regeneration in nerve grafts. Brain Res 679:274-280.

Dailey AT, Avellino AM, Benthem L, Silver J, Kliot M (1998) Complement depletion reduces macrophage infiltration and activation during Wallerian degeneration and axonal regeneration. J Neurosci 18:6713-6722.

Davies SJ, Fitch MT, Memberg SP, Hall AK, Raisman G, Silver J (1997) Regeneration of adult axons in white matter tracts of the central nervous system. Nature 390:680-683.

Deckert-Schluter M, Bluethmann H, Rang A, Hof H, Schluter D (1998) Crucial role of TNF receptor type 1 (p55), but not of TNF receptor type 2 (p75), in murine toxoplasmosis. J Immunol 160:3427-3436.

Elkabes S, Dicicco Bloom EM, Black IB (1996) Brain microglia/macrophages express neurotrophins that selectively regulate microglial proliferation and function. J Neurosci 16:2508-2521.

Engelhardt JI, Tajti J, Appel SH, (1993) Lymphocytic infiltrates in the spinal cord in amyotrophic lateral sclerosis. Arch Neurol 50:30-36.

Ferguson T, Hernandez J, Maria B, Muir D (1997) Neuronal matrix metalloproteinase-2 degrades and inactivates neurite-inhibiting chondroitin sulfate proteoglycan. Soc Neurosci Abst 23:31.

Fernandez-Valle C, Bunge RP, Bunge MB (1995) Schwann cells degrade myelin and proliferate in the absence of macrophages: evidence from in vitro studies of Wallerian degeneration. J Neurocytol 24:667-679.

Franzen R, Schoenen J, Leprince P, Joosten E, Moonen G, Martin D (1998) Effects of macrophage transplantation in the injured adult rat spinal cord: a combined immunocytochemical and biochemical study. J Neurosci Res 51:316-327.

Gehrmann J, Gold R, Linington C, Lannes-Vieira J, Wekerle H, Kreutzberg GW (1992) Spinal cord microglia in experimental allergic neuritis. Evidence for fast and remote activation. Lab Invest 67:100-113.

Gehrmann J, Monaco S, Kreutzberg GW (1991) Spinal cord microglial cells and DRG satellite cells rapidly respond to transection of the rat sciatic nerve. Restor Neurol Neurosci 2:181-198.

Giulian D, Yu J, Li X, Tom D, Li J, Wendt E, Lin SN, Schwarcz R, Noonan C (1996) Study of receptor-mediated neurotoxins released by HIV-1-infected mononuclear phagocytes found in human brain. J Neurosci 16:3139-3153.

Graeber MB, Kreutzberg GW (1986) Astrocytes increase in glial fibrillary acidic protein during retrograde changes of facial motor neurons. J Neurocytol 15 (1986) 363-374.

Graeber MB, Kreutzberg GW (1988) Delayed astrocyte reaction following facial nerve axotomy. J Neurocytol 17:209-220.

Grosche J, Matyash V, Moller T, Verkhratsky A, Reichenbach A, Kettenmann H (1999) Microdomains for neuron-glia interaction: parallel fiber signaling to Bergmann glial cells. Nature Neurosci 2:139-143.

Hailer NP, Bechmann I, Heizmann S, Nitsch R (1997) Adhesion molecule expression on phagocytic microglial cells following anterograde degeneration of perforant path axons. Hippocampus 7:341-349.

Harrison JK, Jiang Y, Chen S, Xia Y, Maciejewski D, McNamara RK, Streit WJ, Salafranca MN, Adhikari S, Thompson DA, Botti P, Bacon PK, Feng L (1998) Role for neuronally derived fractalkine in mediating interactions between neurons and CX3CR1-expressing microglia. Proc. Nat. Acad. Sci. U.S.A. 95:10896-10901.

Harvey GK, Toyka KV, Hartung HP (1994) Effects of mast cell degranulation on blood-nerve barrier permeability and nerve conduction in vivo. J Neurol Sci 125:102-109.

Herdegen T, Kiessling M, Bele S, Bravo R, Zimmermann M, Gass P (1993) The KROX-20 transcription factor in the rat central and peripheral nervous systems: novel expression pattern of an immediate early gene-encoded protein. Neurosci 57:41-52.

Hirschberg DL, Schwartz M (1995) Macrophage recruitment to acutely injured central nervous system is inhibited by a resident factor: a basis for an immune-brain barrier. J Neuroimmunol 61:89-96.

Jones LL, Doetschman T, Kreutzberg GW, Raivich G (1998) Neuroglial activation in the injured central nervous system: role of transforming growth factor-b1. Soc. Neurosci. Abstr. 28:710.2.

Kaiserling E, Xiao JC, Ruck P, Horny HP (1993) Aberrant expression of macrophage-associated antigens (CD68 and Ki-M1P) by Schwann cells in reactive and neoplastic neural tissue. Light- and electron-microscopic findings. Mod Pathol 6:463-468.

Kiefer R, Streit WJ, Toyka KV, Kreutzberg GW, Hartung H (1995) Transforming growth factor-beta-1: A lesion-associated cytokine of the nervous system. Int J Dev Neurosci 13 331-339.

Klein MA, Möller JC, Jones LL, Bluethmann H, Kreutzberg GW, Raivich G (1997) Impaired neuroglial activation in Interleukin-6 deficient mice. Glia 19:227-233.

Kloss CUA, Werner A, Klein MA, Shen J, Menuz K, Probst JC, Kreutzberg GW, Raivich G, (1999) The integrin family of cell adhesion molecules in the injured brain: regulation and cellular localization in the normal and regenerating mouse facial motor nucleus. J Comp Neurol in press.

Kosel S, Egensperger R, Bise K, Arbogast S, Mehraein P, Graeber MB (1997) Long-lasting perivascular accumulation of major histocompatibility complex class II-positive lipophages in the spinal cord of stroke patients: possible relevance for the immune privilege of the brain. Acta Neuropathol 94 532-538.

Kreutzberg GW, Graeber MB (1998) Glial cell activation in the facial nucleus as a response to nerve lesion. In New Horizons in Facial Nerve Research and Facial Expression (Yanagihara N Murakami S, Eds), Kugler Publications, The Hague, pp.11-14.

Kreutzberg GW, Raivich G (1999) Neurobiology of regeneration and degeneration. In The Facial Nerve (May M, Ed). Thieme, New York, 2nd edition, in press.

Kurkowska-Jastrzebska I, Wronska A, Kohutnicka M, Czlonkowski A, Czlonkowska A (1999) The inflammatory reaction following 1-methyl-4-phenyl-1,2,3,6-tetrahydropyridine (MPTP) intoxication in mouse. Exp Neurol 156:50-61.

La Fleur M, Underwood JL, Rappolee DA, Werb Z (1996) Basement membrane and repair of injury to peripheral nerve: defining a potential role for macrophages, matrix metalloproteinases, and tissue inhibitor of metalloproteinases-1. J Exp Med 184:2311-2326.

Lawson LJ, Frost L, Risbridger J, Fearn S, Perry VH (1994) Quantification of the mononuclear phagocyte response to Wallerian degeneration of the optic nerve. J Neurocytol 23:729-744.

Lawson LJ, Perry VH, Gordon S (1992) Turnover of resident microglia in the normal adult mouse brain. Neurosci 48:405-415.

Lazarov-Spiegler O, Solomon AS, Zeev-Brann AB, Hirschberg DL, Lavie V, Schwartz M (1996) Transplantation of activated macrophages overcomes central nervous system regrowth failure. FASEB J 10:1296-1302.

Li Y, Field PM, Raisman G (1998) Regeneration of adult rat corticospinal axons induced by transplanted olfactory ensheathing cells. J Neurosci 18:10514-10524.

Lindholm D, Heumann R, Meyer M, Thoenen H (1987) Interleukin-1 regulates synthesis of nerve growth factor in non-neuronal cells of rat sciatic nerve. Nature 330:658-659.

Ling EA (1979) Evidence for a haematogenous origin of some of the macrophages appearing in the spinal cord of the rat after dorsal rhizotomy. J Anat 128:143-154.

Liu HM, Yang LH, Yang YJ (1995) Schwann cell properties: 3. C-fos expression, bFGF production, phagocytosis and proliferation during Wallerian degeneration. J Neuropathol Exp Neurol 54:487-496.

Lu X, Richardson PM (1991) Inflammation near the nerve cell body enhances axonal regeneration. J Neurosci 11:972-978.

Lu X, Richardson PM. (1993) Responses of macrophages in rat dorsal root ganglia following peripheral nerve injury. J Neurocytol 22:334-341.

Lucas R, Juillard P, Decoster E, Redard M, Burger D, Donati Y, Giroud C, Monso-Hinard C, De Kesel T, Buurman WA, Moore MW, Dayer JM, Fiers W, Bluethmann H, Grau GE (1997) Crucial role of tumor necrosis factor (TNF) receptor 2 and membrane-bound TNF in experimental cerebral malaria. Eur J Immunol 27:1719-1725.

Lunn ER, Perry VH, Brown MC, Rosen H, Gordon S (1989) Absence of Wallerian degeneration does not hinder regeneration in peripheral nerve. Eur J Neurosci 1:27-33.

MacDonald SM, Mezei M, Mezei C (1981). Effect of Wallerian degeneration on histamine concentration of the peripheral nerve. J Neurochem 36:9-16.

Mallat M, Houlgatte R, Brachet P, Prochiantz A (1989) Lipopolysaccharide-stimulated rat brain macrophages release NGF in vitro. Dev Biol 133:309-311.

Matthews MR, Nelson VH (1975) Detachment of structurally intact nerve endings from chromatolytic neurones of rat superior cervical ganglion during the depression of synaptic transmission induced by post-ganglionic axotomy. J Physiol 245:91-135.

McGeer PL, Kawamata T, Walker DG, Akiyama H, Tooyama I, McGeer EG (1993) Microglia in degenerative neurological disease. Glia 7:84-92.

McGovern FH, Estevez J (1980) The use of cromolyn sodium in the prevention of nerve degeneration in Bell's palsy. Laryngoscope. 90:1640-1645.

Möller JC, Klein MA, Haas S, Jones LL, Kreutzberg GW, Raivich G (1996) Regulation of thrombospondin in the regenerating mouse facial nucleus. Glia 17:121-132.

Molleston MC, Thomas ML, Hickey WF (1993) Novel major histocompatibility complex expression by microglia and site-specific experimental allergic encephalomyelitis lesions in the rat central nervous system after optic nerve transection. Adv Neurol 59:337-348.

Monaco S, Gehrmann J, Raivich G, Kreutzberg GW (1992) MHC-positive, ramified macrophages in the normal and injured rat peripheral nervous system. J Neurocytol 21:623-634.

Moneta ME, Gehrmann J, Topper R, Banati RB, Kreutzberg GW (1993) Cell adhesion molecule expression in the regenerating rat facial nucleus. J Neuroimmunol 45:203-206.

Murphy PG, Borthwick LS, Johnston RS, Kuchel G, Richardson PM (1999) Nature of the retrograde signal from injured nerves that induces interleukin-6 mRNA in neurons. J. Neurosci. 19:3791-3800.

Nathaniel EJH, Pease DC (1963) Degenerative changes in rat dorsal roots during Wallerian degeneration. J Ultrastruc Res 9:511-532.

Nishio Y, Minami A, Kato H, Kaneda K, Nishihira J (1999). Identification of macrophage migration inhibitory factor (MIF) in rat peripheral nerves: its possible involvement in nerve regeneration. Biochim Biophys Acta 1453:74-82.

Ohara S, Ikuta F (1985) On the occurrence of the fenestrated vessels in Wallerian degeneration of the peripheral nerve. Acta Neuropathol 68:259-262.

Olsson Y (1966) The effect of the histamine liberator, Compound 48-80 on mast cells in normal peripheral nerves. Acta Pathol Microbiol Scand 68:563-574.

Pekny M, Johansson CB, Eliasson C, Stakeberg J, Wallen A, Perlmann T, Lendahl U, Betsholtz C, Berthold CH, Frisen J (1999) Abnormal reaction to central nervous system injury in mice lacking glial fibrillary acidic protein and vimentin. J. Cell Biol. 145:503-514.

Penkowa M, Moos T, Carrasco J, Hadberg H, Molinero A, Bluethmann H, Hidalgo J (1999) Strongly compromised inflammatory response to brain injury in interleukin-6-deficient mice. Glia 25:343-357.

Perry VH, Tsao JW, Fearn S, Brown MC (1995) Radiation-induced reductions in macrophage recruitment have only slight effects on myelin degeneration in sectioned peripheral nerves of mice. Eur J Neurosci 7:271-280.

Pesini P, Kopp J, Wong H, Walsh JH, Grant G, Hokfelt T (1999) An immunohistochemical marker for Wallerian degeneration of fibers in the central and peripheral nervous system. Brain Res. 828:41-59.

Phillips MJ, Needham M, Weller RO (1987) Role of cervical lymph nodes in autoimmune encephalomyelitis in the Lewis rat. J. Pathol. 182:457-464.

Powell HC, Myers RR, Costello ML (1980) Increased endoneurial fluid pressure following injection of histamine and compound 48/80 into rat peripheral nerves. Lab Invest 43:564-572.

Prewitt CMF, Niesman IR, Kane CJM, Houle JD (1997) Activated macrophage/microglial cells can promote the regeneration of sensory axons into the injured spinal cord. Exp Neurol 148:433-443.

Pyykonen I, Koistinaho J (1991) c-fos protein like immunoreactivity in non-neuronal cells of rat peripheral nerve after transection. Acta Neuropathol 82:66-71.

Rabchevsky AG, Streit WJ (1997) Grafting of cultured microglial cells into the lesioned spinal cord of adult rats enhances neurite outgrowth. J Neurosci Res 47 34-48.

Raisman G (1985) Specialized neuroglial arrangement may explain the capacity of vomeronasal axons to reinnervate central neurons. Neurosci. 14:237-254.

Raivich G, Bohatschek M, Kloss CUA, Werner A, Jones LL, Kreutzberg GW (1999) The neuroglial activation repertoire in the injured brain: molecular mechanisms and cues to physiological function. Brain Res Rev, 30:77-105

Raivich G, Haas S, Werner A, Klein MA, Kloss CUA, Kreutzberg GW(1998a) Regulation of MCSF receptors on microglia in the normal and injured mouse central nervous system: A quantitative immunofluorescence study using confocal laser microscopy. J Comp Neurol 395:342-358.

Raivich G, Gehrmann J, Kreutzberg GW (1991a) Increase of macrophage colony-stimulating factor and granulocyte-macrophage colony stimulating factor receptors in the regenerating rat facial nucleus. J Neurosci Res 30:682-686

Raivich G., Graeber M.B., Gehrmann J., Kreutzberg G.W. (1991b) Transferrin receptor expression and iron uptake in the injured and regenerating rat sciatic nerve. Eur. J. Neurosci. 3:919-927.

Raivich G, Jones LL, Kloss CUA, Werner A, Neumann H, Kreutzberg GW (1998b) Immune surveillance in the injured nervous system: T-lymphocytes invade the axotomized mouse facial motor nucleus and aggregate around sites of neuronal degeneration. J Neurosci 18:5804-5816.

Raivich G., Kreutzberg G.W. (1987a) Expression of growth factor receptors in injured nervous tissue. I. Axotomy leads to a shift in the cellular distribution of specific ß-nerve growth factor binding in the injured and regenerating PNS. J Neurocytol 16:687-700.

Raivich G., Kreutzberg G.W. (1987b) Expression of growth factor receptors in injured nervous tissue. II. Induction of specific platelet-derived growth factor binding in the injured PNS is associated with a breakdown in the blood-nerve barrier and endoneural interstital oedema. J. Neurocytol. 16:701-711.

Raivich G, Kreutzberg GW (1993) Peripheral nerve regeneration: role of growth factors and their receptors. Int J Dev Neurosci 11:311-324 104.

Raivich G, Kreutzberg GW (1994) Pathophysiology of glial growth factor receptors. Glia 11:129-146

Raivich G, Moreno-Flores MT, Möller JC, Kreutzberg GW (1994) Inhibition of posttraumatic microglial proliferation in a genetic model of macrophage colony-stimulating factor deficiency in the mouse. Eur J Neurosci 6:1615-1618

Ramon-Cueto A, Avila J (1998) Olfactory ensheathing glia: properties and function. Brain Res. Bull. 46:175-187.

Ramon y Cajal S (1928) Degeneration and regeneration of the nervous system. Oxford University Press. London/NY.

Reichert F, Saada A, Rotshenker S (1994) Peripheral nerve injury induces Schwann cells to express two macrophage phenotypes: phagocytosis and the galactose-specific lectin MAC2. J Neurosci 14:3231-3245

Relton JK, Rothwell NJ (1992) Interleukin-1 receptor antagonist inhibits ischaemic and excitotoxic neuronal damage in the rat. Brain Res Bull 29:243-246.

Robey E, Allison JP (1995) T-cell activation: integration of signals from the antigen receptor and costimulatory molecules. Immunol Today 16:306-310.

Saada A, Reichert F, Rotshenker S (1996) Granulocyte macrophage colony stimulating factor produced in lesioned peripheral nerves induces the up-regulation of cell surface expression of MAC-2 by macrophages and Schwann cells. J Cell Biol 133:159-167

Schafer M, Fruttiger N, Montag D, Schachner M, Martini R (1996) Disruption of the gene for the myelin-associated glycoprotein improves axonal regrowth along myelin in C57BL/WLDs mice. Neuron 16:1107-1113

Schmidt RE, Summerfield AL, Hickey WF (1990) Ultrastructural and immunohistologic characterization of guanethidine-induced destruction of peripheral sympathetic neurons. J Neuropathol Exp Neurol 49:150-167

Schreiber R, Krivacic K, Vaccariello S, Mocanu O, Ransohoff R, Zigmond RE (1998) LIF mutant mice have decreased expression of chemokines following axonal injury of the superior cervical ganglion. Soc. Neurosci. Abstr. 28:800.9.

Schreiber RC, Shadiack AM, Bennett TA, Sedwick CE, Zigmond RE (1995) Changes in the macrophage population of the rat superior cervical ganglion after postganglionic nerve injury. J Neurobiol 27:141-153

Schwab ME (1990) Myelin-associated inhibitors of neurite growth and regeneration in the CNS. Trends Neurosci. 13:452-456.

Shy ME, Shi Y, Wrabetz L, Kamholz J, Scherer SS (1996) Axon-Schwann cell interactions regulate the expression of c-jun in Schwann cells. J Neurosci Res 43:511-525

Siebert H, Sachse A, Kuziel WA, Bruck W (1999) Reduced macrophage recruitment after Wallerian degeneration in mice lacking the chemokine receptor CCR2. Proceedings of the 27th Göttingen Neurobiology Conference (Elsner N, Eysel U, eds), Thieme, Stuttgart/NY, Vol II, p.773.

Skoff RP (1975) The fine structure of pulse labeled (3H-thymidine cells) in degenerating rat optic nerve. J Comp Neurol 161:595-611

Stephenson JL, Byers MR (1995) GFAP immunoreactivity in trigeminal ganglion satellite cells after tooth injury in rats. Exp Neurol 131:11-22

Stewart HJ (1995) Expression of c-Jun, Jun B, Jun D and cAMP response element binding protein by Schwann cells and their precursors in vivo and in vitro. Eur J Neurosci 7:1366-75

Stoll G, Trapp BD, Griffin JW (1985) Macrophage function during Wallerian degeneration of rat optic nerve: clearance of degenerating myelin and Ia expression. J Neurosci 9:2327-2335

Tanaka K, Zhang QL, Webster HD (1992) Myelinated fiber regeneration after sciatic nerve crush: morphometric observations in young adult and aging mice and the effects of macrophage suppression and conditioning lesions. Exp Neurol 118:53-61

Thanos S, Mey J, Wild M (1993) Treatment of the adult retina with microglia-suppressing factors retards axotomy-induced neuronal degradation and enhances axonal regeneration in vivo and in vitro. J Neurosci 13:455-466

Toews AD, Barrett C, Morell P (1998) Monocyte chemoattractant protein 1 is responsible for macrophage recruitment following injury to sciatic nerve. J Neurosci Res 53:260-267

Troost D, van den Oord JJ, de Jong JM, Swaab DF (1989) Lymphocytic infiltration in the spinal cord of patients with amyotrophic lateral sclerosis. Clin Neuropathol 8:289-294

Tsacopoulos M, Magistretti PJ (1996) Metabolic coupling between glia and neurons. J. Neurosci. 16:877-885.

Vougioukas VI, Roeske S, Michel U, Bruck W (1998) Wallerian degeneration in ICAM-1-deficient mice. Am J Pathol 152:241-249

Wagner R, Myers RR (1996) Schwann cells produce tumor necrosis factor alpha: expression in injured and non-injured nerves. Neuroscience 73 625-629

Waller A (1850) Experiments on the section of the glossopharyngeal and hypoglossal nerves of the frog, and observations of the alterations produced thereby in the structure of their primitive fibers. Philos Trans 140:423-469

Wang GY, Hirai K, Shimada H, Taji S, Zhong SZ (1992) Behavior of axons, Schwann cells and perineurial cells in nerve regeneration within transplanted nerve grafts: effects of anti-laminin and anti-fibronectin antisera. Brain Res 583:216-226

Werner A, Kloss CUA, Walter J, Kreutzberg GW, Raivich G (1998) Intercellular adhesion molecule-1 (ICAM1) in the regenerating mouse facial motor nucleus. J Neurocytol 27:219-232.

Williams PL, Hall SM (1971) Chronic Wallerian degeneration - an in vivo and ultrastructural study. J Anat 109:487-503

Zammit PS, Clarke JD, Golding JP, Goodbrand IA, Tonge DA (1993) Macrophage response during axonal regeneration in the axolotl central and peripheral nervous system. Neurosci 54:781-789

Zhang Z, Chopp M, Goussev A, Powers C (1998) Cerebral vessels express interleukin 1-beta after focal cerebral ischemia. Brain Res. 784:210-217

11

Glial Response to Injury

S. Hirsch and M. Bähr
University of Tübingen, Tübingen, Germany

I. INTRODUCTION

The limited regenerative capacity of the injured mammalian CNS has absorbed the minds of neuroscientists for more than one hundred years. A phenomenon that attracted much attention early on is the formation of a scar at the site of injury that seemed to be impermeable to regenerative axon growth. Investigation of the scar composition showed that it consisted of astrocytes, macrophages and microglia, and varying amounts of connective tissue elements. These cells are converted into a 'reactive' state following injury by mechanisms that still need to be elucidated. For a long time it was dogma that the glial scar would not allow any growth of neurites and experiments were mainly aimed at preventing scar formation. In recent years it has become accepted that scarring is not a mere failure of mammalian CNS to react to injury in an appropriate way. Instead, the aggregating astrocytes are thought to seal the wound with the effect of reestablishing the blood-brain-barrier and isolating the CNS from toxic influences of the external milieu. In this perspective, inhibition of axon growth is an undesired side effect of wound healing in the CNS. Moreover, evidence is accumulating that reactive astrocytes are not generally nonpermissive, but can be good substrates for nerve regeneration under certain circumstances. Their substrate properties are now being analyzed on the molecular level, and it is clear that reactive astrocytes express both growth promoting and inhibiting proteins. Another player in the scarring process is the connective tissue or meningeal cells. The role of these cells in regeneration has been, for the most part, ignored. But recent experiments have shown that they can negatively influence the permissiveness of the scar and change astrocyte properties towards nonpermissiveness. The activation processes are crucially influenced or even triggered by factors released from macrophages and microglia in the course of their inflammatory response to injury.

In this chapter we describe first the processes that lead to the formation of a glial scar with regard to some region specific differences. To that end, we will review some of the information presented in the previous chapter on inflammatory molecules to point out their specific role in scar formation. Second, we will try to give an overview of the molecules influencing astrocytic substrate properties. Here we discuss recent results concerning the role of astrocytic cell surface and extracellular matrix molecules in neural regeneration. Finally, the role of meningeal cells and oligodendrocytes will be considered. The impact of myelin proteins will not be discussed since it is described in detail in chapters 15 and 16.

II. TRAUMATIC CNS LESIONS

Traumatic brain or spinal cord injuries have two major effects on neuronal cells: On the one hand, they can lead directly to neuronal cell loss. This process is termed primary neuronal cell death and there is little chance of rescue once neurons have been subjected to a lesion affecting their somata. They will die quickly, probably in a necrotic way. On the other hand, trauma may lead to axotomy, i.e., the disruption of axons, without initially affecting the parent somata. If the lesion is close to the soma, secondary cell death may occur within days or weeks after axotomy. In this case the majority of neurons die apoptotically (this volume, chapter by Chaudhary and Sharma). This phenomenon is by far the more interesting to study because there is a chance to rescue neurons from cell death that is a prerequisite for subsequent axonal regeneration.

Indeed, a series of experimental paradigms have been developed to investigate the cellular and molecular events after CNS injury. For example, axotomy can be achieved by transection or crush of isolated nerve bundles like the optic nerve or white matter tracts in the brain. Such systems avoid damage to neuronal cell bodies and therefore allow for the study of secondary changes in the cell's response to injury. A more relevant experimental model is the stab wound made into the cortex or hippocampus, a model in which cell somata and axons are equally affected. Here the investigator has to deal with a more diverse cellular environment, thus the injury induced changes are more complex. Many more sophisticated experimental designs resulting in a slightly varied glial reaction have been used, yet the rough time of glial response to injury remains unchanged.

After axotomy, an as yet undefined signal transduces this event to the cell body and may trigger an apoptotic cascade if the lesion is close to the soma. The onset of apoptosis can be as early as 24 hours after axotomy. In the case of a distant lesion with sparing of collaterals and/or a long axon stump, no secondary cell death may occur, but the cell soma response is less pronounced thus limiting the neuronal regenerative capacity (Hüll and Bähr 1994 a,b; Herdegen et al., 1997). In contrast, changes involving glial cells are usually slower. The distal nerve segments are separated from their cell somata and undergo 'Wallerian degeneration,' i.e., they are degraded and taken up by microglia and macrophages over a period of weeks or months. This process is much slower in the CNS than in the PNS (Perry and Brown, 1992). In the majority of experimental lesions the proximal nerve segments that are still connected to the neuronal cell bodies undergo a process of retraction and degeneration that is termed 'axonal die back' and takes place over a period of weeks. Whenever an axon degenerates its surrounding oligodendrocytes and astrocytes are deprived of neuronal contact. Thus, glial functions depending on neuronal activity can no longer be maintained. On the other hand, there can be substantial sprouting of axons into the lesioned area. Most of the time, however, no lengthy neurite growth is achieved with growth cones retracting again or stopping at the margin of the wound. This process is called 'abortive sprouting' and has been attributed to a disruption of the timing of events such as sealing of the wound, myelin removal, reexpression of growth promoting molecules and axon growth (Lazarov-Spiegler et al., 1996).

Direct injury to glial cells causes them to release a number of cytokines and messenger proteins which in turn induce morphological and physiological changes in the environment. As described in the previous chapter invading macrophages, microglia and blood cells are involved in an inflammatory reaction at the lesion site. Taken together, the evolving 'reactive gliosis' is the result of three main triggering processes: deprivation of glial cells from neuronal contact, cellular injury and inflammation.

It should be noted that the glial environment may react differently to trauma according to its cellular composition and the accessibility of a lesioned area for blood derived cells. Even the extent of neuronal regeneration can vary within certain limits between brain areas. For example in the olfactory bulb, unlike the optic nerve or spinal cord, there is considerable regeneration fostered by the local glia, the olfactory ensheathing cells (this volume, chapter by Plant et al.,). In other parts of the CNS the astrocytic reaction predominates in gray matter lesions whereas oligodendrocytes probably play a more important role in white matter lesions. Meningeal cells are involved in the formation of a glial scar only if the meninges are affected by the lesion. Thus, in deep layers of the cortex there will be less meningeal cell invasion than in superficial cortical layers or in isolated nerve bundles. In the following section we will present the overall morphological characteristics of reactive gliosis that are generally found independent of the CNS location.

III. MORPHOLOGY OF REACTIVE GLIOSIS

While the actual cellular composition of CNS scar tissue is rather heterogeneous, including astrocytes, macrophages, microglia and meningeal cells, the common use of the term 'reactive astrocytosis' in the literature indicates that astrocytes are considered to be the major players in the scarring process. More precisely, the subclass of protoplasmic or type I astrocytes have been shown to represent the majority of reactive astrocytes (Miller et al., 1986). Following a widely accepted definition, 'reactive astrocytes' display four main characteristics: hypertrophic morphology, proliferation, migration, and the upregulation of certain gene products.

Probably the most prominent feature of gliosis is the accumulation of intermediate filaments in astrocytes. The expression level of the major component of astrocytic filaments, glial fibrillary acidic protein (GFAP), increases rapidly (Latov et al., 1979; Condorelli et al., 1990). While GFAP is barely detectable in normal astrocytes of the unlesioned CNS, its protein and mRNA levels are significantly elevated 2 days after injury reaching a maximum after 4-5 days (Cancilla et al., 1992). Immunohistochemical staining for GFAP is therefore routinely used as a sensitive and reliable marker for reactive gliosis. To date it is not known whether GFAP has any physiological function in scar formation or axon growth. The level of GFAP expression, however, does not seem to correlate with the extent of regeneration in different CNS areas. For example, high expression levels of GFAP are observed in the regenerating olfactory bulb as well as in the non-regenerating optic nerve (Anders and Johnson, 1990; McPhilemy et al., 1990; Schmidt-Kastner et al., 1993). Thus, there is no indication of any GFAP-dependent growth regulation.

Similar to GFAP, other structural proteins are upregulated during gliosis. Vimentin is an intermediate filament protein that is normally found in developing astrocytes, while in the normal adult its expression is barely detectable (Schnitzer et al., 1981). The upregulation of vimentin expression in response to injury is thought to reflect a rearrangement of the cytoskeleton and a partial dedifferentiation of reactive astrocytes (Dahl et al., 1982; Calvo et al., 1991; Baldwin and Scheff, 1996).

S100β, a calcium-binding protein, can be detected also in normal astrocytes, but its expression is significantly higher in reactive ones (Malhotra and Shnitka, 1994). S100β has been shown to stimulate astrocyte proliferation and to rescue neurons from axotomy induced cell death (Winningham-Major, 1989; Marshak, 1990; Selinfreund, 1991; Iwasaki et al., 1997). Both astrocytosis and increased neurite formation occur in the hippocampus of mice overexpressing S100β protein (Reeves et al., 1994), suggesting that these processes do not exclude one another. Pathological mechanisms, such as apoptotic death of astrocytes, may be mediated by S100β-induced activation of nitric oxide synthase (Reeves et al., 1994; Hu and van Eldik, 1996).

Reactive astrocytes in general exhibit signs of hypertrophy, swelling of the cytoplasm, which may be due to an accumulation of filaments, as well as enlargement of the nucleus, Golgi and rough endoplasmatic reticulum. The latter changes can be interpreted as prerequisites for the extensive production and secretion of proteins. Also, the content of glycogen increases markedly after injury (Haymaker et al., 1970) and there is reason to believe that this may be aimed at stabilizing neuronal energy metabolism after CNS injury (Sorg and Magistretti, 1992). The resulting hypertrophic phenotype is used as an ultrastructural characteristic to distinguish reactive from normal astrocytes.

There has been a long-standing debate as to whether proliferation and/or migration of glial cells are responsible for the accumulation of glial processes at the lesion site. Convincing evidence for astrocytic proliferation has been provided by the colocalization of GFAP-protein and incorporated ^{3}H-thymidine (Janeczko, 1991; Topp et al., 1989). However, there is evidence that proliferation may precede the upregulation of GFAP-expression in astrocytes, since many of the GFAP-negative dividing cells are observed early after lesion, when their identity could not be determined (Janeczko, 1989). Thus, it is difficult to calculate the actual extent of astrocytic proliferation. Migration seems to be a minor component of the astrocytic reaction to injury *in vivo* although cell culture assays and transplantation studies have shown the ability of astrocytes to migrate over rather great distances of several centimeters (Zhou et al., 1990).

Usually the intact CNS tissue is separated from the vascular system by the blood-brain-barrier. The CNS-face of the barrier is made up of tightly associated astrocytic endfeet, which form the glia limitans or glial limiting membrane. Cells outside of the glia limitans are connected via tight junctions and thus accomplish the actual barrier function. The induction of the barrier function by endothelial cells seems to be due to astroglial influences during development (Risau and Wolburg, 1990). Between the cellular layers a continuous collagenous basal lamina is formed. Whenever the blood-brain-barrier is disrupted by a lesion it has to be rebuilt rapidly to reestablish brain homoeostasis and prevent inflow of blood components. Indeed, the formation of a glia limitans can be observed soon after lesions (Berry et al., 1983; Mathewson and Berry, 1985). In contrast to its normal appearance, the reconstituted glia limitans is not an orderly assembled layer but can be highly irregular and convoluted (Reier, 1986). An explanation for this comes from *in vitro* studies which have shown that a basal lamina forms where astrocytes and meningeal cells make contact (Abnet et al., 1991). Unfortunately, the formation of a basal glial limitans deep inside CNS tissue instead of being confined to its outer surface, can be a major obstacle to regeneration.

IV. FACTORS INFLUENCING GLIOSIS

In this section we will focus on messenger factors that trigger and promote glial scarring. In this regard we will describe molecules secreted by astrocytes themselves, but also by the macrophages and microglia that participate in this process. The latter are capable of producing a large number of different cytokines, a family of modulatory proteins that consists of interleukins, tumor necrosis factors, interferons and colony stimulating factors. Some of these cytokines critically influence astrocytic and neuronal behavior either by stimulating the release of other factors or by acting on astrocytic function (Ridet et al., 1997). It has been postulated that a 'cytokine network' influences the composition of the glial scar and thus regulates regenerative success after CNS injury (Giulian et al., 1994). To give an impression of the complexity of the cytokine network, we will only mention some of the most relevant molecules involved (Table 1). Moreover, we will focus on the non-inflammatory actions of cytokines, particularly those on astrocytes, since the inflammatory response has been described in the previous chapter.

Astrocytes are the major source of various growth factors that can act on astrocytes themselves or other cell types in an auto- or paracrine way. As we shall see later, some of the secreted factors also influence neuronal survival and outgrowth. Here, we concentrate on the molecules that are either involved in the development or released as a consequence of gliosis. The tight association and the high number of feedback loops in the network of different factors makes it almost impossible to predict the effect of a single player. Rather, the influence of a factor on the scarring process seems to depend critically on the timing and distribution of a released factor as well as on the status of the receptor cells.

One of the earliest events after injury - immediately to a few days after lesion - is the release of adenosine and its nucleotides ADP and ATP from dying cells. Infusion of ADP and an adenosine analogue into normal rat cortex increases astrogliosis, i.e., the number of reactive astrocytes at the lesion site (Hindley et al., 1994). Since the observation is based on immunohistochemical staining for GFAP protein, it is unknown whether the underlying mechanism is due to proliferation, migration or differentiation of astrocytes. Interleukin-1 (IL-1), interleukin-6 (IL-6) and TNF-α are low molecular weight factors (<30kD) released by macrophages and reactive astrocytes after injury. With different potencies, these cytokines contribute to the activation and proliferation of astrocytes and thus increase scar formation (Giulian, 1988; Selmaj et al., 1990). In addition, they stimulate the production of multiple factors, generating cytokine cascades. In astrocytes, IL-1 has been shown to induce the secretion of IL-6, TNF-α and TGF-β (Aloisi et al., 1992; Chung and Beneviste, 1990; da Cunha et al., 1993). Moreover, IL-1 stimulates the production of nitric oxide that in turn may mediate neurotoxicity (Chao et al., 1995; Lee et al., 1995). Il-6 is thought to mediate neurotrophic effects, probably due to the induction of nerve growth factor (NGF) production by astrocytes (Frei et al., 1989). TNF-α stimulates its own production as well as that of IL-6 (Frei et al., 1989; Beneviste et al., 1994). In contrast to the above mentioned cytokines, transforming growth factor-β (TGF-β) inhibits astrocyte proliferation (Lindholm et al., 1992). Still it may contribute to gliosis, since it is thought to act as a chemotrophic agent attracting astrocytes from the surrounding tissue (Beneviste et al., 1994). The production of TNF-α is also inhibited by TGF- α (Suzumura et al., 1993).

In response to injury, mRNA levels of fibroblast growth factor (FGF) and its receptor are increased highly in reactive astrocytes (Logan et al., 1992; Tourbah et al., 1992). This factor has been shown to induce astrocyte proliferation and glial scar formation as well as the expression of GFAP in astrocytes (Morrison et al., 1985; Eclancher et al., 1996). Surprisingly, the mitogenic effect of FGF has been shown to be stimulated by TGF-β; TGF-β by itself inhibits astrocyte proliferation (Labourdette et al., 1990).

Furthermore, FGF seems to downregulate the production of the ciliary neurotrophic factor (CNTF) (Carroll et al., 1993), another factor that can be produced by astrocytes. Like other factors, CNTF has to be released from the cells to exert its action upon neighbouring cells and its release from astrocytes has been demonstrated *in vitro* (Kamiguchi et al., 1995). However, no secretion signal sequence is encoded in the CNTF gene. It has therefore been proposed that either the factor is released only upon disruption of the astrocyte membrane or it is secreted by an unknown mechanism. Once in the extracellular space, CNTF seems to stimulate multiple aspects of gliosis in astrocytes, e.g., hypertrophy, proliferation, and expression of the gliosis associated markers GFAP and S100β (Levison et al., 1996; Kahn et al., 1997; Hudgins and Levison, 1998). Another function that may be important concerning the repair of brain injury is the promotion of oligodendrocyte survival (Louis et al., 1993; Mayer et al., 1994). The regulation of CNTF seems to depend on the CNS region injured. After optic nerve crush a decrease of CNTF mRNA and protein was found in astrocytes at the lesion site itself (Kirsch et al., 1998). Contrary results were obtained following trauma in other brain areas such as the cortex, hippocampus or striatum (Ip et al., 1993; Asada et al., 1995).

V. FACTORS INFLUENCING NEURONAL REGENERATION

Following a CNS lesion certain secretory and surface properties of astrocytes change. It had been generally accepted that reactive astrocytes from adult animals have predominantly negative substrate properties and thus prevent regeneration as compared to astrocytes from neonates which support regenerative growth (Przyrembel and Bähr, 1993; Bähr et al., 1995). However, it is now becoming clear that in most cases astrocytes express activities that both promote and inhibit neuronal regeneration. As in the interaction of different cytokines, the mosaic of factors acting on regenerative processes appear to be in a delicate balance. Following minimal shifts in the cellular response, positive or negative influences can predominate either facilitating or inhibiting regeneration. Attempts to compare reactive and normal astrocytes have often failed to detect obvious differences, but there is now a list of candidate molecules that appear capable of influencing regeneration. They can be divided into three main classes: growth factors, cell adhesion molecules and extracellular matrix proteins (Table 1).

Table 1. The effects of different molecules on axon growth, neuron survival, and gliosis are listed as a summary of data provided in the text.

	Axon growth	Neuron survival	Gliosis	References
Cytokines				
IL-1		-	+	Chao et al., 1995; Lee et al., 1995; Giulian, 1988
IL-6		+	+	Frei et al., 1989
TNF-α			+	Selmaj et al., 1990
cell adhesion molecules				
NCAM	+		-	Smith et al., 1990 ; Krushel et al., 1995
ECM-molecules				
Laminin	+			Liesi, 1985; Ard and Bunge, 1988
Fibronectin	+			Matthiessen et al., 1991
Phosphacan	+			Snyder et al., 1996
Biglycan		+		Junghans et al., 1995
Tenascin-C	+/-	+/-		Spring et al., 1989; Faissner and Kruse, 1990; Prieto et al., 1992; Goetz et al., 1996
DSD-1-proteoglycan	-			Faissner et al., 1994
ABAKAN	-			Geisert et al., 1993
NG2	-			Dou and Levine, 1994
Growth factors				
TGF-β			+/-	Lindholm et al., 1992
NGF		+	+	Yokoyama et al., 1993; Hamburger and Yip, 1984; Montero and Hefti, 1988; Siliprandi et al., 1993
CNTF		+		Sendtner et al., 1991; Mey and Thanos, 1993; Levison et al., 1996; Kahn et al., 1997; Hudgins and Levison, 1998
FGF		+	+	Morrison et al., 1986; Cuevas et al., 1995; Peterson et al., 1996; Morrison et al., 1985; Eclancher et al., 1996

Neurite outgrowth is supported by the extracellular matrix molecule laminin and the cell adhesion molecule NCAM (Liesi, 1985; Ard and Bunge, 1988; Smith et al., 1990). From *in vitro* experiments a decreased expression of these molecules after lesion has been inferred (Smith et al., 1990; Smith et al., 1993). However, *in vivo* studies have shown that considerable amounts of both factors are present in CNS scar tissue (McKeon et al., 1991; Alonso and Privat, 1993; Risling et al., 1993; Frisen et al., 1995). How can the scar tissue contain large amounts of growth promoting molecules and yet be impermeable for neurites? A possible interpretation would be that growth promoting activities in glial scar tissue are overridden by inhibitory factors (McKeon et al., 1995). Interestingly, NCAM reduces astrocyte proliferation when infused into CNS wounds (Krushel et al., 1995). Thus, the growth promoting action of NCAM may not only be due to direct axon-glia interactions, but may also be due to its ability to limit the extent of gliosis and its inhibitory aspects.

Good candidates for nonpermissive scar components are certain proteoglycans of the chondroitin sulfate, dermatan sulfate or keratan sulfate families, some of which are associated with glial scars in the CNS (Snow et al., 1990; McKeon et al., 1991; Geisert and Bidanset, 1993; Smith-Thomas et al., 1994; Fok Seang et al., 1995; Geisert et al., 1996). For example, the upregulation of chondroitin sulfate proteoglycan NG2 after injury has an inhibitory effect on neurite outgrowth *in vitro* (Dou and Levine, 1994; Levine 1994). The keratan sulfate proteoglycan ABAKAN is also suspected to have an inhibitory function, since it delineates boundary structures during development and is expressed after cortical injury (Geisert et al., 1993). A further extracellular matrix molecule that is upregulated during astrogliosis is tenascin-C (McKeon et al., 1991; Ajemian et al., 1994; Fruttiger et al., 1995). Here the situation is more complicated, since different regions of the tenascin-C molecule promote or inhibit axonal regeneration. The expression of the respective domains may partly depend on the isoform expressed (Spring et al., 1989; Faissner and Kruse, 1990; Prieto et al., 1992; Goetz et al., 1996). It has been speculated that if the expression of certain isoforms is regionally distinct, then this could explain different substrate properties of scars from one brain area to the other.

Among the family of proteoglycans there are also molecules with positive effects on regeneration. One of them is the chondroitin sulfate proteoglycan DSD-1-PG, whose activity has been confirmed *in vitro* (Faissner et al., 1994). In addition, phosphacan and biglycan, both are upregulated after brain injury (Stichel et al., 1995; Snyder et al., 1996). While phosphacan has been shown to promote axon growth *in vitro* (Snyder et al., 1996) biglycan enhances neuronal survival without any obvious effect on neurite extension (Junghans et al., 1995; Koops et al., 1996).

Concerning growth factors, NGF has been shown to be upregulated in astrocytes after CNS trauma (Lindholm et al., 1992; Goss et al., 1998) and this may be related to stimulation by various factors such as TGF-β, FGF, Il-1 and Il-6 (Lindholm et al., 1990; Yoshida and Gage, 1991; Schwartz et al., 1994; Kossmann et al., 1996). The actions of NGF in the process of wound healing are probably diverse. First, as we have already mentioned NGF stimulates astrocyte proliferation (Yokoyama et al., 1993). Second, in addition to its well charaterized neurotrophic activity on cholinergic neurons of the basal forebrain, NGF has been reported to rescue dorsal root ganglionic neurons and retinal ganglion cells (Hamburger and Yip, 1984; Montero and Hefti, 1988; Siliprandi et al., 1993). Third, NGF has been shown to induce antioxidant enzymes, thus reducing the damage caused by injury-induced free radical formation (Pechan et al., 1991; Nistico et al., 1992).

As described earlier, CNTF is produced by reactive astrocytes in different lesion paradigms. CNTF does not only have effects on glial activation but can also promote neuronal survival. This has been demonstrated for different neuron populations such as motoneurons and retinal ganglion cells (Sendtner et al., 1991; Mey and Thanos, 1993).

Also, FGF is known to support neuronal survival in the spinal cord, cerebral cortex and hippocampus (Morrison et al., 1986; Cuevas et al., 1995; Peterson et al., 1996). Additionally FGF may have indirect positive effects on regeneration by inducing the expression of growth promoting molecules, e.g., NCAM and fibronectin in astrocytes (Mahler et al., 1997). However, FGF also induces the production of tenascin-C in astrocyte cultures and a cleavage of the molecule in the extracellular space (Mahler et al., 1996). Whether the resulting form of tenascin-C enhances or reduces axon growth in this case is not known at present.

Growth factor receptors are an important class of molecules subject to injury induced regulation processes. For example, the expression of Trk-family neurotrophin receptors, most dramatically TrkB, is upregulated in reactive astrocytes (Frisen et al., 1992). Glial cells express the functional form of these receptors, but a truncated version that lacks the intracellular signal transduction domain is more abundant (McKeon et al.,1997). Their suspected function is the regulation of local neurotrophin concentrations in the CNS and perhaps the presentation of neurotrophin molecules to neurons. The overexpression of TrkB-receptors has been demonstrated to inhibit BDNF-induced neurite outgrowth *in vitro* (Fryer et al., 1997). Thus, the local concentration of available neurotrophins may be very low in glia scar tissue and neurite outgrowth may therefore be greatly restricted.

VI. MENINGEAL CELLS

When the meninges are disrupted by a lesion, there is considerable migration of meningeal cells into the CNS tissue at the lesion site. The distribution of these cells, in contrast to astrocytes, is confined to the immediate vicinity of the lesion and no infiltration into the surrounding areas is observed. Meningeal cells express high amounts of growth promoting molecules such as laminin, fibronectin and biglycan (Matthiessen et al., 1991; Franklin et al., 1992; Junghans et al., 1995; Wang et al., 1997). However, consistent with earlier investigations, we could show that axons growing on mixed astrocyte/meningeal cell layers *in vitro* prefer adult reactive astrocytes as a substrate and avoid meningeal cells (David, 1988; Hirsch et al., 1999). In line with this observation we have found a number of molecular determinants that may account for axon growth inhibition by meningeal cells. For example, they express proteoglycans of the chondroitin and keratan sulfate type, and lack the expression of the stimulatory cell adhesion molecule NCAM (Hirsch and Bähr, 1999; Fig. 1, 2). *In vitro* experiments have revealed that meningeal cells negatively influence neighboring astrocytes in that they induce an increased astrocytic expression of chondroitin sulfate proteoglycans and tenascin C (Ness and David, 1997). A rather new finding is that NGF, which is produced by astrocytes in lesioned areas, induces process outgrowth from meningeal cells and may thus contribute to the formation of mixed scars (Frisen et al., 1998).

As we have mentioned in the context of scar morphology, a basal lamina forms at the site of injury. *In vitro* a basal lamina has been shown to develop at the contact sites between meningeal cells and astrocytes (Struckhoff, 1995). In addition, when mixed cultures of astrocytes and meningeal cells are transplanted into the lesioned CNS, meningeal cells form separated clusters and thus fragment the CNS environment (Franklin et la., 1992), a feature that does not provide optimal conditions for regeneration. The basal lamina contains high amounts of collagen-IV that seems to be a major inhibitor of axon growth in gray matter scars. Upon contact with pieces of basal lamina, axonal growth cones have been observed to stop their extension in CNS tissue. Remarkably, considerable regeneration could be induced in transected axon tracts by inhibition of collagen synthesis (Stichel et al., 1999).

VII. OLIGODENDROCYTES

Since the impact of myelin proteins on axonal regeneration is described in detail in Chapters 15 and 16, we will confine this section to the histological aspects of the oligodendrocyte reaction to injury. In contrast to lower vertebrates (this volume, Part I) mammalian oligodendrocytes are not permissive for axonal growth. They do not migrate into the lesion area and most of the oligodendrocytes that are directly affected die apoptotically soon after injury (Crowe et al., 1997). What remains present for a long time at the lesion site is myelin, compacted oligodendrocyte membranes, that is removed only very slowly by macrophages.

Nevertheless, some investigators have reported a 'reactive' response of oligodendrocytes to lesion. The functional regeneration of axon tracts in the CNS requires not only the regrowth of axons but also their remyelination by oligodendrocytes. Since oligodendrocytes at the lesion site do not survive, migration of myelinating cells from the surrounding tissue is required. A few days after lesion, no mRNA of MBP, one of the major CNS-myelin components, is detectable in the lesion center. However, an upregulation occurs at the border of the glial scar (Bartholdi and Schwab, 1998). Thus, it seems that oligodendrocytes undergo cell death in the scar region, while in the surrounding areas they prepare for remyelination. The invasion of oligodendrocytes and their precursors into the scar area,

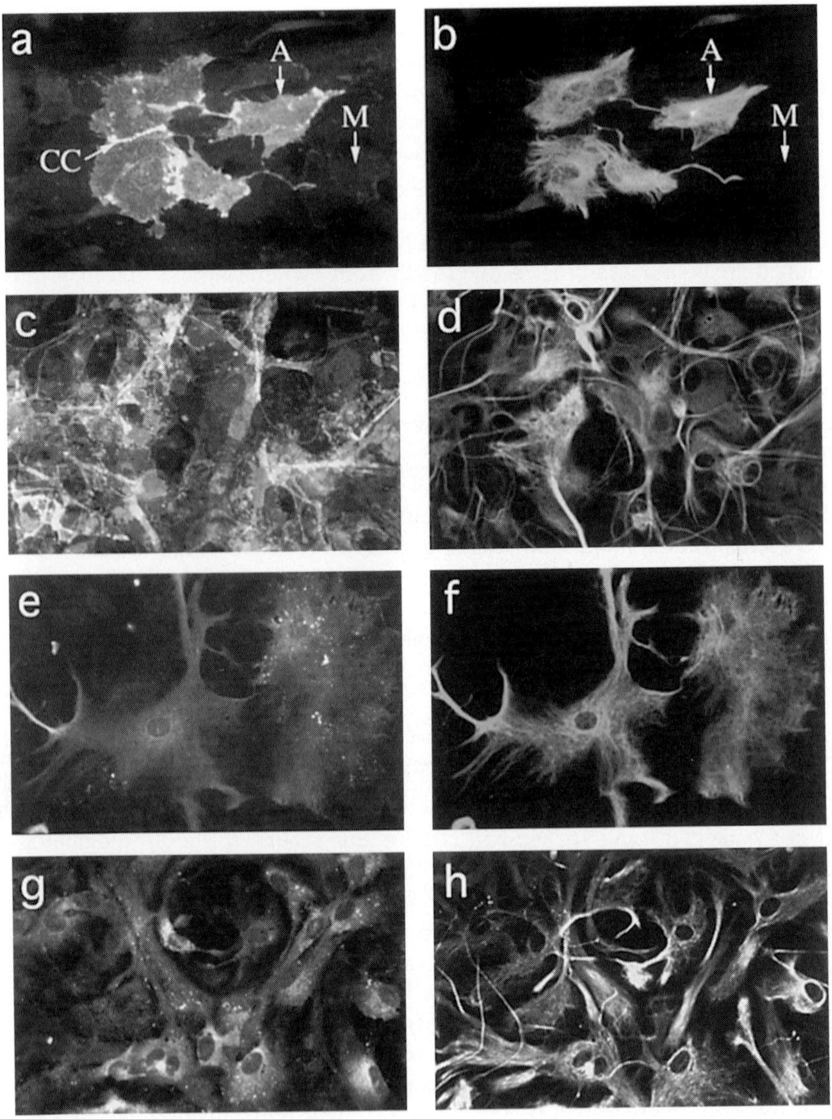

Figure 1 Double immunostaining of reactive adult (a,b,e,f) and neonatal astrocytes (c,d,g,h) for the glial marker protein GFAP (right panel) and the cell adhesion molecules NCAM (a,c) or laminin (e,f). Reactive adult (A) and neonatal astrocytes show intensive staining for NCAM, which is increased at sites of cell-cell contact (cc). In contrast, GFAP-negative meningeal cells (M) express only very weak levels of NCAM. Reactive adult and neonatal astrocytes as well as meningeal cells show comparable levels of laminin immunoreactivity.

however, is prevented by astrocytes. Dense contacts among astrocytes hinder oligodendrocyte migration into the demyelinated tissue (Fok Seang et al., 1995). The cellular contact may be mediated by an interaction of cell adhesion molecules like NCAM and N-Cadherin (Payne et al., 1996). Recently, the effect of cytokines on the migration of oligodendrocytes has been tested. Interestingly, a combination of IL1α and bFGF seems to promote their migration on astrocytes, while TGFβ inhibits this effect (Fok Seang et al., 1998). As has been proposed by other investigators, a mild inflammation with the recruitment of macrophages and microglia that leads to enhanced production of certain cytokines seems to be beneficial for oligodendrocyte migration and remyelination of lesioned axons (Raine and Wu, 1993; Blakemore et al., 1995; Tourbah et al., 1997).

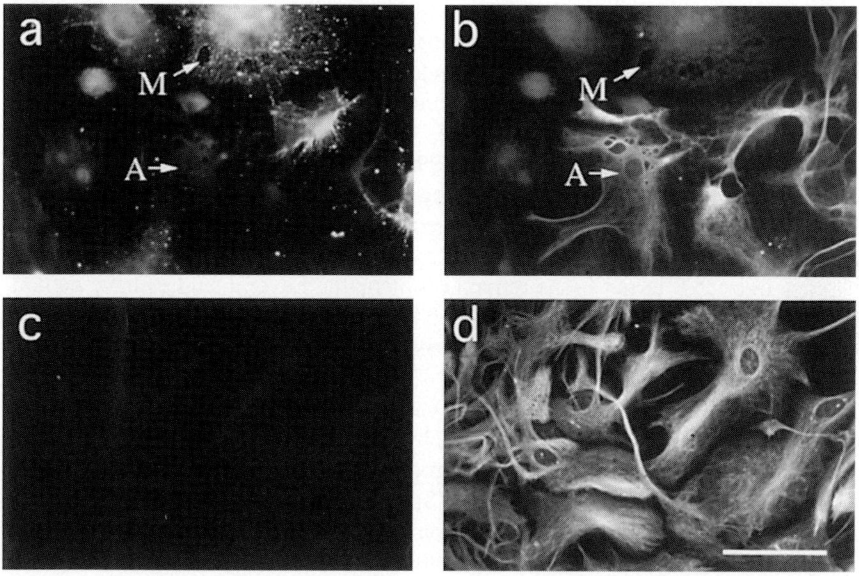

Figure 2. Double immunostaining of reactive adult (a,b) and neonatal astrocytes (c,d) for the glial marker protein GFAP (b,d) and keratan sulfate epitopes (a,c). Keratan sulfate is not expressed by reactive adult (A) nor neonatal astrocytes. In contrast, GFAP-negative meningeal cells (M) express high levels of keratan sulfate.

VIII. FUTURE DIRECTIONS

To overcome the inhibitory aspects of CNS scar formation, several strategies can be pursued. One promising idea first suggested by Cajal (Ramon y Cajal, 1928) is the transplantation of growth promoting cells into the CNS at the site of a lesion. Schwann cells have been used in a great number of studies since they can exert effects that seem to be absent from CNS glial cells. From studies on PNS regeneration it is known that Schwann cells release a number of factors that can not only promote regeneration and survival of PNS neurons, but also of CNS neurons. Furthermore, they participate in myelin removal, a process that is critical for axonal regrowth and that is significantly delayed in the CNS. Schwann cells are also known to remyelinate axons after PNS lesion, a requirement for functional regeneration. Different techniques for introducing Schwann cells into the CNS have been tested, like the use of peripheral nerve grafts (this volume, Chapter by So and Yip), or dissociated Schwann cells in hydrogel matrices or guidance channels together with extracellular matrix. Indeed, transplantation of Schwann cells has been shown to positively influence CNS regeneration in certain lesion paradigms. In some cases, considerable axon growth was observed in the grafts and also a limited remyelination of regenerating axons could be achieved (Raisman, 1997; Baron van Evercooren at al., 1997). In addition to Schwann cells, olfactory bulb ensheathing glia, and to a lesser extent immature astrocytes, have been shown to support CNS regeneration (this volume, Chapter by Plant et al.; Silver, 1988; Smith and Miller, 1991; Franklin et al., 1996; Franklin and Barnett, 1997).

One major obstacle to reestablishing functional connections after transplantation, however, is the inability of regenerating axons to reenter the CNS tissue. Although long distances can be bridged by transplantation techniques the growth of axons into CNS target tissue remain problematic. Several studies have demonstrated very limited success of axons in continuing their growth at the graft border, despite considerable regeneration within the graft (Carter et al., 1989; Brook et al., 1994; Raisman, 1997). Thus, additional strategies must be applied to neutralize growth inhibitors: e.g., myelin inhibitors can be blocked by antibodies (Caroni and Schwab, 1988; this volume, chapter by Schwab), functional substructures removed by enzymatic digestion as in the case of proteoglycans (Zuo et al., 1998) or blockade of synthesis as shown for collagen (Stichel et al., 1999). By comparing nonpermissive and permissive astrocytes several investigators including ourselves are trying to identify the molecular determinants of growth inhibition (Smith et al, 1990; Fok Seang et al., 1995; Fok Seang et al, 1998; Hirsch and Bähr, 1999). Still the major problem is to define the composition of growth inhibitors acting *in vivo*, and it seems likely that more than one molecule will have to be blocked to foster regeneration.

Rather than modifying the components of a glial scar, it seems more promising to interfere with early events in the cascade. One step towards this goal is the finding that certain cytokines can prevent the establishment of an inhibitory astrocytic environment (Fok Seang et al, 1998). Ideally, a different path of astrocyte reaction may be initiated that could even be beneficial for regeneration as in the immature CNS where a simlar gliotic reaction takes place (Trimmer and Wunderlich, 1990; Butt and Colquhoun, 1996), but the scar seems to be only a minor obstacle to axon growth (Berry et al., 1983; Rudge and Silver, 1990).

Only by understanding the mechanisms underlying reactive gliosis will we be able to explain its manifestation and to design effective tools for its prevention. Therefore, further detailed analysis will be necessary. Finally, the best chance to improve CNS regeneration seems to combine anti-gliotic strategies with neurotrophic support and removal of myelin.

REFERENCES

Abnet K, Fawcett JW, Dunnett SB (1991) Interactions between meningeal cells and astrocytes in vivo and in vitro. Brain Res Dev Brain Res 59(2):187-96.

Ajemian A, Ness R, David S (1994) Tenascin in the injured rat optic nerve and in non-neuronal cells in vitro: potential role in neural repair. J Comp Neurol 340(2):233-42.

Aloisi F, Care A, Borsellino G, Gallo P, Rosa S, Bassani A, Cabibbo A, Testa U, Levi G, Peschle C (1992) Production of hemolymphopoietic cytokines (IL-6, IL-8, colony-stimulating factors) by normal human astrocytes in response to IL-1 beta and tumor necrosis factor-alpha. J Immunol 149(7):2358-66.

Alonso G, Privat A (1993) Reactive astrocytes involved in the formation of lesional scars differ in the mediobasal hypothalamus and in other forebrain regions. J Neurosci Res 34(5):523-38.

Anders JJ, Johnson JA (1990) Transection of the rat olfactory nerve increases glial fibrillary acidic protein immunoreactivity from the olfactory bulb to the piriform cortex. Glia 3(1):17-25.

Ard MD, Bunge RP (1988) Heparan sulfate proteoglycan and laminin immunoreactivity on cultured astrocytes: relationship to differentiation and neurite growth. J Neurosci 8(8):2844-58.

Asada H, Ip NY, Pan L, Razack N, Parfitt MM, Plunkett RJ (1995) Time course of ciliary neurotrophic factor mRNA expression is coincident with the presence of protoplasmic astrocytes in traumatized rat striatum. J Neurosci Res 40(1):22-30.

Bähr M, Przyrembel C, Bastmeyer M (1995) Astrocytes from adult rat optic nerves are nonpermissive for regenerating retinal ganglion cell axons. Exp Neurol 131:211-220.

Baldwin SA, Scheff SW (1996) Intermediate filament change in astrocytes following mild cortical contusion. Glia 16(3):266-75.

Baron Van Evercooren A, Avellana Adalid V, Lachapelle F, Liblau R (1997) Schwann cell transplantation and myelin repair of the CNS. Mult Scler 3(2):157-61.

Bartholdi D, Schwab ME (1998) Oligodendroglial reaction following spinal cord injury in rat: transient upregulation of MBP mRNA. Glia 23(3):278-84.

Benveniste EN, Sparacio SM, Norris JG, Grenett HE, Fuller GM (1990) Induction and regulation of interleukin-6 gene expression in rat astrocytes. J Neuroimmunol 30(2-3):201-12.

Berry M, Maxwell WL, Logan A, Mathewson A, McConnell P, Ashhurst DE, Thomas GH (1983) Deposition of scar tissue in the central nervous system. Acta Neurochir Suppl Wien 32:31-53.

Blakemore WF, Crang AJ, Franklin RJ, Tang K, Ryder S (1995) Glial cell transplants that are subsequently rejected can be used to influence regeneration of glial cell environments in the CNS. Glia 13(2):79-91.

Brook GA, Lawrence JM, Shah B, Raisman G (1994) Extrusion transplantation of Schwann cells into the adult rat thalamus induces directional host axon growth. Exp Neurol 126(1):31-43.

Butt AM, Colquhoun K (1996) Glial cells in transected optic nerves of immature rats. I. An analysis of individual cells by intracellular dye-injection. J Neurocytol 25(6):365-80.

Calvo JL, Carbonell AL, Boya J (1991) Co-expression of glial fibrillary acidic protein and vimentin in reactive astrocytes following brain injury in rats. Brain Res 566(1-2):333-6.

Cancilla PA, Bready J, Berliner J, Sharifi Nia H, Toga AW, Santori EM, Scully S, deVellis J (1992) Expression of mRNA for glial fibrillary acidic protein after experimental cerebral injury. J Neuropathol Exp Neurol 51(5):560-5.

Caroni P, Schwab ME (1988) Antibody against myelin-associated inhibitor of neurite growth neutralizes nonpermissive substrate properties of CNS white matter. Neuron 1(1):85-96.

Carroll P, Sendtner M, Meyer M, Thoenen H (1993) Rat ciliary neurotrophic factor (CNTF): gene structure and regulation of mRNA levels in glial cell cultures. Glia 9(3):176-87.

Carter DA, Bray GM, Aguayo AJ (1989) Regenerated retinal ganglion cell axons can form well-differentiated synapses in the superior colliculus of adult hamsters. J Neurosci 9(11):4042-50.

Chao CC, Hu S, Ehrlich L, Peterson PK (1995) Interleukin-1 and tumor necrosis factor-alpha synergistically mediate neurotoxicity: involvement of nitric oxide and of N-methyl-D-aspartate receptors. Brain Behav Immun 9(4):355-65.

Chung IY, Benveniste EN (1990) Tumor necrosis factor-alpha production by astrocytes. Induction by lipopolysaccharide, IFN-gamma, and IL-1 beta. J Immunol 144(8):2999-3007.

Condorelli DF, Dell'Albani P, Kaczmarek L, Messina L, Spampinato G, Avola R, Messina A, Giuffrida Stella AM (1990) Glial fibrillary acidic protein messenger RNA and glutamine synthetase activity after nervous system injury. J Neurosci Res 26(2):251-7.

Crowe MJ, Bresnahan JC, Shuman SL, Masters JN, Beattie MS (1997) Apoptosis and delayed degeneration after spinal cord injury in rats and monkeys [published erratum appears in Nat Med 1997 Feb; 3(2):240]. Nat Med 3(1):73-6.

Cuevas P, Carceller F, Gimenez Gallego G (1995) Acidic fibroblast growth factor prevents death of spinal cord motoneurons in newborn rats after nerve section. Neurol Res 17(5):396-9.

da Cunha A, Jefferson JA, Jackson RW, Vitkovic L (1993) Glial cell-specific mechanisms of TGF-beta 1 induction by IL-1 in cerebral cortex. J Neuroimmunol 42(1):71-85.

Dahl D, Bignami A, Weber K, Osborn M (1981) Filament proteins in rat optic nerves undergoing Wallerian degeneration: localization of vimentin, the fibroblastic 100-A filament protein, in normal and reactive astrocytes. Exp Neurol 73(2):496-506.

Dou CL, Levine JM (1994) Inhibition of neurite growth by the NG2 chondroitin sulfate proteoglycan. J Neurosci 14(12):7616-28.

Eclancher F, Kehrli P, Labourdette G, Sensenbrenner M (1996) Basic fibroblast growth factor (bFGF) injection activates the glial reaction in the injured adult rat brain. Brain Res 737(1-2):201-14.

Faissner A, Clement A, Lochter A, Streit A, Mandl C, Schachner M (1994) Isolation of a neural chondroitin sulfate proteoglycan with neurite outgrowth promoting properties. J Cell Biol 126(3):783-99.

Faissner A, Kruse J (1990) J1/tenascin is a repulsive substrate for central nervous system neurons. Neuron 5(5):627-37.

Fok Seang J, DiProspero NA, Meiners S, Muir E, Fawcett JW (1998) Cytokine-induced changes in the ability of astrocytes to support migration of oligodendrocyte precursors and axon growth. Eur J Neurosci 10(7):2400-15.

Fok Seang J, Mathews GA, Ffrench Constant C, Trotter J, Fawcett JW (1995) Migration of oligodendrocyte precursors on astrocytes and meningeal cells. Dev Biol 171(1):1-15.

Fok Seang J, Smith Thomas LC, Meiners S, Muir E, Du JS, Housden E, Johnson AR, Faissner A, Geller HM, Keynes RJ, et al (1995) An analysis of astrocytic cell lines with different abilities to promote axon growth. Brain Res 689(2):207-23.

Fok Seang J, Smith Thomas LC, Meiners S, Muir E, Du JS, Housden E, Johnson AR, Faissner A, Geller HM, Keynes RJ, et al (1995) An analysis of astrocytic cell lines with different abilities to promote axon growth. Brain Res 689(2):207-23.

Franklin RJ, Barnett SC (1997) Do olfactory glia have advantages over Schwann cells for CNS repair? J Neurosci Res 50(5):665-72.

Franklin RJ, Crang AJ, Blakemore WF (1992) The behaviour of meningeal cells following glial cell transplantation into chemically-induced areas of demyelination in the CNS. Neuropathol Appl Neurobiol 18(2):189-200.

Franklin RJ, Gilson JM, Franceschini IA, Barnett SC (1996) Schwann cell-like myelination following transplantation of an olfactory bulb-ensheathing cell line into areas of demyelination in the adult CNS. Glia 17(3):217-24.

Frei K, Malipiero UV, Leist TP, Zinkernagel RM, Schwab ME, Fontana A (1989) On the cellular source and function of interleukin 6 produced in the central nervous system in viral diseases. Eur J Immunol 19(4):689-94.

Frisen J, Haegerstrand A, Risling M, Fried K, Johansson CB, Hammarberg H, Elde R, Hokfelt T, Cullheim S (1995) Spinal axons in central nervous system scar tissue are closely related to laminin-immunoreactive astrocytes. Neuroscience 65(1):293-304.

Frisen J, Risling M, Korhonen L, Zirrgiebel U, Johansson CB, Cullheim S, Lindholm D (1998) Nerve growth factor induces process formation in meningeal cells: implications for scar formation in the injured CNS. J Neurosci 18(15):5714-22.

Frisen J, Verge VM, Cullheim S, Persson H, Fried K, Middlemas DS, Hunter T, Hokfelt T, Risling M (1992) Increased levels of trkB mRNA and trkB protein-like immunoreactivity in the injured rat and cat spinal cord. Proc Natl Acad Sci U S A 89(23):11282-6.

Fruttiger M, Schachner M, Martini R (1995) Tenascin-C expression during wallerian degeneration in C57BL/Wlds mice: possible implications for axonal regeneration. J Neurocytol 24(1):1-14.

Fryer RH, Kaplan DR, Kromer LF (1997) Truncated trkB receptors on nonneuronal cells inhibit BDNF-induced neurite outgrowth in vitro. Exp Neurol 148(2):616-27.

Geisert EE, Jr., Bidanset DJ (1993) A central nervous system keratan sulfate proteoglycan: localization to boundaries in the neonatal rat brain. Brain Res Dev Brain Res 75(2):163-73.

Geisert EE, Jr., Bidanset DJ, Del Mar N, Robson JA (1996) Up-regulation of a keratan sulfate proteoglycan following cortical injury in neonatal rats. Int J Dev Neurosci 14(3):257-67.

Giulian D, Li J, Li X, George J, Rutecki PA (1994) The impact of microglia-derived cytokines upon gliosis in the CNS. Dev Neurosci 16(3-4):128-36.

Giulian D, Woodward J, Young DG, Krebs JF, Lachman LB (1988) Interleukin-1 injected into mammalian brain stimulates astrogliosis and neovascularization. J Neurosci 8(7):2485-90.

Goss JR, O'Malley ME, Zou L, Styren SD, Kochanek PM, DeKosky ST (1998) Astrocytes are the major source of nerve growth factor upregulation following traumatic brain injury in the rat. Exp Neurol 149(2):301-9.

Gotz B, Scholze A, Clement A, JOESTER A, SCHUTTE K, WIGGER F, Frank R, SPIESS E, EKBLOM P, Faissner A (1996) Tenascin C contains distinct adhesive, anti adhesive, and neurite outgrowth promoting sites for neurons. JOURNAL OF CELL BIOLOGY 132(4):681-699.

Hamburger V, Yip JW (1984) Reduction of experimentally induced neuronal death in spinal ganglia of the chick embryo by nerve growth factor. J Neurosci 4(3):767-74.

Haymaker W, Miquel J, Ibrahim MZ (1970) Glycogen accumulation following brain trauma. Bibl Psychiatr 143:71-86.

Herdegen T, Skene P, Bahr M (1997) The c-Jun transcription factor--bipotential mediator of neuronal death, survival and regeneration. Trends Neurosci 20(5): 227-31.

Hindley S, Herman MA, Rathbone MP (1994) Stimulation of reactive astrogliosis in vivo by extracellular adenosine diphosphate or an adenosine A2 receptor agonist. J Neurosci Res 38(4):399-406.

Hirsch S, Bähr M (1999) Immunocytochemical characterization of reactive optic nerve astrocytes and meningeal cells. GLIA in press

Hu J, Van Eldik LJ (1996) S100 beta induces apoptotic cell death in cultured astrocytes via a nitric oxide-dependent pathway. Biochim Biophys Acta 1313(3):239-45.

Hudgins SN, Levison SW (1998) Ciliary neurotrophic factor stimulates astroglial hypertrophy in vivo and in vitro. Exp Neurol 150(2):171-82.

Hüll M, Bähr M (1994a) Regulation of immediate-early gene expression in rat retinal ganglion cells after axotomy and during regeneration through a peripheral nerve graft. J Neurobiol 25:92-105.

Hüll M, Bähr M (1994b) Differential regulation of c-JUN expression in rat retinal ganglion cells after proximal and distal optic nerve transection. Neurosci Lett 178:39-42.

Ip NY, Wiegand SJ, Morse J, Rudge JS (1993) Injury-induced regulation of ciliary neurotrophic factor mRNA in the adult rat brain. Eur J Neurosci 5(1):25-33.

Iwasaki Y, Shiojima T, Kinoshita M (1997) S100 beta prevents the death of motor neurons in newborn rats after sciatic nerve section. J Neurol Sci 151(1):7-12.

Janeczko K (1989) Spatiotemporal patterns of the astroglial proliferation in rat brain injured at the postmitotic stage of postnatal development: a combined immunocytochemical and autoradiographic study. Brain Res 485(2):236-43.

Janeczko K (1993) Co-expression of GFAP and vimentin in astrocytes proliferating in response to injury in the mouse cerebral hemisphere. A combined autoradiographic and double immunocytochemical study. Int J Dev Neurosci 11(2):139-47.

Junghans U, Koops A, Westmeyer A, Kappler J, Meyer HE, Muller HW (1995) Purification of a meningeal cell-derived chondroitin sulphate proteoglycan with neurotrophic activity for brain neurons and its identification as biglycan. Eur J Neurosci 7(11):2341-50.

Kahn MA, Ellison JA, Chang RP, Speight GJ, de Vellis J (1997) CNTF induces GFAP in a S-100 alpha brain cell population: the pattern of CNTF-alpha R suggests an indirect mode of action. Brain Res Dev Brain Res 98(2):221-33.

Kamiguchi H, Yoshida K, Sagoh M, Sasaki H, Inaba M, Wakamoto H, Otani M, Toya S (1995) Release of ciliary neurotrophic factor from cultured astrocytes and its modulation by cytokines. Neurochem Res 20(10):1187-93.

Kirsch M, Schneider T, Lee MY, Hofmann HD (1998) Lesion-induced changes in the expression of ciliary neurotrophic factor and its receptor in rat optic nerve. Glia 23(3):239-48.

Koops A, Kappler J, Junghans U, Kuhn G, Kresse H, Muller HW (1996) Cultured astrocytes express biglycan, a chondroitin/dermatan sulfate proteoglycan supporting the survival of neocortical neurons. Brain Res Mol Brain Res 41(1-2):65-73.

Kossmann T, Hans V, Imhof HG, Trentz O, Morganti Kossmann MC (1996) Interleukin-6 released in human cerebrospinal fluid following traumatic brain injury may trigger nerve growth factor production in astrocytes. Brain Res 713(1-2):143-52.

Krushel LA, Sporns O, Cunningham BA, Crossin KL, Edelman GM (1995) Neural cell adhesion molecule (N-CAM) inhibits astrocyte proliferation after injury to different regions of the adult rat brain. Proc Natl Acad Sci U S A 92(10):4323-7.

Labourdette G, Janet T, Laeng P, Perraud F, Lawrence D, Pettmann B (1990) Transforming growth factor type beta 1 modulates the effects of basic fibroblast growth factor on growth and phenotypic expression of rat astroblasts in vitro. J Cell Physiol 144(3):473-84.

Latov N, Nilaver G, Zimmerman EA, Johnson WG, Silverman AJ, Defendini R, Cote L (1979) Fibrillary astrocytes proliferate in response to brain injury: a study combining immunoperoxidase technique for glial fibrillary acidic protein and radioautography of tritiated thymidine. Dev Biol 72(2):381-4.

Lazarov Spiegler O, Solomon AS, Zeev Brann AB, Hirschberg DL, Lavie V, Schwartz M (1996) Transplantation of activated macrophages overcomes central nervous system regrowth failure. FASEB J 10(11):1296-302.

Lee SC, Dickson DW, Brosnan CF (1995) Interleukin-1, nitric oxide and reactive astrocytes. Brain Behav Immun 9(4):345-54.

Levine JM (1994) Increased expression of the NG2 chondroitin-sulfate proteoglycan after brain injury. J Neurosci 14(8):4716-30.

Levison SW, Ducceschi MH, Young GM, Wood TL (1996) Acute exposure to CNTF in vivo induces multiple components of reactive gliosis. Exp Neurol 141(2):256-68.

Liesi P (1985) Laminin-immunoreactive glia distinguish regenerative adult CNS systems from non-regenerative ones. EMBO J 4(10):2505-11.

Lindholm D, Castren E, Kiefer R, Zafra F, Thoenen H (1992) Transforming growth factor-beta 1 in the rat brain: increase after injury and inhibition of astrocyte proliferation. J Cell Biol 117(2):395-400.

Lindholm D, Hengerer B, Zafra F, Thoenen H (1990) Transforming growth factor-beta 1 stimulates expression of nerve growth factor in the rat CNS. Neuroreport 1(1):9-12.

Logan A, Frautschy SA, Gonzalez AM, Baird A (1992) A time course for the focal elevation of synthesis of basic fibroblast growth factor and one of its high-affinity receptors (flg) following a localized cortical brain injury. J Neurosci 12(10):3828-37.

Louis JC, Magal E, Takayama S, Varon S (1993) CNTF protection of oligodendrocytes against natural and tumor necrosis factor-induced death. Science 259(5095):689-92.

Mahler M, Ben Ari Y, Represa A (1997) Differential expression of fibronectin, tenascin-C and NCAMs in cultured hippocampal astrocytes activated by kainate, bacterial lipopolysaccharide or basic fibroblast growth factor. Brain Res 775(1-2):63-73.

Mahler M, Ferhat L, Gillian A, Ben Ari Y, Represa A (1996) Tenascin-C mRNA and tenascin-C protein immunoreactivity increase in astrocytes after activation by bFGF. Cell Adhes Commun 4(3):175-86.

Marshak DR (1990) S100 beta as a neurotrophic factor. Prog Brain Res 86:169-81.

Mathewson AJ, Berry M (1985) Observations on the astrocyte response to a cerebral stab wound in adult rats. Brain Res 327(1-2):61-9.
Matthiessen HP, Schmalenbach C, Muller HW (1991) Identification of meningeal cell released neurite promoting activities for embryonic hippocampal neurons. J Neurochem 56(3):759-68.
Mayer M, Bhakoo K, Noble M (1994) Ciliary neurotrophic factor and leukemia inhibitory factor promote the generation, maturation and survival of oligodendrocytes in vitro. Development 120(1):143-53.
McKeon RJ, Hoke A, Silver J (1995) Injury-induced proteoglycans inhibit the potential for laminin-mediated axon growth on astrocytic scars. Exp Neurol 136(1):32-43.
McKeon RJ, Schreiber RC, Rudge JS, Silver J (1991) Reduction of neurite outgrowth in a model of glial scarring following CNS injury is correlated with the expression of inhibitory molecules on reactive astrocytes. J Neurosci 11(11):3398-411.
McKeon RJ, Silver J, Large TH (1997) Expression of full-length trkB receptors by reactive astrocytes after chronic CNS injury. Exp Neurol 148(2):558-67.
McPhilemy K, Mitchell LS, Griffiths IR, Morrison S, Deary AW, Sommer I, Kennedy PG (1990) Effect of optic nerve transection upon myelin protein gene expression by oligodendrocytes: evidence for axonal influences on gene expression. J Neurocytol 19(4):494-503.
Mey J, Thanos S (1993) Intravitreal injections of neurotrophic factors support the survival of axotomized retinal ganglion cells in adult rats in vivo. Brain Res 602(2):304-17.
Miller RH, Abney ER, David S, Ffrench Constant C, Lindsay R, Patel R, Stone J, Raff MC (1986) Is reactive gliosis a property of a distinct subpopulation of astrocytes? J Neurosci 6(1):22-9.
Montero CN, Hefti F (1988) Rescue of lesioned septal cholinergic neurons by nerve growth factor: specificity and requirement for chronic treatment. J Neurosci 8(8):2986-99.
Morrison RS, de Vellis J, Lee YL, Bradshaw RA, Eng LF (1985) Hormones and growth factors induce the synthesis of glial fibrillary acidic protein in rat brain astrocytes. J Neurosci Res 14(2):167-76.
Morrison RS, Sharma A, de Vellis J, Bradshaw RA (1986) Basic fibroblast growth factor supports the survival of cerebral cortical neurons in primary culture. Proc Natl Acad Sci U S A 83(19):7537-41.
Ness R, DAVID S, Author) (1997) Leptomeningeal cells modulate the neurite growth promoting properties of astrocytes in vitro. Glia 19(1):47-57.
Nistico G, Ciriolo MR, Fiskin K, Iannone M, De Martino A, Rotilio G (1992) NGF restores decrease in catalase activity and increases superoxide dismutase and glutathione peroxidase activity in the brain of aged rats. Free Radic Biol Med 12(3):177-81.
Payne HR, Hemperly JJ, Lemmon V (1996) N-cadherin expression and function in cultured oligodendrocytes. Brain Res Dev Brain Res 97(1):9-15.
Pechan P, Cizkova D, Murgacova M, Malatova Z (1991) Effect of nerve growth factor on lesioned PC12 cells. Cell Biol Int Rep 15(6):527-35.
Perry VH, Brown MC (1992) Role of macrophages in peripheral nerve degeneration and repair. Bioessays 14(6):401-6.
Peterson DA, Lucidi Phillipi CA, Murphy DP, Ray J, Gage FH (1996) Fibroblast growth factor-2 protects entorhinal layer II glutamatergic neurons from axotomy-induced death. J Neurosci 16(3):886-98.
Prieto AL, Andersson Fisone C, Crossin KL (1992) Characterization of multiple adhesive and counteradhesive domains in the extracellular matrix protein cytotactin. J Cell Biol 119(3):663-78.

Przyrembel C, Bähr M (1993) Reactive changes of glial cells after optic nerve axotomy in adult rats. Neurosci Lett 163:227-230.

Raine CS, Wu E (1993) Multiple sclerosis: remyelination in acute lesions. J Neuropathol Exp Neurol 52(3):199-204.

Raisman G (1997) Use of Schwann cells to induce repair of adult CNS tracts. Rev Neurol Paris 153(8-9):521-5.

Ramon y Cajal (1928) Degeneration and regeneration of the nervous system. Oxford University Press.

Reeves RH, Yao J, Crowley MR, Buck S, Zhang X, Yarowsky P, Gearhart JD, Hilt DC (1994) Astrocytosis and axonal proliferation in the hippocampus of S100b transgenic mice. Proc Natl Acad Sci U S A 91(12):5359-63.

Reier PJ. AnonymousAstrocytes. Academic Press Inc. 1986;Gliosis Following CNS Injury: The Anatomy of Astrocytic Scars and their Influences on Axonal Elongation. p. 263-324.

Ridet JL, Malhotra SK, Privat A, Gage FH (1997) Reactive astrocytes: cellular and molecular cues to biological function. Trends Neurosci 20(12):570-7.

Risau W, Wolburg H (1990) Development of the blood-brain barrier [see comments]. Trends Neurosci 13(5):174-8.

Risling M, Fried K, Linda H, Carlstedt T, Cullheim S (1993) Regrowth of motor axons following spinal cord lesions: distribution of laminin and collagen in the CNS scar tissue. Brain Res Bull 30(3-4):405-14.

Rudge JS, Silver J (1990) Inhibition of neurite outgrowth on astroglial scars in vitro. J Neurosci 10(11):3594-603.

Schmidt Kastner R, Wietasch K, Weigel H, Eysel UT (1993) Immunohistochemical staining for glial fibrillary acidic protein (GFAP) after deafferentation or ischemic infarction in rat visual system: features of reactive and damaged astrocytes. Int J Dev Neurosci 11(2):157-74.

Schnitzer J, Franke WW, Schachner M (1981) Immunocytochemical demonstration of vimentin in astrocytes and ependymal cells of developing and adult mouse nervous system. J Cell Biol 90(2):435-47.

Schwartz JP, Nishiyama N (1994) Neurotrophic factor gene expression in astrocytes during development and following injury. Brain Res Bull 35(5-6):403-7.

Selinfreund RH, Barger SW, Pledger WJ, Van Eldik LJ (1991) Neurotrophic protein S100 beta stimulates glial cell proliferation. Proc Natl Acad Sci U S A 88(9):3554-8.

Selmaj KW, Farooq M, Norton WT, Raine CS, Brosnan CF (1990) Proliferation of astrocytes in vitro in response to cytokines. A primary role for tumor necrosis factor. J Immunol 144(1):129-35.

Sendtner M, Arakawa Y, Stockli KA, Kreutzberg GW, Thoenen H (1991) Effect of ciliary neurotrophic factor (CNTF) on motoneuron survival. J Cell Sci Suppl 15:103-9.

Siliprandi R, Canella R, Carmignoto G (1993) Nerve growth factor promotes functional recovery of retinal ganglion cells after ischemia. Invest Ophthalmol Vis Sci 34(12):3232-45.

Silver J (1988) Transplantation strategies using embryonic astroglial cells to promote CNS axon regeneration in neonatal and adult mammals. Clin Res 36(3):196-9.

Smith GM, Jacobberger JW, Miller RH (1993) Modulation of adhesion molecule expression on rat cortical astrocytes during maturation. J Neurochem 60(4):1453-66.

Smith GM, Miller RH (1991) Immature type-1 astrocytes suppress glial scar formation, are motile and interact with blood vessels. Brain Res 543(1):111-22.

Smith GM, Rutishauser U, Silver J, Miller RH (1990) Maturation of astrocytes in vitro alters the extent and molecular basis of neurite outgrowth. Dev Biol 138(2):377-90.

Smith Thomas LC, Fok Seang J, Stevens J, Du JS, Muir E, Faissner A, Geller HM, Rogers JH, Fawcett JW (1994) An inhibitor of neurite outgrowth produced by astrocytes. J Cell Sci 107(Pt 6):1687-95.

Snow DM, Lemmon V, Carrino DA, Caplan AI, Silver J (1990) Sulfated proteoglycans in astroglial barriers inhibit neurite outgrowth in vitro. Exp Neurol 109(1):111-30.

Snyder SE, Li J, Schauwecker PE, McNeill TH, Salton SR (1996) Comparison of RPTP zeta/beta, phosphacan, and trkB mRNA expression in the developing and adult rat nervous system and induction of RPTP zeta/beta and phosphacan mRNA following brain injury. Brain Res Mol Brain Res 40(1):79-96.

Sorg O, Magistretti PJ (1992) Vasoactive intestinal peptide and noradrenaline exert long-term control on glycogen levels in astrocytes: blockade by protein synthesis inhibition. J Neurosci 12(12):4923-31.

Spring J, Beck K, Chiquet Ehrismann R (1989) Two contrary functions of tenascin: dissection of the active sites by recombinant tenascin fragments. Cell 59(2):325-34.

Stichel CC, Kappler J, Junghans U, Koops A, Kresse H, Muller HW (1995) Differential expression of the small chondroitin/dermatan sulfate proteoglycans decorin and biglycan after injury of the adult rat brain. Brain Res 704(2):263-74.

Stichel CC, Hermanns S, Luhmann HJ, Lausberg F, Niermann H, D'Urso D, Servos G, Hartwig H-G, Müller HW (1999) Inhibition of collagen IV deposition promotes Eur J Neurosci 11(2):632-647.

Struckhoff G (1995) Cocultures of meningeal and astrocytic cells--a model for the formation of the glial-limiting membrane. Int J Dev Neurosci 13(6):595-606.

Suzumura A, Sawada M, Yamamoto H, Marunouchi T (1993) Transforming growth factor-beta suppresses activation and proliferation of microglia in vitro. J Immunol 151(4):2150-8.

Topp KS, Faddis BT, Vijayan VK (1989) Trauma-induced proliferation of astrocytes in the brains of young and aged rats. Glia 2(3):201-11.

Tourbah A, Linnington C, Bachelin C, Avellana Adalid V, Wekerle H, Baron Van Evercooren A (1997) Inflammation promotes survival and migration of the CG4 oligodendrocyte progenitors transplanted in the spinal cord of both inflammatory and demyelinated EAE rats. J Neurosci Res 50(5):853-61.

Trimmer PA, Wunderlich RE (1990) Changes in astroglial scar formation in rat optic nerve as a function of development. J Comp Neurol 296(3):359-78.

Wang X, Messing A, David S (1997) Axonal and nonneuronal cell responses to spinal cord injury in mice lacking glial fibrillary acidic protein. Exp Neurol 148(2):568-76.

Winningham Major F, Staecker JL, Barger SW, Coats S, Van Eldik LJ (1989) Neurite extension and neuronal survival activities of recombinant S100 beta proteins that differ in the content and position of cysteine residues. J Cell Biol 109(6 Pt 1):3063-71.

Yokoyama M, Black IB, Dreyfus CF (1993) NGF increases brain astrocyte number in culture. Exp Neurol 124(2):377-80.

Yoshida K, Gage FH (1991) Fibroblast growth factors stimulate nerve growth factor synthesis and secretion by astrocytes. Brain Res 538(1):118-26.

Zhou HF, Lee LH, Lund RD (1990) Timing and patterns of astrocyte migration from xenogeneic transplants of the cortex and corpus callosum. J Comp Neurol 292(2):320-30.

Zuo J, Hernandez YJ, Muir D (1998) Chondroitin sulfate proteoglycan with neurite-inhibiting activity is up-regulated following peripheral nerve injury. J Neurobiol 34(1):41-54.

12

Axonal Sealing Following Injury

George D. Bittner
University of Texas, Austin, Texas

Harvey M. Fishman
University of Texas Medical Branch, Galveston, Texas

I. GENERAL SIGNIFICANCE OF AXONAL SEALING

Complete repair of severed (cut or crushed) axonal processes depends upon the successful execution of a series of events, some occurring within seconds and others possibly not until years after the initial injury. These include an initial rapid sealing of damaged axolemmal membranes, followed by recovery of axonal functions (e.g., action potentials, axonal transport), and eventual functional reconnection with the original target. A damaged axolemma leads to the rapid loss of essential axoplasmic substances and the entry into the neuron of potentially deleterious substances such as Ca^{2+}. If the axon is not sealed rapidly (seconds to hours), these changes in axoplasmic composition may induce rapid (hours to days) and complete degeneration of both proximal and distal segments of the axon (Schlaepfer, 1974; Zimmerman and Schlaepfer, 1984; Pant, 1988; Raabe et al., 1995, 1996). Clearly, rapid and complete degeneration of distal or proximal axonal segments eliminates any further role they might otherwise play in axonal repair.

The distal nerve segment in mammals normally undergoes complete dissolution (Wallerian degeneration) within several days and the remnants of the axoplasm and axolemma are engulfed by macrophages (this volume, chapter by Raivich and Kreutzberg). In contrast, in many invertebrates and some lower vertebrates the sealed distal stump often degenerates very slowly, and may survive for weeks or even years (Bittner, 1973, 1981,1988, 1991). Such long-term survival of sealed distal segments is often associated with release of trophic substances by surviving PNS distal segments to maintain postsynaptic muscle fibers (Bittner, 1973; Boone and Bittner, 1974; Velez et al., 1981) and release of trophic substances by surviving CNS distal segments to maintain postsynaptic CNS neurons (Viancour et al., 1981, 1987, 1988). Hence, an ability to retard the degeneration of distal axonal segments in mammals (perhaps by inducing more rapid or more complete axolemmal sealing, or by cooling, or by cyclosporin A), might be part of a strategy for repair of damaged PNS or CNS axons (Sea et al., 1995; Sunio and Bittner, 1997; Lore et al., 1999; Bittner et al., 1999), perhaps to increase the survival of postsynaptic cells whose maintenance depends upon continuous release of trophic substances (Murray, 1997).

Successful complete repair of mammalian neurons normally involves initial sealing of cut proximal segments, changes in gene expression by axotomized neurons, and regenerative sprouting from proximal segments which may eventually make functional synapses with denervated target tissues after weeks to years (this volume, chapter by Fernandes and Tetzlaff). In contrast, in many invertebrates, neuritic outgrowths from the sealed proximal axonal stump often selectively and rapidly (within days) contact and produce action potentials in the appropriate sealed and surviving distal segment by cytoplasmic and axolemmal fusion (Dereimer et al., 1983), gap junction formation (Muller and Carbonetto, 1979; Birse and Bittner, 1981), chemical synapse formation (Fernandez and Fernandez, 1974; Nordlander and Singer, 1976), or ephaptic current spread (Bouton and Bittner, 1981). [Even if the surviving distal segment is not activated by outgrowth from the proximal segment, it can guide neurites from the proximal stump to eventually form synapses with appropriate denervated postsynaptic elements (Bittner, 1973; Bouton and Bittner, 1981)]. Conceivably, keeping sealed distal segments patent could allow for the rapid (within minutes) induction of morphological continuity between surviving proximal and distal axonal segments in mammals *in vivo* by use of polyethyene glycol (PEG), as has recently been demonstrated for mammalian PNS and CNS axons *in vitro* and for invertebrate axons *in vivo* (Lore et al., 1999; Bittner et al, 1999). The longer sealed proximal and distal segments can be induced to survive, the longer is the time window for possibly reconnecting their two severed ends by PEG-induced fusion, i.e. to induce rapid and complete repair of severed mammalian axons (see speculations, this chapter).

Because of the intrinsic experimental advantages of large invertebrate axons (e.g., availability, ability to manipulate axoplasmic composition, relative ease of morphological observation), most of the data discussed in this review have been obtained from myelinated (earthworm) or unmyelinated (cockroach, crayfish, squid) giant axons (GAs). However, most studies suggest that cellular/molecular mechanisms for axonal sealing have experienced a very conservative evolution (Ballinger et al., 1997), rather similar to that described for other essential cellular mechanisms such as DNA transcription, RNA translation, exocytosis, and generation of action potentials (Alberts et al., 1994). Hence, it is likely that data on natural or induced mechanisms for sealing (initial repair) and functional reconnection (eventual complete repair) derived from invertebrate GAs will be applicable to repair of non-giant mammalian axons.

II. MEASURES OF AXOLEMMAL SEALING

The integrity of the axolemma or other portions of the neuronal plasmalemma has traditionally been assessed by determining the membrane potential (V_m) and/or input resistance (R_i) as functional measures of the formation of a barrier to entry of ions (an ionic seal) (Meiri et al., 1981; Yawo and Kuno, 1983, 1985; Lucas et al., 1985; Spira et al., 1993) or by observing the ability of the axolemma to exclude fluorescent dyes or other tracers as a measure of a barrier to entry of larger molecules (Xie and Barrett, 1991). However, more recent studies (Krause et al., 1994a,b; Eddleman et al, 1998b) have shown that each of these measures, taken by itself, provides a very ambiguous assessment of the effectiveness of restored barriers to entry of ions or molecules.

Measures of V_m and/or R_{in} provide a poor assessment of the functional state of an ionic seal, largely because of the distributed cable properties of axons (Krause et al 1994a,b). For example, calculations (Krause et al., 1994b) made from mathematical models of axonal resistance and measurements made on analog circuits with discrete resistances equivalent to a squid GA show that V_m and R_{in} are *very* insensitive to large changes in the seal resistance of the damaged membrane (Fig. 1), even when measured within one one-hundredth of a space constant from the damaged membrane (a nearly impossible physical constraint). Furthermore, values for V_m and R_{in} depend upon changes in the space constant (Fig. 1C,D) which, in turn, depends upon the activation of voltage-sensitive ion channels in the intact membrane and changes in the diameter or length of the intact or injured portions of the axon (Krause et al., 1994b).

A much more reliable assessment of the functional state of an ionic seal is provided by extracellular measures of injury current density (I_i) since I_i does *not* depend upon axonal cable properties (Krause et al., 1994a, b). However, additional information is necessary to interpret the decay of I_i to (baseline) levels in the uninjured, intact axon as a measure of a complete axonal seal. In a damaged axon, a decline of I_i to baseline values could reflect either an increase in the resistance to entry of ions (i.e., a successful ionic seal) or a decline in V_m (i.e., electrical dysfunction of the axon). These two interpretations can be distinguished if I_i declines to baseline by determining whether V_m recovers to control values previously measured in the intact, uninjured axon. A recovery of V_m in addition to a return of I_i to baseline strongly suggests that a *functional* seal has been restored. When these measures are used to assess sealing of GAs transected in physiological saline, then unmyelinated crayfish medial giant axons (MGAs) and myelinated earthworm MGAs (Krause et al., 1994a; Eddleman et al., 1997; Godell et al., 1997) form a complete ionic seal within 30 - 60 minutes posttransection (Fig. 2B, F-H: closed symbols), whereas unmyelinated squid GAs (Krause et al., 1994; Go-

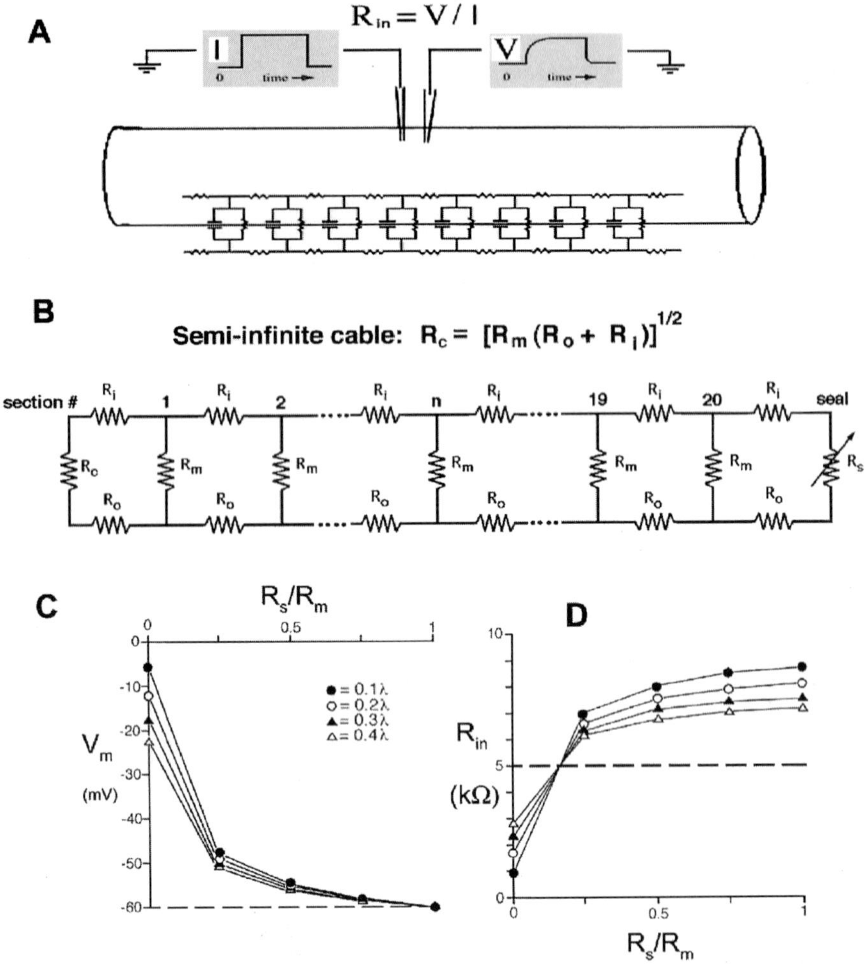

Figure 1 (A) Diagram of conventional microelectrode impalement of an axon for intracellular determination of V_m and R_{in}. The tips of the two microelectrodes are in close proximity so that the recorded voltage response (V) to an applied rectangular current pulse

dell et al., 1997) do not form an ionic seal within 120 minutes posttransection (Fig. 2A, C-E: open symbols).

Measures of dye exclusion at the cut ends of severed axons, in some instances, also provide an ambiguous assessment of the functional state of a barrier to entry of larger molecules. If crayfish MGAs are transected in the presence of various dyes, then negatively, but not positively, charged dye molecules of the same molecular weight are excluded at the cut ends (Eddleman et al., 1998b). Furthermore, axoplasmic outflow at cut axonal ends can exclude the uptake of dyes that are uncharged (e.g., Texas Red-dextran, Sulphorhodamine 101) or negatively charged (e.g., FITC-dextran, pyrene, pyranine) when these dyes are added to the bath saline (Eddleman et al., 1998b). Finally, assessments of barrier formation can depend on the molecular size of the dye molecule used to probe the barrier. For example, electroporated squid GAs exclude Texas Red-dextran (40kDa, uncharged), but not Sulforhodamine 101 (0.65 kDa, uncharged), when both are added to the bath saline (Gallant and Galbraith, 1997).

(I) occurs at the same spatial point, corresponding to location *n* for the electrical resistance model (B) of an axon.

(B) Electrical resistance model of a transected axon (from Fig. 1 of Krause et al., 1994b). Lumped electrical element (resistance) circuit model of the passive DC cable-like electrical properties of an axon with *n* identical repeating sections terminated by a section representing the transection site (seal). Each repeating section is comprised of three resistors: an intracellular resistance (R_{in}), an extracellular resistance (R_o), and an axolemmal resistance (R_m). The resistance of the uncut end is represented by the equivalent resistance of a semi-infinite cable (R_c); the resistance of a seal at the cut end is represented by a variable resistor (R_s).

(C, D) Dependence of V_m (C) and R_{in} (D) on changes in seal resistance R_s (from Figure 2 of Krause et al., 1994b). V_m and R_{in} were measured from the analog electrical model in B using established values (Krause et al., 1995) that simulated the cable-like electrical properties of a transected squid GA. V_m and R_{in} were measured at various distances [0.1 λ (filled circle); 0.2 λ (hollow circle), 0.3 λ (filled triangle); 0.4 λ (hollow triangle)] from a transected end whose seal resistance (R_s) was expressed as a fraction of axolemmal resistance (R_m): $R_s/R_m = 1$ for a completely sealed axon. Dashed lines show the value of V_m and R_{in} in an infinitely long (intact) GA (C, D).

All curves in C and D have an asymptotic character as R_s/R_m goes from 0 to 1. The sensitivity of R_{in} to changes in R_s greatly diminishes as R_s/R_m approaches 1. R_{in} increase very little as $R_s >> R_m$ (data not shown).

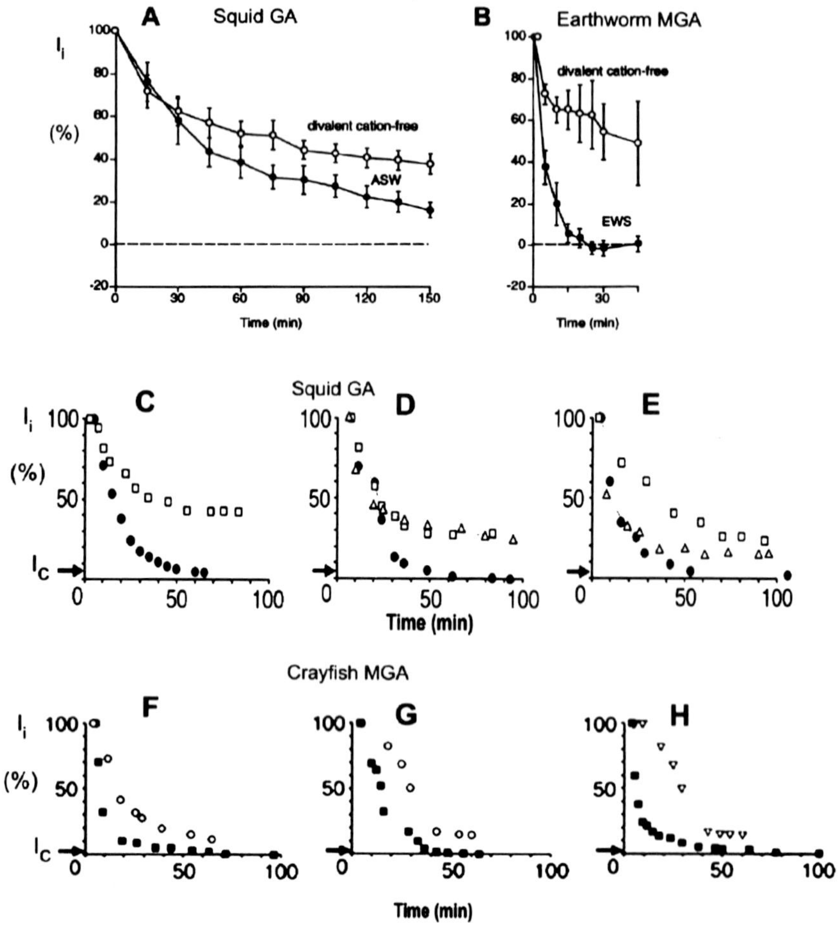

Figure 2 Time course of decay of injury current density (I_i) after transection of squid GAs (A, C - E), earthworm MGAs (B) and crayfish MGAs (F - H), as determined by vibrating probe measurements at cut ends. I_i plotted as % of initial I_i (set to 100%) obtained within 3 - 5 min after transection. Dashed line (A, B) or arrow (C - H) on the ordinate denotes the baseline current (I_c) of the intact axon prior to its transection.

Morphological observations have also produced ambiguous assessments of seal formation. Historically, the presence of a seal has most often been assessed morphologically by examining phase-contrast images (Yawo and Kuno, 1983) or electron micrographs (Kao et al., 1983; Spira et al., 1993). However, the former method lacks the resolution necessary to determine whether the plasmalemma is intact, and the latter has not been used to examine whether the axolemma is intact in electron micrographs of sufficient magnification or in more than a few sections through the lesion site.

In summary, current data suggest that a combination of measures (V_m, I_i, exclusion of positively or uncharged dyes, many high-magnification electron micrographs taken through the lesion site) are necessary to assess the functional and morphological state of a seal with reasonable confidence. Furthermore, since the exclusion of various dyes at cut axonal ends typically occurs in about half the time needed for I_i to return to baseline levels, measures of the state of an ionic seal *vs.* a seal to larger molecules almost certainly do *not* assess the same functional permeation properties of the barrier (Ballinger et al., 1997; Eddleman, 1999). No differences have been noted in proximal vs distal segments for any functional or morphological measure of axonal sealing.

III. POSSIBLE CELLULAR MECHANISMS OF AXOLEMMAL SEALING

Cut axonal ends could seal by a rearrangement of the existing axolemma at the cut end, e.g., a complete collapse of the severed axolemmal leaflets which then fuse to form a continuous membrane at the cut end (Fig. 3A). Until actual observations were made (Krause et al., 1994a), this intuitive assumption was by far the most commonly proposed mechanism (Kelley, 1985) for axolemmal sealing following transection of various invertebrate Gas [cockroach GA (Meiri et al., 1981) and

---

(A) I_i decay after transection of GAs in physiological saline (EWS) and in divalent cation-free saline (from Fig. 1 of Krause et al., 1994a).
(B) I_i decay after transection of earthworm MGAs in physiological saline (ASW) and in divalent cation-free saline (from Fig. 1 of Krause et al, 1994a).
(C, D, E) I_i decay in individual squid GAs transected in physiological saline (open squares) and physiological saline containing 0.02 units/ml calpain (filled circles) or 10 μg/ml chymotrypsin (open triangles) (from Fig. 1 of Godell et al, 1997).
(F, G, H) I_i decay in individual crayfish MGAs transected in physiological saline (filled squares) or physiological saline containing 200 μg/ml leupeptin (open circles) or 100 μg/ml calpeptin (open triangles) (from Fig. 1 of Godell et al., 1997).

squid GA (Gallant, 1988)], non-giant invertebrate axons [Aplysia (Spira et al., 1993)] or mammalian axons [spinal (Kao et al., 1977,1983) and septal (Xie and Barrett, 1991)]. As one alternative to a collapse and fusion of the transected axolemma, Yawo and Kuno (1985) proposed that new membrane of unspecified origin might form a partition-like structure near the cut end (Fig. 3B) to seal transected cockroach GAs. As a second alternative, Fishman et al., (1990) proposed that injury-induced vesicles, which form and accumulate rapidly at sites of axolemmal injury in squid GAs, might somehow be involved in axonal repair (Fig. 3C - F). This latter suggestion has been documented in a set of recent studies (Krause et al., 1994; Ballinger et al., 1997; Eddleman et al., 1997, 1998a; Godell et al., 1997). As described in greater detail in following sections, injury-induced vesicles and other membranous structures (e.g., myelin delaminations) accumulate and interact in various (but not all possible, Fig. 3C,E) ways to seal holes in the axolemma (Fig. 3D) or to seal transected axons (Fig. 3F- H).

A. Current evidence for axonal sealing by injury-induced membranous structures

Although vesicles and other membranous structures have long been known to accumulate near sites of axonal injury (Ramon y Cajal, 1928; Levi and Meyer, 1945; Lubinska, 1956; Zelena et al., 1968; Kao et al., 1977), only recently has it been proposed that they may play a role in axonal repair or regeneration (Fishman et al., 1990). This proposal is based, in part, on photomicrographs (Fig. 4A: inset, B), electron micrographs (Fig. 4A, C, D), and confocal fluorescence images (Figs. 5 - 7), all showing that small holes or complete transections are sealed by single or multi-layered vesicles that arise from the axolemma and/or glialemma in unmyelinated axons as well as the myelin sheath in myelinated axons. A dye barrier forms amidst these membranous structures that migrates and accumulates at the lesion site (Krause et al.,1994a; Ballinger et al., 1997; Eddleman et al., 1997, 1998a; Godell et al., 1997). Specifically, when hydrophilic dyes are added to the bath 15 - 90 minutes after transecting an axon, a dye barrier located amidst an accumulation of membranous structures excludes the dye in >90% of the cases (Figs. 5 - 7). If similar experiments are performed 5 minutes posttransection many fewer and less densely packed vesicles are seen at the injury site and <5% of the axons exclude the dye. (No differences in dye exclusion have been noted for distal vs proximal ends of crayfish, squid or earthworm axons severed in physiological salines.)

When one hydrophilic dye is injected into an unmyelinated crayfish MGA and another dye is added to the bath at 15 - 90 minutes posttransection, confocal images show that the boundaries of the two dyes are each abrupt (no more than 2 μm wide), and the two boundaries coincide (Fig. 5A,B). When a styryl dye (e.g., FM1-43) is then added to the bath, many labeled vesicles accumulate at the dye boundaries at the cut end (Figs. 5C,E - G). [Styryl dyes placed in the bath are readily incorporated into myelin, glialemmal, and axoplasmic membranes, but do not cross the plasma membranes, and fluoresce substantially only when incorporated into a membrane (Betz et al., 1992; Eddleman et al., 1997, 1998).] Within minutes after transection in physiological saline, 1 to 20 μm diameter vesicles accumulate at the cut end, which narrows to a small opening (pore) that is a fraction (3 - 20%) of the original axon diameter of 80 - 150 μm (Figs. 4A, 5C, E-G). The small opening at the cut end of a crayfish axon never completely closes (Fig. 4A), i.e., the severed axolemmal leaflets never completely collapse as had once been hypothesized (Fig. 3A). The glial sheath does not completely cover the cut end, but rather terminates at the pore-like opening (Fig. 4A). At 60 minutes post-transection, the axolemma and glialemma are both disrupted and axoplasm mixes with gliaplasm for 100 - 200 μm proximal to the porelike opening.

For unmyelinated crayfish MGAs [or squid GAs exposed to exogenous calpain (Godell et al., 1997)], many of the vesicles which accumulate at the seal appear to arise by endocytosis of the axolemma or glialemma shortly after transection (Eddleman et al., 1997, 1998a). This conclusion is based on the following data: when (1) the axolemma and glialemma are pulse-labeled with a styryl (FM) dye prior to transection (and the styryl dye removed prior to transection), (2) a hydrophilic dye is injected into the axon before transection, and (3) another hydrophilic dye is placed in the bath shortly after transection, then the membrane of the vesicles which form shortly after transection are labeled in a ring-like pattern by the styryl dye and the vesicle contents are labeled in a disc-like pattern by the hydrophilic dye added to the bath but not by the hydrophilic dye placed in the axoplasm (Fig. 6A - D). When the hydrophilic dye is removed from the bath, most of the styryl dye-labeled membranous structures continue to contain that hydrophilic dye (Fig. 6E, F) and do not take up an additional hydrophilic dye added to the bath saline. These data suggest that most of the membranous structures are vesicles completely surrounded by axoplasm rather than invaginations of the axolemma or glialemma.

In similar experiments, when the glial cytoplasm was selectively loaded with calcein-AM and the fluorophore calcein was activated after glial esterases cleaved the AM moiety (Eddleman et al., 1995), most of the injury-induced vesicles did not contain calcein (Fig. 6G, H). Time-lapse confocal images (Fig. 7) show that many such structures appear to arise from the axolemma by endocytosis and then migrate toward the cut end of the MGA (Fig. 6A - C). All these data are consistent with the hypothesis that most of these membranous structures at the cut end of unmyelinated crayfish MGAs are single-walled vesicles which arise from the axolemma by endocytosis, although some membranous structures appear to arise from the glialemma and mix with these axoplasmic structures near the cut end at regions where the axolemma and glialemma are no longer continuous (Eddleman et al., 1997, 1998a).

Many aspects of the sealing of myelinated earthworm MGAs (Krause et al., 1994a; Ballinger et al., 1997) are similar to those described above for unmyelinated crayfish MGAs (Eddleman et al., 1997, 1998a). For example, the proximal and distal ends of a transected earthworm MGA do not completely collapse at any time after severance (Fig. 4B), the cut ends fill with membranous structures

(Figs.4B - F), the barrier to dye exclusion at the cut end is < 2 µm wide and is located within an accumulation of multilayered vesicles (Fig. 5A - D), and the axolemma and adaxonal glialemma are disrupted for about 100 µm from a cut end at 60 minutes postseverance. In contrast to the unmyelinated crayfish MGA, the glial sheath in the myelinated earthworm MGA is greatly delaminated for 100 µm from the cut ends and most membranous structures in the axoplasm are multilayered and contain desmosomes similar to those observed in the myelin sheath (Fig. 4B - F). These and other data suggest that a cut end of the proximal or distal segment of an earthworm MGA is sealed by membranous material, much of which arises from the delaminating (pseudo)myelin of the glial sheath (Ballinger et al., 1997).

B. Multiple roles of calcium in axonal sealing

Many studies have reported that plasmalemmal repair does not occur (Yawo and Kuno, 1983; Xi and Barrett, 1991; Krause et al., 1994a; Steinhardt et al., 1994; Bi et al., 1995; Ballinger et al., 1997; Eddleman et al., 1997, 1998a; Terasaki et al., 1997) and vesicles or other membranous structures do not form (Krause et al., 1994a; Ballinger et al., 1997; Eddleman et al., 1997, 1998a) unless Ca^{2+} is present in the bath saline. For example, when earthworm (Fig. 2B) or crayfish MGAs (Table 1) are severed in divalent-cation-free saline, I_i does *not* decline to baseline (control) levels for measurement intervals lasting 120 minutes posttransection (Krause et al., 1994a; Eddleman et al., 1997).

The injury-induced formation of vesicles and other membranous structures which mediate seal formation depends on the level of internal [Ca^{2+}] in microdialyzed squid GAs (Fishman & Metuzals, 1993; Eddleman et al., 1998a) and in microinjected crayfish MGAs (Eddleman, 1999). Elevation of axoplasmic [Ca^{2+}] above 100 µM by microdialysis of intact squid GAs bathed in Ca^{2+}-free saline (Fig 8A, B) induces formation of vesicles and other membranous structures, suggesting that a 1000-fold increase in intracellular [Ca^{2+}] above nominal intracellular levels (about 100 nM) is the specific trigger to form injury-induced membranous structures. A threshold dependence on [Ca^{2+}] instead of a graded dependence also suggests that injury-induced membranous structures are not solely produced by upregulation of an existing low-level process (e.g., endocytosis). Furthermore, micropipette injection of Ca^{2+} (1 mM) into intact crayfish MGAs bathed in Ca^{2+}-free saline also induces formation of many vesicles at the injection site (Fig. 8C, D). These data agree with other reports that extracellular [Ca^{2+}] must be raised to at least 100 µM to induce sealing of severed septal neurites in tissue culture (Xie and Barrett, 1991) and that intracellular [Ca^{2+}] reaches µM to mM levels following axotomy of axons in the lamprey spinal cord (Strautman et al., 1990), squid GAs (Fishman et al, 1995) and *Aplysia* axons *in vitro* (Ziv and Spira, 1995).

An abnormally high level of intracellular [Ca^{2+}], after axonal injury, could be due to entry of extracellular Ca^{2+} through voltage-dependent ion channels in the axolemma (Sattler et al., 1996; George et al., 1995), to release of Ca^{2+} from inter

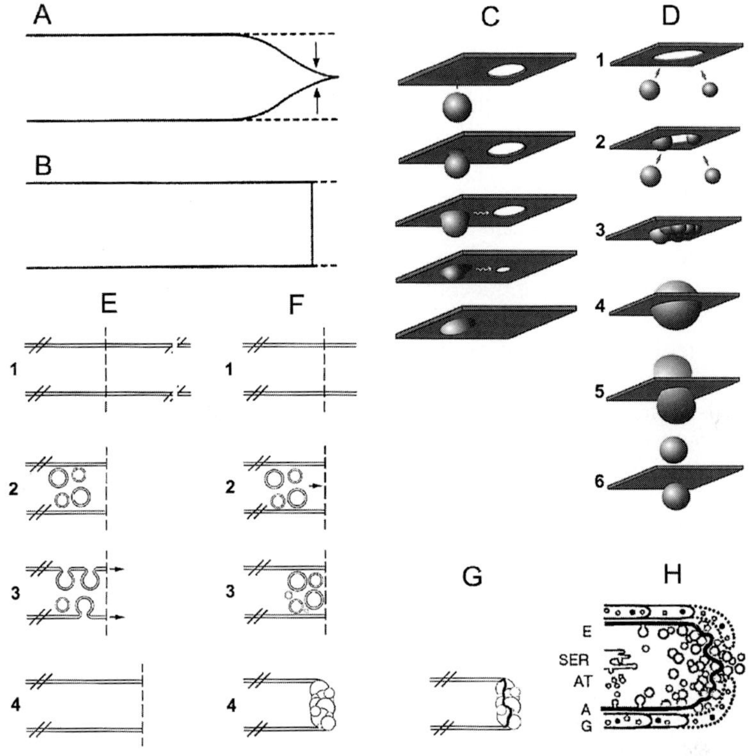

Figure 3 Topological models showing how vesicles might seal a complete transection (A, B, E - G) of an axon or a small hole (C, D) in the plasmalemma of a nerve axon or any other eukaryotic cell (modified from Fig. 4 of Eddleman et al., 1997)
(A) Complete collapse and fusion at an axonal cut end.
(B) Formation of a partition-like structure near an axonal cut end.
(C) Sealing of a small hole in a plasmalemmal membrane.(E - G) Complete transection represented by dashed line that could be repaired by an aggregation of vesicles (F_4) which may also help form a continuous membrane (represented by a darker solid line in G).
(H) Schematic drawing of a transected crayfish MGA in which vesicles that interact to help form a seal at the cut end may arise from endocytosis of the plasmalemma or glialemma (E), budding from the smooth endoplasmic reticulum (SER), axonal transport vesicles (AT), other glial membranes (G), etc. Dotted line represents disrupted glialemma or axolemma; solid line represents an intact, undamaged glialemma; heavy solid line (A) represents a newly-formed continuous membrane at a cut axonal end. These membranes and/or interactions between vesicles form part of the seal at a cut end of a transected MGA.

nal stores, to extracellular Ca^{2+} entering at the lesion site, or to a combination of the above mechanisms. Recent data suggest that the increase in accumulated Ca^{2+} is primarily due to Ca^{2+} at the cut axonal end: (1) the temporal changes in the pattern of luminescence of a Ca^{2+} indicator (aequorin) in severed squid GAs (Fishman et al., 1995) and (2) temporal variations of fluorescence intensity in severed lamprey spinal cord axons loaded with Fura-2 (Strautman et al., 1990) or *Aplysia* ax ons loaded with mag-Fura-2 (Ziv and Spira, 1995) are as expected for Ca^{2+} entry at the cut end rather than entry of extracellular Ca^{2+} through depolarized voltage-sensitive ion channels which span the axolemma.

In addition to increasing intracellular [Ca^{2+}], axolemmal damage should increase intracellular [Na^+] and [Cl^-], and reduce [K^+]. In fact, Na^+ and Ca^{2+} are the predominant ionic carriers of inwardly-directed injury currents at the cut ends of lamprey spinal cords (Borgens et al., 1980) or squid GAs (Fishman et al., 1995). Increases by microdialysis of [Na^+] and [Cl^-] does induce the formation of membranous structures (Eddleman et al., 1998a), but at much higher internal con centrations (> 100 mM) and on a reduced scale compared to increases of axoplasmic [Ca^{2+}] (>100 μM). Such an increase in internal [Ca^{2+}] is an appropriate cellular signal to initiate emergency repair of the axolemma by membranous structures because normally in intact cells [Ca^{2+}] is so low (<100 nM), Ca^{2+} is in much greater electrochemical disequilibrium than any other ion, and changes in internal [Ca^{2+}] greatly affect other cellular processes (e.g., endocytosis, exocytosis, membrane fusion) involving membranous structures. These data are also all consistent with the hypothesis that elevated intracellular [Ca^{2+}], rather than injury *per se*, is the necessary trigger to form injury-induced membranous structures and an axonal barrier (seal) to various dyes and ions.

Figure 4 (A) Electron micrograph or photomicrograph (inset) of longitudinal sections of a crayfish MGA severed in physiological saline and fixed 60 min later (from Fig. 3 of Eddleman et al., 1997). Cut axonal end is to the right of the figure. Small pore at cut end enlarged in boxed area of inset . V = remnants of larger vesicles (> 2 μm in diameter) often observed to burst when MGAs severed in physiological saline were exposed to fixative and imaged with DIC. Scale bar = 0.5 μm for A and 20 μm for its inset.

(B) Photomicrograph of longitudinal section of an earthworm MGA fixed at 1 hr posttransection (from Fig. 8 of Krause et al., 1994a). Cut axonal end (identified by two large arrows) is to the right of the figure. Note that the cut end is slightly constricted and that large intra-axonal vesicles (v) can be seen along the axolemma and accumulated at the cut end. Scale bar = 10 μm.

(C – F) Electron micrographs of longitudinal sections of MGAs fixed at 30 min posttransection (from Fig. 3 of Ballinger et al., 1997). C shows axoplasmic single- and multi-layered vesicles in MGA axoplasm. D shows vesicles in close apposition to each other. E shows a desmosome and delaminating pseudomyelin extending into the axoplasm at a cytoplasmic plaque. F shows desmosomal remnants in axoplasm. cp = cytoplasmic plaque; f = focal contacts between vesicles; dr = desmosomal remnants. Scale bar = 1.3 μm for C, 0.2 μm for D, and 0.3 μm for E - F.

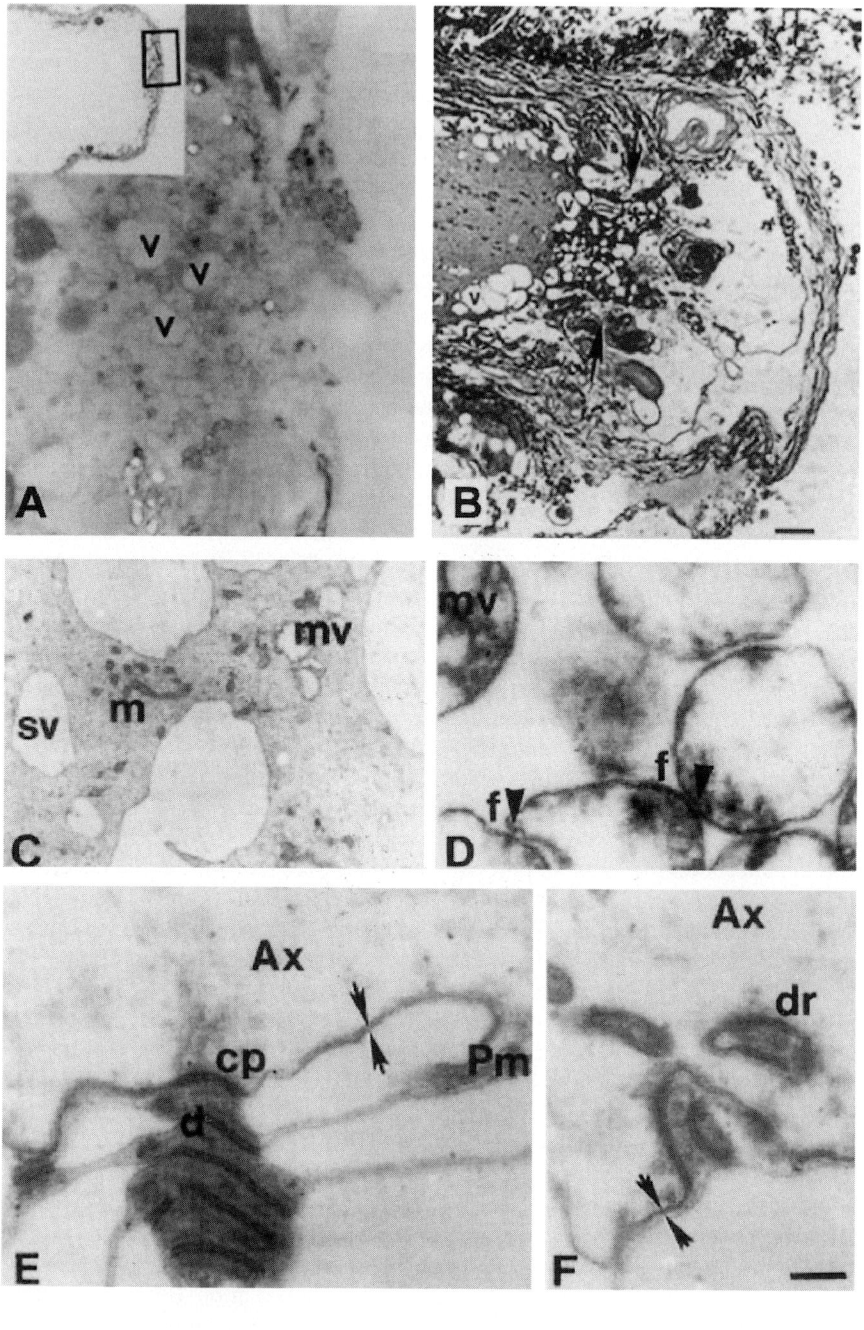
v
v
v
A
v
v
B
mv
m
sv
C
mv
f
f
D
Ax
cp
Pm
d
E
Ax
dr
F

C. Calpain and other compounds that enhance or inhibit plasmalemmal sealing

In both mammalian (Xie and Barrett, 1991) and crayfish axons (Godell et al., 1997), inhibitors of calpain and other proteases prevent axonal sealing; in squid axons calpain and other proteases induce transected squid GAs to seal (Godell et al., 1997). That is, in the absence of exogenous calpain, squid GAs do not seal for observation intervals up to 120 minutes post-severance (Krause et al., 1994a; Godell et al., 1997) according to measures of injury current decay (Fig. 2A, C-E, open symbols) or dye exclusion examined by confocal fluorescence imaging (Godell et al., 1997). The morphology of the cut ends of squid GAs transected in physiological salines is similar in many respects to crayfish MGAs. For example, the cut ends of squid GAs are not completely closed and contain loosely-packed, single-layered vesicles 0.1 - 50 μm in diameter at 60 - 120 minutes posttransection and the axolemma and glialemma are both disrupted for 50 - 200 μm from the cut end. In contrast to GAs transected in physiological saline, I_i for GAs transected in exogenous calpain decays to control levels within 90 minutes post-transection section (Fig. 2C-E, closed symbols) and V_m recovers to levels at 90 minutes post transection that do not differ significantly ($p > 0.05$) from control values (Godell et al, 1997). The time course (60 min) of sealing of crayfish MGAs transected in physiological saline (Fig. 2F-H, closed symbols) is somewhat faster than the time course (90 min) of sealing of squid GAs transected in calpain (Fig. 2C-E. closed symbols). The time course (60 min) of sealing of squid GAs injected with calpain prior to transection in physiological saline is very similar to that of crayfish MGAs transected in physiological saline, suggesting that increased endogenous calpain activity in the axoplasm expedites sealing. Squid GAs transected and maintained in calpain for 90 - 120 minutes contain larger vesicles somewhat more densely packed at or near the cut end, compared to GAs transected in physiological saline. With the exception that a small pore-like structure does not form at the cut end of squid GAs, the morphology of sealed squid and crayfish MGAs are very similar.

According to electrical (Fig. 2) or dye-exclusion (Fig. 5, Table 1) measures, chymotrypsin or low-activity calpain do not induce sealing in squid GAs (Godell et al., 1997). The initial decay of I_i and the final value of I_i for squid GAs transected in exogenous chymotrypsin (Fig. 2D, E: open triangles) is comparable to that for squid GAs transected in physiological saline (Fig.2C - E: open squares). Vesicles are obviously present in the axoplasm and at the cut end. Dye is not excluded at the cut ends of transected squid GAs exposed to chymotrypsin (Table 1). In contrast to calpain-treated squid GAs, which have a very gel-like axoplasm at the cut end, the axoplasm of chymotrypsin-treated GAs is not viscous and flows out the cut end (Godell et al., 1997).

The small, but significantly greater than baseline, values of I_i in crayfish MGAs transected in physiological salines containing calpain *inhibitors* (Fig. 2F-H; leupeptin, open circles; calpeptin, open inverted triangles) at 60-120 min posttransection, indicate that calpain inhibition results in a *very* incomplete seal, i.e., a

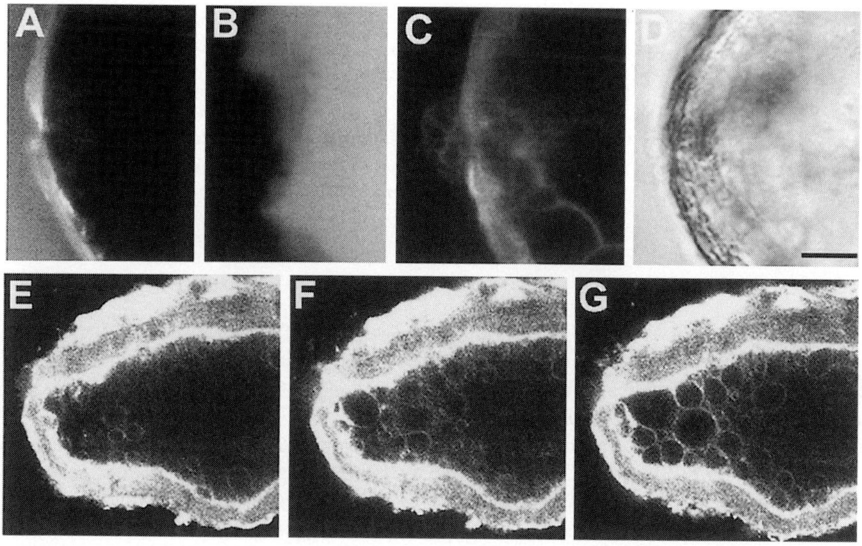

Figure 5 Confocal fluorescence images of the cut end of an MGA transected in physiological saline with one hydrophilic dye placed extracellularly (A) and another placed intracellularly (B) showing the abrupt inner and outer dye boundaries at vesicular accumulations, vesicles labeled with a membrane-incorporating styryl dye placed extracellularly (C), and the DIC image (D) (from Fig. 2 of Eddleman et al., 1997)
(A, B) long-axis midsection fluorescence images both obtained at 90 min posttransection. (A) image of 0.1% Texas Red-dextran added to physiological saline 60 min posttransection and (B) image of 0.1% FITC-dextran in intracellular saline injected into MGA prior to transection.
(C) Fluorescence image at 120 min posttransection of an MGA following addition of FM1-43 to the bath at 95 min posttransection. The fluorescence of the FITC-dextran was greatly reduced (photobleached) by prior illumination and was much less than the fluorescence intensity of the FM1-43 which was incorporated into the membranes of the vesicles at the cut end.
(D) DIC image taken simultaneously with C.
(E - G) Series of time-lapse fluorescence images (from Fig. 7 of Eddleman et al., 1998a) in the same optical section of a severed MGA showing the movement toward, and accumulation at, the cut end of vesicles formed by endocytosis (see Fig. 7A - C) of the axolemma. The MGA was pulse-labeled with FM1-43 and then transected. The cut end of the MGA is oriented to the left. Successive images acquired at 3, 8, and 13 min posttransection (E-G), respectively and are representative of a larger set of images acquired every 6 s. Scale bar (in *D*): 40 μm for A-C and 15 μm for E – G.

substantial opening at the cut end (Godell et al., 1997). Furthermore, in crayfish MGAs transected in physiological salines containing leupeptin, calpeptin or calpastatin (Table 1; Calpains are the only proteases inhibited by leupeptin, calpeptin *and* calpastatin), I_i rarely declines to baseline values of I_i within 120 minutes posttransection.

The conclusion that *inhibitors* of calpain activity prevent sealing is based not only on electrophysiological data described above, but also on optical observations made at 60 minutes posttransection (Table 1). The optical data show that dye is rarely excluded by MGAs placed in leupeptin (50 - 200 μg), calpeptin, en-

---

Figure 6 Confocal images taken 50 μm from the cut ends of lesioned MGAs exposed to fluorescent dyes (from Fig. 4 of Eddleman et al, 1998a)
(A, B) Membranous structures identified in DIC images (not shown) in the axoplasm of an MGA injected with 0.01% FITC-dextran prior to transection and viewed 10 min posttransection. Absence of fluorescence ("black holes") indicates membranous structures whose contents do not include FITC-dextran. Fluorescent area (white region) at the top of panels A and B delineates the axoplasm (a) just interior to the axolemma; the black region at the bottom of the panels is the extracellular space. Black holes were not observed in the axoplasm before transecting the MGA.
(C) Same axoplasmic region shown in A, but imaged for fluorescence of Texas Red-dextran placed in the bath after black holes had formed. Many of the black holes in A remain unlabeled, indicating that they are axoplasmic vesicles. Fluorescent area delineates the extracellular bath (b).
(D) Same axoplasmic region shown in B, but imaged for fluorescence of Texas Red-dextran placed in the bath after black holes had formed. The black holes in B are dye-filled in D, indicating that they are invaginations connected to the extracellular space.
(E) Ring-shaped fluorescence of injury-induced membranous structure in axoplasm 10 min after transection of an MGA that was pulse-labeled with FM 4-64 (25 μM for 10 min) prior to transection.
(F) Same axoplasmic region shown in E, but imaged for fluorescence of FITC-dextran placed in the bath 2 min after transection and washed off at 10 min posttransection. After dye wash out from the bath, the membranous structure retained the dye indicating its isolation from the bath saline, i.e., this structure was an axoplasmic vesicle. The images in E and F are consistent with that of a vesicle that formed from FM-labeled plasmalemmal membrane after an axolemmal invagination that subsequently budded off to become an axoplasmic vesicle.
(G) Image of a membranous structure invaginating into the axoplasm. The contents of this structure filled with Texas Red-dextran, which was added to the bath saline at 10 min posttransection.
(H) Same optical section as in G, but imaged for calcein (glial cytosolic marker, Eddleman et al., 1995) showing no evagination of the glial cell associated with the axoplasmic invagination in G. These images in G and H are consistent with an axolemmal invagination *not* associated with a glialemmal evagination. Scale bar (in H): 5 μm for A - D, 1 μm for E and F and 15 μm for G and H.

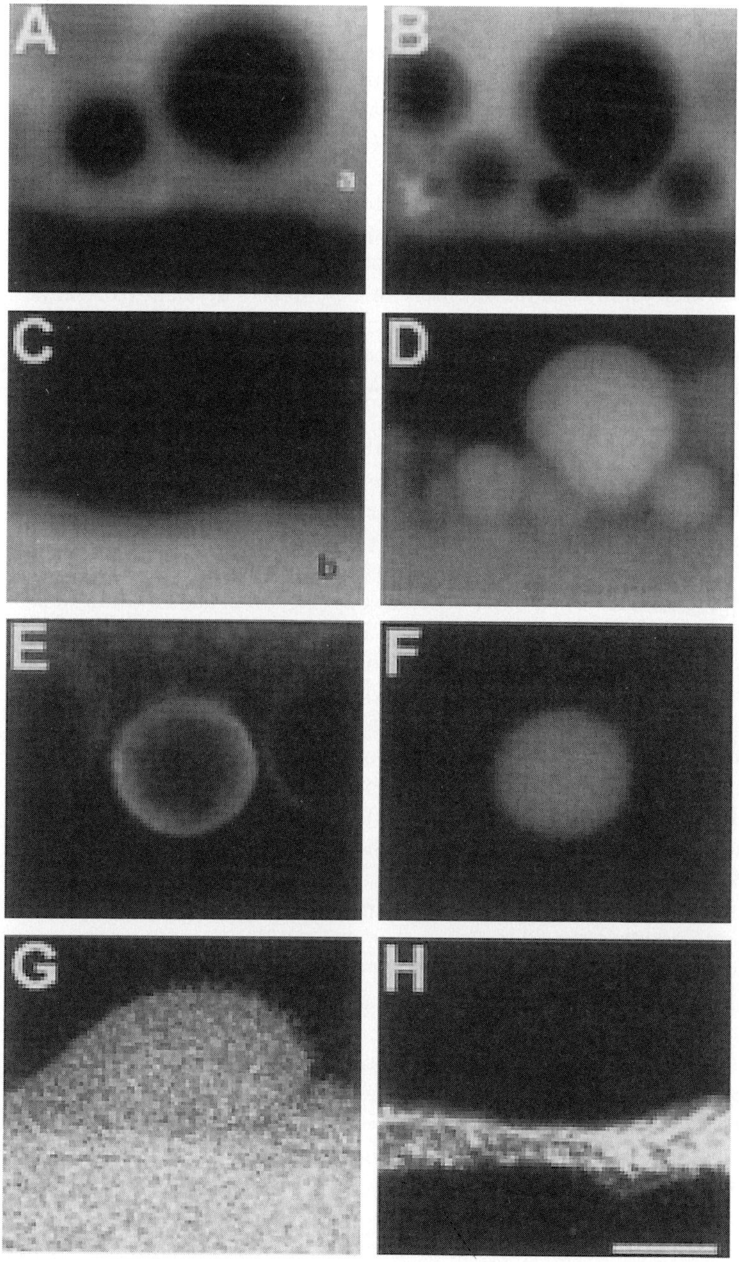
A
B
a
C
D
b
E
F
G
H

dogenous rabbit calpastatin, iodoacetamide, or a monoclonal antibody to calpain (Table 1). In addition, the cut ends of leupeptin-treated MGAs incompletely close to form a pore-like structure, which is filled with vesicles, and the rate of vesicle migration to the cut end in leupeptin-treated crayfish MGAs is not obviously less than MGAs transected in physiological saline (Godell et al., 1997). When other proteases [which are not as dependent on Ca^{2+} as is calpain for activation] are added to divalent-free salines or Ca^{2+}-free salines, crayfish MGAs usually seal within 60 minutes when transected and maintained for 20 minutes in salines containing these proteases (Table 1). All these proteases (bromelian, papain, trypsin, dispase, and chymotryspin) behave similarly in Ca^{2+}-free *vs* divalent-free salines, except for dispase which requires Mg^{2+} for activation. Dispase always induces sealing in Ca^{2+}-free salines containing Mg^{2+}, but dispase does not always induce sealing in divalent-free salines containing EDTA, a chelator of Mg^{2+} (Godell et al., 1997).

These observations are in agreement with a previous report (Xie and Barrett, 1991) that several proteases (papain, dispase, and trypsin) enhance sealing in Ca^{2+}-free salines of severed mammalian septal axons in tissue culture. This study suggested that calpain and several exogenous proteases enhance sealing by promoting the complete collapse of the axon and fusion of the apposed axolemmal leaflets at the cut end. However, other observations (Godell et al., 1997) show that the cut axonal ends are *not* completely closed when transected squid GAs seal in exogenous calpain or when transected crayfish MGAs seal in physiological salines. Furthermore, inhibitors of calpain activity (e.g., leupeptin) do not inhibit sealing in crayfish MGAs by preventing pore formation or partial constriction of the cut end. Finally, various stabilizers of microtubules (20 mM taxol) or destabilizers of F-actin (6 μg/ml cytochalasin E)--compounds which should stabilize or reduce axonal diameter--do not significantly affect the sealing of crayfish MGAs (Table 1), whereas taxol, cytochalasin E, and phalloidin inhibit sealing and colchicine promotes sealing of mammalian septal axons (Xie and Barrett, 1991).

In contrast to the above, Gitler and Spira (1998) report that inhibition of calpain prevents growth cone formation rather than sealing in severed axons of cultured Aplysia neurons. Whether inhibition of calpain affects sealing depends on a proper assessment of sealing. As discussed earlier, the measures of V_m and R_{in}, used by Gitler and Spira (1998) are ambiguous functional measures of the extent of seal formation. Consequently, their data are equivocal with respect to whether sealing is affected by calpain inhibition.

Considering all these data, it appears that Ca^{2+} entry at sites of plasmalemmal damage has at least two major roles: (a) Ca^{2+} entry elevates axoplasmic $[Ca^{2+}]$, which induces or facilitates processes (e.g., endocytosis, vesiculation, myelin delamination and fusions) necessary for the rapid repair of axolemmal damage (Eddleman et al., 1997; 1998a; Ballinger et al, 1997) and (b) Ca^{2+} entry activates Ca^{2+}-dependent proteases (e.g., calpain), which promote processes (e.g., vesicular interactions) that are essential for axonal seal formation.

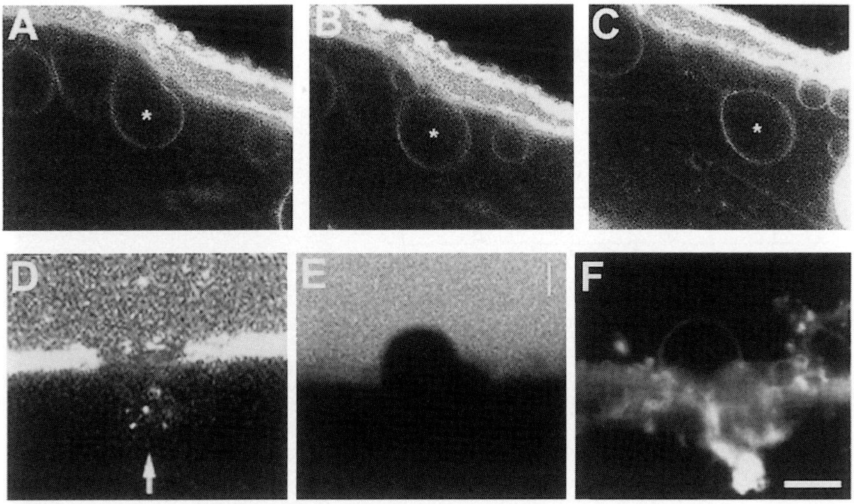

Figure 7. (A - C) Series of time-lapse confocal fluorescence images in the same optical midsection about 100 μm from the cut end showing stages of injury-induced endocytosis beginning with an invagination of FM-labeled membrane and ending with a vesicle moving in the axoplasm toward the cut end of a transected MGA (from Fig. 6 of Eddleman et al.,1998a). In all panels, the axon is at the bottom of the figure, the bath is at the top, and the cut end is toward the right. The plasmalemmal membranes of an intact MGA were pulse-labeled with FM 1-43. The MGA was transected and imaged for FM1-43 fluorescence starting at 11 min posttransection without changing the confocal plane or the position of the micrometer stage. Successive images A - C were acquired at 36 s intervals and taken from a larger set of images acquired every 6 s. An asterix marks the same vesicle in every frame. Note that vesicles are sometimes joined by a fluorescent line (in C), presumably a tether of membranous material.
(D - F) Confocal images of MGAs micropunctured in Ca^{2+}-free salines (D) or Ca^{2+}- containing salines (E, F) or showing dye uptake (D) or showing dye exclusion amidst an accumulation of Ca^{2+}-induced vesicles and other membranous structures (E, F) (from Fig. 8 of Eddleman et al., 1998a). All MGAs were incubated in calcein-AM for 5-30 min before being micropunctured. In panels D-F, the axon is at the top of the figure, the bath is at the bottom, and the micropuncture is approximately in the center. D. Image of calcein hydrophilic dye leaking out of an MGA at the micropuncture site (arrow) at 3 min postpuncture, i.e., prior to formation of a barrier (seal) to hydrophilic dyes. E. Image of calcein fluorescence showing membranous structures identified in DIC (not shown) at the micropuncture site in an MGA at 25 min postpuncture. F. Same confocal plane as D and E, but imaged at 50 min postpuncture for FM1-43, which was added to the bath at 40 min postpuncture. The styryl dye incorporated into the membranes of the structures at the injury site and did not label membranes in the interior of the MGA, i.e. a barrier to the FM dye formed amidst a collection of vesicles at the micropuncture site. Scale bar (in F): 10 μm for A - C, 15 μm for D - F.

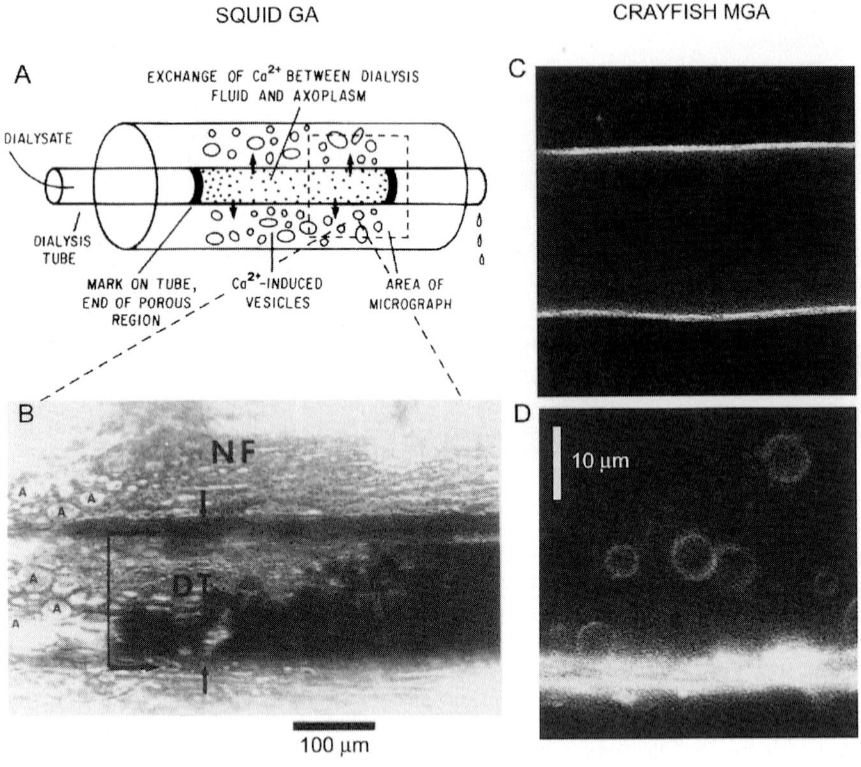

Figure 8 (A) Diagram of internal dialysis of squid GAs (from Fig. 1 of Fishman and Metuzals, 1993) with a dialysis tube having a porous section indicated by two thick black lines. (B) Micrograph of portion, within dashed lines of diagram in A, of squid giant nerve fiber (NF) bathed in control solution (isosmotic potassium glutamate containing 2.5 mM EGTA), 30 min after internal dialysis with control solution plus 3.5 mM $CaCl_2$ (free $[Ca^{2+}]$ = 1 mM). Arrows in B mark the porous/non-porous transition region of the dialysis tube (DT). Notice the presence of axoplasmic vesicles and membranous structures (labeled A) only in the porous region. (C, D) Induction of vesiculation in an intact crayfish MGA (from Fig. 3 of Eddleman, 1999). C. Intact crayfish MGA pulse-labeled with FM1-43 for 10 min and maintained in a calcium-free saline. Notice that no vesicles are present that are labeled with the FM dye. D. 5 min after injection of ~1 mM Ca^{2+} buffered internal saline into an intact crayfish MGA bathed in a Ca^{2+}-free saline. Also notice that vesicles were induced to form even though the axon was intact and maintained in a bath lacking Ca^{2+}. Scale bar (in D) = 75 μm for C.

D. Conservative evolution of mechanisms for sealing membrane damage

As originally described in Eddleman et al. (1997), most eukaryotic cells almost certainly repair plasmalemmal damage by variations in an evolutionarily conserved process involving Ca^{2+}-induced formation of membranous structures that interact with each other, the plasmalemma, and/or with other existing membranous structures. The details of this repair vary with the type of lesion, the morphological configuration of the injured plasmalemma, the type of injured cell and the relationship of a cell to nearby cells.

Despite the lack of information on the molecular mediators (e.g., protein receptors) of membranous processes (e.g., docking and fusion) that result in the formation of an ionic seal after plasmalemmal damage, topological models of vesicular repair of plasma membranes, based on minimization of surface free energy of lipid bilayers, are useful to conceptualize various ways that vesicles might repair plasmalemmal lesions. Two distinct classes of models have been proposed (Eddleman et al, 1997) to repair a small hole (ranging in size from less than a micrometer to tens of micrometers) in the plasmalemma of a spherically shaped cell. In indirect repair models, vesicular fusion with an intact portion of plasma membrane (i.e., exocytosis, Steinhardt et al., 1994; Bi et al., 1995) near a plasmalemmal hole supplies extra lipid to the plasma membrane necessary for hole closure (Fig. 3C). In direct repair models (Fig. 3D), vesicles accumulate and interact with the boundary of the hole to form a tightly packed plug, which may constitute a sufficient ionic seal (Fig. $3D_1$ -$3D_3$), or be an intermediate stage of a more elaborate process that leads to reestablishment of plasmalemmal continuity (Fig. $3D_4$ – D_6). Many variations of the direct repair model are possible. For example, Wohlfarth-Botterman and Stokem (1970) and Terasaki et al. (1997) suggest that plasmalemmal holes are repaired by vesicles which fuse to form a single "wound vesicle" prior to its interaction with the hole boundary.

The morphological configuration of the damaged cell membrane combined with the type of lesion also help determine the repair mechanism. In spherical or non-spherical cells, the mechanisms described in Figure 3C and D can repair a small hole in the plasmalemma. In spherical cells, these mechanisms can also repair a complete transection of the plasmalemma. However, assuming that the addition of lipid/protein molecules to the plasmalemmal bilayer is not subjected to bending forces arising from disrupted or degraded cytoskeletal elements, these mechanisms cannot repair a completely transected portion of a cell that is non-spherical, e.g., an axon, muscle fiber, or pseudopod (Fig. 3E). That is, membranous structures (Fig. $3E_2$) which fuse with a non-spherical plasmalemma that is completely transected (Fig. $3E_3$) only extend the plasmalemma while the completely severed end remains open (Fig. $3E_4$). In contrast (Fig. 3F), if membranous structures (Fig. $3F_2$) move toward the severed end (Fig. $3F_3$), aggregate and inter act (form junctional complexes) with each other and/or the plasmalemma to form a tightly-packed plug (Fig. $3F_4$), then a barrier to diffusion of large molecules

Table 1 The sealing of squid GAs and crayfish MGAs 90-120 min after transection in physiological saline as measured by the percent of axons in which I_i decayed to control current density (I_c), or by the percent of axons which excluded dye as assessed by fluorescence imaging

Experimental Conditions	Measures of Sealing		
	Electrophysiological	Optical	
Substances Added	(% decay of I_i to I_c)	(% dye exclusion)	
		Fluorescence	Confocal
	Squid GAs		
None (control)	0% (n = 14)	0% (n = 14)	0% (n = 11)
Calpain (0.02 au/ml)	100% (n = 5)*	100% (n = 4)*	88% (n = 8)*
Chymotrypsin (0.01 au/ml)	0% (n = 5)	20% (n = 5)	20% (n = 5)
	Crayfish MGAs		
None (control)	100% (n = 6)	93% (n = 42)	95% (n = 37)
Leupeptin (200 μg/ml)	--	0% (n = 2)*	0% (n =30)*
(100 μg/ml)	14% (n = 14)*	20% (n = 30)*	8% (n = 12)*
(50 μg/ml)	--	--	25% (n = 4)*
Calpeptin (100 μg/ml)	0% (n = 3)*	0% (n = 8)*	0% (n = 5)*
Human calpastatin (100 μM)	--	0% (n = 16)*	--
Rabbit calpastatin (0.04 au/ml)	0% (n = 3)*	25% (n = 16)*	0% (n = 5)*
Calpain antibody (1:50 dilution)	--	17% (n = 28)*	--
Iodoacetamide (10 mM)	--	0% (n = 9)*	--
Taxol (20 mM)	--	93% (n = 14)	--
Cytochalasin E (6 μg/ml)	--	92% (n = 12)	--
OCa^{2+} saline	--	21% (n = 43)*	--
plus bromelian (1mg/ml)	--	100% (n = 4)	--
Divalent-free saline	--	17% (n = 12)*	--
plus bromelian (1mg/ml)	--	88% (n = 8)	--
plus papain (140 μg/ml)	--	100% (n = 8)	--
plus trypsin (2.5 mg/ml)	--	100% (n = 4)	--
plus dispase (340 μg/ml)	--	50% (n=10)*	--
plus chymotrypsin (0.01 au/ml)	--	75% (n = 4)	--

*Significally different ($p < 0.05$, chi-square test) from controls. Data are from proximal and distal cut ends examined except, iodoacetamide treated MGAs where data are from proximal cut ends only. Au = activity units.. (modified from Godell et al., 1997).

and/or an ionic seal can be established at the severed end. Alternatively, membranous structures might fuse with each other and with the plasmalemma (including large plasmalemmal invaginations) to form a continuous membrane barrier which seals off the severed end to large molecules and to ions (Fig. $3F_5$). One of these two repair mechanisms (Fig. $3F_4$ *vs* $3F_5$) occurs in all completely transected unmyelinated and myelinated axons studied to date (Krause et al., 1994a; Eddleman et al., 1997, 1998a; Ballinger et al., 1997; Godell et al., 1997).

The type of cell and its relationship to nearby cells determines the membranous sources from which vesicles are derived and the processes by which vesicles are formed. The origin of Ca^{2+}-induced vesicles probably depends on readily available sources. For example, in unfertilized oocytes, pre-formed vesicles (cortical granules) docked at the plasmalemma may repair small holes by Ca^{2+}-induced exocytosis (Steinhardt et al., 1994; Bi et al., 1995; Terasaki et al., 1997; McNeil and Steinhardt, 1997). However, most eukaryotic cells (including axons) do not have large numbers of membranous structures pre-docked at the plasmalemma. Rather, in most eukaryotic cells, membranous structures are induced upon elevation of intracellular Ca^{2+} by inflow after injury (Lubinska, 1956; Yawo and Kuno, 1983; Fishman et al., 1990; Krause et al., 1994a; Miyake and McNeil, 1995; Tanner et al., 1995; Eddleman et al., 1997,1998a; Ballinger et al., 1997; Godell et al., 1997). In squid giant axons and crayfish MGAs (Eddleman et al., 1997, 1998a), Ca^{2+}-dependent endocytosis of axolemmal membrane induced after injury is a significant source of vesicular membrane (Figs. 5 - 6). In earthworm MGAs, myelin delaminations, evaginations, and other membranous structures from glia adjacent to the injury site contribute most significantly to vesicle formation and/or to other membranes that accumulate at the cut ends (Krause et al., 1994a; Ballinger et al., 1997). This multi-source origin of membrane postulated for injury-induced vesicles is in agreement with the presence of non-axolemmal ion channels in patch clamps of injury-induced vesicles extruded from transected squid giant axons (Fishman et al., 1990).

In summary, cells probably use whatever membrane sources are at their disposal, recycling and/or redistributing existing or injury-induced endogenous membrane or exogenous membrane from adjacent supporting cells to produce membranous structures that repair damage to the plasmalemma. The dye barriers that are formed are always located amidst an accumulation of this membranous material. Such dye barriers are always sharply defined (< 2 μm wide) and are always coincident for internal *vs.* external dye barriers. Such membranous structures and dye barriers only form when $[Ca^{2+}]$ exceeds about 100 μM. This requirement for elevated $[Ca^{2+}]$ holds for Ca^{2+}-induced endocytotic vesicles in unmyelinated axons (Eddleman et al., 1998a) and for Ca^{2+}-induced pseudomyelin delaminations in earthworm MGAs (Ballinger et al., 1997). This latter process appears to be very similar to a Ca^{2+}-induced myelin vesiculation reported for mammalian myelinated axons (Schlaepfer, 1977; Smith et al., 1985), perhaps because degradation of neurofilament proteins by calpain (Raabe et al., 1995) dislodge desmosomes that hold concentric layers of myelin in place (Roots and Lane, 1983).

The conservative evolution of vesicles and/or other membranous structures to repair plasmalemmal damage in eukaryotes may share some molecular mechanisms with the conserved vesicular mechanisms responsible for intracellular protein transport such as axonal transport or vesicular traffic in the Golgi apparatus (Rothman and Wieland, 1996), release of transmitters at nerve synapses (Südhof, 1995), and growth of regenerating axons (Cheng and Reese, 1988; Ashery et al., 1996). In support of this hypothesis, we note that botulinum toxin B, which disrupts docking of vesicles to the presynaptic membrane (Südhof, 1995), also prevents vesicular sealing of plasmalemmal damage in sea urchin eggs (Steinhardt et al., 1994) and crayfish MGAs (Bittner and Fishman, unpublished observations).

E. Induction of axolemmal fusion (rapid repair) by polyethylene glycol (PEG)

Various strategies have been attempted to re-establish functional connections of severed axons. For PNS axons, nerve grafts (Jenq and Coggeshall, 1986), connective tissue matrices (Herbert et al., 1996, 1998) and nerve growth guides (Aebischer et al., 1990), have been used to enhance the number of severed axons which regenerate at 1-2 mm/day from proximal stumps (for reviews see Das and Wallace, 1986; Lundberg, 1990). However, even if they eventually reestablish some functions, these PNS axons usually take months to years to reach denervated target tissues in larger mammals such as humans (Das and Wallace, 1986; Bittner, 1988, 1991). To try to re-establish functional connections after severance of CNS axons that normally do not regenerate, strategies such as donor transplants of peripheral nerve sheaths (David and Aguayo, 1981; this volume, chapter by So) or embryonic tissues (Giovanni et al., 1997: Miya et al., 1997) and introduction of antibodies to oligodendrocytic inhibitors of axonal outgrowth (Schnell and Schwab, 1990; this volume, chapter by Schwab) have been designed to induce regeneration from proximal stumps. However, as is the case for regeneration of PNS axons, strategies that rely on axonal outgrowth of 1-2 mm/day cannot avoid waiting weeks to years for any functional regeneration of CNS connections in mammals.

As an alternate and novel strategy to more rapidly reestablish function following severance of PNS or CNS axons in mammals *in vivo*, Ca^{2+}-free PEG solutions were initially used *in vitro* to induce fusion between the severed ends of myelinated MGAs in the CNS of earthworms (Krause and Bittner, 1990; Krause et al., 1991) or unmyelinated MGAs in the CNS of crayfish or mammalian NG 108-15 cells in tissue culture (Bittner et al., 1986). As described in greater detail in the following section, PEG solutions appear to produce incomplete joining of severed axolemmal ends, leaving many holes in the fused membranes. These holes are then sealed by vesicles when the fused membranes are again placed in a Ca^{2+}-containing saline. Most recently, Lore et al. (1999) have used Ca^{2+}-free PEG solutions that induce functional and morphological continuity (PEG-induced fusion) within minutes *in vitro,* between the cut or crushed ends of myelinated sciatic or spinal axons in rats (Fig. 9A, B, D). A PEG-based hydrogel that binds to connective tissue to provide mechanical strength at the lesion site and is nontoxic to nerve tissues in earthworms and mammals *in vivo* is also used to permanently maintain earthworm myelinated MGAs whose functional and morphological integrity is restored by PEG-induced fusion following axonal severance. In all these *in vitro* or *in vivo* procedures, the success of PEG-induced fusion of sciatic or spinal axons and MGAs is measured by the restored conduction of action potentials through the lesion site (Fig. 9A - C), the presence of intact axonal profiles in electron micrographs taken at the lesion site, and/or the intra-axonal diffusion of fluorescent dyes across the lesion site (Fig. 9D). Finally, when the PEG-based hydrogel is applied to connective tissue sheaths of PEG-fused MGAs *in vivo*, then MGAs PEG-fused *in vivo* remain functionally and morphologically intact for at least 20 days in non-anesthetized earthworms, and MGA-mediated behaviors are permanently re-established.

III. SPECULATIONS ON MOLECULAR MECHANISMS OF AXONAL SEALING

We speculate that following axon transection, membranous structures form a dye barrier by fusing to produce a continuous membrane, by forming junctional complexes, and/or by packing more densely (Eddleman et al., 1997, 1998a). A change in the nature of the interactions among membranous structures could account for differences in the times for exclusion of dextran-conjugated fluorescent dyes *vs* ions. For example, the formation of more junctional complexes between membranous structures or a tighter packing density of membranous structures could produce a more restricted diffusion pathway for dyes or ions. Alternatively, if a continuous membrane forms the barrier amidst the membranous material at the cut end, then the restricted diffusion pathway might be due to small pores that decrease in diameter with time, membrane channels which decrease in number with time, and/or membrane channels which close because the membrane potential is repolarized by plasmalemmal transport of ions and/or organelle sequestration of ions. For comparably-sized injuries, such a dye barrier appears to form gradually over several minutes in axons (Krause et al., 1994a; Eddleman et al., 1997, 1998a; Ballinger et al., 1997, ; Godell et al., 1997) rather than within seconds as in sea urchin oocytes (Steinhardt et al., 1994; Bi et al., 1995; Terasaki et al., 1997; McNeil and Steinhardt, 1997).

We speculate further that endogenous calpain helps induce plasmalemmal sealing in squid GAs, crayfish MGAs, and other cells by enhancing interactions of vesicles with other vesicles, the plasmalemma, and/or other membranous structures, perhaps by promotion of membrane fusion (Hayashi et al., 1992; Kwak et al., 1993; Balcerak et al., 1995) or activation of various kinases (Shea et al., 1994, 1995; Eto et al., 1995). Inhibitors of protease activity some of which are specific for calpain (e.g., calpain antibody, human calpastatin peptide, and endogenous rabbit calpastatin) inhibit seal formation by inhibiting these calpain-activated processes. In fact, squid GAs may possess all the necessary components of the multistage sealing process *except* for a sufficient level of calpain activity since squid GAs contain endogenous calpain (Pant et al., 1980).

Finally, we speculate that a recently developed technique (Lore et al., 1999) using polyethylene glycol (PEG) to rapidly repair (rejoin) the severed ends of PNS or CNS axons in invertebrates or mammals depends upon axolemmal sealing mechanisms for its success. A fusiogen like PEG induces the ends of cut or crushed axons to fuse by removing water from hydrophilic groups on the plasmalemmal surface (Sowers, 1987; Lee and Lentz, 1997). Ca^{2+}-free salines containing EGTA prevent the cut axonal ends axons from sealing by inhibiting their constriction and the formation of injury-induced vesicles and other membranous strutures.

Figure 9. Compound action potentials (CAPs) from a strip of sciatic axons (A) or spinal axons (B) or individual action potentials (APs) from earthworm MGAs (C) in intact and PEG-fused preparations extracellularly recorded using double sucrose gap (A, B) or conventional (C) techniques. A - C from Figure 1 and D from Figure 4 of Lore et al. (1999).
(A, B) CAPs recorded from control rat spinal or sciatic axons (traces labeled "i") prior to replacing the rat physiological saline (Krebs solution) with Ca^{2+}-free Krebs containing 1 mM EGTA (trace labeled "OCa^{2+} ") at ~25° C. The sciatic or spinal axons were then transected to eliminate the CAP (traces labeled "t"). PEG was applied to the apposed cut ends, and the preparation was again perfused with Krebs. Within 10 min, the CAP again appeared in PEG-fused sciatic or spinal axons (traces labeled "f"), and remained for = 30 min. The CAP was again eliminated when the sciatic or spinal axons were re-transected at the original lesion site (traces labeled "rt"). The sciatic nerve or strip of spinal axons was always extracellularly stimulated by a maximal voltage (e.g., ~6 V for the preparation shown in A and ~10 V in B) that reliably produced a CAP with the greatest peak amplitude .
(C) Individual MGA and LGA APs recorded conventionally using the single chamber device of Krause et al. (1991). Control (intact) MGA (m) and LGA (L) APs (trace 1) placed in physiological earthworm saline stimulated by a rostral electrode and recorded from rostrally (r) and caudally (c) placed electrodes prior to cutting the axons between the two recording electrodes to eliminate the APs from the caudal electrode (trace 2). The VNC was placed in Ca^{2+}-free earthworm saline and PEG was applied to the apposed cut ends of the MGA, but not the LGA, to induce PEG-fusion only of the MGA and the preparation was again perfused with earthworm saline . PEG hydrogel was then applied to the lesion site. Within 10 min, the MGA (but not LGA) AP was again recorded for 1 - 24 hrs on the caudal side of the lesion site (trace 3).Scale bars: A, B = 1 mV, 0.5 msec; C = 0.5 mV, 1 msec.
(D) Confocal fluorescence image (photomicrograph) of cut sciatic axons subsequently PEG-fused and injected with sulforhodamine 101 at 24 hr prior to viewing. The figure is oriented so that the injected segment is at the bottom of the panel and the injection site is about 3 mm from the lesion site (marked by a bar). Image obtained using 10X Leica lens showing some dye-filled axons traversing the lesion site. For this cut sciatic nerve, the peak amplitude of the CAP was 6.2 mV prior to transection, 4.0 mV in Ca^{2+}-free saline with 1.0 mM EGTA, 0 mV after transection, 1.9 mV within 10 min after PEG-induced fusion, and 0 mV when re-transected. Scale bar = 110 μm.

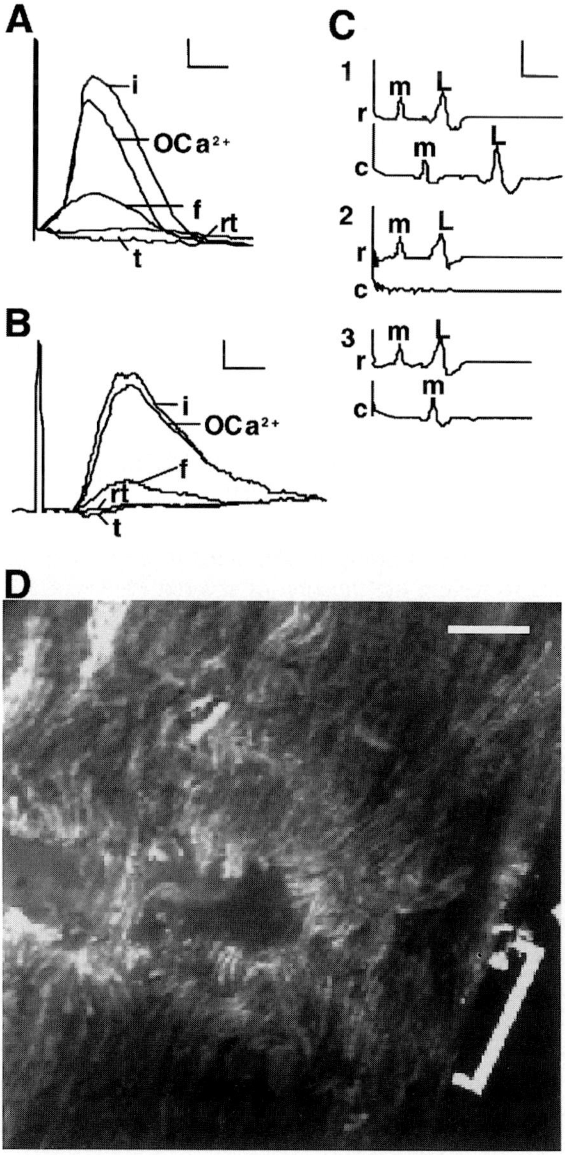
A
i
OCa2+
f
rt
t
B
i
OCa2+
f
rt
t
C
1
m
L
r
m
L
c
2
m
L
r
c
3
m
L
r
m
c
D

That is, two open axonal ends not filled with vesicles can be more easily fused than two constricted ends filled with membranous structures and closely apposed axons incompletely fused by PEG intially have many plasmalemmal discontinuities. When subsequently placed in Ca^{2+}-containing physiological saline, Ca^{2+} inflow at the plasmalemmal discontinuities induces the formation of endocytotic vesicles and other membranous structures that, in turn, seal those discontinuities (Krause et al., 1994a; Ballinger et al., 1997; Eddleman et al., 1997, 1998a). This plasmalemmal repair takes seconds to hours, depending on the size and type of membrane lesion (Krause et al., 1994a; Steinhardt et al., 1994; Ballinger et al., 1997; Eddleman et al., 1997, 1998a). Calpain facilitates the sealing of cut axonal ends (Xie and Barrett, 1991; Eddleman et al., 1997; Godell et al., 1997). In contrast, leupeptin (an inhibitor of calpain) inhibits sealing of severed axonal ends (Eddleman et al., 1997; Godell et al., 1997).

IV. SPECULATIONS ON CLINICAL APPLICATIONS OF SUBSTANCES THAT AFFECT AXOLEMMAL SEALING

Lore et al., (1999) have considered several problems that need to be solved for successful use of PEG solutions to restore the function of severed PNS or CNS axons in mammals *in vivo.*

First, the cut nerve ends would have to be perfectly aligned and all axons successfully PEG-fused to restore the original connectivity of a bundle of severed PNS or CNS axons. Clinically, axonal regeneration is not high unless the ends of severed PNS fascicles are carefully aligned by microsurgery (Lundborg, 1990; Seckel, 1990). [This problem is less severe for crush injuries to CNS or PNS axons since crushed ends often remain aligned (Blight, 1989; Lundborg, 1990; Seckel, 1990).] However, if partial restoration of function is a goal, then the survival or regeneration of only 10% of CNS axons in mammals produces significant behavioral recovery (Eidelberg et al., 1977; Das and Wallace, 1986. Furthermore, successful PEG-induced fusion of carefully aligned PNS axons would restore function much more rapidly (within minutes) compared to regeneration by growth cone outgrowth at 1 - 2 mm/day.

Second, axonal fusion is not induced by PEG solutions unless the severed axonal ends are tightly apposed. However, various surgical procedures (Das and Wallace, 1986) bring cut CNS or PNS nerve ends into close apposition and crushed axonal ends can be opened and brought into close apposition using Ca^{2+}-free, slightly hypotonic salines (Krause and Bittner, 1990; Krause et al., 1991).

Third, the mechanical strength at the site of PEG-fusion is not high because PEG solutions do not reconnect severed connective tissue elements which give mechanical strength to nerve bundles. However, the PEG hydrogel provides high mechanical strength at the lesion .

Fourth, mammalian distal stumps usually degenerate within hours to a few days after axonal severance (Ramón y Cajal, 1928; Das and Wallace, 1986; Bittner, 1991). In such cases, PEG-induced fusion would have to be induced within several hours after injury. However, *in vivo* cooling to 13°C (Sea et al., 1995) or injection of cyclosporin A (Sunio and Bittner, 1997) allows the distal stumps of many myelinated axons to survive for at least 6 - 10 days in rats, as does injection of antibodies to complement 3 receptors (Lunn et al., 1989).

Finally, PEG-induced fusion techniques might be combined with other techniques such as microsurgery, nerve growth guides (Jenq and Coggeshall, 1986; Aebischer et al., 1990; Herbert et al., 1996), transplants of peripheral nerve sheaths (David and Aguayo, 1981) or embryonic tissues (Giovanini et al., 1997; Miya et al., 1997) or injections of antibodies to oligodendritic inhibitors of CNS axonal outgrowth (Schnell and Schwab, 1990). Compared to the use of any single strategy, such a combined approach might produce more rapid and more complete restoration of function to severed mammalian PNS and/or CNS axons (Bittner et al., 1999).

ACKNOWLEDGEMENTS

We wish to thank Mr. Martis Ballinger and Dr. Christopher S. Eddleman for significant contributions toward understanding axonal sealing and for their help in the preparation of this chapter. Supported by NIH Grants NS31256 and HD31484 and TATP grants.

REFERENCES

Aebischer P, Guenard V, Valentini RF (1990) The morphology of regenerating peripheral nerves is modulated by the surface microgeometry of polymeric guidance channels. Brain Res 531:211-218.

Alberts B, Bray D, Lewis J, Raff M, Roberts K, Watson JD (1994) The cell (Third ed). New York: Garland Publishers.

Ashery U, Penner R, Spira ME (1996) Acceleration of membrane recycling by axotomy of cultured *Aplysia* neurons. Neuron 16:641-651.

Balcerzak D, Poussard S, Brustis, JJ, Elamrani N, Soriano M, Cottin P, Ducastaing A (1995) An antisense oligodeoxyribonucleotide to m-calpain mRNA inhibits myoblast fusion. J Cell Sci 108:2077-2082.

Ballinger ML, Blanchette AR, Krause TL, Smyers ME, Fishman HM, Bittner GD (1997) Delaminating myelin membranes help heal the cut ends of severed earthworm giant axons. J Neurobiol 33:945-960.

Betz WJ, Mao F, Bewick GS (1992) Activity-dependent staining and destaining of living vertebrate motor nerve terminals. J Neurosci 12:363-375.

Bi G, Alderton JM, Steinhardt RA (1995) Calcium-regulated exocytosis is required for cell membrane resealing. J Cell Biol 131:147-1758.

Birse SC, Bittner GD (1981) Regeneration of earthworm giant axons following transection or ablation. J. Neurophysiol. 45: 724-742.

Bittner GD (1973) Degeneration and regeneration in crustacean neuromuscular systems. Am Zool 13: 379-408.

Bittner GD (1981) Trophic interactions of crustacean giant axons. Comp Biochem Physiol 68A:299-306.

Bittner GD (1988) Long term survival of severed distal axonal stumps in vertebrates and invertebrates Am Zool 28:1165-1179.

Bittner GD (1991) Long term survival of anucleate axons and its implications for nerve regeneration. Trends Neurosci 14:188-193.

Bittner GD, Ballinger, ML, Raymond, MA (1986) Reconnection of severed nerve axons with polyethylene glycol. Brain Res. 367:351-365.

Bittner GD, Schallert T, Peduzzi JD (1999) Degeneration, trophic interactions and repair of severed axons: a reconsideration of some common assumptions. The Neuroscientist, In press.

Blight AR (1989) Effect of 4-Aminopyridine on axonal conduction-block in chronic spinal cord injury. Brain Res Bul 22:47-52.

Borgens R, Jaffe L, Cohen H (1980) Large and persistent electrical currents enter the transected lamprey spinal cord. Proc Natl Acad Sci USA 77:1209-1213.

Bouton MS, Bitner GD (1981) Regeneration of motor axons in crayfish limbs: distal stump activation followed by synaptic reformation. Cell Tiss Res 219:379-392.

Cheng TP, Reese TS (1998) Compartmentalization of anterogradely and retrogradely transported organelles in axons and growth cones from chick optic tectum. J Neurosci 8:3190-3199.

Das GD, Wallace RB (1986) Neural transplantation and regenration. New York: Springer.

David S., Aguayo AJ (1981) Axonal elongation into peripheral nervous system "ridges" after central nervous system injury in adult rats. Science 241:931-933.

Deriemer SA, Elliot EJ, Macagno ER, Muller KJ (1983) Morphological evidence that regenerating axons can fuse with severed axon segments. Brain Res 272:157-161.

Eddleman CS (1999) Vesicular repair of axonal injury. Ph.D. dissertation, Moody Medical Library, University of Texas Medical Branch, Galveston, Texas.

Eddleman CS, Ballinger ML, Smyers ME, Fishman HM, Bittner GD (1998a) Endocytotic formation of vesicles and other membranous structures induced by Ca^{2+} and axoplasmic injury J Neurosci 18:4029-4041.

Eddleman CS, Ballinger ML, Smyers ME, Godell CM, Fishman HM, Bittner GD (1997) Repair of plasmalemmal lesions by vesicles. PNAS 94:4745-4750.

Eddleman CS, Godell CM, Fishman HM, Tytell M, Bittner GD (1995) Fluorescent labelling of the glial sheath of giant nerve fibers. Biol Bull 189:218-219.

Eddleman CS, Smyers ME, Lore A, Fishman HM, Bittner GD (1998b) Anomalies associated with dye exclusion as a measure of axolemmal repair. Neurosci Lett 256:123-125

Eidelberg E, Straehley D, Erspamer R, Watkins CJ (1977) Relationship between residual hindlimb-assisted locomotion and surviving axons after incomplete spinal cord injuries. Exp Neurol 56:312-322.

Eto A, Akita Y, Saido TC, Suzuki K, Kawashima S (1995) The role of the calpain-calpastatin system in thyrotropin-releasing hormone-induced selective down-regulation of a protein kinase C isozyme, nPKC epsilon, in rat pituitary GH4C1 cells. J Biol Chem 270:25115-25120.

Fernandez J, Fernandez MS (1974) Morphological evidence for an experimentally induced synaptic field. Nature 251:428-430.

Fishman HM, Krause TL, Miller AL, Bittner GD (1995) Retardation of the spread of extracellular Ca^{2+} into transected, unsealed squid giant axons. Biol Bull 189:208-209.

Fishman HM, Metuzals J (1993) Ca^{2+}-induced axosome formation in internaly dialized giant axons of *Loligo pealei.* Biol Bull 185:292-293.
Fishman HM, Tewari KP, Stein PG (1990) Injury-induced vesiculation and membrane redistribution in squid giant axon. Biochim Biophys Acta 1023:421-435.
Gallant PE (1998) Effects of the external ions and metabolic poisoning on the constriction of the squid giant axon after axotomy. J Neurosci 8:1479-1484.
Gallant PE, Gailbraith JA (1997) Axonal structure and function after axolemmal leakage in the squid giant axon. J Neurotrauma 14:811-822.
Gallant PE, Hammar K, Reese TS (1995) Cytoplasmic constriction and vesiculation after axotomy in the squid giant axon. J Neurocytol 24:943-954.
George EB, Glass JD, Griffin JW (1995) Axotomy-induced axonal degeneration is mediated by calcium influx through ion-specific channels. J Neurosci 15:6449-6452.
Giovanini MA, Reier PJ, Eskin TA, Wirth E, Anderson DK (1997) Characteristics of human fetal spinal cord grafts in the adult rat spinal cord: influences of lesion and grafting conditions. Exp Neurol 148:523-543.
Gitler D, Spira ME (1998) Real time imaging of calcium-induced localized proteolytic activity after axotomy and its relation to growth cone formation. Neuron. 20:1123-1135.
Godell CM, Ballinger M, Eddleman CS, Smyers ME, Fishman HM, Bittner, GD (1997) Calpain promotes the sealing of severed giant axons. PNAS 94:4751-4756.
Hayashi M, Saito Y, Kawashima S (1992) Calpain activation is essential for membrane fusion of erythrocytes in the presence of exogenous Ca2+. Biochem. Biophys Res Commun 182:939-946.
Herbert CB, Bittner GD, Hubbell JA (1996) Effects of fibrinolysis on neurite growth from dorsal root ganglia cultured in two- and three-diemensional fibrin gels. J Comp Neurol 365:380-391.
Herbert CB, Nagaswami, C, Bittner GD, Hubbell JA, Weisel JW (1998) Effects of fibrin micro-morphology on neurite growth from dorsal root ganglia cultured within three-dimensional fibrin gels. J Biomed Materials Res 40:441-449.
Jenq C-B, Coggeshall RE (1986) The effects of an autologous transplant on patterns of regeneration in rat sciatic nerve. Brain Res 364:45-56.
Kao CC, Chang LW, Bloodworth JMB (1997) Electron microscopic observation of the mechanism of terminal club formation in transected spinal cord axons. J Neuropathol Exp Neurol 36:140-156.
Kao CC, Wrathall JR, Kyoshimov K (1983) Axonal reaction to transection. In: Spinal cord reconstruction (Kao CC, Bunge RP, Reier PJ, eds), pp 41-57. New York: Raven.
Kelly JP (1985) Reaction of neurons to injury. In: Principles of neural science (Kandel ER, Schwartz JH eds), pp 979 . Amsterdam: Elsevier/North Holland.
Krause TL, Bittner GD (1990) Rapid morphological fusion of severed myelinated axons by polyethylene glycol PNAS 87:1471-1475.
Krause TL, Fishman HM, Ballinger ML, Bittner GD (1994a) Extent and mechanism of sealing in transected giant axons of squid and earthworms. J Neurosci 14:6638-6651.
Krause TL, Fishman HM, Bittner GD (1994b) Axolemmal and septal conduction in the impedance of the earthworm medial giant nerve fiber. Biophys J 67:692-695.
Krause TL, Marquis RM, Lyckman AW, Ballinger ML, Bittner GD (1991) Rapid artificial restoration of electrical continuity across a crush lesion of a giant axon. Brain Res 561:350-353.
Kwak KB, Kambayashi J, Kang M, Ha DB, Chung CH (1993) Cell-penetrating inhibitors of calpain block both membrane fusion and filamin cleavage in chick embryonic myoblasts. FEBS Lett 323:151-154.

Lee J, Lentz BR (1997) Evolution of lipidic structures during model membrane fusion and the relation of this process to cell membrane fusion. Biochemistry 36:6251-6259.
Levi G, Meyer H (1945) Reactive, regressive and regenerative processes of neurons cultivated in vitro and injured with the micromanipulator. J Exp Zool 99:141-181.
Lore AB, Hubbell JA, Bobb DS Jr, Ballinger ML, Loftin KL, Smith JW, Smyers ME, Garcia HD, Bittner GD (1999) Rapid induction of functional and morphological continuity between severed ends of mammalian or earthworm myelinated axons. J Neurosci 19:2442-2454.
Lubinska L (1956) Outflow form cut ends of nerve fibers. Exp Cell Res 10:40-47.
Lucas JH, Gross GW, Emery DG, Gardner CR (1985) Neuronal survival or death after dendrite transection close to the perikaryon: correlation with electrophysiologic, morphologic and ultrastructural changes. Cent Nerv Syst Trauma 2:231-255.
Lundborg G (1990) Nerve regeneration problems in a clinical perspective. Rest Neurol Neurosci 1:297-302.
Lunn ER, Perry VH, Brown MC, Rosen H, Gordon S (1989) Absence of Wallerian degeneration does not hinder regeneration in peripheral nerve. Eur J Neurosci 1:27-33.
McNeil PL, Steinhardt RA (1997) Loss, restoration, and maintenance of plasma membrane integrity. J Cell Biol 137:1-4.
Meiri H, Spira M, Parnas I (1981) Membrane conductance and action potential of a regenerating axon tip. Science 211:709-712.
Miya D, Giszter S, Mori F, Adipudi V, Tessler A, Murray M (1997) Fetal transplants alter the development of function after spinal cord transection in newborn rats. J Neurosci 17:4856-4872.
Miyake K, McNeil PL (1995) Vesicle accumulation and exocytosis at sites of plasma membrane disruption. J Cell Biol 131:1737-1745.
Muller KH, Carbonetto S (1979) The morphological and physiological properties of a regenerating synapse in the CNS of the leech. J Comp Neurol 185:485-516.
Murray M (1997) Strategies and mechanisms of recovery after spinal cord injury. Advances Neurol 72:219-225.
Nordlander RH, Singer M (1972) Electron microscopy of severed motor fibers in the crayfish. Z Zellforsch 1256:157-181.
Pant HC (1988) Dephosphorylation of neurofilament proteins enhances their susceptibility to degradation by calpain. Biochem J 256:665-668.
Pant HC, Gainer, H (1980) Properties of a calcium-activated protease in squid axoplasm which selectively degrades neurofilament proteins. J Neurobiol 11:1-12.
Raabe TD, Nguyen T, Archer C, Bittner, GD (1996) Mechanisms for the maintenance and eventual degradation of neurofilament proteins in the distal segments of severed goldfish Mauthner axons. J Neurosci 16:1605-1613.
Raabe TD, Nguyen T, Bittner GD (1995) Calcium activated proteolysis of neurofilament proteins in goldfish Mauthner axons. J Neurobiol 26:253-261.
Ramon y Cajal S (1928) Degeneration and regeneration of the nervous system. London: Oxford UP.
Roots BI, Lane NJ (1983) Myelinating glia of earthworm giant axons: thermally induced intramembranous changes. Tissue Cell 15:695-709.
Rothman JE, Wieland FT (1996) Protein sorting by transport vesicles. Science 272:227-234.
Sattler, R. Tymianski, M., Feyaz, I., Hafner, M., and Tator, C.H. (1996)Voltage sensitive calcium channels mediate calcium entry into cultured mammalian sympathetic neurons following neurite transection. Brain Res. 719, 239-246.

Schlaepfer WW (1974) Calcium-induced degeneration of axoplasm in isolated segments of rat peripheral nerve. Brain Res 69:203-215.

Schlaepfer WW (1977) Vesicular disruption of myelin simulated by exposure of nerve to calcium ionophor. Nature (Lond) 265:734-736.

Schnell L, Schwab ME (1990) Axonal regeneration in the rat spinal cord produced by an antibody against myelin-associated neurite growth inhibitors. Nature 343:269-272.

Sea T, Ballinger ML, Bittner GD (1995) Cooling of peripheral myelinated axons retards Wallerian degeneration. Exp Neurol 133:85-95.

Seckel B (1990) Enhancement of peripheral nerve regeneration. Muscle Nerve 13:785-800.

Shae TB, Beermann ML, Griffin WR, Leli U (1994) Degradation of protein kinase C alpha and its free catalytic subunit, protein kinase M, in intact neuroblastoma cells and under free conditions. Evidence that PKM is degraded by mM calpain-mediated proteolysis at a faster rate than PKC. FEBS Lett 350:223-229.

Shae TB, Cressman CM, Spencer MJ, Beermann ML, Nixon RA (1995) Enhancement of neurite outgrowth following calpain inhibition is mediated by protein kinase C. J Neurochem 65:517-527.

Smith KJ, Hall SM, Schauf CL (1985) Vesicular demyelination induced by raised intracellular calcium J Neurosci 71:19-37.

Sowers AE (1987) Cell fusion. New York: Plenum.

Spira ME, Benbassat D, Dormann A (1993) Resealing of the proximal and distal cut ends of transected axons: electrophysiological and structural analysis. J Neurobiol 24:300-316.

Steinhardt RA, Bi G, Alderton JM (1994) Cell membrane resealing by a vesicular mechanism similar to neurotransmitter release. Science 263:390-393.

Strautman AF, Cork RJ, Robinson KR (1990) The distribution of free calcium in transected spinal axons and its modulation by applied electric fields. J Neurosci 10:3564-3575.

Südhof TC (1995) The synaptic vesicle cycle: a cascade of protein-protein interactions. Nature 375:645-653.

Sunio A, Bittner GD (1997) Cyclosporin retards the Wallerian degeneration of peripheral mammalian axons. Exp Neurol 146:46-56.

Tanner SL, Storm EE, Bittner GD (1995) Protein transport in intact and severed (anucleate) crayfish medial giant axons. J Neurochem 64:1491-1501.

Terasaki M, Miyake K, McNeil PL (1997) Large plasma membrane disruptions are rapidly resealed by Ca^{2+}-dependent vesicle-vesicle fusion events. J Cell Biol . 139:63-74.

Velez S, Bittner, GD, Govind GK, Atwood HL (1981) Trophic reactions of crayfish muscle fibers and nerve synapses following denervation, tenotomy, and immobilization. Exp Neurol 71:307-325.

Viancour TA, Bittner GD, Ballinger, ML (1981) Selective transfer of Lucifer Yellow CH from axoplasm to adaxonal glia. Nature 293:65-67.

Viancour TA, Seshan KR, Bittner GD, Sheller RA (1987) Organization of axoplasm in crayfish giant axons. J Neurocytol 16:557-566.

Viancour TA, Sheller, RA, Bittner, GD, Seshan KR (1988) Protein transport between crayfish lateral giant axons. Brain Res 439:211-221.

Wohlfarth-Bottermann KE, Stockem W (1970) Die Regeneration des Plasmalemms von Physarum polycephalum. Wihelm Roux' Archiv. 164:321-340

Xie X, Barrett JN (1991) Membrane resealing in cultured rat septal neurons after neurite transection: evidence for enhancement by Ca^{2+}-triggered protease activity and cytoskeletal disassembly. J Neurosci 11:3257-3267.
Yawo H, Kuno M (1983) How a nerve fiber repairs its cut end: involvement of phospholipase A_2. Science 222:1351-1353.
Yawo H, Kuno M (1985) Calcium dependence of membrane sealing at the cut end of the cockroach giant axon. J Neurosci 5:1626-1632.
Zelená J, Lubinska L, Gutmann E (1968) Accumulation of organelles at the ends of interrupted axons. Z. Zellforsch 91:200-219.
Zimmerman U-JP, Schlaepfer WW (1984) Calcium-activated neutral proteases (CANP) in brain and other tissues. Prog Neurobiol 23:63-78.
Ziv NE, Spira, ME (1995) Axotomy induces a transient and localized elevation of the free intracellular calcium concentration to the millimolar range. J Neurophysiol 75: 2635-2647.

13

N-Terminal Arginylation of Proteins and Transcellular Transfer of Small Molecules in Regenerating Nerves

Nicholas A. Ingoglia and Nan Zhang
New Jersey Medical School-UMDNJ, Newark, New Jersey

I. INTRODUCTION

Perhaps one of the least understood discoveries of the last 30 years in the cell biology of neurons is the function of the relatively high concentrations of transfer RNA found to be present within axons. The inability to ascribe function to axonal tRNAs has been due primarily to the failure to observe the reactions in which these RNAs participate *in vivo*, and when those reactions have been studied *in vitro,* they occur at such low levels that characterization of the products, and thus an understanding of their role in normal axonal metabolism, has proved extremely difficult. Following nerve injury and during the subsequent regeneration of a nerve, however, the reactions in which axonal tRNAs appear to be utilized, i.e., as amino acid donors in the posttranslational modification of nerve proteins, increase by several orders of magnitude in the portion of nerve just proximal to injury, and in the advancing tips of regenerating axons. The first part of this chapter will describe research into the putative role these reactions play in the ability of a nerve to regrow a severed axon.

In the second part of this chapter another novel phenomenon of axonal physiology, the ability of intact and regenerating axons to transport axonally and then transfer a variety of small molecules to adaxonal cells, will be described. In this area too, knowledge of the physiological role this system plays in intact or regenerating axons has not progressed much further than a description of the phenomenon (Droz et al., 1978; Ingoglia et al., 1982). However, recent data from several laboratories on the ways that cells communicate and regulate gene expression have offered some tantalizing possible explanations for the original observations and these data may be relevant to mechanisms involved in nerve regeneration.

II. N-TERMINAL ARGINYLATION AND NERVE REGENERATION

A. Transfer RNAs are present in axons

The original demonstration that transfer RNAs are present in axons was performed by extruding axoplasm from squid and *Myxicola* giant axons, extracting the RNA using conventional techniques and analyzing the product by SDS PAGE (Lasek et al., 1973). The RNA extracted from these pure samples of axoplasm was found to be composed primarily (>85%) of 4S RNA, the size of transfer (t) RNA. Subsequent experiments demonstrated that the tRNA could be charged by a variety of amino acids and fulfilled several other criteria confirming their identity as tRNAs (Black and Lasek, 1977; Ingoglia et al., 1983). Since it is extremely difficult to extrude axoplasm from vertebrate axons and be certain of its purity (i.e. assurance that it is not contaminated by glial/Schwann cell cytoplasm), similar extrusion experiments could not be performed convincingly in higher organisms. However, radioactive tracer experiments in chick (Por et al., 1978), goldfish (Ingoglia and Tuliszewski, 1976) and rat (Lindquist et al., 1981) nerves were completely consistent with the findings in extruded axoplasm. While evidence for other RNA species in axons (e.g., Capano et al., 1987; Koenig and Martin, 1996; Chun et al., 1997) and for limited axonal protein synthesis (e.g., Giuditta et al., 1968, 1977; Eng et al., 1999) has been reported, the fact remains that the vast majority of the RNA in axons is tRNA and that it is likely functioning in a role separate from protein synthesis.

B. Transfer RNAs are found in axons and growth cones of regenerating nerves

The conclusions concerning the presence of tRNAs in axoplasm of vertebrate nerves were solidified by the electron microscopic autoradiographic results of Pierluigi Gambetti and colleagues. Initial experiments in the optic nerves of rabbits indicated that following injection of labeled uridine into the eye, more than 80% of the radioactive RNA along distal regions of the optic nerve was in surrounding glia and not in optic axons (Gambetti et al., 1973). At the same time, our laboratory was finding large increases in the axonal transport of label associated with RNA in optic nerves of goldfish that were regenerating following injury, some of which appeared, by light autoradiograhy, to be present in regenerating axons (Ingoglia et al., 1975). When our labs collaborated on an EM

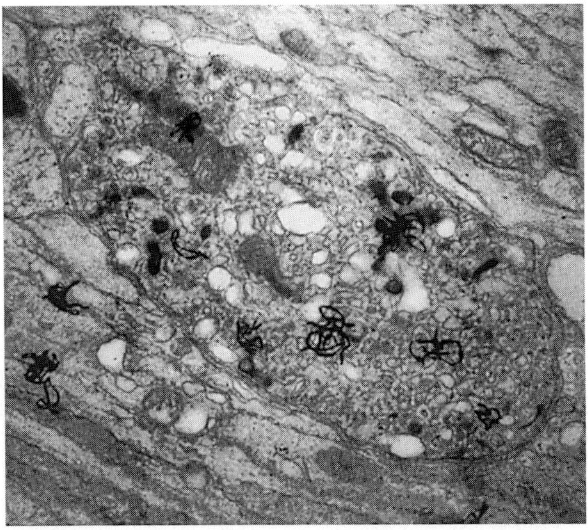

Figure 1 Electron microscopic autoradiogram of a growth cone in the goldfish optic tectum following intraocular injection of ^{3}H-uridine, and during regeneration of retinal ganglion cell axons. Silver grains represent molecules of ^{3}H-tRNA (see Gambetti, et al., 1978; Ingoglia, 1979 for details).

autoradiographic analysis of the distribution of RNA associated radioactivity, more than 50% of the silver grains in the goldfish optic tectum were found to be within regenerating axons (Gambetti et al., 1978). Further, a significant portion of the silver grains could be clearly localized to axonal growth cones (Fig. 1). Thus, the most advanced tip of regenerating optic axons of goldfish contained molecules of transfer RNA.

C. Axonal tRNAs mediate the posttranslational amino acid modification of proteins

Transfer RNAs had been shown to be able to serve as amino acid donors in the posttranslational modification of proteins by adding amino acids to the N-terminus of acceptor proteins (Kaji et al., 1968; Soffer, 1980). While this seemed a reasonable role for tRNA in axons and growth cones, the only tRNA reported to be able to carry out this function in liver extracts was $tRNA^{arg}$ (Soffer,1990). However, we (Ingoglia et al., 1983) and others (Giuditta et al., 1968; Black and Lasek, 1977) had shown that axoplasm of squid contained multiple species of tRNA and not just $tRNA^{arg}$. When we tested the hypothesis that not only Arg, but other amino acids as well, could be transferred from tRNA to protein, we found that this was true only if low molecular weight inhibitors were removed from *in vitro* preparations of axoplasm extracts (Fig. 2; Ingoglia et al., 1983).

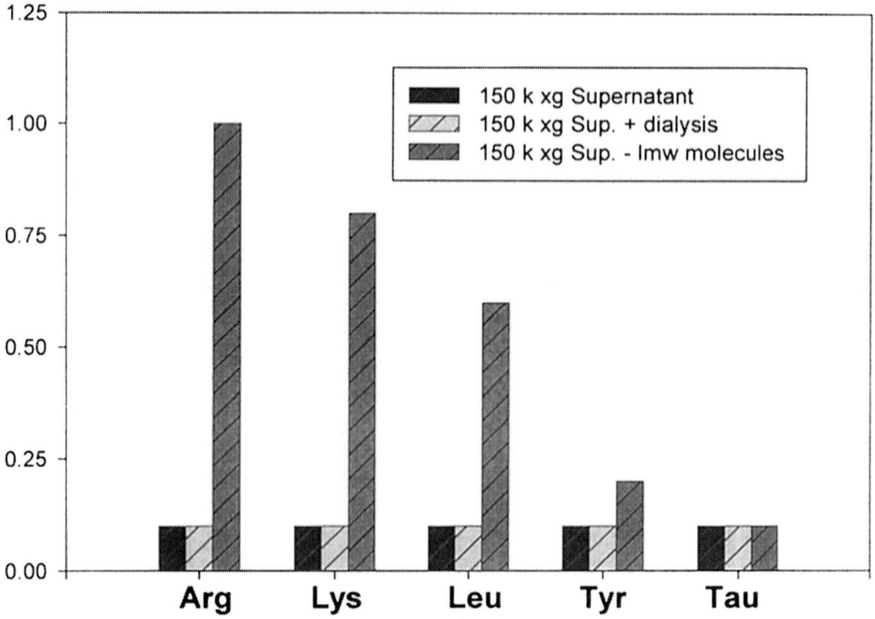

Figure 2 Posttranslational incorporation of several amino acids into protein in 150k xg supernatants of axoplasm taken from the giant axon of squid. Values have been normalized to those obtained for arginine. No activity was found in the unfractionated or dialyzed supernatant, suggesting the presence of a low molecular weight (lmw) inhibitor. Following removal of molecules < approx. 120k D covalent incorporation was observed. Taurine (Tau) a sulfonic amino acid not incorporated into protein and lacking a cognate tRNA was used as a control and showed no incorporation under any of the conditions (taken from Ingoglia et al., 1983).

While this was also found to be the case in vertebrate nerves, what was more intriguing and important in the latter case, was the effect of nerve injury on the expression of these reactions. Transection of sciatic nerve axons increased posttranslational amino acid addition 10-fold within the first two hours of injury in the nerve segment just proximal to the site of injury, whereas the distal segment (separated from the cell body) and the more proximal (noninjured) portion of the nerve showed no activation of the reaction (Shyne-Athwal et al., 1988). The data indicate that a significant and very early increase in the addition of amino acids to nerve proteins occurs in the region of the nerve where axoplasm has been exposed to the extracellular environment by injury and where regrowth of axonal sprouts originates (Fig. 3).

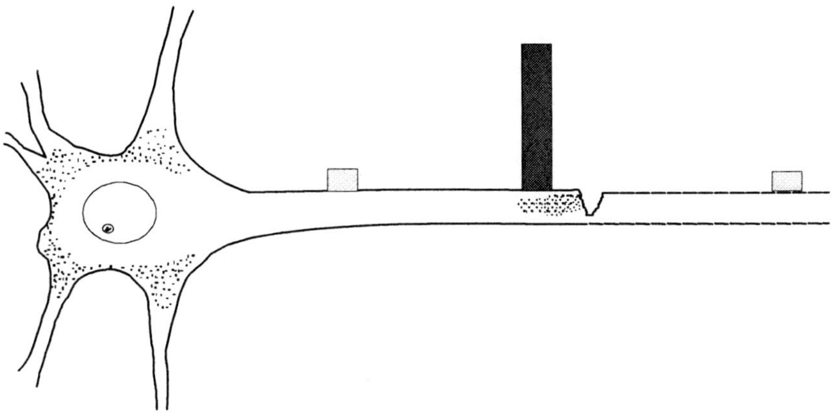

Figure 3 Schematic drawing of a ventral horn of a rat showing site of axonal injury and the area of activation of posttranslational amino acid addition. Ten fold increases were found in the area immediately proximal to the injury but not in more proximal nor distal regions (taken from Zanakis et al., 1984).

D. Amino acid modification of proteins increases in the proximal stump of an injured peripheral nerve capable of regeneration but not in an injured central nerve which cannot regenerate

When the same experiments were performed in optic nerves of rats, increases in the posttranslational addition of amino acids to endogenous proteins were significantly delayed, occurring 6 days after nerve injury compared with 2 hours following sciatic nerve injury (Shyne-Athwal et al., 1986). This finding is significant for several reasons. First, it is one of the earliest post-injury biochemical differences reported between peripheral and central nerves. Second, it implies that whatever function these reactions serve in a peripheral nerve, they are also capable of performing that function in a central nerve. Thus, several questions arise: 1) What functions do these reactions play in the response of a nerve to injury? 2) Why are they delayed in optic nerves? 3) Does the delayed response play a role in the ability of the optic nerve to regenerate following injury?

E. Attempts to determine the function of amino acid modification of proteins focus on N-terminal arginylation

Complete answers to all of the questions posed above are not known. However, a possible reason for the delayed expression of the reactions in mammalian optic nerves has been recently explored. These experiments and their potential role in determining the ability of a nerve to regenerate will be discussed at the end of this chapter.

The answer to the first question posed, the physiological role played by these reactions following nerve injury, remains unknown despite investigations over the past 10 years. The endogenous substrates for modification by Arg and Lys (the two amino acids showing highest levels of posttranslational incorporation) in regenerating sciatic nerves of rats were examined using 2 dimensional SDS PAGE and approximate molecular weights and isoelectric points were determined (Luo et al., 1990). However, further characterization of the amino acid modified proteins has not been possible because the level of labeling was too low (picomoles/mg protein). A testable hypothesis for the function of one of the amino acids, Arg, emerged when experiments in reticulocyte lysates showed that the presence of Arg at the N-terminus of a protein led to its rapid degradation (Bachmair et al., 1986). This suggested that the $tRNA^{arg}$ modification of a protein might be a signal to the cell to degrade that protein.

F. N-terminal arginylation is implicated in the ubiquitin mediated degradation of damaged proteins – the N-end rule

Ubiquitin (Ub) is a highly conserved 76 amino acid peptide found in eukaryotic but not in prokaryotic cells. The covalent conjugation of Ub to a protein generally leads to the attachment of additional Ub moieties and the subsequent degradation of the modified protein by the 26S proteasome (reviewed in Varshavsky, 1997a). The enzyme mediating the transfer of Arg from tRNA to protein, arginyl transferase (R-transferase), is, like Ub, found only in eukaryotes (other transferases appear to serve similar functions in prokaryotes). Further association of R-transferase and Ub was discovered when it was shown that proteins to which Arg had been added by molecular engineering (Bachmair et al., 1986) or which had undergone enzymatic arginylation (Ferber and Ciechanover, 1987), were rapidly degraded by the Ub pathway. The presence of other amino acids in the N-terminus could also be destabilizing, but at least in some cases, this was due to their conversion to acidic amino acids (the only N-terminal residues capable of accepting Arg) or to selective N-terminal deamidation exposing an acidic residue (Baker and Varshavsky 1995). These findings form the basis for a rule governing the degradation of some cytosolic proteins, "The N-end rule." The essence of this proposal is that the nature of the N-terminal amino acid regulates the half-life of a protein; the primary destabilizing amino acid was Arg and it was transferred to the N-terminus from $tRNA^{arg}$ using R-transferase (Varshavsky et al., 1998).

The N-end rule hypothesis suggested a function for the activation of posttranslational arginylation following nerve injury. In this scheme, we reasoned that nerve injury leads to interruption of the axonal membrane with damage to intra-axonal proteins (primarily free radical induced oxidation of susceptible protein residues). While the axon membrane is still open and the axoplasm is in equilibrium with the extracellular fluids, cytosolic reactions cannot be activated.

But, following resealing and reestablishment of intracellular homeostasis, damaged proteins are identified and targeted for degradation (damaged proteins are one of the targets for the Ub pathway, Varshavsky, 1997a). This hypothesis predicts that oxidatively damaged proteins would be targets for arginylation and ubiquitination.

G. Failure to observe conclusive evidence of an association between oxidative damage and N-terminal arginylation of a protein in crude extracts of rat brain

Experiments were designed to test the hypothesis that oxidatively damaged proteins could be targets for N-terminal arginylation. This hypothesis would be inconsistent with prior studies demonstrating that only those proteins with acidic residues in their N-termini could be substrates for arginylation (Soffer 1980). However, several factors made this a reasonable series of experiments to attempt. First, the idea that only proteins with acidic N-terminals could be arginylated seemed too restrictive to be completely true *in vivo* . This was especially clear in light of the evidence that the substrates for the reaction changed during development (Hallak et al., 1985) and that the reaction could be activated following nerve injury (Shyne-Athwal et al., 1986). Second, while evidence from experiments using purified components indicated that only Arg participates in these reactions (Soffer 1980), we had found that a variety of amino acids could modify proteins under the appropriate *in vitro* conditions (Fig. 2). Third, when we attempted experiments in which the aminoacylating high molecular weight, multi-enzyme complex was fractionated and the components reconstituted, we found a precipitous loss of activity (Zanakis et al., 1984). The latter findings suggested that the activity of the posttranslational modifications were maximal when components were left in their multi-enzyme states (presumably similar to their physiological state) and that reducing them to their component parts resulted in a significant loss of activity. Thus, we studied arginylation in a crude fraction of tissue with the hope that it would retain some of its physiologically relevant activity.

The system we chose as a source of arginylating enzymes was a crude extract of rat brain that lacked protein synthetic activity (105k xg supernatant) and lacked molecules of less than 10k D (the inhibitor of arginylation in rat brain had been shown to be a peptide of approx. 3.5k D; Yu et al., 1993). To this we added radioactive Arg, ATP and a series of test proteins and peptides. In an initial series of experiments we found suggestive evidence for the arginylation of oxidized proteins when both oxidized bovine serum albumin and oxidized RNase were found to be substrates for arginylation (Zhang et al., 1998). More definitive evidence of this association was found when the oxidized A-chain of insulin was added to the extract. Here we could isolate the A-chain following incubation in the arginylating extract and show that radioactive Arg was associated with the purified (by reversed phase-HPLC) oxidized A-chain of insulin (Zhang et al., 1998). While these data were encouraging, less than 1 % of the A-chain was found to be arginylated and we could not distinguish between the possibility that Arg had been added to the N-terminal residue of the insulin A-chain (Gly) (supporting our hypothesis of *oxidation induced arginylation*) or whether the A-chain had undergone N-terminal cleavage exposing the 4th Glu residue and it was arginylated (supporting the *acidic N-terminus induced arginylation* hypothesis).

Experiments were also conducted in which the microtubule associated protein Tau was oxidized and examined for its ability to serve as a substrate for arginylation. Arginylation of tau was found. But it was not specific to the oxidized form of the molecule and the level of Arg associated with oxidized tau was in the low picomole range (Steinberg et al., 1997). As was the case with the oxidized A-chain, radioactive Arg labeling was so low (we estimated that approximately 1 in 10,000 molecules of tau had been arginylated) that it was not possible to determine if arginylation had been to the non-acidic N-terminal amino acid or to a truncated form of tau which contained an acidic N-terminal amino acid.

H. Studies with synthetic peptides fail to show oxidized residues or proteins with N-terminal acidic amino acids as signals for arginylation

To try to circumvent the problems described above, we constructed a synthetic peptide that contained no acidic residues but did contain several residues capable of being oxidized. If the *oxidation induced arginylation* hypothesis was correct this 10 amino acid peptide, when oxidized, should be arginylated. We also constructed the same peptide with a Glu in the N-terminus. If the *acidic residue induced arginylation* hypothesis was correct this peptide should be a substrate for arginylation. Neither peptide showed evidence of arginylation, despite confirmation that the oxidized A-chain of insulin (22 amino acid) was arginylated under identical conditions (Ingoglia et al., 1999; Fig. 4). Our tentative conclusion is that in these crude extracts of brain, and likely *in vivo* as well, the attributes of a protein that make it a target for arginylation are more complex than either the presence of an acidic N-terminal amino acid, or the presence of an oxidatively damaged residue. We are now trying to uncover the properties of a neuronal protein which make it a substrate for arginylation in an attempt to understand the function of this reaction following nerve injury.

I. Failure to find a correlation between N-terminal arginylation and ubiquitination

In trying to understand what leads to the arginylation of a protein, our ultimate goal was to test the hypothesis that once arginylated, a protein becomes a substrate for ubiquitination and degradation according to the "N-end Rule" (see above). To date, we have been unable to demonstrate this association with any degree of certainty. This is despite attempts (using Western blots of arginylated proteins and probing with a monoclonal antibody to ubiquitin) to observe this association with arginylated oxidized BSA, ribonuclease and the A-chain of insulin (Zhang et al., 1998), arginylated oxidized tau (Steinberg 1997) and recent experiments examin-

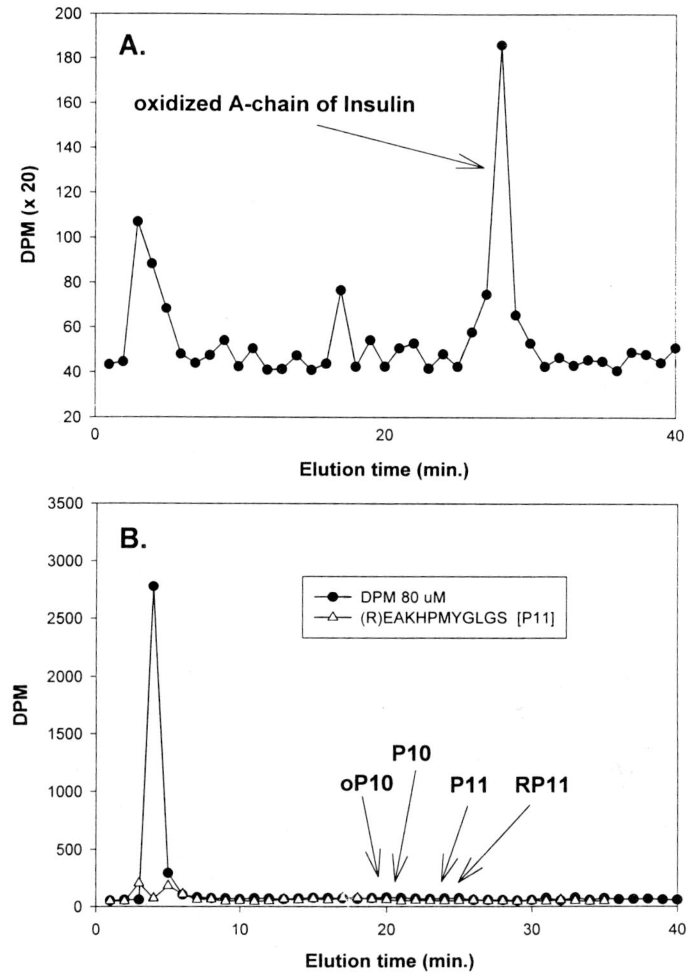

Figure 4 Arginylation of the oxidized A-chain of insulin in a crude extract of a rat brain homogenate (A) and the failure to arginylate synthetic peptides in the same extract (B). P10 is a construct containing several oxidized residues (oP10) and P11 is a peptide containing an acidic amino acid in the N-terminus. Peptides were separated by reverse phase HPLC and the arrows indicate the position where each eluted from the columns. RP 11 is the position of migration of the P11 peptide with Arg in its N-terminal (see Zhang et al., 1998 and Ingoglia et al., 2000, for details).

ing oxidatively damaged proteins in synaptosomes (Ramanathan et al., 1998). In the latter series of experiments we could demonstrate an association between oxidative damage and ubiquitination of synaptosomal proteins (Ramanathan et al., 1999), but failed to show that the proteins that were oxidized were substrates for arginylation prior to their ubiquitination. Thus, our original hypothesis is not supported by the experimental data. This may be because the levels of arginylation and ubiquitination are too low for us to detect, because the experimental conditions have not been optimized to observe the phenomena or because the hypothesis is incorrect. Without completely abandoning the possibility of a link between nerve injury induced up-regulation of arginylation and ubiquitination, we are currently investigating the possibility that arginylation, and other posttranslational amino acid modifications (e.g., by Lys/Leu; Shyne-Athwal 1986, 1988) play roles in the response of nerves to injury which we have not yet considered.

III. TRANSFER OF SMALL MOLECULES FROM AXONS TO PERIAXONAL CELLS

One of the difficulties encountered in demonstrating the intra-axonal localization of RNA in vertebrate nerves (see above) was that following the *in vivo* injections of ^{3}H-uridine or adenosine into the vicinity of a nerve cell body, the nucleosides (or their derivatives) were exported into the axon and released to cells surrounding the axon where they were then utilized by periaxonal cells in the synthesis of RNA (Por et al., 1978; Ingoglia and Tuliszewski, 1976; Lindquist et al., 1981). Thus, nerves contained locally synthesized RNA from adaxonal cells as well as putative intra-axonal tRNA. This was completely unexpected since similar experiments performed using radioactive amino acids had all shown that while radioactive proteins were transported axonally and could be transferred to postsynaptic neurons, free amino acids were not transported, nor did cells along the length of the axons show any evidence of the presence of labeled proteins (reviewed in Grafstein and Forman, 1980). What made this finding intriguing was that during regeneration of the optic nerve of goldfish (Ingoglia et al., 1982) or the sciatic nerve of rats (Lindquist et al., 1981), there were large increases in the levels of free nucleosides transported and transferred to surrounding cells where they were utilized for RNA synthesis.

A. Nucleosides(tides) are transferred from axons to Schwann cells and incorporated into RNA in Schwann cell cytoplasm

Following injections of ^{3}H-uridine into the spinal cord to label ventral horn cells giving rise to the motor axons of the sciatic nerve, radioactivity moves along the axon at approximately the rate of the slow component B (3-4 mm/day) of axonal transport, predominantly labeling the cytoplasm of surrounding Schwann cells (Fig. 5; Lindquist et al., 1981). The label is present as all species of RNA (demonstrated by SDS PAGE, Lindquist et al., 1981), indicating that Schwann cells used axonal precursors for RNA synthesis. We have never been able to see this kind of labeling following local injections into the nerve itself (unpublished), nor following systemic injections. Based on these and other data we proposed that

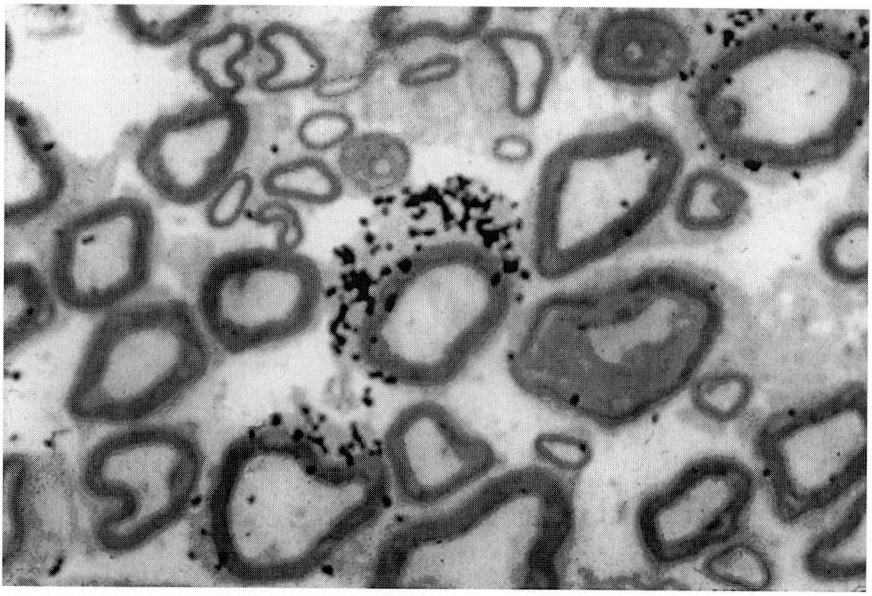

Figure 5 Light microscopic autoradiogram of a histological section taken from the sciatic nerve of a rat removed from a region proximal to a nerve crush and 10 days after the intraspinal injection of ^{3}H-uridine. Radioactivity was confirmed as ribosomal and transfer RNA. Note the heavy concentration of grains over Schwann cell cytoplasm (Lindquist et al., 1981).

axons supply at least a portion of the nuclesosides (nucleotides) needed to support RNA synthesis in Schwann and glial cells and that this was a mechanism whereby axons could influence glial metabolism (Ingoglia et al., 1982). While this still seems a likely possibility, other roles for transferred purines and their derivatives have been reported recently and will be discussed below.

B. Polyamines are transferred from axons to Schwann cells and are located over Schwann cell cytoplasm and nuclei

When identical experiments were performed using radioactive putrescine or the polyamines spermidine and spermine, similar results were obtained; i.e., polyamines are transported at approximately 3-4 mm/d, the amount transported increases in regenerating nerves and they are not confined to the axon, but rather are transferred to periaxonal cells (Ingoglia et al., 1982; Lindquist et al., 1985). The difference in distribution was that labeled polyamines were frequently found over myelin and over Schwann cell nuclei (Fig 6).

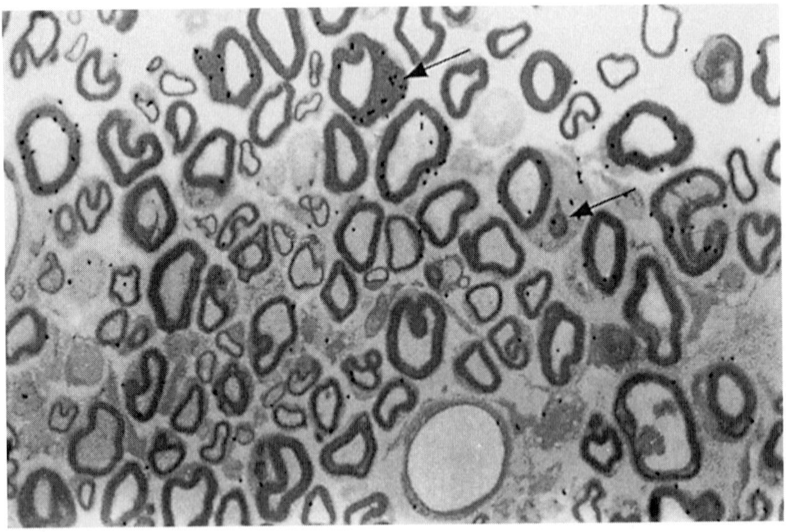

Figure 6 Light microscopic autoradiogram of the sciatic nerve of a rat taken approximately 20 mm from the spinal cord and 3 days after the intraspinal injection of ^{3}H-putrescine. Radioactivity was confirmed as primarily spermine and spermidine. Note the silver grains over myelin and Schwann cell cytoplasm and nuclei (arrows) (Lindquist et al., 1985).

C. Lipids are transferred from axons to Schwann cell myelin and cytoplasm

Using either ^{3}H-glycerol (Droz et al., 1978) or ^{3}H-choline (Gould et al., 1982) it has been shown that lipid precursors, like nucleotides and polyamines can be transported axonally, transferred to surrounding myelin and Schwann cell cytoplasm and utilized there for lipid biosynthesis (Haley and Ledeen, 1979). In all of the studies cited above it was clear that the processes being examined were not the result of simple diffusion nor were they true for all small molecules, but represented active axonal transport and intercellular transfer processes of specific substances and were therefore likely to be physiologically relevant events (Ingoglia et al., 1982). The functional questions raised by these findings have for the most part, still not been answered. However, recent studies may indicate fruitful areas for further experimentation and help to answer questions concerning the role played by these processes in nerve regeneration.

D. The transfer of small molecules from axons to Schwann cells may be mediated by paranodal, axon-Schwann cell networks

One of the first questions raised by the findings described above was how these small molecules can be transferred from axons to surrounding cells. A recently investigated prime candidate for mediating this transfer is the membrane specialization found at the paranodal region of the nodes of Ranvier of myelinated axons. These areas of interdigitating axonal and Schwann cell membranes (axon-Schwann cell networks, ASNs), were first described in feline ventral root fibers (Berthold, 1968). A function for these morphological specializations was found by Gatzinsky et al., when they showed that fluorescent latex microspheres which were introduced into the terminals of damaged (Persson and Gazinsky, 1993) or intact (Gatzinsky, Persson and Berthold, 1997) motor axons of rats were, following their retrograde axonal transport, transferred to surrounding Schwann cell cytoplasm. These paranodal regions contain large concentrations of lysosomes (Gatzinsky and Berthold,1990) and mitochondria (Rydmark et al., 1998) and have been proposed to be sites where the axon can eliminate retrogradely transported foreign substances and debris before reaching the perikaryon. The function of ASNs in transferring anterogradely transported molecules has not been investigated. However, they must be considered as prime candidates for the anatomical substrates responsible for the transcellular transfer of nucleosides, polyamines and lipid precursors.

E. Small molecules transferred from axons to surrounding cells may regulate periaxonal gene expression and/or metabolism

Schwann cell gene expression is dependent, in part, on its association with axons. Following axotomy, Schwann cells in the distal nerve segment which have lost contact with their axons, increase expression of NGF and the p75 NGF receptor (Heumann et al., 1987), glial maturation factor β (Bosch et al., 1989) and N-CAM (Jensen et al., 1987). While evidence indicates that axon membrane contact may be required to activate some Schwann cell genes, the regulation of $p75^{NGFR}$ and myelin P_0 expression has been shown to be independent of membrane contact, but rather, to be under the control of diffusible molecules released from axons (Bolin and Shooter, 1993). These molecules have not as yet been identified, but both nucleosides and polyamines or their derivatives released from axons to surrounding cells may be candidates for regulators of gene expression in Schwann cells.

In studies examining the signals for myelination in cultured dorsal root ganglion cells it was shown that low frequency neural impulses reduced myelination and that the inhibition of myelination correlated with a decrease in the expression of the cell adhesion molecule, L1 (Stevens et al., 1998a). Subsequent experiments showed that the transcription factor released from axons was likely to be ATP, or a derivative of ATP (Stevens et al., 1998b). Thus, axonally derived adenosine or a derivative may regulate myelination by controlling Schwann cell gene expression. Another purine derivative (AIT-082) has been reported to enhance neurite outgrowth from PC12 cells (Middlemiss et al., 1995) and stimulate genes involved in regenerative repair (press release from NeoTherapeutics, Irvine Calif, July 27, 1998). Finally, synthetic polyamides containing N-methylimidazole and N-methylpyrrole amino acids have been shown to be able to penetrate cell membranes and bind with a specific region of DNA (Gottesfeld et al., 1997). While these experiments have been performed with synthetic polyamides, it may be that *in vivo* the polyamines play a similar role and can work as activators or inhibitors of transcription. Thus, polyamines (or derivatives) released from axons may regulate gene expression in intact and regenerating nerves.

A possible non-genetic role for polyamines may be related to the regulation of ion channel activity. Recent studies have shown that in glia, polyamines can act as modulators of inward rectifying K channels, performing an important role in sequestering excess extracellular K^+. These experiments also show that glia have a low capacity for synthesizing their own polyamines since under normal conditions ornithine decarboxylase, (required for polyamine synthesis) is expressed in very low amounts (Biedermann et al., 1998). Thus, it may be that one of the functions of the transfer of polyamines from axons to glia is to regulate glial K channels thereby regulating the sequestration of extracellular K^+ .

IV. FUTURE DIRECTIONS

The questions raised above concerning: 1) the function of the tRNA mediated posttranslational protein modifications in nerve regeneration and 2) whether the delay in the activation of these reactions in injured central nerves (Shyne-Athwal et al., 1986) is related to their failure to regenerate remain unanswered. However, recent experiments may shed light on why the reactions were delayed in injured central compared with peripheral nerves. In these experiments, we reasoned that if cut optic axons failed to reseal in the same time as cut peripheral nerves (this volume, chapter by Bittner and Fishman), then a delay in re-establishing the internal milieu of the axon could result in an environment not suitable for the reactions we were studying or any other cytosolic reactions for that matter. If the axons eventually did reseal, then the reactions might be able to be activated and this would be consistent with our earlier data (Shyne-Athwal et al., 1986). This hypothesis has been tested in the laboratory of Sansar Sharma. Using a dye exclusion technique to estimate the length of time needed for resealing (this volume, chapter by Bittner and Fishman), dorsal root ganglion cell axons cut *in vivo*, were found to completely exclude the dye by about 10 hours after injury, while optic axons transected under the same experimental procedure, did not exclude the dye for more than 24 hours after axotomy (Ahmed, Ingoglia and Sharma, submitted). Thus, damaged optic nerve axons appear to have an impaired ability to close severed axons when compared with peripheral nerve axons. This may be the reason why cell death is so prominent following optic nerve injury (this volume, chapter by Chaudary and Sharma) and suggests that a possible interventional strategy following optic nerve damage in humans would be immediate attempts to create an environment at the site of injury that would promote resealing.

With respect to studies on the effect of transcellularly transferred small molecules, what seems clear is that these molecules, that have been demonstrated unequivocally to be delivered from axons to glia/Schwann cells, may affect transcription, ion channel activity and the general metabolism of cells surrounding the axons. The specific details of their action and how the transfer of these small molecules to surrounding cells aids in the successful regeneration of a nerve are likely to be fruitful areas for further experiments.

REFERENCES

Bachmair A, Finley D, Varshavsky A (1986) In vivo half-life of a protein is a function of its amino-terminal residue.Science 234:179-186.

Baker RT, Varshavsky A (1995). Yeast N-terminal amidase: a new enzyme and component of the N-end rule pathway. J Biol Chem 270:12065-12074.

Berthold CH (1968). Ultrastructure of the node-paranode region of mature feline ventral lumbar spinal-root fibres. Acta Soc Med Uppsala 73:(Suppl 9) 37-78.

Biedermann B, Sketchkov SN, Brunk I, Bringmann A, Pannicke T, Bernstein HG, Faude F, Germer A, Veh R, Reichenbach A. (1998). Spermine/spermidine is expressed by retinal glial (Muller) cells and controls distinct K^+ channels of their membrane. Glia 23:209-220.

Black MM and Lasek RJ (1977). The presence of transfer RNA in the axoplasm of the squid giant axon. J Neurobiol 8:229-237.

Bolin LM, Shooter EM (1993). Neurons regulate Schwann cell genes by diffusible molecules. J Cell Biol 123:237-243.

Bosch EP, Zhong PW, Lim R (1989). Axonal signals regulate expression of glial maturation factor in Schwann cells: an immunohistochemical study of injured sciatic nerves and cultured Schwann cells. J Neurosci 9:3690-3698.

Capano CA, Giuditta A, Castigli E, Kaplan BB (1987). Occurrence and sequence complexity of polyadenylated RNA in squid axoplasm. J Neurochem 49:698-704.

Chun JT, Gioio AE, Crispino M, Eyman M, Giuditta A, Kaplan BB (1997). Molecular cloning and characterization of a novel mRNA present in the squid giant axon. J Neurosci Res 49:144-153.

Droz B, DiGiamberardino L, Koenig HL, Boyenval J, Hassig R (1978). Axon-myelin transfer of phospholipid components in the course of their axonal transport as visualized by radioautography. Brain Res 155:347-353.

Eng H, Lund K, Campenot RB (1999). Synthesis of α tubulin, actin, and other proteins in axons of sympathetic neurons in compartmented cultures. J Neurosci 19:1-9.

Ferber S, Ciechanover A (1987). Role of arginine-tRNA in protein degradation by the ubiquitin pathway. Nature 326:808-811.

Gambetti P, Autilio-Gambett L, Shafer B, Pfaff L (1973). Quantitative autoradiographic study of labeled RNA in rabbit optic nerve after intraocular injection of ^{3}H-uridine. J Cell Biol 59:677-684.

Gambetti P, Ingoglia NA, Autilio-Gambetti L, Weis P (1978). Distribution of [^{3}H]RNA in goldfish optic tectum following intraocular or intracranial injection of [^{3}H]uridine.

Evidence of axonal migration of RNA in regenerating optic fibers. Brain Res 154:285-300.

Gatzinsky KP, Berthold CH (1990). Lysosomal activity at nodes of Ranvier during retrograde axonal transport of horseradish peroxidase in alpha-motor neurons of the cat. J Neurocytol 19:989-1002.

Gatzinsky KP, Persson GH, Berthold CH (1997). Removal of retrogradely transported material from rat lumbosacral alpha-motor axons by paranodal axon-Schwann cell networks. Glia 20:115-126.

Giuditta A, Dettban WD, Brzin M (1968). Protein synthesis in the isolated giant axon of the squid. Proc Nat Acad Sci USA 59:1284-1287.

Giuditta A, Metafora S, Felsami A, Del Rio, A (1977). Factors of protein synthesis in the axons of squid giant axons. J Neurochem 28: 1393-1395.

Gould RM, Spivack WD, Sinatra RS, Lindquist TD, Ingoglia NA (1982). Axonal transport of choline lipids in normal and regenerating rat sciatic nerve. J Neurochem 39:1569-1578.

Gottesfeld JM, Neely L, Trauger JW, Baird EE, Dervan PB (1997) Regulation of gene expression by small molecules. Nature 387:202-205.

Grafstein B, Forman D.S. (1980) Intracellular transport in neurons. Physiol. Rev. 60: 1167-1283.

Haley JE, Ledeen RW (1979) Incorporation of axonally transported substances into myelin lipids. J Neurochem 32:735-742.

Hallak ME, Barra HS, Caputto R (1985) Post-translational incorporation of [^{14}C] arginine into rat brain proteins. Acceptor changes during development. J Neurochem 44:665-669.

Heumann R, Lindholm D, Brandtlow C, Meyer M Radeke MJ, Misko TP, Shooter EM, Thoenen H (1987) Differential regulation of mRNA encoding nerve growth factor and its receptor in rat sciatic nerve during development, degeneration and regeneration; role of macrophages. Proc Natl Acad Sci USA 84:8735-8739.

Ingoglia, NA (1979). 4S RNA is present in regenerating optic nerves of goldfish. Science, Vol. 206, 73-75.

Ingoglia NA, Chakraborty G, Yu M, Luo D, Liu C (1990) Posttranslational modification of nerve proteins by amino acids. Restorative Neurology and Neuroscience 1:245-252.

Ingoglia NA, Giuditta A, Zanakis MF, Babigian A, Tasaki I, Chakratorty G, Sturman J (1983). Incorporation of ^{3}H-amino acids into proteins in a partially purified fraction of axoplasm: evidence for transfer RNA mediated, posttranslational protein modification in squid giant axons. J Neurosci 3:2463-2473.

Ingoglia NA, Ramanathan M, Zhang N, Tzeng, B, Mathur G, Opuni K, Donnelly R (2000). What is the signal for the posttranslational arginylation of proteins? Neurochem Res. 25:51-58.

Ingoglia NA, Sharma SC, Pilchman J, Baranowski K, Sturman JA (1982). Axonal transport and transcellular transfer of nucleosides and polyamines in intact and regenerating optic nerves of goldfish: speculation on the axonal regulation of periaxonal cell metabolism. J Neurosci 2:1412-1423.

Ingoglia NA, Tuliszewski R. (1976): Transfer RNA may be axonally transported during regeneration of goldfish optic nerves. Brain Res 112:371-381.

Ingoglia NA, Weis P, Mycek J (1975) Axonal transport of RNA during regeneration of optic nerves of goldfish. Brain Res 112:371-381.

Jensen KR, Mirsky R, Morgan L (1987). Myelinated, but not unmyelinated axons, reversibly down regulate N-CAM in Schwann cells. J Neurocytol 16:681-688.

Kaji H, Novelli GD, Kaji AA (1963). A soluble amino acid incorporating system from rat liver. Biochem. Biophys. Acta. 76:1034-1040.

Koenig E, Martin R (1996). Cortical plaque-like structures identify ribosome-containing domains in the Mauthner cell axon. J Neurosci 16:1400-1411.

Lasek RJ, Dabrowski C, Nordlander R (1973). Analysis of axonal RNA from invertebrate giant axons. Nature, New Biology 144: 162-165.

Lindquist TD, Ingoglia NA, Gould R (1981). 4S RNA is transported axonally in normal and regenerating axons of the sciatic nerve of rats. Brain Res 230:181-194.

Lindquist TD, Sturman JA, Gould RM, Ingoglia NA (1985). Axonal transport of polyamines in intact and regenerating axons of the rat sciatic nerve. J Neurochem 44:1913-1919.

Luo D, Chakraborty G, Ingoglia NA (1990). Post-translational modification of proteins by arginine and lysine following crush injury and during regeneration of rat sciatic nerves. Restorative Neurology and Neuroscience 2:53-61.

Middlemiss PJ, Glasky AJ Rathbone MP, Werstuik E, Hindley S, Gysbers J (1995). AIT-082, a unique purine derivative, enhances nerve growth facotr mediated neurite outgrowth from PC12 cells. Neurosci Lett 199(2):131-134.

Persson H, Gazinsky KP (1993). Distribution of retrogradely transported fluorescent latex microspheres in rat lumbosacral ventral root axons following peripheral crush injury: a light and electron microscopic study. Brain Res 630:115-124.

Por SB, Komiya Y, McGregor A, Jeffrey PL, Gunning PW, Austin L (1978). The axoplasmic transport of 4S RNA within the sciatic nerve of the chicken. Neurosci Lett 8:165-169.

Ramanathan M, Zhang N, Ingoglia NA (1998). Oxidative stress in synaptosomes. II. Ubiquitination of synaptosomal proteins. Soc. Neurosci. Abstr Vol 24: 2157.

Ramanathan M, Hassanian M, Levitt M, Seth A, Tolman JS, Fried AF, Ingoglia NA (1999). Oxidative stress increases ubiquitin-protein conjugates in synaptosomal proteins. NeuroReport 10:3797-3802.

Rydmark M, Berthold CH, Gatzinsky KP (1998). Paranodal Schwann cell mitochondria in spinal roots of the cat. An ultrastructural morphometric analysis. J Neurocytol 27:99-108.

Shyne-Athwal S, Chakraborty G, Gage E, Ingoglia NA (1988). Comparison of posttranslational protein modification by amino acid addition after crush injury to sciatic and optic nerves of rat. Exp Neurol 99:281-295

Shyne-Athwal S, Riccio RV, Chakraborty G. Ingoglia NA (1986). Protein modification by amino acid addition is increased in crushed sciatic but not optic nerves. Science 231:603-605.

Soffer RL (1980). Biochemistry and biology of amino acyl tRNA protein transferases, in: *Transfer RNA: Biological Aspects* (Soll D, Abelson JN and Schimmel PR eds.) Monograph No.93, Cold Spring Harbor Laboratory, Cold Spring Harbor, NY, pp, 493-505.

Steinberg, D.J. and Ingoglia, N.A. (1997) Tau: Oxidation, arginylation and ubiquitination. Soc. Neurosci Abstr V23 p. 1643.

Stevens B, Tanner S, Fields RD (1998). Control of myelination by specific patterns of neural impulses. J Neurosci 18:9303-9311.

Stevens B, Fields RD (1998) Neural impulse activity induces CREB phosphorylation in Schwann cells. Soc. Neurosci. Abstr Vol 24: 49.

Varshavsky A (1997a). The ubiquitin system. Trends Biochem Sci 22:383-387.

Varshavsky A (1997b). The N-end rule pathway of protein degradation. Genes Cells 2:13-28.

Varshavsky A, Byrd C, Davydov IV, Dohmen RJ Du F, Ghislain M, Gonzalex M, Grigoryev S, Johnson ES, Johnsson N, Johston JA, Kwon YT, Levy F, Lomovskaya O, Madura K, Ota, I, Rumenapf T, Shrader TE, Suzuki T, Turner,G, Waller PRH, Webster A. (1998). The N-end rule pathway, p223-278. In: *Ubiquitin and the Biology of the Cell.* Peters JM, Harris JR, and Finley D (eds) Plenum Press, New York, N.Y.

Yu, M., Grabow, M. and Ingoglia, N.A. (1993). Isolation of a peptide which inhibits the posttranslational arginylation of protein in rat brain. Journal of Molecular Neuroscience, 4 (3): 195-203.

Zanakis MF, Chakraborty G, Sturman JA, Ingoglia NA (1994) Posttranslational protein modification by amino acid addition in intact and regenerating axons of the rat sciatic nerve. J Neurochem 43:1286-1294.

Zhang N, Donnelly R, Ingoglia NA (1998) Evidence that oxidized proteins are substrates for N-terminal arginylation. Neurochemical Research 23:1411-1420.

14

Gene Expression in Degenerating/Regenerating Nerves

Clemens Gillen
University of Düsseldorf, Düsseldorf, Germany

I. INTRODUCTION

The analysis of gene expression in injured peripheral nerves plays an important role in the understanding of nerve regeneration and has led to a plethora of reports during the last decade. The major interest in the molecular mechanisms of peripheral nerve regeneration and degeneration is based on several principles. The scientific interpretation of expression data can be linked to a well-established sequence of histopathological reactions, known as Wallerian degeneration (for review see Schwartz, 1987). These cellular reactions include the complete degeneration of the axon distal to the lesion, myelin breakdown, dedifferentiation, and proliferation of Schwann cells as well as other non-neuronal cells. Macrophages invade the injured nerve (Stoll and Müller, 1986) phagocytose and degrade axon and myelin membrane, and stimulate the proliferation of Schwann cells. As a consequence the distal segment of an injured nerve provides a supportive environment for axonal regeneration and nerve maturation. Regenerative reactions include axonal regrowth, reestablishment of axon-Schwann cell contacts, redifferentiation of Schwann cells and myelination of axons, and eventually reinervation of the target. The regenerative potency of degenerated peripheral nerve stumps was demonstrated by David and Aguayo (1981) who showed that peripheral nerve grafts could induce axonal regeneration of CNS neurons. These stereotyped and reproducible reactions are the result of intricate interactions among different cell populations including neurons, Schwann cells, endoneurial fibroblasts and endothelial cells normally present in peripheral nerves as well as hematogenous cells (e.g. macrophages) that infiltrate the damaged nerve. Therefore it is likely that this stereotyped sequence of cellular events reflects the differential and coordinate expression of specific genes. The regeneration of peripheral nerves is a striking example of plasticity within the nervous system and findings herein may help to elucidate other plasticity-associated processes such as nervous system development, memory or learning. There are well-established animal models of peripheral nerve lesion, which are easy to perform, yield reproducible results and allow the distinction between degenerative and regenerative events due to different lesion paradigms. Whereas regeneration occurs after a crush injury, regeneration is prevented when both stumps of transected nerves are ligated. In addition these models allow not only the temporal analysis of gene expression but also a spatial expression analysis due to the proximodistal direction of the regenerative response originating from the site of the injury.

The molecular analyses performed with these animal models serve several purposes. Genes identified by other means, that harbor an interesting function could be tested for a potential role in nerve regeneration or degeneration. For genes with unknown function the expression analysis can help to elucidate their function. Based on the fidelity of this model, several systematic cloning strategies were used in order to isolate new regeneration-associated genes and have led to the identification of several relevant genes (De Leon et al., 1991; Gillen et al., 1995). Taken together, these studies represent further steps towards a deeper understanding of the molecular basis of peripheral nerve regeneration. In this chapter I describe and compare the distinct time courses and cellular origins of expression of these gene/gene products and further discuss their established or putative molecular interrelationships and functions with respect to the molecular regeneration program of the PNS.

II. REGULATION OF NEUROTROPHIC FACTORS AND THEIR RECEPTORS SHOW COMPLEX PATTERNS

A. Neurotrophins

The neurotrophin family includes NGF, BDNF, neurotrophin-3 (NT-3) and NT-4/5, which bind to high affinity tyrosine kinase receptors (trkA-C) and a low affinity NGF receptor, p75 (for review see Mendell, 1995). All neurotrophins, except NT-3 are upregulated in the distal stump after axotomy (Table 1). NGF mRNA is regulated in a biphasic manner. While normally expressed at very low concentrations, it is strongly upregulated within the first 12 hours after injury, and a second upregulation at 3 days after injury correlates with invasion of macrophages. Interleukin-1 released by these invading macrophages is thought to be the most essential mediator of this effect. The sustained up-regulation of NGF mRNA after axotomy contrasts with a decline during remyelination that takes place in the regenerating nerve. The role of NGF during nerve regeneration is still in question. The upregulated $p75^{NGFR}$ in Schwann cells has been suggested to present NGF to high affinity receptors on regenerating NGF-sensitive axons (Johnson et al., 1990). However, the downregulation of Trk receptors and $p75^{NGFR}$ on axotomized dorsal root ganglia (DRG) neurons and the reduced transport of neurotrophins by regenerating axons (Raivich et al., 1991; Raivich and Kreutzberg, 1993) support an autocrine role for NGF in Schwann cells. The regeneration-enhancing effect of NGF appears to be more indirect by promoting Schwann cell migration (Anton et al., 1994), increasing cell adhesion via upregulation of the L1 molecule on Schwann cells and neurites (Seilheimer and Schachner, 1987; Friedlander et al., 1986) and enhancing angiogenesis (Santos et al., 1991).

BDNF mRNA rises slowly in non-neuronal cells at 7 days after injury, when the regenerating axons are growing into the distal stump, and reaches its maximum 4 weeks later (Funakoshi et al., 1993; Meyer et al., 1992). The temporal and spatial pattern of expression of BDNF is different from NGF, and correlates with a different mechanism of regulation. BDNF is effective in promoting the survival and growth of not only sensory and sympathetic neurons but also motoneurons (Sendtner et al., 1992b) and thus could complement the effect of NGF.

NT-3 mRNA, which is clearly detected in the intact sciatic nerve, is downregulated within 6-12 hours after nerve transection in the distal segment, then returns progressively to control levels 2 weeks after injury (Funakoshi et al., 1993). A similar expression pattern for NT-3 after sciatic nerve crush did not correlate with an axon-regulated expression (Chai et al., 1998).

NT-4/5 mRNA decreases 6-12 hr after axotomy in the distal segment of sciatic nerves, but increases progressively thereafter, reaching levels eightfold higher than control after 2 weeks (Funakoshi et al., 1993).

Expression of trkA mRNA is not detectable in the injured sciatic nerve either proximal or distal to the lesion. TrkB and trkC mRNAs increase in Schwann cells proximal to the lesion, but decrease in the distal segment of the injured nerve (Funakoshi et al., 1993). On the other hand, $p75^{NGFR}$ mRNA is up-regulated in Schwann cells in proximal, as well as in distal nerve segments, but this receptor is downregulated in sensory and motoneurons after axotomy (Heumann et al., 1987a, 1987b; Zhou et al., 1996). Besides its role in accumulating neurotrophins at the Schwann cell membrane there is now evidence that $p75^{NGFR}$ may be involved in apoptosis, and that NGF binding prevents $p75^{NGFR}$ -mediated apoptosis. This is also supported by a recent report of increased neuronal survival and regeneration capacity in $p75^{NGFR}$ -knock out mice (Ferri et al., 1998).

B. Neuropoietic cytokines

Neurotrophic factors of the cytokine family include ciliary neurotrophic factor (CNTF), interleukin-6 (IL-6) and leukemia inhibitory factor (LIF). They bind to receptors that have both common (gp130, LIFR-β) and specific (CNTFRα, IL-6Rα) transmembrane subunits and signal using the JAK/STAT pathway. CNTF mRNA is present in Schwann cells of adult sciatic nerves (Friedman et al., 1992). After axotomy, CNTF mRNA levels fall dramatically in the distal stump and do not recover until axons regenerate (Sendtner et al., 1992a). CNTF is believed to act as a "lesion factor," since it lacks the secretory signal sequence and is not likely to be released unless the Schwann cells are damaged. Consistent with this hypothesis, it has been shown that CNTF is released by non-neuronal cells in the facial nerve after lesion, in quantities sufficient to prevent the degeneration of motoneurons (Friedman et al., 1992) and peripheral nerve axotomy enhances retrograde transport of CNTF (Curtis et al., 1993).

IL-6 is induced within hours of nerve injury (Bolin et al., 1995, Reichert et al., 1996). It remains elevated for 3 weeks in degenerating nerves of mice (Reichert et al., 1996) but not in crushed rat nerves (Bolin et al., 1995). It is expressed predominantly in fibroblasts and macrophages but also, to a lesser extent in Schwann cells. Synthesis of IL-6 in these cells may be stimulated by IL-1 (Ng et al., 1994), LIF (Villiger et al., 1993) and IL-6 itself (Bolin et al., 1995). Although the precise role of IL-6 in the distal stump is presently unknown its early upregulation in fibroblasts suggests a role in promoting the infiltration of hematogenous cells into the degenerating nerve stump.

Within 24 hours after rat sciatic nerve injury, the mRNA of LIF increases in Schwann cells adjacent to the lesion site and remains high for about 1 week (Curtis et al., 1994). LIF acts as a neurotrophic factor for sensory neurons and motoneurons and induces the expression of neuropeptides, such as vasoactive intestinal peptide (VIP), somatostatin, and substance P (Ip et al., 1992; Patterson, 1994). A prominent role in nerve regeneration is also supported by the enhanced retrograde transport and accumulation of LIF in sensory neurons and motoneurons (Curtis et al., 1994).

C. Fibroblast growth factors

The lesion-induced decline in FGF expression (Eckenstein et al., 1991; Ishikawa et al., 1992) is in contrast to the regeneration-enhancing function of FGFs, e.g., by inducing mitosis of Schwann cells and by promoting angiogenesis. Similar to CNTF, the FGFs lack the signal peptide sequence necessary for secretion.

D. Glia-cell-line derived neurotrophic factors (GDNF)

The GDNF-family includes Artemin, GDNF, Neurturin and Persephin and is distantly related to the TGF-β family. They signal through a multicomponent receptor system composed of a high-affinity binding component (GFRα1-GFRα4) and a common signaling component (RET). After nerve injury the GDNF mRNA is upregulated in Schwann cells proximal as well as distal to the injury site and expression of this mRNA remains at high levels for at least 5 month (Hammarberg et al., 1996). GDNF exhibits a strong trophic effect on Schwann cells and has been shown to be the most potent survival–promoting–factor for adults motoneurons *in vivo* (Li et al., 1995). Artemin is a survival factor for sensory and sympathetic nerves *in vitro* and was found to be upregulated in the distal segment of the sciatic nerve following transection (Baloh et al., 1998). Concomitantly the GFRα-mRNA is upregulated in the distal but not in proximal parts of the sciatic nerve or in spinal cord.

E. Glia Growth Factors (GGFs)

The Glia growth factors (GGF-I, GGF-II, GGF-III) are alternatively spliced members of the neuregulin family that act as potent mitogens by binding to the erbB receptors (Marchionni et al, 1993; Minghetti et al., 1996). After axotomy both GGF and erbB2 and erbB3 are coordinately upregulated in the Schwann cells of the distal stump (Carroll et al., 1997).

F. Insulin-like growth factors (IGFs) and their receptors

Within 3 days after axotomy the mRNA of IGF–I and of IGF-I receptors increase significantly in the distal nerve segment. The mRNA of IGF-I reaches a maximum between day 4 and 6 postinjury and declines during the following 24 hours (Cheng et al., 1996; Pu et al., 1995). This expression pattern parallels the proliferation of nonneuronal cells after nerve injury, suggesting that IGF-I acts as a mitogen. In contrast, due to its late expression in distal nerve segments, IGF-II has been suggested to be involved in the establishment of neuromuscular junctions (Pu et al., 1995).

G. Transforming growth factors (TGFs)

The low TGF-β1 mRNA level rapidly increases to maximum levels within 4 days after axotomy of rat sciatic nerves, whereas the high level of TGF-β3 mRNA in non-injured nerves decreases markedly postlesion (Scherer et al., 1993). As TGFβ1-mRNA is detected in Schwann cells and its expression pattern correlates with Schwann cell proliferation, TGF-β may be released and induce Schwann cell mitosis via an autocrine pathway (Ridley et al., 1989; Scherer et al., 1993). TGFβ resembles cAMP dependent mitogens in inducing the premyelinating status of Schwann cells, including the down-regulation of $p75^{NGFR}$ and upregulation of NgCAM/L1, NCAM and SCIP (Einheber et al., 1995; Mews and Meyer, 1993).

H. Other growth factors

GMF-β is synthesized in the distal nerve segment after injury (Bosch et al., 1989) and increases the number of regenerating axons when applied to the lesion site (Harman et al., 1991). The mRNA of the sulfated glycoprotein SGP-1, the rat homologue of the human prosaposin is upregulated after nerve injury (Gillen et al., 1995). Proteolytic cleavage of prosaposin leads to the saposins A-D that activate different sphingolipid hydrolases. Additional functions in regeneration can be assumed, because prosaposin shows neurotrophic activity *in vitro* (O'Brien et al., 1994) and facilitates peripheral nerve regeneration *in vivo* (Kotani et al., 1996).

Several neurotrophic factors that are expressed in the distal nerve stump appear to promote the survival of injured neurons. These trophic activities have mostly been observed *in vitro* studies, but this role has not been confirmed *in vivo* after nerve crush. There is evidence that most of the regeneration-promoting effect is due to indirect paracrine and autocrine effects on nonneuronal cells in the distal nerve stump, rather than a direct effect on regenerating axons. Since most studies have investigated the effect of growth factors independently of each other, the effect of combinations of growth factors and the differentiation status of the target cells are variables that have not yet been investigated.

III. INFILTRATING MACROPHAGES CONTRIBUTE TO SUCCESSFUL REGENERATION

The role of macrophages in peripheral nerve damage and repair is a central question in current neural regeneration research. The hematogenous macrophages invade the distal nerve stump 2-3 days after nerve lesion by a still unknown mechanism of recruitment. The importance of their role is based on several effects, that are reflected by the expression of relevant genes. Macrophages participate in myelin phagocytosis and in the process remove inhibitory substances. These phagocytosing macrophages express the C3b complement receptor MAC-1 and the Fc receptor that are involved in the opsonin-dependent myelin phagocytosis (Reichert et al., 1994). In addition they express the galactose-specific lectin MAC-2 that is responsible for the opsonin-independent phagocytosis of the galactolipid-rich myelin (Reichert et al., 1994). Macrophages secrete several cytokines that stimulate the synthesis of growth factors and adhesion molecules by nonneuronal cells of the nerve sheath. For example macrophage derived IL-1β induces synthesis of NGF and GM-CSF in sheath cells, that in turn supports macrophage function related to myelin breakdown. The rapid increase of IL-1β mRNA within 24 hours after sciatic nerve crush (Gillen et al., 1998) suggests that Schwann cells are most likely the initial source of IL1β and macrophages contribute later. Simultaneously with induction of IL1β mRNA, increased levels of IL10-mRNA were detectable within 1 day after nerve crush (Jander et al., 1996; Gillen et al., 1998). At present there is no known function of IL10 in nerve biology. IL12p40 mRNA showed a biphasic response after nerve injury with maxima at 1 day and a second more prominent peak at 7-14 days after lesion (Gillen et al., 1998) when myelin phagocytosis by macrophages is maximal (Stoll et al., 1989). Transcripts coding for the tumor necrosis factor-α (TNF-α) showed a biphasic pattern of expression in the distal segment of crushed nerves. TNF-α mRNA is induced maximally by one day post-injury, is downregulated at day 2 and then maintained at a high steady-state level for 10 days (La Fleur et al., 1996) with an expression confined to Schwann cells and macrophages (Stoll et al., 1993). TNF-α may have a role in the induction of NGF in Schwann cells and fibroblasts and in tissue remodeling by induction of TIMP-1 expression, the tissue inhibitor of metalloproteases. It is interesting to note that endoneurial injected TNF-α produces neuropathic pain (Wagner and Myers, 1996) and that successful treatment of neuropathic pain in mice by IL-10 application correlates with reduced TNF-α levels (Wagner et al., 1998). Macrophages contribute to tissue remodeling by a coordinated secretion of proteinases and their inhibitors. After nerve crush, the matrix metalloproteinase gelatinase B is increased within 2 days after injury and is expressed in neutrophils, macrophages and perhaps in Schwann cells (La Fleur et al., 1996). The mRNA of TIMP-1, is increased 10-fold after nerve crush, and could help to prevent proteolysis of the basal membrane (La Fleur et al., 1996). The prominent role of macrophages in nerve regeneration is convincingly shown by the findings that in macrophage invasion deficient C57BL/Wld mice, Wallerian degeneration and regeneration are delayed after nerve injury (Hall, 1993; Myers et al., 1996).

IV. LIPID METABOLISM AND TRANSPORT IS IMPORTANT IN MEMBRANE REPAIR

During nerve degeneration, biological membranes, such as the myelin sheath and axonal membranes, are degraded, and large amounts of lipids are stored in macrophages and reutilized during regeneration for membrane biogenesis (Ignatius et al., 1987; Spreyer et al., 1990; Rothe and Müller, 1991). The importance of enhanced lipid transport and recycling is seen on the molecular level by the synchronized and marked increase in the amount of several lipid carrier proteins. The protein concentration of the apolipoproteins Apo D, ApoE, Apo A-I, and Apo A-IV increased to maximum levels at 2-3 weeks after crush injury of rat sciatic nerve and declined afterwards (Müller et al., 1985; Boyles et al., 1989; Boyles et al., 1990; Le Blanc and Poduslo, 1990; Spreyer et al., 1990). ApoE was expressed by infiltrating macrophages in the distal stump (Stoll and Müller; 1986) and could be identified in endoneurial lipoprotein complexes together with ApoD (Spreyer et al., 1990; Rothe and Müller, 1991) The apolipoproteins Apo A-I and Apo A-IV are not expressed in nonneuronal sheath cells, but enter the nerve as components of high-density lipoproteins (Boyles et al., 1989). ApoD mRNA was found to be expressed in endoneurial fibroblasts (Spreyer et al., 1990). Beside a function for ApoD in lipid transport and recycling, another role has been suspected. ApoD is a member of the α_{2U}-microglobin-superfamily that is known to carry small hydrophobic proteins, like retinol or purpurin. It was suggested that ApoD binds to billirubin and therefore fulfills antioxidative functions during nerve regeneration (Peitsch and Bogulski, 1990). After nerve lesion the recycling of cholesterol is accompanied by a down-regulation of 3-hydroxy-3-methylglutaryl-CoA (HMG-CoA)-reductase, the rate–limiting enzyme of cholesterol synthesis (Goodrum, 1990).

V. SCHWANN CELL RESPONSES CONTRIBUTE TO SUCCESSFUL REGENERATION

Schwann cells appear to be crucial for the regenerative capacity of peripheral nerves (this volume, chapter by Grumet). Injury induces a sequence of dramatic changes in the morphological and molecular phenotype of Schwann cells that include dedifferentiation, proliferation, formation of Hanke-Büngner bands, a second burst of axonally-induced proliferation and finally redifferentiation of Schwann cells, all of which are based on the differential expression of specific genes. As a consequence, Schwann cells promote axonal regeneration in three ways, (I) by synthesis of cell surface adhesion molecules, (II) by elaboration of a basement membrane with various extracellular matrix molecules, and (III) by production of neurotrophic factors and their receptors.

In parallel to axonal degradation, the myelin sheath is fragmented within 2 days, and the resulting debris is phagocytosed by Schwann cells and invading macrophages. The dedifferentiation of the myelin-forming Schwann cells is reflected by a marked downregulation of myelin-specific mRNAs, including myelin-associated glycoprotein (MAG) (Gupta et al., 1990), myelin basic protein (MBP) (Gupta et al., 1990), P0 Protein (LeBlanc and Poduslo, 1990a), periaxin (Scherer et al., 1995a), peripheral myelin protein 22 kD (PMP22) (Spreyer et al., 1991), Plasmolipin (Gillen et al., 1996), the fatty-acid binding protein P2 (Narayanan et al., 1988), the enzyme UDP-galactose:ceramid-galctosyltransferase (Stahl et al., 1994), and the β_4-integrin subunit (Feltri et al., 1994). The steady state levels of all these transcripts appear to be down-regulated within 2 days after nerve lesion. Dedifferentiation of Schwann cells is followed by a massive proliferation, showing a maximum at postlesion days 3-4 and leading to steadily increasing Schwann cell numbers up to day 14 after injury. Factors that stimulate Schwann cell proliferation include those released by macrophages and other inflammatory response cells, or substances (e.g. heparin-binding proteins) on the surface of the degenerating nerve fibers in the distal stump. Consistent with the cytoskeletal rearrangement in proliferating Schwann cells, an increased expression of the genes encoding γ-actin, α-tubulin, and intermediate filaments, like vimentin and GFAP, was shown in lesioned peripheral nerve (Gillen et al., 1995). The dedifferentiated Schwann cells up-regulate the expression of several molecules that are normally detected in non-myelinating Schwann cells, including $p75^{NGFR}$, L1/NgCAM, NCAM, GAP-43 (Plantinga et al., 1993), endopeptidase 24.11, and the transcription factors Pax3, and SCIP.

Schwann cell-$p75^{NGFR}$ has been suggested to present NGF to high affinity receptors but other functions are under discussion (see above).

Endopeptidase-24.11 is a cell surface glycoprotein that is upregulated in regenerating nerve (Kioussi et al., 1995a) and plays a key role in the hydrolysis of physiologically active peptides, like calcitonin gene-related peptide, enkephalins, or tachykinins. Concomitantly, CGRP and preprotachykinin are also upregulated after injury (Arvidsson et al., 1990; Nielsch and Keen, 1989).

Pax-3, a paired domain-containing transcription factor, has been implicated in the establishment of the myelinating Schwann cell phenotype. During development of the PNS, Pax3 is expressed in embryonic Schwann cells and remains in the non-myelinating Schwann cells but is downregulated in myelinating Schwann cells (for review see Kioussi and Gruss, 1996). Consistent with this observation, Pax3 overexpression in Schwann cell cultures correlates with enhanced NCAM, L1/NgCAM, and p75NGFR protein levels and decreased MBP expression, whereas the level of S100 protein is unaffected (Kioussi et al., 1995b).

SCIP is a POU-domain transcription factor that is expressed during development in myelinating Schwann cells for a very short time and is down-regulated in the Schwann cells that maintain a myelin sheath (Kioussi and Gruss, 1996). *In vitro*, SCIP acts as a repressor of myelin genes, like P0, and MBP (Monuki et al., 1990). Because of their roles during development, Pax3 and SCIP are likely to be involved in dedifferentiation and redifferentiation of Schwann cells after peripheral nerve lesion.

As a result of these processes, the degenerated distal stump contains columns of dedifferentiated Schwann cells, Büngner bands, surrounded by basal lamina. After a second burst of proliferation induced by the ingrowing axons, Schwann cells begin to redifferentiate by establishing a new myelin sheath. This process is reflected on the molecular level by the downregulation of the molecules specific for non-myelinating Schwann cells as described above, and the upregulation of the myelin-specific genes that were downregulated after injury. The upregulation of the myelin genes occurs between 2 and 4 weeks after lesion and their time-course and sequence of expression recapitulates myelination that is observed during nerve development.

VI. CONNEXINS COORDINATE SCHWANN CELL RESPONSES

The connexins are a family of transmembrane proteins that build up the hexameric gap junction channels involved in cell-cell communication. Connexin 32 is normally present in myelinating Schwann cells at the nodes of Ranvier and Schmidt-Lantermann incisures and its mRNA-expression pattern follows the established myelin genes (Scherer et al., 1995b; Söhl et al., 1996). The mRNA encoding connexin 46 is upregulated after nerve injury in proliferating Schwann cells, and may coordinate the response of these cells by gap junctional communication (Chandross et al., 1996). Connexin 43 may have similar functions since it shows increased mRNA expression 3 days after crush that may be confined to endoneurial fibroblasts (Chandross et al., 1996).

VII. BASAL LAMINA PROVIDES GUIDANCE FOR REGENERATING AXONS

The importance of the basal membranes with their extracellular matrix (ECM) molecules for axon regeneration has been widely appreciated (for review see Reichardt, 1991; Martini, 1994). The continuous basal lamina tubes provide regenerating axons with an appropriate space in the form of a tunnel through which to grow, and in addition, serves as a scaffold for regenerating axons. Although the basal lamina surrounding the Schwann cells is severed only at the lesion site, the expression level of several ECM-molecules e.g., laminin, fibronectin, F-spondin, tenascin, and collagen I, III and IV is altered after peripheral nerve injury.

Laminin, a glycoprotein composed of three polypeptide chains (A, B1, and B2) is one of the most effective promotors of neurite extension *in vitro* (Bixby and Harris, 1991). Laminin is present in nervous systems that are able to regenerate and absent in those, that are not, suggesting that laminin is a prerequisite for successful axonal regeneration (Hopkins et al., 1985; Liesi, 1985). After nerve crush, the mRNA steady state levels of the B1 and B2 chains are rapidly downregulated in the distal segment within 1 day and slowly increase to control levels within 28 days postcrush. In transected nerves that were prevented from regenerating, the B1 and B2 mRNA steady state levels remained at a low level (Doyu et al., 1993). It is important to note that the corresponding A-chain was not detectable in peripheral nerve, assuming that it may replaced by Merosin, a A-chain homologue that was reported to be present in Schwann cell derived basal lamina (Leivo and Engvall, 1988). Interestingly, the newly synthesized laminin is not predominantly incorporated into the Schwann cell basal lamina, but consistent with its axon growth-promoting function, is accumulated at axon-Schwann cell contact sites (Kuecherer-Ehret et al., 1990).

Fibronectin is a glycoprotein of the ECM that supports the attachment, spreading, and migration of neural crest cells and potently promotes neurite outgrowth. After peripheral nerve injury, fibronectin synthesis is increased (Siironen et al., 1992a), and the protein is distributed around endoneurial tubes and in the perineurium. The expression follows a spatial gradient with highest concentrations at the lesion site (Lefcort et al., 1992). There it may serve a dual function. As a chemoattractant and mitogen, fibronectin could induce migration and proliferation of Schwann cells to the site of injury which, in turn could promote neurite outgrowth, e.g., through release of laminin. Fibronectin could further support neural adhesion and neurite extension and, thus partly substitute for the lost nerve sheath at the lesion site. Interestingly, the fibronectin protein synthesized after nerve injury includes embryonic isoforms generated by alternative splicing (Matthews and ffrench-Constant, 1995).

Tenascin-C is normally confined to the extracellular matrix around the node of Ranvier and the perineurium (Daniloff et al., 1989; Martini et al., 1990). After lesion, tenascin-C is upregulated in the distal as well as in the proximal stump, including the lesion site (Martini et al., 1990) and tenascin-C immunoreactivity is associated with the basal lamina of Schwann cells. Expression of tenascin is closely related to Schwann cell proliferation. Nonmyelinating Schwann cells that reach their peak of proliferation a day earlier than myelinating Schwann cells (Clemence et al., 1989), begin to express tenascin-C a day earlier than myelinating Schwann cells (Fruttiger et al., 1995).

F-Spondin is an ECM molecule with adhesive properties normally expressed in floorplate of spinal cord or embryonal Schwann cells. After axotomy a massive upregulation of mRNA and protein distal to the lesion was shown (Burstyn-Cohen et al., 1998). F-Spondin can bind to axons by interaction with the $\alpha_3\beta_1$ integrin.

Collagen type I, III, and IV are components of the basal lamina, and their mRNAs are coordinately up-regulated after nerve injury, with a peak of expression two weeks after lesion (Siironen et al., 1992a; Siironen et al., 1992b). These collagens are either expressed by Schwann cells (collagen type IV) or by endoneurial fibroblasts (type I) and play a role in the remodeling of the endoneurial space after nerve injury. Because of the identical expression patterns in the degenerating and regenerating nerve, respectively, this remodeling process seems to be a stereotypical response to nerve lesion.

VIII. CELL ADHESION MOLECULES (CAMS) REGULATE AXONAL GROWTH

The lesion-induced switch of Schwann cells from the myelinating to the nonmyelinating phenotype is accompanied by the enhanced expression of cell adhesion molecules. These molecules are involved in adhesion between axons and Schwann cells and thereby regulate axonal growth in the distal nerve segment.

A. Immunoglobulin Superfamily

In the adult peripheral nerve the cell adhesion molecules L1 and N-CAM are expressed mainly in unmyelinated fibers on the plasma membranes of axons and Schwann cells where they are in contact with each other (Martini, 1994). Myelinated fibers show only a trace of N-CAM and L1 at the axon-Schwann cell contact and at the nodes of Ranvier (Martini et al., 1994). After nerve injury L1 and N-CAM are upregulated in Schwann cells and localized on the surfaces of columns formed by Schwann cells where they are in contact with each other (Martini and Schachner, 1988). When the regenerating axons enter the distal stump and grow along the Schwann cell columns, L1 and N-CAM are localized on the plasma membrane at contact sites between Schwann cells and the ingrowing axon (Nieke and Schachner, 1985; Martini et al., 1994; Martini, 1994). L1 and N-CAM are downregulated concurrent with re-expression of MAG at begin of myelination when Schwann cells have made one or two turns of cytoplasmic processes around the axon (Martini, 1994).

B. Cadherin Family

N-Cadherin is a member of a multigene family that mediates homophilic Ca^{2+}-dependent cell adhesion. In the non-injured peripheral nerve, N-Cadherin is localized on membranes of all Schwann cells where they contact other Schwann cells and the membranes of nonmyelinated axons (Shibuya et al., 1995). After nerve injury N-Cadherin is expressed in proliferating Schwann cells (Cifuentes-Diaz et al., 1994). When axons regenerate into the distal stump, N-cadherin immunoreactivity is localized to the axon and Schwann cell membrane at sites of axon-axon and axon-Schwann cell contacts. Therefore N-cadherin, in addition to L1 and N-CAM, is thought to be involved in axonal growth by mediating adhesion between axons and Schwann cells (Shibuya et al, 1995).

C. Integrin Family

Integrins are heterodimeric receptors that consist of an α and a β subunit and mediate the interactions of cells with ECMs and other cells (for review, see Hynes, 1992). The α_5-subunit interacts only with the RGD-sensitive major cell attachment site of fibronectin. Protein levels of the α_5-subunit increase after nerve lesion, and the protein localizes with axons, growth cones and dedifferentiated Schwann cells (Lefcort et al., 1992). The elevated expression of $\alpha_5\beta_1$ on both Schwann cells and regenerating axons could facilitate their motility through a fibronectin-rich region.

Taskinen and coworkers (1995) demonstrated enhanced immunoreactivity of the β-subunit after sciatic nerve injury. In peripheral nerve, the β_1-subunit is known to interact either with α_5, yielding a fibronectin receptor (see above), or with the α_6-subunit. The $\alpha_6\beta_1$ integrin is found on dedifferentiated Schwann cells *in vivo* and *in vitro* and could potentially be involved in Schwann cell proliferation because $\alpha_6\beta_1$ binds to laminin that acts as a potent Schwann cell mitogen in vitro (McGarvey et al., 1984). In addition a role in the initiation of myelination has been assumed because $\alpha6\beta1$ is replaced by $\alpha6\beta4$ at the beginning of myelination and anti-β_1 integrin antibodies inhibit myelination *in vitro* (Fernandez-Valle et al., 1994).

The β_4-integrin subunit interacts only with α_6. The resulting $\alpha_6\beta_4$-heterodimer was shown to interact with laminin-5 in the basal membrane/extracellular-matrix (Wagner et al., 1997), a laminin isoform whose expression in peripheral nerve has not yet examined. In contrast to the above mentioned integrin subunits, the expression of β_4 correlates with the expression of myelin genes. Within 4 days after injury, β_4 mRNA is downregulated and is reexpressed up to control levels 8 weeks after lesion (Feltri et al., 1994). In addition, β_4 is localized on the abaxonal Schwann cell membrane and shows a myelin-associated expression in nerve development and *in vitro* (Feltri et al., 1994). Therefore, the β_4 subunit could play a role in the establishment of cellular polarity of the myelinating Schwann cell by interacting with the basal lamina. There is compelling evidence that Schwann cell deposition of a basal lamina is a prerequisite for ensheathment and myelination of axons. In turn, the full assembly of the Schwann cell basal lamina requires axon-Schwann cell contact (Clark and Bunge, 1989). However, a similar upregulation of β_4 was found in permanently interrupted nerve segments, suggesting additional roles of this integrin subunit (Feltri et al., 1994).

D. Ninjurin

Ninjurin (Nerve injury induced protein) is a recently identified adhesion molecule protein that mediates homophilic interactions. Ninjurin mRNA was found to be upregulated in Schwann cells of the distal stump after axotomy (Araki and Milbrandt, 1996). An important role of ninjurin during nerve regeneration was suggested because it promotes neurite extension of dorsal root ganglia (DRG) neurons.

IX. FUTURE DIRECTIONS

During the last decade, an impressive number of regulated genes with identified or putative functions in peripheral nerve regeneration and degeneration have been characterized. The regulated expression of such genes and the coordinate interactions of their proteins participate in the structural reorganization of injured peripheral nerves. However, our knowledge of the regulatory mechanisms and signaling cascades underlying the complex molecular regeneration program is still very limited. The systematic identification of all expressed genes by the genome-projects, the massive parallel analysis of gene expression by the cDNA array/chip technology and the enhanced capabilities to discover gene function by e.g., antisense-strategies, knock-out animals or yeast two-hybrid-system can be expected to have a great impact on our understanding of these processes. The accumulating information from all these techniques will surely lead to a more complete understanding of the gene program of nerve regeneration and degeneration and will cause improvements in diagnosis and therapy of PNS disorders.

Table 1. Expression of genes after peripheral nerve injury.

Regulated Gene	Expression at different time points after lesion								Cell Type	Reference
	Ctr	1d	2d	4d	1w	2w	4w	8w		
Neurotrophins										
NGF							–	–	Schwann cells	Heumann et al., 1987a; 1987b
							–	–		
NGRFp75							–	–	Schwann cells	Heumann et al., 1987a; 1987b
							–	–		
BDNF	–	–	–	–	–	–	–	–	Schwann cells	Meyer et al., 1992
							–	–		
NT-3							–	–	Schwann cells	Chai et al., 1998
							–	–		Funakoshi et al., 1993
NT-4	–	–	–	–	–	–	–	–	Non-neuronal cells	Funakoshi et al., 1993
							–	–		
TrkB, trkC	–	–	–	–	–	–	–	–	Schwann cells	Funakoshi et al., 1993
							–	–		
Neuropoetic Cytokines										
CNTF									Schwann cells	Sendtner et al., 1992a
GM-CSF							–	–	Fibroblasts	Saada et al., 1996
	–	–	–	–	–	–	–	–		
IL-6							–	–	Non-neuronal cells	Bolin et al., 1995; Reichert et al, 1996
	–	–	–	–	–	–	–	–		
LIF								–	Schwann cells	Curtis et al; 1994
	–	–	–	–	–	–	–	–		
Cytokines										
IL-1β								–	Macrophages,	Gillen et al., 1998
	–	–	–	–	–	–	–	–	(Schwann cells)	
IL-10								–	Schwann cells	Gillen et al., 1998
	–	–	–	–	–	–	–	–		
IL-12								–	?	Gillen et al., 1998
	–	–	–	–	–	–	–	–		
TNFα							–	–	Macrophages,	La Fleur et al., 1996
	–	–	–	–	–	–	–	–	Schwann cells	

Table 1 Time course of expression of genes encoding neurotrophins, neuropoetic cytokines, and cytokines after nerve injury. The first row for each gene describes the expression pattern in regenerating nerves, (crush-injury or transection without ligation), the second row describes the expression pattern in degenerating nerves (transection with ligation of both stumps). The level of expression is given for the time points indicated at which a higher expression level is reflected by a darker grey level. A hyphen indicates the time points not measured. The cells types that express the corresponding gene(s) are indicated.

REFERENCES

Anton ES, Weskamp G, Reichardt LF, Matthew WD (1994) Nerve growth factor and its low-affinity receptor promote Schwann cell migration. Proc Natl Acad Sci USA 91:2795-2799.

Araki T and Milbrandt J (1996). Ninjurin, a novel adhesion molecule, is induced by nerve injury and promotes axonal growth. Neuron 17:353-361.

Arvidsson U, Johnson H, Piehl F et al., (1990) Peripheral nerve sections induces increased levels of calcitonin gene-related peptide (CGRP)-like immunoreactivity in axotomized motoneurons. Exp Brain Res 79:212-216.

Baloh RH, Tansey MG, Lampe PA, Fahrner TJ, Enemoto H, Simburger KS, Leitner ML, Raki T, Johnson Jr. EM, Milbrandt J (1998) Artemin, a novel member of the GDNF ligand family, supports peripheral and central neurons and signals through the GFRα3-RET receptor complex. Neuron 21:1291-1302.

Bixby JL and Harris WA (1991) Molecular mechanisms of axon growth and guidance. Ann Rev Cell Biol 7:117-159.

Bolin LM, Verity AN, Silver JE, Shooter EM, Abrams JS (1995) Interleukin-6 production by Schwann cells and induction in sciatic nerve injury. J Neurochem 64:850-858.

Bosch EP, Zhong W, Lim R (1989) Axonal signals regulates expression of glia maturation factor-β in Schwann cells: Immunohistochemical study of injured sciatic nerve and cultured Schwann cells. J Neurosci 9:3690-3698.

Boyles JK, Nottterpek LM, Anderson LJ (1990) accumulation of apolipoproteins in the regenerating and remyelinating mammalian peripheral nerve. J Biol Chem 265:17805-17815.

Boyles JK, Zoelnner CD, Anderson LJ, et al., (1989) A role for apolipoprotein E, apolipoprotein A-I and the low density lipoprotein receptors in the cholesterol transport during regeneration and remyelination of the rat sciatic nerve. J Clin Invest 83:1015-1031.

Burstyn-Cohen T, Frumkin A, Xu Y-T, Scherer SS, Klar A (1998) Accumulation of F-Spondin in injured peripheral nerve promotes the outgrowth of sensory axons. J Neurosci 18:8875-8885.

Carroll SL, Miller ML, Frohnert PW, Kim SS, Corbett JA (1997) Expression of neuregulins and their putative receptors is induced during Wallerian degeneration. J Neurosci 17:1642-1659.

Chai F, Tomlinson DR, Fernyhuogh P (1998) Effect of sciatic nerve crush on local and target tissue production of neurotrophin-3 transcripts in rats. Neurosci Lett 252:45-48.

Chandross KJ, Kessler JA, Cohen RI, Simburger E, Spray DC, Bieri P, Dermietzel R (1996) Altered connexin expression after peripheral nerve injury. Mol Cell Neurosci 7:501-518.

Cheng H-L, Randolph A, Yee D, Delafontaine P, Tenekoon G, Feldman EL (1996) Characterization of insulin-like growth factor-I and its receptor and binding proteins in transected nerves and cultured Schwann cells. J Neurochem 66:525-536.

Cifuentes-Diaz C, Nicolet M, Goudou D, Rieger F, Mege RM (1994) N-Cadherin expression in developing, adult and denervated chicken neuromuscular system: accumulations at both the neuromuscular junction and the node of Ranvier. Development 120:1-11.

Clark MB and Bunge MB (1989) Cultured Schwann cells assemble normal-appearing basal lamina only when they ensheath axons. Dev Biol 133:393-404.

Clemence A, Mirsky R, Jessen KR (1989) Non-myelin-forming Schwann cells proliferate rapidly during Wallerian degeneration in the rat sciatic nerve. J Neurocytol 18:185-192.

Curtis R, Adryan KM, Zhu Y, Harkness PJ, Lindsay RM, DiStefano PS (1993) Retrograde axonal transport of ciliary neurotrophic factor is increased by peripheral nerve injury. Nature 365:253-255.

Curtis R, Scherer SS, Somogyi R et al., (1994) Retrograde axonal transport of LIF is increased by peripheral nerve injury: correlation with increased LIF expression in distal nerve. Neuron 12: 191-204.

Daniloff JK, Crossin KL, Pincon-Raymond M, Murawsky M, Rieger F, Edelman GM (1989) Expression of cytotactin in normal and regenerating neuromuscular junction. J Cell Biol 108:625-635.

David S and Aguayo AJ (1981) Axonal elongation into peripheral nervous system bridges after central nervous system injury in adult rats. Science 214:931-933.

De Leon M, Welcher AA, Suter U, Shooter EM (1991) Identification of transcriptionally regulated genes after sciatic nerve injury. J Neurosci Res 29:437-448.

Doyu M, Sobue G, Ken E et al. (1993) Laminin A, B1, and B2 chain gene expression in transected and regenerating nerves: regulation by axonal signals. J Neurochem 60:543-551.

Eckenstein FP, Shipley GD, Nishi R (1991) Acidic and basic fibroblast growth factors in the nervous system: distribution and differential alteration of levels after injury of central versus peripheral nerve. J Neurosci 11:412-419.

Einheber S, Hannocks M-J Metz CN, Riffkin DB, Salzer JL (1995) Transforming growth factor-β1 regulates axon/Schwann cell interactions. J Cell Biol 129:443-458.

Feltri L, Scherer SS, Nemni R, Kamholz J, Vogelbacker H, Scott MO, Canal N, Quaranta V, Wrabetz L (1994) β4 integrin expression in myelinating Schwann cells is polarized, developmentally regulated and axonal dependent Development 120:1287-1301.

Fernandez-Valle C, Gwynn L, Wood P, Carbonetto W, Bunge MB (1994). Anti β1 integrin antibody inhibits Schwann cell myelination.. J Neurobiol 25:1207-1226.

Ferri CC, Moore FA, Bisby MA (1998) Effects of facial nerve injury on mouse motoneurons lacking the p75 low-affinity neurotrophin receptor. J Neurobiol 34:1-9.

Friedlander DR, Grumet M, Edelman GM (1986) Nerve growth factor enhances expression of neuron-glia cell adhesion molecule in PC12 cells. J Cell Biol 102: 413-419.

Friedman B, Scherer SS, Rudge JS, Helgren M, Morrisey D, McClain J, Wang D-Y, Wiegand SJ, Furth ME, Lindsay RM, Ip NY (1992) Regulation of ciliary neurotrophic factor expression in myelin-related Schwann cells in vivo. Neuron 9:295-305.

Fruttiger M, Schachner M, Martini R (1995) Tenascin-C expression during Wallerian degeneration in C57BL/Wlds mice: possible implications for axonal regeneration. J Neurocytol 24:1-14.

Funakoshi H, Frisen J, Barbany G et al., (1993) Differential expression of mRNAs for neurotrophins and their receptors after axotomy of the sciatic nerve. J Cell Biol 123:455-465.

Gillen C, Gleichmann M, Greiner-Petter R, Zoidl G, Kupfer S, Bosse F, Auer J, Müller HW (1996) Full length cloning, expression and cellular localization of rat plasmolipin mRNA, a proteolipid of PNS and CNS. Eur J Neurosci 8:405-414.

Gillen C, Gleichmann M, Spreyer P and Müller HW (1995) Differentially expressed genes after peripheral nerve injury. J Neurosci Res 42:159-171.

Gillen C, Jander S, Stoll G (1998) Sequential expression of mRNA for proinflammatory cytokines and interleukin-10 in the rat peripheral nervous system: comparison between immune-mediated demyelination and Wallerian degeneration. J Neurosci Res 51:489-496.

Gimenez-Gallego G and Cuevas P (1994) Fibroblast growth factors, proteins with a broad spectrum of biological activities. Neurol Res 16:313-316.

Goodrum JF (1990) Cholesterol synthesis is down-regulated during regeneration of peripheral nerve. J Neurochem 54:1709-1715.

Gupta SK, Poduslo JF, Dunn R, Roder J, Mezei C (1990) Myelin-associated glycoprotein gene expression in the presence and absence of Schwann cell-axonal contact. Dev Neurosci 12: 22-31.

Hall SM (1993) Observations on the progress of Wallerian degeneration in transected peripheral nerves of C57BL/Wld mice in the presence of recruited macrophages. J Neurocytol 22:480-490.

Hammarberg H, Piehl F, Cullheim S, Fjell J, Hökfelt T, Fried K (1996) GDNF mRNA in Schwann cells and DRG satellite cells after chronic sciatic nerve injury. Neuroreport 22:857-860.

Harman K, Katnick J, Lim R, Zaheer A, de la Torre JC (1991) Glia maturation factor and regulation of Schwann cell proliferation in vivo. J Neurosci Res 31: 254-262.

Heumann R, Korsching S, Bandtlow C, Thoenen H (1987b) Changes of nerve growth factor synthesis in nonneuronal cells in response to sciatic nerve transection. J Cell Biol 104:1623-1631

Heumann R, Lindholm D, Bandtlow C, et al., (1987a) Differential regulation of mRNA encoding nerve growth factor and its receptor in rat sciatic nerve during development, degeneration and regeneration: role of macrophages. Proc Natl Acad Sci USA 84:8735-8739

Hopkins JM, Ford-Holevinski TS, McCoy JP, Agranoff BW (1985) Laminin and optic nerve regeneration in the goldfish. J Neurosci 5:3030-3038.

Hynes RO (1992) Integrins: versatility, modulation, and signaling in cell adhesion. Cell 69:11-25.

Ignatius MJ, Shooter EM, Pitas RE, Mahley RW (1987) Lipoprotein uptake by neuronal growth cones. Science 236:959-962.

Ip NY, Nye SH, Boulton TG, Davis S, Taga T, Li Y, Birren SJ, Yasukawa K, Kishimoto T, Anderson DJ, Stahl N, Yancopoulos GD (1992) CNTF and LIF act on neuronal cells via shared signaling pathways that involve the IL-6 signal transducing receptor component gp130. Cell 69:1121-1132.

Ishikawa R, Nishikori K, Furukawa Y, Hayashi K, Furukawa S (1992) Injury induced reduction of acidic fibroblast growth factor levels in the distal parts of the rat sciatic nerves. Neurosci Lett 135: 113-116.

Jander S, Pohl J, Gillen C, Stoll G (1996) Differential expression of Interleukin-10 mRNA in Wallerian degeneration and immune-mediated inflammation of the rat peripheral nervous system. J Neurosci Res 43:254-259.

Johnson EM, Taniuchi M, DiStefano PS (1990) Expression and possible function of nerve growth factor receptors on Schwann cells. Trends Neurosci 11:299-304.

Kioussi C, Gross MK, Gruss P (1995b) Pax3: a paired domain gene as a regulator in PNS myelination. Neuron 15:553-562.

Kioussi C and Gruss P (1996) Making a Schwann. Trends in Genet 12:84-86

Kioussi C, Mamalaki A, Jessen KR, Mirsky R, Hersh LB, Matsas R (1995a) Expression of endopeptidase-24.11 (common acute lymphoblastic leukemia antigene CD10) in the sciatic nerve of adult rats after lesion and during regeneration. Eur J Neurosci 7: 951-961.

Kotani Y, Matsuda S, Suganaka M, Kondoh K, Ueno S, Sano A (1996) Prosaposin facilitates sciatic nerve regeneration in vivo. J Neurochem 66:2019-2025.

Kuecherer-Ehret A, Graeber MB, Edgar D, Thoenen D (1990) Immunoelectron microscopic localization of laminin in normal and regenerating mouse sciatic nerve. J Neurocytol 19:101-109.

La Fleur et al. (1996) Basement membrane and repair of injury to peripheral nerve: Defining a potential role for macrophages, matrix, metalloproteinases, and tissue inhibitor of metalloproteinases-1. J Exp Med 184:2311-2326.

Le Blanc AC and Poduslo JF (1990a) Axonal modulation of myelin gene expression in the peripheral nerve. J Neurosci Res 26:317-326.

Le Blanc AC and Poduslo JF (1990b) Regulation of apolipoprotein E gene expression after injury of the rat sciatic nerve. J Neurosci Res 25:162-171.

Lefcort F, Venstrom K, McDonald JA, Reichardt LF (1992) Regulation of expression of fibronectin and its receptor $\alpha 5\beta 1$ during development and regeneration of peripheral nerve. Development 116:767-782.

Leivo I and Engvall E (1988) Merosin, a protein specific for basement membranes Schwann cells, striated muscle, and trophoblasts, is expressed late in muscle and nerve development. Proc Natl acad Sci USA 85:1544-1548.

Liesi P (1985) Laminin immunoreactive glial cells distinguish regenerative CNS systems from nonregenerative ones. EMBO J 4:2502-2511.

Marchionni MA, Goodearl AD, Chen MS et al., (1993) Glia growth factors are alternatively spliced erbB2 ligands expressed in the nervous system. Nature 362:312-318.

Martini R (1994) Expression and functional roles of neural cell surface molecules and extracellular matrix components during development and regeneration of peripheral nerves. J Neurocyt 23:1-28.

Martini R and Schachner M (1988) Immunelectron microscope localization of neural cell adhesion molecules (L1, N-CAM, and MAG) in regenerating mouse sciatic nerve. J Cell Biol 106:1735-1746.

Martini R, Schachner M, Faissner A (1990) Enhanced expression of the extracellular matrix molecule J1/tenascin in the regenerating adult mouse sciatic nerve. J Neurocytol 19:601-616.

Martini R, Xin Y, Schachner M (1994) Restricted localization of L1 and N-CAM at sites of contact between Schwann cells and neurites in culture. Glia 10:70-74.

Matthews GA, ffrench-Constant C (1995) Embryonic fibronectins are up-regulated following peripheral nerve injury in rats. J Neurobiol 26:171-188.

Mc Garvey ML, Baron-Van Evercooren A, Kleinman HK, Dubois-Dalcq M (1984) Synthesis and effects of basement membrane components in cultured rat Schwann cells. Dev Biol 105:18-28.
Mendell LM (1995) Neurotrophic factors and the specification of neural function. Neuroscientist 1:26-34.
Mews M and Meyer M (1993) Modulation of Schwann cell phenotype by TGF-β1: inhibition of P_0 mRNA expression and down-regulation of the low affinity NGF receptor. Glia 8:208-217.
Meyer M, Matsuoka I, Wetmore C, Olson L, Thoenen H (1992) Enhanced synthesis of brain-derived neurotrophic factor in the lesioned peripheral nerve: different mechanisms are responsible for the regulation of BDNF and NGF mRNA. J Cell Biol 119:45-54.
Minghetti L, Goodearl AD, Mistry K, Stroobant P (1996) Glial growth factors I-III are specific mitogens for glial cells. J Neurosci Res 43:684-693.
Monuki ES, Kuhn R, Weinmaster G, Trapp BD, Lemke G (1990) Expression and activity of the POU transcription factor SCIP. Science 249:1300-1303.
Müller HW, Gebicke-Haerter PJ, Hangen DH, Shooter EM (1985) A specific 37,000-dalton protein that accumulates in regenerating but not in nonregenerating mammalian nerves. Science 228:499-501.
Myers RR, Heckman HM, Rodriguez M (1996) Reduced hyperalgesia in nerve injured WLD mice: relationship to nerve fiber phagocytosis, axonal degeneration, and regeneration in normal mice. Exp Neurol 141:94-101.
Narayanan V, Barbosa E, Reed R Tennekoon G (1988) Characterization of a cloned cDNA encoding rabbit myelin P2 protein. J Biol Chem 263:8332-8337.
Ng SB, Tan YH, Guy GR (1994) Differential induction of the interleukin-6 gene by tumor necrosis factor and interleukin-1. J Biol Chem 269:19021-19027.
Nieke J and Schachner M (1985) Expression of the neural cell adhesion molecule L1 and N-CAM and their common carbohydrate epitope L2/HNK-1 during development and after transection of the mouse sciatic nerve. Differentiation 30:141-151.
Nielsch U, Keen P (1989) Reciprocal regulation of tachykinin- and vasoactive intestinal peptide-gene expression in rat sensory neurons following cut and crush injury. Brain Res 481:25-30.
O'Brien JS, Carson GS, Seo H-C, Hiraiwa M, Kishimoto Y (1994) Identification of prosaposin as a neurotrophic factor. Proc Natl Acad Sci USA 91:9593-9596.
Patterson PH (1994) Leukemia inhibitory factor, a cytokine at the interface between neurobiology and immunology. Proc Natl Acad Sci USA 91:7833-7835.
Peitsch MC and Bogulski MS (1990) Is apolipoprotein D a mammalian billin-binding protein. New Biol 2:197-206.
Plantinga LC, Verhaagen J, Edwards PM, Hol EM, Bär PR, Gispen WH (1993) The expression of B-50/GAP-43 in Schwann cells is upregulated in degenerating peripheral nerve stumps following nerve injury. Brain Res 602:69-76.
Pu S-F, Zhuang H-X, Ishii DN (1995) Differential spatial-temporal expression of the insulin-like growth factor genes in regenerating sciatic nerves. Mol Brain Res 34:18-28.
Raivich G, Hellweg R, Kreutzberg GW (1991) NGF receptor-mediated reduction in axonal NGF uptake and retrograde transport following sciatic nerve injury and during regeneration. Neuron 7:151-164.
Raivich G and Kreutzberg GW (1993) Peripheral nerve regeneration: role of growth factors and their receptors. Int J Dev Neurosci 11:311-324.

Reichardt LF (1991) Extracellular molecules and their receptors: function in neural development. Ann Rev Neurosci 14:531-570.
Reichert F, Levitzky R, Rothshenker S (1996) Interleukin 6 in intact and injured mouse peripheral nerves. Eur J Neurosci 8:530-535.
Reichert F, Saada A, Rothshenker S (1994) Peripheral nerve injury induces Schwann cells to express two macrophage phenotypes: phagocytosis and the galactose-specific lectin MAC-2. J Neurosci 8: 530-535.
Ridley AJ, Davies JB, Stroobant P, Land H (1989) Transforming growth factors-beta 1 and beta 2 are mitogens for rat Schwann cells. J Cell Biol 109:3419-3424.
Rothe T and Müller HW (1991) Uptake of endoneurial lipoprotein into Schwann cells and sensory neurons is mediated by low density lipoprotein receptors and stimulated after axonal injury. J Neurochem 57:2016-2025.
Saada A, Reichert F, Rothshenker S (1996) Granulocyte macrophage colony stimulating factor produced in lesioned peripheral nerves induces the up-regulation of cell surface expression of MAC-2 by macrophages and Schwann cells. J Cell Biol 1333:159-167.
Santos PM, Winterowd JG, Allen GG, Bothwell MA, Rubel EW (1991) Nerve growth factor: increased angiogenesis without improved nerve regeneration. Otaryngol-Head Neck Surg 105:12-15.
Scherer SS, Deschênes SM, Xu Y-t, Grinspan JB, Fischbeck KH, Paul DL (1995b) Connexin 32 is a myelin-related protein in the PNS and CNS. J Neurosci 15:8281-8294.
Scherer SS, Kamholz, J, Jakowlew SB (1993) Axons modulate the expression of transforming growth factors in Schwann cells. Glia 8:265-276.
Scherer SS, Xu Y-t, Bannermann PGC, Sherman DL, Brophy PJ (1995a) Periaxin expression in myelinating Schwann cells: modulation by axon-glia interactions and polarized localization during development. Development 121:4265-4273.
Schreiner CL, Bauer JS, Danilov YN, Hussein S, Seekan MM, Juliano RL (1989) Isolation and characterization of CHO cell variants deficient in the expression of fibronectin receptor. J Cell Biol 109:3157-3167.
Schwartz M (1987) Molecular and cellular aspects of nerve regeneration. CRC Crit Rev Biochem 22:89-110.
Seilheimer B and Schachner M (1987) Regulation of neural cell adhesion molecule expression on cultured mouse Schwann cells by nerve growth factor. EMBO J 6:1611-1616.
Sendtner M, Holtmann B, Kolbeck R, Thoenen H, Barde Y-A (1992b) Brain-derived neurotrophic factor prevents the death of motoneurons in newborn rats after nerve transection. Nature 360: 757-759.
Sendtner M, Stöckli KA, Thoenen H (1992a) Synthesis and localization of ciliary neurotrophic factor in the sciatic nerve of the adult rat after lesion and during regeneration. J Cell Biol 118: 139-148.
Shibuya Y, Mizoguchi A, Tekeichi M, Schimada K, Die C (1995) Localization of N-cadherin in the normal and regenerating nerve fibers of the chicken peripheral nervous system. Neuroscience 67:253-261.
Siironen J, Sandberg M, Vuorinen V, Röyttä M (1992a) Expression of type I and III collagens and fibronectin after transection of rat sciatic nerve (reinervation compared with enervation). Lab Invest 67:80-87.
Siironen J, Sandberg M, Vuorinen V, Röyttä M (1992b) Laminin B1 and collagen type IV gene expression in transected peripheral nerve: reinervation compared to deinervation. J Neurochem 59:2184-2192.

Söhl G, Gillen C, Bosse F, Gleichmann M, Müller HW, Willecke K (1996) A second alternative transcript of the gap junction gene connexin 32 is expressed in murine Schwann cells and modulated in injured sciatic nerve. Eur J Cell Biol 69:267-275.

Spreyer P, Kuhn G, Hanemann CO, Gillen C, Schaal H, Kuhn R, Lemke G, Müller HW (1991) Axon-regulated expression of a Schwann cell transcript that is homologous to a ′growth arrest-specific′ gene. EMBO J 10: 3661-3668.

Spreyer P, Schaal H, Kuhn G, Rothe T, Unterbeck A, Olek K, Müller HW (1990) Regeneration-associated high level expression of apolipoprotein D mRNA in endoneurial fibroblasts of peripheral nerve. EMBO J 9:2479-2484.

Stahl N, Jurevics H, Morell P, Suzuki K, Popko B (1994) Isolation, characterization, and expression of cDNA clones that encode rat UDP-galactose:ceramide galactosyltransferase. J Neurosci Res 38:234-242.

Stoll G, Griffin JW, Li CY, Trapp BD (1989) Wallerian degeneration in the peripheral nervous system: participation of both Schwann cells and macrophages in myelin degradation. J Neurocytol 18:671-683.

Stoll G, Jung S, Jander S, Van der Meide PH, Hartung H-P (1993) Tumor necrosis factor-α in immune-mediated demyelination and Wallerian degeneration of the rat peripheral nervous system. J Neuroimmunol 45: 175-182.

Stoll G and Müller HW (1986) Macrophages in the peripheral nervous system and astroglia in the central nervous system of rat commonly express apolipoprotein E during development but differ in their response to injury. Neurosci Lett 72:233-238.

Taskinen HS, Heino J, Röyttä M (1995) The dynamics of β1 integrin expression during peripheral nerve regeneration. Acta Neuropath (Berl) 89:144-151.

Villiger PM, Geng Y, Lotz M (1993) Induction of cytokine expression by leukemia inhibitory factor. J Clin Invest 91:1575-158.

Wagner R, Jangjian M, Myers RR (1998) Anti-inflammatory interleukin-10 therapy in CCI neuropathy decreases thermal hyperalgesia, macrophage recruitment, and endoneurial TNF-α expression. Pain 74:35-42.

Wagner R and Myers RR (1996) Endoneurial injection of TNF-α produces neuropathic pain behaviors. Neuroreport 7:2897-2901.

Wagner S, Tagaya M, Koziol JA, Quaranta V, del Zoppio GJ (1997) Stroke 28:858-865.

Zhou X-F, Rush RA, McLachlan EM (1996) Differential expression of the p75 nerve growth factor receptor in glia and neurons of rat dorsal root ganglia after peripheral nerve transection. J Neurosci 16:2901-2911.

15

Inhibition of Axonal Growth by the Myelin-associated Inhibitory Proteins NI-35/250/Nogo-A

Martin E. Schwab
University of Zurich & Swiss Federal Institute of Technology, Zurich, Switzerland

I. INTRODUCTION

In 1911, F. Tello, a collaborator of S. Ramon y Cajal, published the first successful transplantation of a peripheral nerve into the adult CNS of a mammal: previously denervated sciatic nerve pieces were implanted into the cortex of rabbits, and silver staining showed fascicles as well as individual nerve fibers invading these peripheral nerves 2-4 weeks after transplantation (Tello, 1911). "Juice" squeezed out of denervated nerves and sucked up into spongy material (elder pith) also attracted growth cones and neurites following implantation into the cortex. Tello and later Ramon y Cajal (Ramon y Cajal, 1928) concluded from these experiments that peripheral nerve Schwann cells reacted to the loss of their axons by the synthesis of attractive and neurite-promoting factors. These factors would act on peripheral as well as central neurons. They hypothesized further that CNS glia would be devoid of such a reaction. Stimulated by the beautiful demonstration by A. Aguayo's group in the early eighties showing that many types of CNS neurons can regenerate axons over very long distances if offered a peripheral nerve as a substrate (David and Aguayo, 1981; Richardson et al., 1984; Keirstead et al., 1989), we wanted to test the original "lack of trophic factor hypothesis" by exposing perinatal DRG or sympathetic neurons to optic and sciatic nerve explants of adult rats in the presence of trophic factors (NGF). To our surprise, electron microscopic analyses of the explants after 2 weeks in culture showed that no or extremely few axons could be found in the optic nerves, in contrast to the sciatic nerves most of which were invaded by hundreds of nerve fibers (Schwab and Thoenen, 1985). Repeated freezing and thawing of the explants prior to culture gave the same results, showing that the absence of neurite growth in the adult optic nerve explants was due to an intrinsic property of the adult CNS tissue rather than to reactions to the lesion or the culture conditions.

II. MYELIN IS AN INHIBITORY SUBSTRATE FOR NEURITE GROWTH

The postulated existence of neurite growth inhibitory factors in the adult CNS was subsequently confirmed in several labs by experiments studying neurite growth in relation to various types of glial cells *in vitro* and on tissue sections of developing and adult central and peripheral nervous system. White matter of mammals (in contrast to fish and to peripheral nerves) (Carbonetto et al., 1987; Crutcher, 1989; Savio and Schwab, 1989; Tuttle and Matthew, 1991; Watanabe and Murakami, 1989) and in particular oligodendrocytes (Schwab and Caroni, 1988; Fawcett et al., 1989; Bandtlow et al., 1990; Igarashi et al., 1993; Moorman, 1996), and also subpopulations of astrocytes (Meiners et al., 1995; Fitch and Silver, 1997) were shown to be inhibitory to neurite growth. A first biochemical analysis of rat brain myelin showed two protein constistuents of MW 35 kDa and 250 kDa which were potent neurite growth inhibitors when coated as a tissue culture substrate or added in liposomes to growing nerve fibers (Caroni and Schwab, 1988b). These constituents were called neurite growth inhibitors NI-35/250. In bovine and human spinal cord, only the large MW fraction could be found (bNI-220, hNI-220) (Spillmann et al., 1997; Spillmann et al., 1998). More recently, additional neurite growth inhibitory factors were isolated from CNS myelin, in particular myelin-associated glycoprotein (MAG; see this volume, chapter by David and McKerracher; McKerracher et al., 1994; Mukhopadhyay et al., 1994) and chondroitin-sulfate-proteoglycans. Much of the work currently done in this field concentrates on the full molecular identification of components with neurite growth inhibitory activity, the analysis of their mechanism of action including neuronal receptors and intracellular response mechanisms, the analysis of their spectrum of actions with regard to neuronal types, and their roles in the developing and adult nervous system. Obviously, the relative contribution of these different molecules to the very limited growth capacity of the lesioned adult CNS is a crucial question.

III. IDENTIFICATION OF NI-35/250 – NOGO

Early in the investigations of myelin-associated neurite growth inhibitory activity several neutralizing antisera and monoclonal antibodies were obtained (Caroni and Schwab, 1988a). One monoclonal antibody called inhibitor-neutralizing antibody mAB IN-1 was used extensively for subsequent *in vitro* and *in vivo* experiments. This antibody decreases the inhibitory activity of a crude myelin extract by about 50% and neutralizes highly purified bovine NI-220 (the homologue of rat NI-250) by 80 – 100 % (Spillmann et al., 1998). Unfortunately, mAB IN-1 is not useful for Western-blots due to high background. Gel-purified NI-35 as well as NI-250 was neutralized by IN-1 (Caroni and Schwab, 1988a).

The full purification of NI-35/250 was difficult for two main reasons: the relatively low abundance of these components and the requirement for detergents in all purification steps. Starting with large amounts of bovine spinal cord, Spillmann et al., succeeded in purifying the bovine homologue bNI-220 to homogeneity (single spot on 2-dimensional PAGE) (Spillmann et al., 1998). Six stretches of amino acids obtained by microsequencing, showed the presence of a so far unknown protein. The corresponding cloned cDNA shows the characteristics of a type-II membrane protein and is derived from a gene which gives rise to three mRNAs (Chen et al., 1998; Chen et al., in preparation). This gene has been called *nogo*. The longest transcript, Nogo-A, expressed in COS or CHO cells, gives rise to a protein comigrating with oligodendrocyte NI-250 kDa. Recombinant Nogo-A is an inhibitory substrate for neurite outgrowth *in vitro* (Chen et al., 1998; Chen et al., in preparation). In situ hybrizidation and immunohistochemistry for Nogo-A show its presence in oligodendrocytes and the inner- and outer-most myelin membranes of all regions of the CNS (Huber et al., 1998; Chen et al., in preparation). Nogo-A is also expressed by subpopulations of neurons, especially during development, and also in some peripheral tissues. The smaller splice forms Nogo-B and Nogo-C have expression profiles different from Nogo-A.

Several antisera were raised against peptide sequences or recombinant protein domains. Two of these sera neutralize bovine or rat myelin inhibitory activity as well as the inhibition exerted by living oligodendrocytes, very similar to mAB IN-1. Injection of optic nerve explants with one of these antisera allowed massive ingrowth of axons from co-cultured perinatal DRG neurons.

All these results show that Nogo-A is most probably identical to the activity originally called NI-250 (NI-220). The exact identity of NI-35, which occurs in rat myelin but is not detectable in bovine or human myelin, remains to be established; because several antisera as well as mAB IN-1 neutralize NI-35, we suspect it to be a processing- or breakdown product of Nogo-A/NI-250.

IV. DEVELOPMENTAL CORRELATION OF MYELIN FORMATION AND DOWN REGULATION OF NEURITE GROWTH IN THE CNS

In several classical lesion studies a correlation between the developmental time at which a lesion occurred and the functional outcome or phenomena of regeneration and plasticity were observed (Kennard, 1936; Schwab and Bartholdi, 1996; Kapfhammer, 1997 for review). Thus, lesions of the cortical motor system in humans or monkeys occurring perinatally result in a much better functional outcome than lesions of the same areas acquired as adults (Kennard, 1936; Cao et al., 1994;

Rouiller et al., 1998). Defined transections of fiber tracts in newborn opossums, rats, hamsters, cats or E8 – 12 chicken induced regeneration of lesioned and/or compensatory growth of unlesioned fiber systems (Kalil and Reh, 1982; Tolbert and Der, 1987; Hasan et al., 1991; Treherne et al., 1992; Bregman et al., 1993; Saunders et al., 1998). Functional improvements were also observed (Reh and Kalil, 1982; Hasan et al., 1991; Bregman et al., 1993; Saunders et al., 1998). Both anatomical growth and functional improvement ceased to occur when the lesion was made at an age later than 1 - 2 weeks postnatally in rodents or E13 – 15 in chicks. In a developmental correlative study, close parallels between the appearance of myelin and the IN-1 antigen on the one hand and the loss of the growth-associated protein GAP-43 on the other hand were observed in the spinal cord (Kapfhammer and Schwab, 1994a). In the adult CNS the same negative correlation exists; highly myelinated white matter areas have lower or undetectable GAP-43 levels, whereas those grey matter areas known to retain structural plasticity throughout life exhibit high GAP-43 levels along with a low myelin content (Kapfhammer and Schwab, 1994b). Interestingly, a temporal correlation between myelination of layers 4 – 6 of the visual cortex with the end of the critical period for plasticity was also noted (LeVay et al., 1980).

In other studies, growth cones of E13 DRG neurites growing on laminin in the presence of NGF showed only short lasting reactions to NI-250-liposomes, whereas about 70% of the growth cones of E18 and over 90% of newborn or adult rat DRG growth cones collapsed in response to NI-250-liposomes (Bandtlow and Löschinger, 1997). This collapse led to long-lasting growth paralysis. Embryonic chick retinal cells showed a similar developmentally regulated growth cone collapse response. Interestingly, the inhibitory response of DRG cells to another myelin protein, MAG, is also developmentally regulated, although with a different time window (Mukhopadhyay et al., 1994; McKerracher et al., 1994). For newborn rat DRG neurites MAG is an adhesive and growth-promoting substrate. In contrast, neurites from adult DRGs are repulsed and inhibited by MAG. Recent studies show that neurotrophins and intracellular cyclic nucleotide balance play a crucial role in modifying growth cone responses to MAG and also to another developmentally important repulsive guidance molecule, Semaphorin-3 (Song et al., 1998; Cai et al., 1998).

A causal relationship between myelination and neurite growth was established by experiments where developing oligodendrocytes were either killed by X-irradiation or myelin was destroyed by the application of antibodies against GalC and complement (Savio and Schwab, 1990; Keirstead et al., 1992). Transection of fiber tracts (rats) or the entire spinal cord (chicken) resulted in impressive long-distance regeneration at an age where no regeneration can normally be seen (2 – 4 week old rat; newborn chicks) (Savio and Schwab, 1990; Keirstead et al., 1992; Keirstead et al., 1995). In chicks the large majority of the descending tracts showed successful anatomical regeneration which led to a high degree of recovery of locomotory functions (Keirstead et al., 1992; Keirstead et al., 1995). Sprouting of intact fiber systems into denervated territory after partial lesions (a phenomenon that occurs perinatally but not at later ages) (Schwegler et al., 1995) was documented in the rat spinal cord for incoming dorsal root axons as well as corticospinal fibers (Schwegler et al., 1995; Vanek et al., 1998). All these experiments demonstrate that the perinatal state allowing regeneration and compensatory growth in response to CNS lesions can be extended to later stages by the prevention of oligodendrocyte differentiation and myelin formation.

V. THE ANTIBODY IN-1 ENCOURAGES REGENERATION *IN VIVO*

Over the last 9 years, a large number of experiments were performed in which mAB IN-1 (or its recombinant Fab' fragment) (Bandtlow et al., 1996) were applied to the lesioned CNS of young or adult rats. A technical problem relating to mAB IN-1 made special ways of application necessary: mAB IN-1 is an IgM which is rather unstable upon purification. The best way of application, therefore, was the implantation of living mouse hybridoma cells, either encapsulated or as small tumors (Schnell and Schwab, 1990; Cadelli and Schwab, 1991; Z'Graggen et al., 1998). These hybridoma tumors grow slowly, are highly vascularized, produce large amounts of antibody and are resorbed upon withdrawl of the necessary immunosuppressive treatment. Recently, some of these earlier results were reproduced by pump application of a highly purified, bacterially produced, partially humanized recombinant IN-1 Fab-fragment (Brösamle et al., 1998).

The presence of IN-1 antibodies in the CSF greatly facilitates regeneration of lesioned corticospinal axons (spinal cord), optic nerve axons and cholinergic septohippocampal fibers (Schnell and Schwab, 1990; Cadelli and Schwab, 1991; Schnell and Schwab, 1993; Weibel et al., 1994, Bregman et al., 1995; Brösamle et al., in preparation). Embryonic spinal cord implants in adult rat thoracic spinal cord lesions or of NT-3 (but not BDNF) enhanced sprouting of the lesioned corticospinal axons, but, in our experiments, did not induce long-distance regeneration unless combined with mAB IN-1 (Schnell and Schwab, 1993; Schnell et al., 1994). Impressive sprouting and regeneration up to several millimeter in grey matter were observed in recent experiments where NT-3 was locally released over many days from transfected implanted fibroblasts (Grill et al., 1997). Reconstructions of serial sections showed that the corticospinal fibers and their sprouting collaterals often circumvent the bilateral dorsal hemisection lesion by growing through a ventral or ventrolateral grey or white matter bridge (von Meyenburg, 1998). Regenerating axons, which demonstrate a typical irregular course, grow down the spinal cord over distances which vary between 2 and 20 mm (Schnell and Schwab, 1990; Schnell and Schwab, 1993). They are observed to give off collaterals which branch profusely in grey matter and are decorated with bouton-like varicosities (von Meyenburg, 1998) (Brösamle et al., in preparation). Many of these axons elongate in positions which are abnormal for CST axons; a third of the axons, however, were found to grow towards and into the original CST territory after having crossed the lesion site (Brösamle et al., in preparation). Ongoing experiments also show reactions of rubrospinal axons to the presence of mAB IN-1: after unilateral lesions, extensive sprouting of the lesioned rubrospinal axons, together with massive compensatory fiber growth of the unlesioned, contralateral tract was observed (O. Raineteau, personal communication).

Corticospinal tract transections at the level of the medulla oblongata, immediately rostral to the pyramidal decussation, leads, in the presence of mAB IN-1, to extensive sprouting with reinnervation of the dorsal column nuclei (Thallmair et al., 1998; Z'Graggen et al., 1998; Raineteau, 1999). However, long distance regeneration is minimal, probably largely due to the apparant inability of the regenerating fibers to navigate through the pyramidal decussation (Raineteau, 1999). Thus, this unilateral lesion paradigm was ideally suited to study the compensatory axon growth/plasticity of unlesioned corticospinal and corticobulbar fibers in response to mAB IN-1. In the adult spinal cord, the remaining, intact tract was seen to sprout across the midline and to innervate the dorsal as well as the ventral horn of the denervated side of the spinal cord (Thallmair et al., 1998). In the brainstem, the cortico-rubral and cortico-pontine fibers of that cortex which has lost its access to the spinal cord by the lesion sent collaterals across the midline and established a bilateral innervation (Z'Graggen et al., 1998). (Cortico-rubral and cortico-pontine projections in the rat are almost completely ipsilateral in normal animals). Sprouting across the midline and innervation of the red nucleus, pons and striatum by intact cortico-fugal fibers was also observed following complete unilateral motor cortex aspiration lesions and application of mAB IN-1 in adult rats (Wenk et al., 1999). These results show that a high degree of compensatoy growth and plasticity can be established in adult spinal cord and brain stem by mAB IN-1 which is otherwise only observed following lesions in neonates. In all of the anatomical analyses a potent barrier effect of large lesion scars was evident (Brocke et al., 1993; Schnell et al., 1994; von Meyenburg, 1998). Sprouting fibers unable to cross the lesion or the macrophage filled debris zones were frequently observed.

Behavioral studies in mAB IN-1 treated rats with large spinal cord lesions showed functional recovery of various locomotion related motor functions (Bregman et al., 1995). A detailled analysis of skilled forelimb movements was done in pyramidal tract lesioned animals (Thallmair et al., 1998; Z'Graggen et al., 1998). These animals, which showed pronounced compensatory axon growth in the brain stem and spinal cord in response to mAB IN-1 treatment, exhibited almost complete recovery of food pellet reaching, a behavior which was severely and permanently affected in the lesioned control antibody treated rats.

VI. REGENERATION OF NEURITES CAN OCCUR IN ADULT CNS WHITE MATTER

When neurons were transplanted into the adult CNS, long-distance regeneration could be observed in several types of experiments under particular conditions. When embryonic aminergic neurons were implanted into spinal cord lesions, fiber growth was obtained over several millimeters, but was largely restricted to grey matter (Nornes et al., 1983; Privat et al., 1989). Regeneration up to the centimeter range was observed by Wictorin and Björklund when they transplanted human early neuroblasts into the rat striatum (Wictorin et al., 1990). Interestingly, transplanted rat or mouse embryo neurons did not elongate over the usual short distances of about 1 mm under the same conditions. Nevertheless, embryonic mouse hippocampal neurons transplanted as single cells or microtransplants into hippocampal white matter, the corpus callosum or the spinal cord did show successful long-distance growth (Davies et al., 1993; Li and Raisman, 1993; Davies et al., 1997). In the spinal cord, microtransplants of embryonic or adult dorsal root ganglion cells also resulted in long-distance regeneration in many cases (J. Silver, personal communication). Small transplants and small lesions were a prerequisite for successful regeneration; no long-distance neurite growth was observed with large lesions, which caused strong astrocyte reactivity and accumulation of chondroitin sulfate immunoreactive material (Davies et al., 1997). All these results suggest that the responsiveness of neurons to myelin-associated inhibitory factors can be modulated in important ways. Such modulations have indeed been shown by *in vitro* studies.

In the case of the transplantation experiments outlined above, the effects of axotomy, dissociation and implantation into an inflammed lesion site may well influence the neuronal response to environmental molecules and cues, including growth inhibitory proteins. Downregulation of receptors for inhibitory proteins, changes in the intracellular signaling machinery, or growth promotion overriding the inhibitory environmental effects are possible mechanisms that should be studied on the cellular and molecular level.

VII. FUTURE DIRECTIONS

A. Cellular and molecular mechanisms

Much of the available evidence indicates that Nogo-A/NI-220/250 is part of a signalling system composed of extracellular ligands and receptor(s). In fact, defined second messenger steps (in particular the release of calcium from intracellular stores) have been shown to be involved in growth cone collapse and growth inhibition (Bandtlow et al., 1993; Igarashi et al., 1993; Moorman, 1996). As a top priority, the binding partner/receptor of Nogo-A on the neuronal cell surface needs to be identified. Further, the intracellular signaling pathway and its lateral interactions with pathways of other (negative or positive) guidance signals should be analyzed. Regulation of the level of receptor expression and on various levels of the signal transduction cascade are important aspects determining the neuronal response(s) to Nogo-A. It is also not excluded that Nogo-A plays additional roles, especially during development, which may not be related to neurite growth inhibition. Such dual roles have been shown recently for the guidance molecule families of the Netrins and the Semaphorins, and broad pleiotropic actions are well known e.g., for the neurotrophin family (Tessier-Lavigne and Goodman, 1996; Caroni, 1998).

The role of inflammatory cells in the axonal reactions at lesion sites needs to be evaluated. Most of the neuroanatomical studies disregard the fact that a dynamic and very complex inflammatory reaction creates a very specific mixture of factors and a very different extracellular milieu at sites of CNS compared with PNS lesions (Schwab and Bartholdi, 1996). Results suggesting that inflammatory cells can modify myelin-associated neurite growth inhibitory activity have, in fact, been shown (David et al., 1990; Hirschberg et al., 1994).

B. IMPORTANCE OF NI-250/NOGO-A FOR REGENERATION IN THE ADULT CNS

The experiments using the neutralizing antibody IN-1 *in vivo* were among the first to show successful long-distance regeneration of lesioned axons in the adult rat CNS. They indicate that, at least for the fiber tracts studied (corticospinal tract, optic nerve, septohippocampal fibers), Nogo-A plays an important and crucial role in restricting the spontaneously occurring regeneration attempts. Still, the percentage of successfully regenerating fibers was in the range of about 10 % in these experiments. The scar and the large debris zones and cysts forming at spinal cord lesions, are major and long recognized obstacles to regeneration. Other important local factors could be the occurrence of additional neurite growth repulsive or inhibitory molecules as discussed in the following chapters. The cell body response to axotomy, which in many adult neurons is a spontaneous switch to a growth program resulting in local sprouting and, in the appropriate environment, in neurite elongation, may also vary in subpopulations of neurons. Treatment with appropriate neurotrophic factors or factor combinations can enhance the regenerative response and counteract cell death. Some of the beneficial effects of implanted cells, e.g., Schwann cells or the very successful olfactory ensheathing cells (see this volume, chapter by Plant), probably result from a combination of trophic factor release, synthesis of local growth-promoting substrates, formation of bridges across the lesion site and, in the case of olfactory glia, highly migratory, invasive behavior along spinal cord pathways (Xu et al., 1993; Li et al., 1997; Ramon-Cueto et al., 1998). Thus, combinatorial treatments may be an important way to maximize regeneration and hopefully functional recovery in animal models. When planning their transfer to the human level, however, one has to bear in mind that the safety requirements for any invasive treatment in paraplegic patients have to be extremely high.

REFERENCES

Bandtlow, C.E. and Löschinger, J. (1997). Developmental changes in neuronal responsiveness to the CNS myelin-associated neurite growth inhibitor NI-35/250. Europ.J.Neurosci. *9*, 2743-2752.

Bandtlow, C., Schiweck, W., Tai, H.-H., Schwab, M.E., and Skerra, A. (1996). The Escherichia coli-derived Fab fragment of the IgM/kappa antibody IN-1 recognizes and neutralizes myelin-associated inhibitors of neurite growth. Eur.J.Biochem. *241*, 468-475.

Bandtlow, C.E., Schmidt, M.F., Hassinger, T.D., Schwab, M.E., and Kater, S.B. (1993). Role of intracellular calcium in NI-35-evoked collapse of neuronal growth cones. Science *259*, 80-83.

Bandtlow, C.E., Zachleder, T., and Schwab, M.E. (1990). Oligodendrocytes arrest neurite growtn by contact inhibition. J.Neurosci. *10*, 3837-3848.

Bregman, B.S., Kunkel-Bagden, E., Reier, P.J., Dai, H.N., McAtee, M., and Gao, D. (1993). Recovery of function after spinal cord injury: mechanisms underlying transplant-mediated recovery of function differ after spinal cord injury in newborn and adult rats. Exp.Neurol. *123*, 3-16.

Bregman, B.S., Kunkel-Bagden, E., Schnell, L., Dai, H.N., Gao, D., and Schwab, M.E. (1995). Recovery from spinal cord injury mediated by antibodies to neurite growth inhibitors. Nature *378*, 498-501.

Broesamle, C., Huber, A., Fiedler, M., Skerra, A., and Schwab, M.E. (1998). A recombinant humanized IN-1 Fab-fragment promotes axonal regeneration of lesioned corticospinal fibers in adult rat. Soc.Neurosci. *24*, -1559(Abstract)

Broesamle, C., Huber, A.B., Fiedler, M., Skerra, A. and Schwab, M.E. (1999). Nerve fiber regeneration in the adult CNS induced by a recombinant, humanized antibody fragment. (Submitted).

Cadelli, D. and Schwab, M.E. (1991). Regeneration of lesioned septohippocampal acetylcholinesterase-positive axons is improved by antibodies against the myelin-associated neurite growth inhibitors NI-35/250. Europ.J.Neurosci. *3*, 825-832.

Cai, D., Shen, Y., De Bellards, M.E., Tang, S., and Filbin, M.T. (1998). Prior exposure to neurotrophins blocks inhibition of axonal regeneration by MAG and myelin via a cAMP-dependent mechanism. Neuron *22*, 89-101.

Cao, Y., Vikingstad, E.M., Huttenlocher, P.R., Towle, V.L., and Levin, D.N. (1994). Functional magnetic resonance studies of the reorganization of the human hand sensorimotor area after unilateral brain injury in the perinatal period. Proc.Natl.Acad.Sci.USA *91*, 9612-9616.

Carbonetto, S., Evans, D., and Cochard, P. (1987). Nerve fiber growth in culture on tissue substrata from central and peripheral nervous systems. J.Neurosci. *7*, 610-620.

Caroni, P. (1998). Driving the growth cone. Science *281*, 1465-1466.

Caroni, P. and Schwab, M.E. (1988a). Antibody against myelin-associated inhibitor of neurite growth neutralizes nonpermissive substrate properties of CNS white matter. Neuron *1*, 85-96.

Caroni, P. and Schwab, M.E. (1988b). Two membrane protein fractions from rat central myelin with inhibitory properties for neurite growth and fibroblast spreading. J.Cell Biol. *106*, 1281-1288.

Chen, M.S., Huber, A.B., van der Haar, M.E., Frank, M., Spillmann, A.A., Christ, F., and Schwab, M.E. (1998). Neurite outgrowth inhibitory factors in CNS myelin: molecular characterization of Nogo (NI-35/250). Soc.Neurosci. *24*, -1766(Abstract)

Crutcher, K.A. (1989). Tissue sections from the mature rat brain and spinal cord as substrates for neurite outgrowth in vitro: extensive growth on gray matter but little growth on white matter. Exp.Neurol. *104*, 39-54.

David, S. and Aguayo, A.J. (1981). Axonal elongation into peripheral nervous system "bridges" after central nervous system injury in adult rats. Science *214*, 931-933.

David, S., Bouchard, C., Tsatas, O., and Giftochristos, N. (1990). Macrophages can modify the nonpermissive nature of the adult mammalian central nervous system. Neuron *5*, 463-469.

Davies, S.J.A., Field, P.M., and Raisman, G. (1993). Long fiber growth by axons of embryonic mouse hippocampal neurons microtransplanted into the adult rat fimbria. Europ.J.Neurosci. *5*, 95-106.

Davies, S.J.A., Fitch, M.T., Memberg, S.P., Hall, A.K., Raisman, G., and Silver, J. (1997). Regeneration of adult axons in white matter tracts of the central nervous system. Nature *390*, 680-683.

Fawcett, J.W., Rokos, J., and Bakst, I. (1989). Oligodendrocytes repel axons and cause axonal growth cone collapse. J.Cell Science *92*, 93-100.

Fitch, M.T. and Silver, J. (1997). Glial cell extracellular matrix: boundaries for axon growth in development and regeneration. Cell Tissue Res. *290*, 379-384.

Grill, R., Murai, K., Blesch, A., Gage, F.H., and Tuszynski, M.H. (1997). Cellular delivery of neurotrophin-3 promotes corticospinal axonal growth and partial functional recovery after spinal cord injury. J.Neurosci. *17*, 5560-5572.

Hasan, S.J., Nelson, B.H., Valenzuela, J.I., Keirstead, H.S., Shull, S.E., Ethell, D.W., and Steeves, J.D. (1991). Functional repair of transected spinal cord in embryonic chick. Rest.Neurol.Neurosci. *2*, 137-154.

Hirschberg, D.L., Yoles, E., Belkin, M., and Schwartz, M. (1994). Inflammation after axonal injury has conflicting consequences for recovery of function: rescue of spared axons is impared but regeneration is supported. J.Neuroimmunol. *50*, 9-16.

Huber, A.B., Chen, M.S., van der Haar, M.E., and Schwab, M.E. (1998). Developmental expression pattern and functional analysis of Nogo (formerly NI-35/250), a major inhibitor of CNS regeneration. Soc.Neurosci. *24*, -1559(Abstract)

Igarashi, M., Strittmatter, S.M., Vartanian, T., and Fishman, M.C. (1993). Mediation by G proteins of signals that cause collapse of growth cones. Science *259*, 77-79.

Kalil, K. and Reh, T. (1982). A light and electron microscopic study of regrowing pyramidal tract fibers. J.Comp.Neurol. *211*, 265-275.

Kapfhammer, J.P. (1997). Restriction of plastic fiber growth after lesions by centarl nervous system myelin-associated neurite growth inhibtors. In Brain Plasticity, Advances in Neurology. H.-J. Freund, B.A. Sabel, and O.W. Witte, eds. (Philadelphia: Lippincott-Raven Publ.), pp. 7-27.

Kapfhammer, J.P. and Schwab, M.E. (1994a). Increased expression of the growth-associated protein GAP-43 in the myelin-free rat spinal cord. Europ.J.Neurosci. *6*, 403-411.

Kapfhammer, J.P. and Schwab, M.E. (1994b). Inverse pattern of myelination and GAP-43 expression in the adult CNS: neurite growth inhibitors as regulators of neuronal plasticity? J.Comp.Neurol. *340*, 194-206.

Kartje, G.L., Schulz, M.K., Lopez, A., Schnell, L. and Schwab, M.E. (1999). Corticostriatal plasticity is restricted by myelin-associated neurite growth inhibitors in the adult rat. Ann. Neurol., 45(6):778-786.

Keirstead, H.S., Dyer, J.K., Sholomenko, G.N., McGraw, J., Delaney, K.R., and Steeves, J.D. (1995). Axonal regeneration and physiological activity following transection and immunological disruption of myelin within the hatchling chick spinal cord. J.Neurosci. *15*, 6963-6974.

Keirstead, H.S., Hasan, S.J., Muir, G.D., and Steeves, J.D. (1992). Suppression of the onset of myelination extends the permissive period for the functional repair of embryonic spinal cord. Proc.Natl.Acad.Sci.USA *89*, 11664-11668.

Keirstead, S.A., Rasminsky, M., Fukada, Y., Carter, D.A., Aguayo, A.J. and Vidal-Sanz, M. (1989). Electrphysiologic responses in hamster superior colliculus evoked by regenerating retinal axons. Science *246*, 255-257.

Kennard, M. A. Age and other factors in motor recovery from precentral lesions in monkeys. Am.J.Physiol. *115*, 138-146. 1936.

LeVay, S., Wiesel, T.N., and Hubel, D.H. (1980). The development of ocular dominance columns in normal and visually deprived monkeys. J.Comp.Neurol. *191*, 1-51.

Li, Y., Field, P.M., and Raisman, G. (1997). Repair of adult rat corticospinal tract by transplants of olfactory ensheathing cells. Science *277*, 2000-2002.

Li, Y. and Raisman, G. (1993). Long axon growth from embryonic neurons transplanted into myelinated tracts of the adult rat spinal cord. Brain Res. *629*, 115-127.

McKerracher, L., David, S., Jackson, D.L., Kottis, V., Dunn, R.J., and Braun, P.E. (1994). Identification of myelin-associated glycoprotein as a major myelin-derived inhibitor of neurite growth. Neuron *13*, 805-811.

Meiners, S., Powell, E.M., and Geller, H.M. (1995). A distinct subset of tenascin/CS-6-PG-rich astrocyte restricts neuronal growth in vitro. J.Neurosci. *15*, 8096-8108.

Moorman, S.J. (1996). The inhibition of motility that results from contact between two oligodendrocytes in vitro can be blocked by pertussis toxin. Glia *16*, 257-265.

Mukhopadhyay, G., Doherty, P., Walsh, F.S., Crocker, P.R., and Filbin, M.Y. (1994). A novel role of myelin-associated glycoprotein as an inhibitor of axonal regeneration. Neuron *13*, 1-20.

Nornes, H., Björklund, A., and Stenevi, U. (1983). Reinnervation of the denervated adult spinal cord of rats by intraspinal transplants of embryonic brain stem neurons. Cell Tissue Res. *230*, 15-35.

Privat, A., Mansour, H., Rajaofetra, N., and Geffard, M. (1989). Intraspinal transplants of serotonergic neurons in the adult rat. Brain Res.Bull. *22*, 123-129.

Raineteau, O., Z'Graggen, W.J, Thallmair, M. and Schwab, M.E. (1999). Sprouting and regeneration after pyramidotomy and blockade of the myelin-associated neurite growth inhibitors NI-35/250 in adult rats. Europ.J.Neurosci. 11(4): 1486-1490.

Ramon-Cueto, A., Plant, G.W., Avila, J., and Bunge, M.B. (1998). Long-distance axonal regeneration in the transected adult rat spinal cord is promoted by olfactory ensheathing glia transplants. J.Neurosci. *18*, 3803-3815.

Ramon y Cajal, S. (1928). Degeneration and Regeneration of the Nervous System. (1959). (New York: Hafner).

Reh, T. and Kalil, K. (1982). Functional role of regrowing pyramidal tract fibers. J.Comp.Neurol. *211*, 276-283.

Richardson, P.M., Issa, V.M.K., and Aguayo, A.J. (1984). Regeneration of long spinal axons in the rat. J.Neurocytol. *13*, 165-182.

Rouiller, E.M., Yu, X.H., Moret, V., Tempini, A., Wiesendanger, M., and Liang, F. (1998). Dexterity in adult monkeys following early lesion of the motor cortical hand area: the role of cortex adjacent to the lesion. Europ.J.Neurosci. *10*, 729-740.

Saunders, N.R., Kitchener, P., Knott, W.G., Nicholls, J.G., Potter, A., and Smith, T.J. (1998). Development of waling, swimming and neuronal connections after complete spinal cord transection in the neonatal Opossum, Monodelphis domestica. J.Neurosci. *18*, 339-355.

Savio, T. and Schwab, M.E. (1989). Rat CNS white matter, but not gray matter, is nonpermissive for neuronal cell adhesion and fiber outgrowth. J.Neurosci. *9*, 1126-1133.

Savio, T. and Schwab, M.E. (1990). Lesioned corticospinal tract axons regenerate in myelin-free rat spinal cord. Proc.Natl.Acad.Sci.USA *87*, 4130-4133.

Schnell, L., Schneider, R., Kolbeck, R., Barde, Y.-A., and Schwab, M.E. (1994). Neurotrophin-3 enhances sprouting of corticospinal tract during development and after adult spinal cord lesion. Nature *367*, 170-173.

Schnell, L. and Schwab, M.E. (1990). Axonal regeneration in the rat spinal cord produced by an antibody against myelin-associated neurite growth inhibitors. Nature *343*, 269-272.

Schnell, L. and Schwab, M.E. (1993). Sprouting and regeneration of lesioned corticospinal tract fibers in the adult rat spinal cord. Europ.J.Neurosci. *5*, 1156-1171.

Schwab, M.E. and Bartholdi, D. (1996). Degeneration and regeneration of axons in the lesioned spinal cord. Physiol.Rev. *76*, 319-370.

Schwab, M.E. and Caroni, P. (1988). Oligodendrocytes and CNS myelin are nonpermissive substrates for neurite growth and fibroblast spreading in vitro. J.Neurosci. *8*, 2381-2393.

Schwab, M.E. and Thoenen, H. (1985). Dissociated neurons regenerate into sciatic but not optic nerve explants in culture irrespective of neurotrophic factors. J.Neurosci. *5*, 2415-2423.

Schwegler, G., Schwab, M.E., and Kapfhammer, J.P. (1995). Increased collateral sprouting of primary afferents in the myelin-free spinal cord. J.Neurosci. *15*, 2756-2767.

Song, H., Ming, G., He, Z., Lehmann, M., McKerracher, L., Tessier-Lavigne, M., and Poo, M.-M. (1998). Conversion of neuronal growth cone responses from repulsion to attraction by cyclic nucleotides. Science *281*, 1515-1518.

Spillmann, A.A., Amberger, V.R., and Schwab, M.E. (1997). High molecular weight protein of human central nervous system myelin inhibits neurite outgrowth: an effect which can be neutralized by the monoclonal antibody IN-1. Europ.J.Neurosci. *9*, 549-555.

Spillmann, A.A., Bandtlow, C.E., Lottspeich, F., Keller, F., and Schwab, M.E. (1998). Identification and characterization of a bovine neurite growth inhibitor (bNI-220). J.Biol.Chem. *273*, 19283-19293.

Tello, F. (1911). La influencia del neurotropismo en la regeneracion de los centros nerviosos. Trab.Lab.Invest.Biol. *9*, 123-159.

Tessier-Lavigne, M. and Goodman, C.S. (1996). The molecular biology of axon guidance. Science *274*, 1123-1133.

Thallmair, M., Metz, G.A.S., Z'Graggen, W.J., Raineteau, O., Kartje, G.L., and Schwab, M.E. (1998). Neurite growth inhibitors restrict plasticity and functional recovery following corticospinal tract lesions. Nature Neurosci. *1*, 124-131.

Tolbert, D.L. and Der, T. (1987). Redirected growth of pyramidal tract axons following neonatal pyramidotomy in cats. J.Comp.Neurol. *260*, 299-311.

Treherne, J.M., Woodward, S.K.A., Varga, Z.M., Ritchie, J.M., and Nicholls, J.G. (1992). Restoration of conduction and growth of axons through injured spinal cord of neonatal opossum in culture. Proc.Natl.Acad.Sci.USA *89*, 431-434.

Tuttle, R. and Matthew, W.D. (1991). An in vitro bioassay for neurite growth using cryostat sections of nervous tissue as a substratum. J.Neurosci.Meth. *39*, 193-202.

Vanek, P., Thallmair, M., Schwab, M.E., and Kapfhammer, J.P. (1998). Increased lesion-induced sprouting of corticospinal fibers in the myelin-free rat spinal cord. Europ.J.Neurosci. *10*, 45-56.

von Meyenburg, J. Brösamle C. Metz G. A. S. Schwab M. E. (1998). Regeneration and sprouting of chronically injured corticospinal tract fibers in adult rats promoted by NT-3 and the mAB IN-1, which neutralizes myelin-associated neurite growth inhibitors. Exp.Neurol. 154, 583-594.

Watanabe, E. and Murakami, F. (1989). Preferential adhesion of chick central neurons to the gray matter of the central nervous system. Neurosci.Lett. *97*, 69-74.

Weibel, D., Cadelli, D., and Schwab, M.E. (1994). Regeneration of lesioned rat optic nerve fibers is improved after neutralization of myelin-associated neurite growth inhibitors. Brain Res. *642*, 259-266.

Wenk, C.A., Thallmair, M., Kartje, G.L., and Schwab, M.E. (1999). Increased corticofugal plasticity after unilateral cortical lesions combined with neutralization of the IN-1 antigen in adult rats. J.Comp.Neurol. *410*(1):143-157.

Wictorin, K., Brundin, P., Gustavii, B., Lindvall, O., and Björklund, A. (1990). Reformation of long axon pathways in adult rat central nervous system by human forebrain neuroblasts. Nature *347*, 556-558.

Xu, X.M., Guénard, A., Kleitman, N., and Bunge, M.B. (1997). Schwann cell trasnplants promote axonal regeneration form both the rostral and caudal stumps of transected adult rat spinal cord. J. Neurocytol. *26*, 1-16.

Z'Graggen, W.J., Metz, G.A.S., Kartje, G.L., Thallmair, M., and Schwab, M.E. (1998). Functional recovery and enhanced corticofugal plasticity after unilateral pyramidal tract lesion and blockade of myelin-associated neurite growth inhibitors in adult rats. J.Neurosci. *18*, 4744-4754.

16

Inhibition of Axon Growth by Myelin-Associated Glycoprotein

Samuel David
Centre for Research in Neuroscience, The Montreal General Hospital Research Institute and McGill University, Montreal, Quebec, Canada

Lisa McKerracher
University of Montreal, Montreal, Quebec, Canada

I. INTRODUCTION: MYELIN-ASSOCIATED GLYCOPROTEIN INHIBITS AXON GROWTH *IN VITRO* AND *IN VIVO*

Although neurons in the adult mammalian CNS are unable to regenerate for long distances through adult CNS tissue, they retain the ability to regrow for long distances if provided with an appropriate glial environment. This ability for long distance growth by CNS neurons was first demonstrated in 1981 by David and Aguayo using peripheral nerve grafts transplanted into the CNS. Another important discovery in the field of CNS regeneration was made in 1988 by Caroni and Schwab who showed that a major factor contributing to the failure of axon regeneration through CNS tissue was the axon growth inhibitory properties of CNS myelin. Their work led to the identification of the first neurite growth inhibitor (NI-35/250) recognized by the monoclonal antibody IN-1 (Caroni and Schwab, 1988a, b). The characterization and influence of this inhibitor on axon regeneration are discussed in the preceding chapter. In this chapter we discuss the evidence that led to the identification and functional characterization of myelin-associated glycoprotein (MAG) as an inhibitor of axon growth. We also review a number of other studies done over the past five years that have extended our understanding of the specificity and mechanism of action of MAG in inhibiting axon growth.

II. MAG IS AN INHIBITOR OF NEURITE GROWTH

In 1994 two laboratories using different experimental approaches showed that MAG has strong neurite growth inhibitory activity (Mukhopadhyay et al., 1994; McKerracher et al., 1994).

A. Studies with Bovine CNS Myelin

As work on myelin-derived axon growth inhibition progressed through the early 1990s it became evident that inhibitors in addition to NI-35/250 were likely to be present in CNS myelin. This reasoning was based on the finding that while the IN-1 antibody was able to stimulate some axon regrowth following axotomy in the CNS, the number of axons growing past the lesion site was extremely limited (Schnell and Schwab, 1990). To search for additional myelin-derived neurite growth inhibitors we purified myelin from bovine white matter, extracted the myelin with detergent and separated the myelin proteins by DEAE anion exchange chromatography (McKerracher et al., 1994). Proteins eluted from this column were tested for neurite growth inhibitory activity using an *in vitro* neurite growth assay. Several of the 25-30 fractions eluted from the DEAE column possessed neurite growth inhibitory activity which resolved into two well-defined peaks. Western blots showed that the first peak, which was the larger of the two, contained MAG. Immunodepletion of MAG from fractions contributing to the first inhibitory peak resulted in a marked loss of neurite growth inhibition strongly suggesting that MAG contributes to the inhibitory activity in these fractions. Additional confirmation of the neurite growth inhibitory effect of MAG was obtained by testing purified recombinant MAG (described in the next section). The contribution of MAG to the overall neurite growth inhibition by myelin was estimated by immunodepleting MAG from total CNS myelin extracts. A significant amount of the inhibitory activity associated with myelin was removed by this procedure. The precise contribution of MAG to myelin-derived inhibition of axon regeneration *in vivo* still remains to be determined. However, the evidence available at present shows that MAG contained in CNS myelin is indeed capable of inhibiting neurite growth *in vitro*.

B. Studies with Recombinant MAG

Filbin's group was the first to show that neurite growth from primary neurons was markedly inhibited on CHO cells expressing MAG, but was normal on untransfect ed CHO cells or cells expressing Po, another myelin protein (Mukhopadhyay et al., 1994). The recombinant MAG expressed by these cells was found to be similar to native MAG in its molecular weight and glycosylation. Neurite growth on

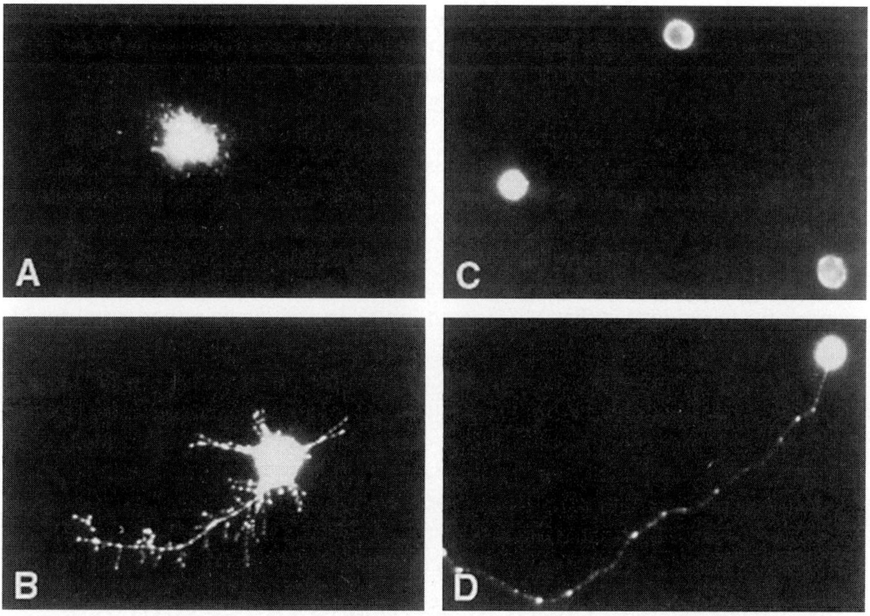

Figure 1 MAG inhibits neurite growth. Neurite growth from embryonic day 19 rat hippocampal neurons (**A**) and neonatal rat cerebellar neurons (**C**) is inhibited when plated on MAG-coated substrates for 18 hours. On a control substrate, hippocampal (**B**) and cerebellar (**D**) neurons extend long neurites. Note that the cerebellar neurons on MAG remain rounded while the hippocampal neurons have very short processes.

MAG-expressing CHO cells was reduced by 70% from rat cerebellar neurons and by about 40% from dorsal root ganglion (DRG) neurons (DeBellard et al., 1996). Furthermore, this effect of MAG could be reversed by approximately 50% with anti-MAG antibodies (Mukhopadhyay et al., 1994). Retinal, hippocampal, spinal and superior cervical ganglion (SCG) neurons from neonatal rats were also similarly inhibited from extending neurites on CHO cells expressing MAG (DeBellard et al., 1996). Inhibition of neurite growth was also detected on Schwann cells expressing recombinant MAG (Tang et al., 1997b). In other work, we also showed that the percentage of neurons extending neurites was drastically reduced when NG108-15 cells, neonatal rat cerebellar neurons or embryonic day 19 rat hippocampal neurons were plated directly onto a tissue culture substrate coated with purified recombinant MAG (McKerracher et al., 1994; Li et al., 1996). On these purified recombinant MAG substrates, cerebellar neurons often appeared rounded while hippocampal neurons had small processes that were generally less than one cell body diameter in length (Figure 1). The apparently stronger inhibition on purified recombinant MAG-coated substrates as compared to MAG expressing CHO cells, may reflect the presence of adhesion molecules present on the cell membrane of CHO cells which may modulate some of the inhibitory effects of MAG. Nevertheless, even on these complex cellular substrates neurite growth as measured by neurite length was severely reduced in the order of 40%-70% depending on the type of neuron.

In addition to its inhibitory effects when presented as a substrate-bound molecule, soluble MAG-Fc chimeric protein was also found to inhibit neurite growth when added to cerebellar neurons plated on substrates coated with the cell adhesion molecule L1, or on 3T3 cells expressing L1, N-CAM or N-cadherin (Tang et al., 1997b). The evidence that soluble MAG can inhibit neurite growth provides further evidence that MAG is an inhibitory molecule rather than providing a nonpermissive substrate. Interestingly, Tang et al., (1997b) also showed that the proteolytic fragment of MAG consisting of its entire extracellular domain (referred to as dMAG) can also inhibit neurite growth when added in solution to cultures of rat cerebellar neurons. Soluble dMAG is generated in the CNS *in vivo* (Möller et al., 1996; Stebbins et al., 1998) and could potentially diffuse and exert its effects at a distance from the site of origin. It is therefore possible that soluble dMAG may also inhibit axon growth and regeneration *in vivo.*

III. NEURONAL RESPONSIVENESS TO MAG VARIES WITH NEURONAL TYPE AND DEVELOPMENTAL AGE

Not all neurons were inhibited to the same extent when plated on CHO cells expressing MAG. Postnatal day 2 (P2) SCG neurons were inhibited by about 70% while P3 DRG neurons were only inhibited by 40% (DeBellard et al., 1996). A variety of CNS neurons were also found to be inhibited between 50%-90% (DeBellard et al., 1996). Such differences in the percentage of inhibition may be due in part to the varying length to which these neurons extend neurites on untransfected CHO cells. Interestingly, MAG stimulated neurite growth from P1 rat DRG neurons, while DRG neurons from P3 and older rats were inhibited by 40% as noted above (Mukhopadhyay et al., 1994; DeBellard et al., 1996). The timing of this change in responsiveness to MAG corresponds to the onset of myelination in the dorsal columns of the spinal cord where the central processes of the DRG neurons extend on their way to the dorsal column nuclei (Schwab and Schnell, 1991). The responsiveness of DRG neurons to MAG at P3 may thus serve to prevent abnormal sprouting of dorsal column sensory fibers within the spinal cord. Developmental differences in responsiveness to MAG may also occur with spinal cord neurons (DeBellard et al., 1996; Turnley and Bartlett, 1998). MAG was shown to stimulate neurite growth of spinal cord neurons from embryonic day 17 mouse (Turnley and Bartlett, 1998), while inhibiting neurite growth from P2 and P9 rats (DeBellard et al., 1996). The testing for such differences for other types of neurons (retinal, cerebellar, hippocampal and SCG) was only done with neurons at P2 and P9 (DeBellard et al., 1996). It is possible that developmental differences may be detected at earlier embryonic ages. Developmental differences in the responsiveness to several cell adhesion molecules such as N-CAM, N-cadherin and integrins have also been observed for a variety of neurons (Doherty et al., 1992; Carbonetto and David, 1993). Such precisely timed recruitment of various adhesion and inhibitory mechanisms are likely needed to stimulate and guide axons to their appropriate targets during development.

IV. AXONS AND DENDRITES RESPOND DIFFERENTLY TO MAG

The question as to whether the reduction of neurite growth on MAG containing substrates is due to the inhibitory effects of MAG or the lack of a sufficiently permissive growth substrate was directly examined by assessing the effects of MAG on growth cones. The behavior of growth cones of newborn rat hippocampal neurons was studied when grown in the presence of polystyrene beads coated with MAG (Shibata et al., 1998; Li et al., 1996). The coupling of MAG to polystyrene beads allowed the discrete delivery of substrate-bound molecules to the growth cone. Furthermore, hippocampal pyramidal neurons were chosen because these neurons develop clearly identifiable axonal and dendritic processes *in vitro* (Craig and Banker, 1994). Using this approach it was found that the majority of growth cones which prior to contact with the polystyrene beads displayed a spread lamellipodium with long filopodia collapsed upon contact with MAG-coated beads (Figure 2) (Li et al., 1996; Shibata et al., 1998). The collapse resulted in retraction of the lamellipodium and filopodia and left the growth cone immotile.

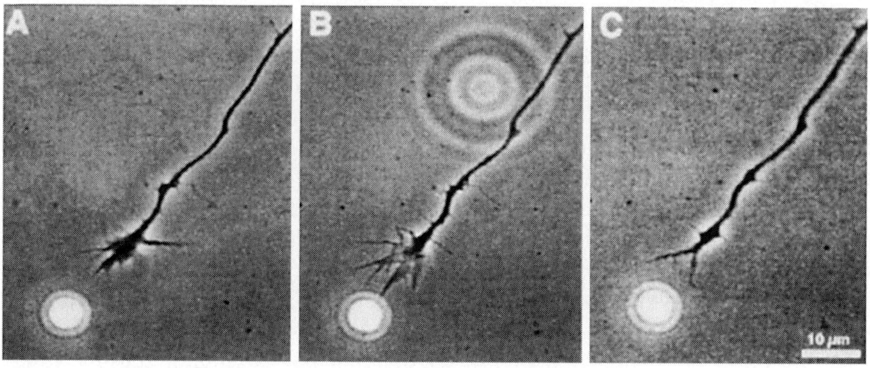

Figure 2 MAG causes collapse of axonal growth cones. **A**. Axonal growth cone of a neonatal rat hippocampal neuron displays a normal, spread morphology of the lamellipodium and long filopodia before contacting recombinant MAG-coated bead (bottom left side). **B**. The elongating growth cone contacts the bead with a few filopodia. **C**. After 17 minutes the lamellipodium has collapsed, as have most of the filopodia. The growth cone has retracted from the MAG-coated bead (Reproduced from Li et al, 1996).

Interestingly, axonal and dendritic growth cones behaved differently. About 72% of the MAP-2-negative axonal growth cones collapsed after contact with MAG-coated beads, while a similar number of MAP-2-positive dendritic growth cones did not collapse under the same conditions (Shibata et al., 1998). Fifty percent of the axonal growth cones that collapsed retracted about 20 μm after contacting MAG-coated beads. These results show clearly that MAG acts preferentially on axonal rather than dendritic growth cones. A similar difference in axonal and dendritic responses was also seen with oligodendrocytes (Shibata et al., 1998). In contrast to differentiated axonal and dendritic growth cones, the majority of the growth cones of minor processes, which are the earliest undifferentiated neuronal processes, are also inhibited by oligodendrocytes (67.6%) but not by MAG-coated beads (Shibata et al., 1998). These findings indicate that MAG acts specifically to inhibit and paralyze the motility of differentiated axonal rather than dendritic growth cones. It also suggests that other inhibitors associated with oligodendrocytes mediate the collapse response of the minor processes. Whether similar responses occur with other types of neurons is still to be established. This differential ability of axonal and dendritic growth cones to respond to MAG is likely to be dependant upon the presence of appropriate MAG receptors and intracellular molecules which will be discussed later.

The growth of axonal and dendritic processes has also been shown to be differentially regulated by astrocytes *in vitro*. For example, dendritic growth from mesencephalic dopaminergic neurons is favored on homotypic (mesencephalic) astrocytes, while axonal outgrowth was stimulated on heterotypic (striatal) astrocytes (Denis-Donini et al., 1984; Prochiantz, 1995). LeRoux and Reh (1994) have also shown that axonal but not dendritic growth is influenced by the developmental age of the cultured astrocytes. Substrate-bound and secreted molecules may underlie these responses. The finding that axonal but not dendritic processes are inhibited by mature oligodendrocytes and the inhibitors associated with myelin, such as MAG and NI-35/250, adds another source of substrate-bound molecules that can differentially influence axonal and dendritic process outgrowth. The combined influence of these myelin and astrocyte associated substrate-bound molecules together with diffusible inhibitory and neurotrophic factors serve to sculpt the dendritic arborization and axonal projections that are unique to different populations of neurons. During development, the ability of axonal growth cones to be inhibited by myelin-associated inhibitors may play a role, for example, in restricting the growth of axons of later developing fiber pathways to their own territory. This was demonstrated for the rat corticospinal tract which develops after the onset of myelination of the surrounding dorsal column sensory fibers (Schwab and Schnell, 1991). In the mature CNS, such responsiveness of axonal growth cones to myelin-derived inhibitors appear to be an important cause of the failure of regeneration of the long fiber tracts (Schwab et al., 1993; David, 1998).

V. MAG HAS INHIBITORY EFFECTS ON AXON GROWTH *IN VIVO*

A. MAG-Deficient Mice

Several studies have examined the axon growth inhibitory properties of myelin in MAG-/- mice (Bartsch et al., 1995; Li et al., 1996; Shen et al., 1998). As for the *in vitro* work on myelin membranes purified from MAG+/+ and MAG-/- mice, one study failed to detect any difference in the inhibitory activity (Bartsch et al., 1995), another study found a trend toward reduced inhibition (Li et al., 1996) and a third study reported significant differences (Shen et al., 1998). The differences between these studies may lie in the sensitivity of the assay used for analysis of neurite growth and the test neurons used. Measurement of the length of the neurites (Shen et al., 1998) is much more sensitive at detecting differences than estimation of the percentage of neurons that extend neurites. The latter authors have also reported that the methods used to purify myelin can lead to loss of inhibitory activity due to the proteolytic production of soluble dMAG which would be removed when the myelin membranes are prepared (Shen et al., 1998). This may account for the high degree of variability we observed with our myelin preparations (Li et al., 1996). On the other hand, we found that testing detergent-solubilized myelin proteins after separation by DEAE chromatography revealed that the major neurite growth inhibitory peak (first peak) which normally contains MAG is reduced significantly in the MAG-knockout mice (Li et al., 1996). In an *in vivo* model of spinal cord injury, we detected a small improvement in regeneration of corticospinal tract fibers in MAG-deficient mice (Li et al., 1996), while another group did not see any improvement in a similar model (Bartsch et al., 1995). These *in vivo* results are consistent with the presence of or compensatory increase in other axon growth inhibitors in the myelin of MAG-deficient mice that mask the absence of MAG.

Interestingly, the inhibitory effect of MAG *in vivo* was most clearly demonstrated in the regenerating peripheral nerve in MAG-deficient mice crossbred with the C57BL/Wld^S mice (Schäfer et al., 1996). The C57BL/Wld^S mutant has a deficiency in macrophage recruitment and activation after peripheral nerve injury (Brown et al., 1992). As a result, the clearance of myelin during Wallerian degeneration after peripheral nerve injury is markedly delayed in this mutant and this is accompanied by a reduction in axon regeneration (Brown et al., 1992; Chen and Bisby, 1993). In contrast, axon regeneration after peripheral nerve injury is significantly enhanced in C57BL/Wld^S mice that have been crossbred with MAG-deficient mice. Myelin is still not cleared after nerve injury in these double-mutant mice but it lacks MAG (Schäfer et al., 1996). These findings clearly point to MAG exerting a substantial inhibitory effect on axon regeneration *in vivo*.

B. Other Studies on Peripheral Nerve Regeneration

After peripheral nerve injury a large number of sprouts emerge from the cut end of the nerve. How is the excessive number of sprouts eliminated so as to achieve normal innervation of the target? This was tested in mice in which segments of peripheral nerve that were lesioned 7 days earlier were grafted by placing them close to the distal end of the proximal portion of a freshly cut sciatic nerve (Torigoe and Lundborg, 1998). Under these conditions regeneration of axons or axon sprouts was inhibited. However, if the cut axons were allowed to regenerate for 3 days to allow the regenerating axons to become ensheathed by Schwann cells, the growth of these axons was not inhibited by placing a 7-day lesioned nerve graft in close proximity. On the other hand if the cut axons were only allowed 2 days to regenerate, the regenerating axon sprouts which are naked at this stage (i.e., unensheathed by Schwann cells) are eliminated by the 7-day lesioned nerve graft. This inhibitory effect on axon sprouts could be blocked completely with antibodies against MAG (Torigoe and Lundborg, 1998). It has therefore been suggested that after crush injury or transections and reapposition of a peripheral nerve the regenerating axon sprouts that immediately enter Schwann cell basal lamina tubes distal to the injury will be maintained, while the growth of the sprouts that appear later or are unensheathed by Schwann cells will be inhibited by MAG.

The absence in the adult mammalian CNS of properly aligned growth promoting cells such as Schwann cells, the presence of 10-fold more MAG in the CNS than in peripheral nerves, and the evidence that a variety of CNS neurons are inhibited by MAG *in vitro* suggests that MAG may also play a significant role in inhibiting axon regeneration in the CNS *in vivo*. However, direct *in vivo* evidence for a strong inhibitory role for MAG in the CNS has yet to be obtained.

VI. MAG HAS MULTIPLE FUNCTIONAL DOMAINS

Myelin-associated glycoprotein is an integral membrane protein that is highly glycosylated, and has a molecular weight of approximately 100 kDa (Arquint et al., 1987; Lai et al., 1987; Salzer et al., 1987). It has five immunoglobulin (Ig)-like extracellular domains, a transmembrane and a cytoplasmic domain (Figure 3). The extracellular domain consists of one N-terminal V-type Ig domain followed by 4 C2-type Ig domains (Arquint et al., 1987 ; Lai et al., 1987; Salzer et al., 1987). MAG is expressed by oligodendrocytes and Schwann cells and is about one-tenth as abundant in peripheral nerve myelin as it is in CNS myelin (Trapp, 1990). In CNS myelin it is localized to the periaxonal region where it comes in contact with the axonal membrane (Bartsch et al., 1989). In peripheral nerves it has also been localized to the periaxonal membrane, outer mesaxon and basal lamina (Trapp, 1990; Martini and Schachner, 1986). Two isoforms exist that are generated by alternative RNA splicing. These two isoforms are similar in the extracellular and transmembrane regions but differ in their cytoplasmic domain. The

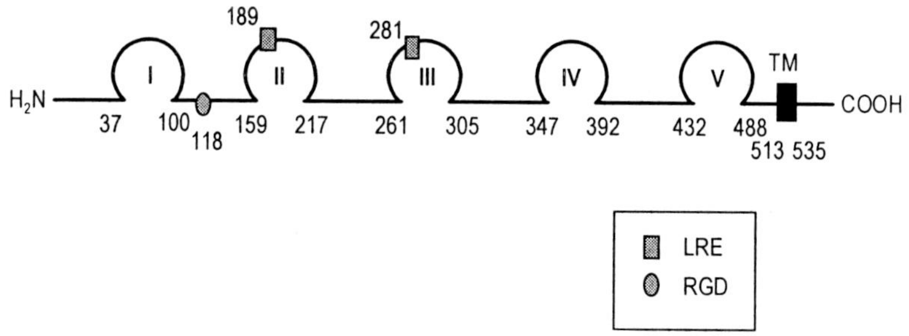

Figure 3 Schematic diagram showing the structure of MAG. Note the 5 Ig-like domains, transmembrane (TM) and cytoplasmic domains. The location of the LRE and RGD epitopes are indicated. Figure adapted from Meyer-Franke et al., (1995).

large isoform referred to as (L-MAG) and the small isoform referred to as (S-MAG) have molecular weights of 72 and 67 kDa, respectively, after deglycosylation, and are differentially expressed during development (Frail and Braun, 1983; Tropak et al., 1988). The functional differences of these two isoforms are still not known. Based on its structure and adhesive properties MAG was initially postulated to be important for myelination, but recent studies on MAG-null mutant mice indicate that it is not essential for myelination (Li et al., 1994; Montag et al., 1994), but may be required for the formation and maintenance of the periaxonal region and optimal production of myelin (Fruttiger et al., 1995; Li et al., 1998).

Myelin-associated glycoprotein is also a member of the sialic acid-binding immunoglobulin superfamily called siglecs (Crocker et al., 1998). In this group, MAG is classified as siglec-4a (Crocker et al., 1998). The functional topography of MAG is partly known, in large part due to epitope mapping of anti-MAG antibodies (Fahrig et al., 1993; Meyer-Franke et al., 1995; Pedraza et al., 1995; Tropak et al., 1995; Tang et al., 1997a). Electron microscopy of rotary-shadowed fragments showed that the molecule is bent in two so that the N-terminal region folds over toward the transmembrane domain (Fahrig et al., 1993). This finding is supported by biophysical data (sedimentation analysis and gel chromatography) that indicate that MAG is not an extended molecule but likely to be a bent rod (Attia et al., 1993). Mapping of monoclonal antibody 513 binding to MAG also supports the idea that MAG is a bent rod. The 513 antibody has a conformationally-sensitive epitope (Tropak et al., 1995), and electron microscopic studies demonstrated that 513 binds to the hinge region (Fahrig et al., 1993). Deletion analysis studies also support the contention that 513 binds to the middle of the MAG molecule (Meyer-Franke et al., 1995).

The antibody 513 blocks binding of MAG liposomes to neurons (Johnson et al., 1989a), and binding of soluble MAG-Fc chimeric proteins to neurons (Tang et al., 1997a). However, 513 does not block growth inhibition by recombinant MAG expressed on the surface of CHO cells. One possible explanation for these findings is that inhibition of neurite growth likely occurs in two steps: first, adhesion has to occur between MAG and the neuronal cell surface followed by neurite growth inhibition (Tang et al., 1997a). Therefore, neurite growth inhibition by MAG can be prevented by disruption of the adhesive event, such as occurs when the 513 antibody prevents binding of soluble MAG-Fc to the cell surface. It is therefore likely that there is a yet to be characterized growth inhibitory domain that is separate from the cell adhesion domain recognized by the 513 antibody that mediates inhibition by substrate-bound MAG (Tang et al., 1997a).

The mapping of binding sites for other members of the immunoglobulin superfamily has demonstrated multiple functional domains (Ranheim et al., 1996; Appel et al., 1993). Similarly, the available evidence suggests that MAG has cell adhesion sites in domains I to III and the growth inhibitory site is in domains IV or V (Tang et al., 1997a). CHO cells expressing domains III, IV and V were incapable of cell binding (Tropak and Roder, 1997), implicating domains I and II in cell adhesion. MAG has an RGD sequence (arginine, glycine, aspartic acid) in domain I or domain II, depending on predicted protein folding models (Pedraza et al., 1995; Fahrig et al., 1993). The RGD sequence is directly implicated in integrin-mediated cell adhesion to extracellular matrix proteins, and therefore, it is a good candidate for the cell adhesion site of MAG. However, it was proposed that the RGD sequence may be buried inside the first domain because an anti-peptide antibody directed to a 20mer containing the RGD site was not able to bind to native protein, only to denatured protein (Pedraza et al., 1995). While these results suggest the antibody recognized a hidden epitope, it is not certain that the RGD sequence itself is hidden. Tang et al., (1997a) have used mutational analysis to demonstrate that R118, the arginine in the RGD sequence, is required for neuronal binding to MAG. Mutation of R118 to either alanine or aspartate abolished neuronal binding to MAG, but the mutated MAG expressed in CHO cells retained its growth inhibitory activity. Therefore, R118 is important for cell adhesion by MAG, but it is not yet established if only R118 is needed, or if the binding site is the entire RGD sequence which is not conformationally hidden. In addition, cell binding sites that are distinct from R118 are likely to exist. Experiments with other function-blocking antibodies suggest that there is a separate cell binding site in domain III (Meyer-Franke et al., 1995). It is known that MAG does not bind well to sialic acid-containing ligands when domains IV and V are missing (Schnaar et al., 1998).

Less is known about the inhibitory sequence of MAG. MAG contains 2 LRE (leucine, arginine, glutamic acid) sequences, one in domain II and another in domain III (Arquint et al., 1987). The LRE sequence is important in motor neuron binding to S-laminin at the neuromuscular junction, and both soluble and substrate-bound LRE peptides inhibit neurite growth from motor neurons (Hunter et al., 1991). However, LRE-dependent adhesion is thought to be motor neuron specific (Hunter et al., 1991), whereas inhibition by MAG is not. Also, deletion mapping has shown that the dominant growth inhibitory domain is likely to reside in domain IV or domain V because a truncated MAG -Fc missing domains IV and V was not able to inhibit neurite outgrowth (Tang et al., 1997a). Therefore, it seems likely that the LRE sequence is not a dominant inhibitory domain of MAG, and that the growth inhibitory sequence in domains IV or V has yet to be identified.

VII. MAG BINDS TO SIALIC ACID CONTAINING GANGLIOSIDES ON THE NEURONAL SURFACE

MAG is considered to be a lectin because it is a sialic acid binding protein (Kelm et al., 1994; Crocker et al., 1998). Experiments with MAG-transfected fibroblasts have demonstrated that MAG exhibits heterophilic interactions (Afar et al., 1991), which is not unexpected because neurons do not express MAG. Ligands that bind MAG are glycoconjugates that are sialylated, and they may be gangliosides, which are sialic acid-containing glycosphingolipids (Collins et al., 1997a, b; Yang et al., 1996). A specific glycoprotein receptor has not yet been found. Binding of MAG-transfected CHO cells to sialic-acid expressing cells and inhibition of neurite outgrowth by MAG are both reduced when neurons or target cells are desialylated with neuraminidase (Tropak and Roder, 1997; Schnaar et al., 1998; Shen et al., 1998). By contrast, neuraminidase treatment of the MAG-expressing CHO cells increases binding to MAG (Tropak and Roder, 1997). The construction and analysis of multiple glycosylation site mutations in MAG demonstrated that the N-linked glycosylation sites in MAG are not required for MAG-mediated cell binding (Tropak and Roder, 1997), and removal of sialic acid from MAG enhances its binding activity (Collins et al., 1997b). Also, recombinant MAG produced in the baculovirus system, which is poorly glycosylated, retains potent inhibitory activity (McKerracher et al., 1994; Johnson et al., 1989b). Therefore, sialylation of the neuronal cell surface ligand, but not of MAG itself, is the major regulator of MAG binding to neurons.

Several different MAG binding partners have been identified (Kelm et al., 1994; Yang et al., 1996; Collins et al., 1997a, b), and specific neuronal receptors to MAG are likely to exist. MAG preferentially binds to 2,3-linked sialic acids on O-linked glycans and gangliosides (Kelm et al., 1994; Yang et al., 1996; Schnaar et al., 1998). Molecules that act as ligands for MAG are gangliosides, with GD1a, GT1b, GQ1b being the best binding partners (Collins et al., 1997b; Schnaar et al., 1998). Chimeric MAG-Fc with only domains I, II and III, thought to contain the binding site (Tropak and Roder, 1997; Tang et al., 1997a), is able to bind ganglioside GQ1b , but does not recognize other gangliosides that bind full-length MAG (Schnaar et al., 1998). These results suggest that there are multiple ganglioside recognition domains in MAG.

VIII. cAMP AND Rho PLAY A ROLE IN INTRACELLULAR SIGNALLING BY MAG

While the neuronal receptor to MAG is not known, we now have a better understanding about the intracellular pathways that are involved in neurite growth inhibition by MAG. Several recent reports have implicated adenosine 3', 5'-monophosphate (cAMP) as a second messenger that regulates the neuronal response to MAG (Song et al., 1998; Cai et al., 1999). When Xenopus spinal neurons are placed in culture and exposed to a microscopic gradient of soluble recombinant MAG, the growth cones turn and grow away from the MAG. This growth cone repulsion by soluble MAG can be converted into attraction by elevation of intracellular cAMP levels to activate protein kinase A (PKA) (Song et al., 1998). Similarly, Cai et al., (1999) demonstrated that the addition of dibutyryl cAMP to cerebellar or DRG neurons in culture is sufficient to overcome growth inhibition by MAG or myelin. These results suggest that upon neuronal interaction with MAG, levels of cyclic nucleotides are kept low and PKA is relatively inactive. Cai et al., (1999) provide evidence that MAG activates a pertussis-toxin sensitive heterotrimeric G-protein that prevents neurotrophin-induced increases in cAMP. They found that priming neurons with neurotrophins blocked MAG-induced neurite growth inhibition by increasing cAMP levels and activating PKA. However, treatment with pertussis toxin alone did not affect inhibition of neurite growth by MAG, but it eliminated the need for priming with neurotrophins to overcome growth inhibition, i.e., neurotrophins could be effective if added at the same time as exposure to MAG. These authors also noted a similar response with myelin (Cai et al., 1999). However, it has also been shown that the pertussis toxin subunit, which does not inactivate heterotrimeric G-proteins, can cause growth cones to lose the ability to follow guidance cues provided by laminin, possibly because it binds to cell surface carbohydrates (Kindt and Lander, 1995). Therefore, further work is needed to establish and clarify the involvement of heterotrimeric G proteins in growth cone collapse and in repressing the elevation of cAMP.

Recent data suggest that the Rho pathway is a key target for regulating growth cone motility and growth cone collapse (Jalink et al., 1994; Tigyi et al., 1996b; Strittmatter, 1997; Katoh et al., 1998; Jin and Strittmatter, 1997). Experiments with non-neuronal cells have implicated cAMP in the regulation of Rho because PKA directly phosphorylates Rho on Ser188 (Lang et al., 1996). While this phosphorylation does not affect nucleotide exchange, phosphorylation decreases the ability of Rho kinase ROK to interact with activated Rho (Dong et al., 1998). In neurons, the small lipid mediator lysophosphatidic acid causes growth cone collapse by activation of Rho (Tigyi et al., 1996a). In PKA deficient PC12 cells, elevation of cAMP fails to protect neurites from the activation of Rho by lysophosphatidic acid (Tigyi et al., 1996a). These results demonstrate that the activation of PKA by cAMP is necessary to prevent neurite retraction induced by Rho, probably through the ability of PKA to phosphorylate Rho. It is likely that

PKA-dependent regulation of Rho may also be an important regulator of neurite growth and growth cone collapse in primary neurons.

Recently, our studies have shown that Rho is important in regulating the response of neurons to MAG and myelin (Selles-Navarro et al., 1998; Lehmann et al., 1999). First, Rho can be detected by immunocytochemistry in DRG neuron growth cones (Renaudin et al., 1998). Second, PC12 cells transfected with a dominant negative RhoA were able to grow on MAG substrates but not on myelin substrates. Endogenous Rho is not completely inactivated by a dominant negative mutation, and we suggest that inactivation of all forms of Rho is necessary to overcome the multiple growth inhibitory proteins that are present in myelin (Lehmann et al., 1999). We have also made use of the C3 enzyme from *Clostridium botulinum* that selectively ADP-ribosylates Rho in its effector domain to inactivate Rho. We found that treatment of PC12 cells or retinal neurons with C3 allowed neurite growth on inhibitory MAG or myelin substrates (Figure 4).

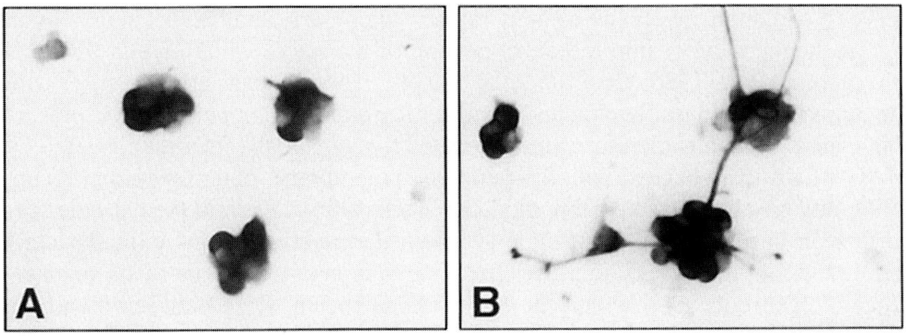

Figure 4 Treatment of retinal neurons with C3 to inactivate Rho promotes neurite growth on MAG-coated substrates. **A**. Retinal neurons triturated with PBS and plated on MAG do not extend neurites. **B**. Retinal neurons triturated with C3 enzyme before plating on MAG substrates show significantly more cells extending long neurites. Neurons were detected by immunocytochemistry with an anti-III tubulin antibody.

Finally, the treatment of injured rat optic nerve with C3 *in vivo* allowed a robust but short-lived regenerative growth. After C3 treatment of injured optic nerve, anterogradely labeled RGC axons extended past the site of the crush injury into the myelinated distal segment of the nerve (Selles-Navarro et al.,1998; Lehmann et al., 1999). Therefore, it seems likely that the neuronal interaction with MAG activates Rho leading to inhibition of axon growth, and that inactivation of Rho with C3 overrides growth inhibition by both MAG and myelin.

IX. ADHESION MOLECULES CAN OVERRIDE MAG AND MYELIN-DERIVED INHIBITION OF NEURITE GROWTH

There is now evidence that certain adhesion molecules can override the inhibitory effects of myelin and MAG. Although peripheral nerve myelin is as inhibitory as CNS myelin, this inhibition can be overridden by the presence of laminin (Bähr and Przyrembel, 1995; David et al., 1995). Peripheral nerve myelin purified using two different protocols was found to yield myelin that either contains very little laminin or abundant amounts of laminin (David et al., 1995). The former myelin preparation was as inhibitory as CNS myelin, while the latter preparation stimulated extensive neurite growth. Blocking the laminin in the latter myelin preparation with an anti-laminin antibody resulted in a reduction in neurite growth (David et al., 1995). The laminin in these preparations is likely derived from the Schwann cell basal lamina. MAG appears to be an important inhibitor in peripheral nerve myelin, since NI-35/250 which is recognized by the IN-1 monoclonal antibody is not expressed in peripheral nerves (Rubin et al., 1994). Furthermore, laminin can also override the neurite growth inhibitory effects of recombinant MAG (David et al., 1995).

What role could laminin play *in vivo* in overriding inhibitors in peripheral nerves? Although myelin is cleared rapidly after peripheral nerve injury, axon sprouts begin to grow into the distal portion of the nerve while myelin debris is still present (Hall, 1986; Goodrum et al., 1994). These sprouts are in contact with the Schwann cell basal lamina and plasma membrane. Laminin which is present in the basal lamina is therefore ideally located to override the inhibition exerted by MAG which is associated with the periaxonal membrane, outer mesaxon (Trapp, 1990) and basal lamina (Martini and Schachner, 1986). Even in the extreme scenario seen in the C57BL/Wld^S mice in which the myelin remains virtually intact during the first few weeks after peripheral nerve injury, an average of 1.6 regenerating axon sprouts grew within the basal lamina sheath, lying between it and the intact myelin, in about 15-25% of the axons counted. This growth may be due to the effects of laminin to override some of the myelin-derived inhibition. The cell adhesion molecule L1 which is present on the Schwann cell membrane has also been shown to be capable of overriding the inhibitory effects of myelin (Mohajeri et al., 1996) and may work in concert with laminin in the peripheral nerve to minimize the effects of inhibitors after peripheral nerve injury.

Laminin is also able to override the inhibitory effects of CNS myelin *in vitro* (Bähr and Przyrembel, 1995; David et al., 1995). Adding 1.5 μg of laminin to 8 μg of CNS myelin was sufficient to override about 80% of the inhibitory activity (David, et al., 1995). In these experiments laminin was distributed evenly in the mixed myelin/laminin substrates as punctate dots. The growth cones of the neurons plated on such a substrate likely extend from one spot of laminin to the next. This may involve intracellular changes within the growth cone to override the effects of the inhibitors associated with the myelin, as has been shown in another culture model using polystyrene beads coated with adhesion molecules (Kuhn et al., 1995). When the spots of laminin are more widely separated from each other, as happens with the lower concentrations of laminin, the growth cones appear unable to negotiate the larger distances between laminin spots. The findings that laminin can override the inhibitory effects of myelin were further supported by the work of Tang et al., (1997b) who showed that soluble dMAG is not able to inhibit neurite growth from cerebellar neurons plated on laminin-coated substrates but is able to do so when the neurons are grown on fibronectin or poly-L-lysine. In these experiments laminin was able to completely abrogate the inhibitory effects of dMAG.

There is also evidence that the cell adhesion molecule L1 can override the inhibitory effects of CNS myelin. Earlier studies have shown that neurite growth is very poor on unfixed cryostat sections of the adult rat optic nerve (Carbonetto et al., 1987; David et al., 1990). However, the optic nerves of transgenic mice over expressing L1 are able to support better neurite growth than their wild-type controls (Mohajeri et al., 1996). L1 therefore appears to be able to override the inhibitory effects of CNS myelin. Whether other cell adhesion molecules can block myelin-derived inhibitors is not yet known.

Certain cell adhesion molecules can therefore override the inhibitory effects of CNS myelin *in vitro*. It remains to be seen whether such an approach can be used to neutralize myelin-derived inhibitors *in vivo* to promote axon regeneration in the adult mammalian CNS.

X. NEUROTROPHINS CAN OVERRIDE MAG AND MYELIN-DERIVED INHIBITION OF NEURITE GROWTH

As discussed above, recent studies have shown that MAG and myelin-derived inhibition of neurite growth can also be overridden by priming neurons with neurotrophins or increasing cAMP levels (Cai et al., 1999). Several earlier studies have shown that the addition of neurotrophic factors to cultures at the time of plating did not stimulate neurite growth on myelin-coated substrates. However, Filbin's group recently reported the remarkable finding that the inhibitory effects of MAG and myelin could be completely blocked if the neurons are primed with neurotrophins prior to plating (Cai et al., 1999). Priming of cerebellar neurons overnight with either BDNF or GDNF but not NGF was effective in completely neutralizing the inhibitory effects of MAG. Postnatal day 5 DRG neurons on the other hand were responsive to all three factors under similar conditions. Both types of neurons responded in a like manner when plated onto CNS myelin after being primed with neurotrophins (Cai et al., 1999). These authors raise the possibility that such a mechanism might underlie the unexpected axon growth through myelinated regions of the CNS in two different animals models, one in the optic nerve after implantation of a piece of peripheral nerve into the eye (Berry et al., 1996) and the other in the spinal cord after embryonic CNS transplants and neurotrophin treatment (Bregman, 1998).

The intracellular pathways that might be involved in mediating the overriding of MAG and myelin-derived inhibition of neurite growth by neurotrophins were discussed earlier. Additional experiments testing *in vivo* the effectiveness of neurotrophins in stimulating axon regeneration through myelinated regions after CNS injury need to be performed.

X. FUTURE DIRECTIONS

The growth inhibitory activity of MAG has been well established by several laboratories using different cell culture techniques (McKerracher et al., 1994, Mukhopadhyay et al., 1994, Shibata et al., 1998, Song et al., 1998). Moreover, recent experiments have suggested that *in vivo,* MAG is likely to contribute to growth inhibition by myelin after axonal injury (Schäfer et al., 1996; Torigoe and Lundborg, 1998). While over the last five years our understanding about the growth inhibitory properties of MAG has increased, there are still some important gaps in our knowledge. Future work needs to be focused on identifying the axon growth inhibitory domains of MAG and the neuronal MAG receptors that interact with it. Identification of such domains in MAG and the neuronal receptors will provide the information needed to develop more effective antagonists such as blocking antibodies or peptides that could be delivered more effectively to block the inhibitory effects of MAG. Attention also needs to be directed at a fuller understanding of the intracellular signaling pathways utilized by MAG, and a comparison of these pathways with other growth inhibitory proteins. Such an understanding should lead to the development of strategies to overcome axon growth inhibition by MAG and other inhibitors present in myelin.

ACKNOWLEDGMENTS: This work was supported by grants from the Canadian MRC and the MRC NeuroScience Network.

REFERENCES

Afar DEH, Marius RM, Salzer JL, Stanners CL, Braun PE, Bell JC (1991) Cell adhesion properties of myelin-associated glycoprotein in L cell fibroblasts. J Neurosci Res 29:429-436.

Appel F, Holm J, Conscience J, Schachner M (1993) Several extracellular domains of the neural cell adhesion molecule L1 are involved in neurite outgrowth and cell body adhesion. J Neurosci 13:4764-4775.

Arquint M, Roder J, Chia L, Down J, Wilkinson D, Bayley H, Braun P, Dunn R (1987) Molecular cloning and primary structure of myelin-associated glycoprotein. PNAS 84:600-604.

Attia J, Hicks L, Oikawa K, Kay CM, Dunn RJ (1993) Structural properties of the myelin-associated glycoprotein ectodomain. J Neurochem 61:718-726.

Bähr M, Przyrembel, C (1995) Myelin from peripheral and central nervous system is a nonpermissive substrate for retinal ganglion cell axons. Exp. Neurol. 134: 87-93.

Bartsch U, Bandtlow C, Schnell L, Bartsch S, Spillmann AA, Rubin BP, Hillenbrand R, Montag D, Schwab ME, Schachner S (1995) Lack of evidence that myelin-associated glycoprotein is a major inhibitor of axonal regeneration in the CNS. Neuron 15: 1375-1381.

Bartsch U, Kirchoff F, Schachner S (1989) Immunohistochemical localization of the adhesion molecules L1, N-CAM and MAG in the developing and adult optic nerves of mice. J. Comp. Neurol. 284: 454-462.

Berry M, Carlile J, Hunter A (1996) Peripheral nerve explants grafted into the vitreous body of the eye promote the regeneration of retinal ganglion cell axons severed in the optic nerve. J. Neurocytol. 25: 147-170.

Bregman BS (1998) Transplants and neurotrophins increase regeneration and recovery of function after spinal cord injury. In Frontiers of Neural Development. K. Uyemura, ed., Tokyo: Springer-Verlag.

Brown MC, Lunn ER, Perry VH (1992) Consequences of slow Wallerian degeneration for regenerating motor and sensory axons. J. Neurobiol. 83: 521-536.

Cai D, Shen Y, DeBellard ME, Tang S, Filbin MT (1999) Prior exposure to neurotrophins blocks inhibition of axonal regeneration by MAG and myelin via a cAMP-dependent mechanism. Neuron 22:89-101.

Carbonetto S, David S (1993) Adhesive molecules of the cell surface and extracellular matrix in neural regeneration. In: Gorio, A., ed. Neuroregeneration. New York: Raven Press, pp77-100.

Carbonetto S, Evans D, Cochard P (1987) Nerve fiber growth in culture on tissue culture substrata from central and peripheral nervous systems. J. Neurosci. 7: 610-620.

Caroni P, Schwab ME (1988a) Antibody against myelin-associated inhibitor of neurite growth neutralizes nonpermissive substrate properties of CNS white matter. Neuron 1:85-96.

Caroni P, Schwab ME (1988b) Two membrane protein fractions from rat central myelin with inhibitory properties for neurite growth and fibroblast spreading. J Cell Biol 106:1281-1288.

Chen S, Bisby MA (1993) Impaired motor axon regeneration in the C57BL/Ola mouse. J. Comp. Neurol. 333: 449-454.

Collins BE, Kiso M, Hasegawa A, Tropak MB, Roder JC, Crocker PR, Schnaar RL (1997a) Binding specificities of the sialoadhesion family of I-type lectins. J Biol Chem 272:16889-16895.

Collins BE, Yang LJ-S, Mukhopadhyay G, Filbin MT, Kiso M, Hasegawa A, Schnaar RL (1997b) Sialic acid specificity of myelin-associated glycoprotein binding. J Biol Chem 272:1248-1255.

Crocker PR, Clark EA, Filbin M, Gordon S, Jones Y, Kehrl JH, Le Douarin N, Powell L, Roder J, Schnaar RL, Sgroi DC, Stamenkovic I, Schauer R, Schachner M, van den Berg TK, van der Merwe PA, Watt S, M. (1998) Siglecs: a family of sialic-acid binding lectins. Glycobiology 2:v-vi.

David S (1998) Axon growth promoting and inhibitory molecules involved in regeneration in the adult mammalian central nervous system. Ment. Retard. & Dev. Disabilities Res. Rev. 4: 171-178.

David S, Aguayo AJ (1981) Axonal elongation into peripheral nervous system "bridges" after central nervous system injury in adult rats. Science 214:931-933.

David S, Bouchard C, Tsatas O, Giftochristos N (1990) Macrophages can modify the non-permissive nature of the adult mammalian central nervous system. Neuron 5: 463-469.

David S, Braun PE, Jackson JL, Kottis V, McKerracher L (1995) Laminin overrides the inhibitory effects of PNS and CNS myelin-derived inhibitors of neurite growth. J Neurosci Res 42:594-602.

DeBellard ME, Tang S, Mukhopadhyay G, Shen Y-J, Filbin MT (1996) Myelin-associated glycoprotein inhibits axonal regeneration from a variety of neurons via interaction with a sialoglycoprotein. Molec Cell Neurosci 7:89-101.

Denis-Donini S, Glowinski J, Prochiantz A (1984) Glial heterogeneity may define the three-dimensional shape of mouse mesencephalic dopaminergic neurones. Nature 307: 641-643.

Doherty P, Skaper SD, Moore SE, et al., (1992) A developmentally regulated switch in neuronal responsiveness to NCAM and N-cadherin in the rat hippocampus. Development 115: 885-892.

Dong J, Leung T, Manser E, Lim L (1998) cAMP-induced morphological changes are counteracted by the activated RhoA small GTPase and the Rho kinase ROK . J Biol Chem 273:22554-22562.

Fahrig T, Probstmeier R (1993) Functional topography of the myelin-associated glycoprotein.I. Mapping of domains by electron microscopy. Europ J Neurosci 5:1118-1126.

Frail DE, Braun PE (1983) Two developmentally regulated messenger RNAs differing in their coding region may exist for the myelin-associated glycoprotein. J. Biol. Chem. 259: 14857-14862.

Fruttiger M, Montag D, Schachner M, Martini R (1995) Crucial role for the myelin-associated glycoprotein in the maintenance of axon-myelin integrity. Europ. J. Neurosci. 7:511-515.

Goodrum JF, Earnhardt T, Goines N, Bouldin TW (1994) Fate of myelin lipids during degeneration and regeneration of peripheral nerve: an autoradiographic study. J. Neurosci. 14: 357-367.

Hall SM (1986) The effects of inhibiting Schwann cell mitosis on the reinnervation of acellular autografts in the peripheral nervous system of the mouse. Neuropathol. Appl. Neurobiol. 12:401-414.

Hunter DD, Cashman N, Morris-Valero R, Bulock JW, Adams SP, Sanes JR (1991) An LRE (leucine-arginine-glutamate)-dependent mechanism for adhesion of neurons to S-laminin. J Neurosci 11:3960-3971.

Jalink K, van Corven EJ, Hengeveld T, Morii N, Narumiya S, Moolenaar WH (1994) Inhibition of lysophosphatidate-and thrombin-induced neurite retraction and neuronal cell rounding by ADP ribosylation of the small GTP-binding protein Rho. J Cell Biol 126:801-810.

Jin Z, Strittmatter SM (1997) Rac1 mediates collapsin-1-induced growth cone collapse. J Neurosci 17:6256-6263.

Johnson PW, Abramow-Newerly W, Seilheimer B, Sadoul R, Tropak MB, Arquint M, Dunn RJ, Schachner S, Roder JC (1989a) Recombinant myelin-associated glycoprotein confers neural adhesion and neurite outgrowth function. Neuron 3: 377-385.

Johnson PW, Attia J, Richardson CD, Roder JC, Dunn RJ (1989b) Synthesis of soluble myelin-associated glycoprotein in insect and mammalian cells. Gene 77:287-296.

Katoh H, Aoki J, Ichikawa A, Negishi M (1998) p160 RhoA-binding kinase ROK induces neurite retraction. J Biol Chem 273:2489-2492.

Kelm S, Pelz A, Schauer R, Filbin MT, Tang S, DeBellard ME, Schnaar RL, Mahoney JA, Hartnell A, Bradfield P, Crocker PR (1994) Sialoadhesion, myelin-associated glycoprotein and CD22 define a new family of sialic acid-dependent adhesion moelcules of the immunoglobulin superfamily. Curr Biol 4:965-972.

Kindt RM, Lander AD (1995) Pertussis toxin specifically inhibits growth cone guidance by a mechanism independent of direct G protein inactivation. Neuron 15:79-88.

Kuhn TB, Brown MD, Wilcox CL, Raper JA, Bamburg JR (1999) Myelin and collapsin-1 induce motor neuron growth cone collapse through different pathways: inhibition of collapse by opposing mutants of Rac1. J Neurosci 19:1965-1975.

Kuhn TB, Schmidt MF, Kater SB (1995) Laminin and fibronectin guideposts signal sustained but opposite effects to passing growth cones. Neuron 14: 275-285

Lang P, Gesbert F, Delespine-Carmagnat M, Stancou R, Pouchelet M, Bertoglio J (1996) Protein kinase A phosphorylation of RhoA mediates the morphological and functional effects of cyclic AMP in cytotoxic lymphocytes. EMBO J 15:510-519.

Lehmann M, Fournier AE, Selles-Navarro I, Dergham P, Leclerc N, Tigyi G, McKerracher L (1999) Inactivation of the small GTP-binding protein Rho promotes CNS axon regeneration. Submitted

Li M, Shibata A, Li C, Braun PE, McKerracher L, Roder J, Kater SB, David S (1996) Myelin-associated glycoprotein inhibits neurite/axon growth and causes growth cone collapse. J. Neurosci. Res. 46: 404-414.

Li C, Tropak MB, Gerlai R, Clapoff S, Abramow-Newerly W, Trapp B, Peterson A, Roder JC (1994) Myelination in the absence of myelin-associated glycoprotein. Nature 369: 747-750.

Li C, Trapp B, Ludwin S, Peterson A, Roder J (1998) Myelin associated glycoprotein modulates glia-axon contact in vivo. J. Neurosci. Res. 51: 210-217.

Martini R, Schachner M (1986) Immunoelectron microscopic localization of neural cell adhesion molecules (L1, M-CAM and MAG) their shared carbohydrate epitope and myelin basic protein in developing sciatic nerve. J. Cell Biol. 103: 2439-2448.

McKerracher L, David S, Jackson JL, Kottis V, Dunn R, Braun PE (1994) Identification of myelin-associated glycoprotein as a major myelin-derived inhibitor of neurite outgrowth. Neuron 13:805-811.

Meyer-Franke A, Tropak MB, Roder JC, Fischer P, Beyreuther K, Probstmeir R, Schachner M (1995) Functional topography of myelin-associated glycoprotein. II. Mapping of domains on molecular fragments. J Neurosci Res 41:311-323.

Möller JR (1996) Rapid conversion of myelin-associated glycoprotein to a soluble derivative in primates Brain Res. 741: 27-31.

Montag D, Giese KP, Bartsch U, Martini R, Lang Y, Bluthmann H, Karthigasan J, Kirschner DA, Wintergerst ES, Nave K-A, Zielasek J, Toyka KV, Lipp H-P, Schachner S (1994) Mice deficient for myelin-associated glycoprotein show subtle abnormalities in myelin. Neuron 13: 229-246

Mukhopadhyay G, Doherty P, Walsh FS, Crocker PR, Filbin MT (1994) A novel role for myelin-associated glycoprotein as an inhibitor of axonal regeneration. Neuron 13: 757-767.

Pedraza L, Spagnol G, Latov N, Salzer JL (1995) Biosynthesis and regulation of expression of the HNK-1 epitope on myelin-associated glycoprotein in a transfected cell model system. J of Neurosci Res 40:716-727.

Prochiantz A (1995) Neuronal polarity: giving neurons heads and tails. Neuron 15: 743-746.

Ranheim TS, Edelman GM, Cunningham BA (1996) Homophilic adhesion mediated by the neural cell adhesion molecule involves multiple immunoglobulin domains. PNAS 93:4071-4075.

Renaudin A, Lehmann M, McKerracher L (1998) Organization of point contacts in neuronal growth cones. J Neurosci Res 55:458-471.

Rubin BP, Dusart J, Schwab ME (1994) A monoclonal antibody (IN-1) which neutralizes growth inhibitory proteins in the rat central nervous system recognizes antigens localized in CNS myelin. J. Neuocytol. 23: 209-217.

Schäfer M, Fruttiger M, Montag D, Schachner M, Martini R (1996) Disruption of the gene for the myelin-associated glycoprotein improves axonal regrowth along myelin in C57BL/Wlds mice. Neuron 16:1107-1113.

Schnaar RL, Collins BE, Wright LP, Kiso M, Tropak MB, Roder JC, Crocker PR (1998) Myelin-associated glycoprotein binding to gangliosides. Structural specificity and functional implications. In: Sphingolipids as signaling modulators in the nervous system. (Anonymouspp 92-105. NY: NY Academy of Sci.

Schnell, L. and Schwab, M.E. (1990). Axonal regeneration in the rat spinal cord produced by an antibody against myelin-associated neurite growth inhibitors. Nature *343*, 269-272.

Schwab ME, Kapfhammer JP, Bandtlow CE (1993) Inhibitors of neurite growth. Annu Rev Neurosci 16: 565-595

Schwab ME, Schnell L (1991) Channeling of developing rat corticospinal tract axons by myelin-associated neurite growth inhibitors. J. Neurosci. 11: 709-721.

Selles-Navarro I, Fournier A, Dergham P, Lehmann M, McKerracher L (1998) Regeneration of adult rat retinal ganglion cell (RGC) axons after microlesion and inactivation of the GTPase Rho by treatment with C3 enzyme. Soc Neurosci Abstr 24:1560.

Shen YJ, DeBellard ME, Salzer JL, Roder J, Filbin MT (1998) Myelin-associated glycoprotein in myelin and expressed by Schwann cells inhibits axonal regeneration and branching. Molec Cell Neurosci 12:79-91.

Shibata A, Wright MV, David S, McKerracher L, Braun PE, Kater SB (1998) Unique responses of differentiating neuronal growth cones to inhibitory cues presented by oligodendrocytes. J Cell Biol 142:191-202.

Song H, Ming G, He Z, Lehmann M, McKerracher L, Tessier-Lavigne M, Poo M (1998) Conversion of growth cone responses from repulsion to attraction by cyclic nucleotides. Science 281:1515-1518.

Stebbins JW, Jaffe H, Möller JR (1998) Characterization of myelin-associated glycoprotein (MAG) proteolysis in the human central nervous system. Neurochem. Res. 23: 1005-1010.

Tang S, Shen YJ, DeBellard ME, Mukhopadhyay G, Salzer JL, Crocker PR, Filbin MT (1997a) Myelin-associated glycoprotein interacts with neurons via a sialic acid site at ARG118 and a distinct neurite inhibition site. J Cell Biol 138:1355-1366.

Tang S, Woodhall RW, Shen YJ, DeBellard ME, Saffell JL, Doherty P, Walsh FS, Filbin MT (1997b) Soluble myelin-associated glycoprotein (MAG) found in vivo inhibits axonal regeneration. Molec Cell Neurosci 9:333-346.

Tigyi G, Fischer DJ, Sebok A, Marshall F, Dyer DL, Miledi R (1996a) Lysophophatidic acid-induced neurite retraction in PC12 cells: neurite-protective effects of cyclic AMP signaling. J Neurochem 66:549-558.

Tigyi G, Fischer DJ, Sebok A, Yang C, Dyer DL, Miledi R (1996b) Lysophosphatidic acid-induced neurite retraction in PC12 cells: control by phosphoinositide - Ca^{+2} signaling and Rho. J Neurochem 66:537-548.

Torigoe K, Lundborg G (1998) Selective inhibition of early axonal regeneration by myelin-associated glycoprotein. Exp. Neurol. 150: 254-262.

Trapp BD (1990) Myelin-associated glycoprotein: location and potential functions. Ann. NY Acad. Sci., 605: 29-43.

Tropak MB, Jansz GF, Abramow-Newerly W, Roder JC (1995) Conservation of functionally important epitopes on myelin associated glycoprotein (MAG). Comp Biochem Physiol 112B:345-354.

Tropak MB, Johnson PW, Dunn RJ, Roder JC (1988) Differential splicing of MAG transcripts during CNS and PNS development. Mol. Brain Res. 4: 143-155

Tropak MB, Roder JC (1997) Regulation of myelin-associated glycoprotein binding by sialylated *cis*-ligands. J Neurochem 68:1753-1763.

Turnley AM, Bartlett PF (1998) MAG and MOG enhance neurite outgrowth of embryonic mouse spinal cord neurons. NeuroReport 9: 1987-1990.

Yang LJ-S, Zeller CB, Shaper NL, Kiso M, Hasegawa A, Shapiro RE, Schnaar RL (1996) Gangliosides are neuronal ligands for myelin-associated glycoprotein. Proc Natl Acad Sci USA 93:814-818.

17

Axonal Growth in a Glial Environment

Geoffrey Raisman

The Norman and Sadie Lee Research Centre, Division of Neurobiology, National Institute for Medical Research, MRC, London, United Kingdom

I. INTRODUCTION

Nerve cells are arranged in a way which is unique among all tissues – they interact with each other through long axonal processes which carry the myriad individual signals whose total comprises the function of the nervous system. In the adult CNS, these axonal processes are bundled into myelinated (white matter) tracts. Because of this arrangement, nervous tissue also presents a unique situation with regard to injury. When white matter tracts are cut, the axons lose their functional role as message carriers, but the neuronal cell bodies survive. During this period, the severed ends of the cut nerve fibers form local sprouts, but are unable to regenerate to their original destinations.

This period provides us with a window of opportunity, through which we glimpse the tantalizing prospect of devising methods for encouraging nerve fibers to regenerate, re-establish their former contacts, and therefore restore the lost functions. To learn how to achieve such a repair would be of profound significance for patients with spinal injury, as well as other axonal injuries, such as stroke.

In the course of this chapter I shall cherry-pick some of the studies from my lab group in Oxford and later in London, not necessarily in a chronological order, but re-arranged with the benefit of hindsight, so as to illustrate a viewpoint on the problem of axon repair in the adult brain and spinal cord.

II. THE REASONS FOR STUDYING THE GLIAL STRUCTURE OF TRACTS

During axonal elongation in development or in culture, the expanded, motile surfaces provided by the plasma membranes of the growth cone and filopodia at the tip of advancing axons act as a sensory structure, exploring the environment, and detecting and responding to molecular signals that determine advance, collapse, or turning of the axon (Mason, Wang, 1997; Tessier-Lavigne, Goodman, 1996; Fan, Raper, 1995). From this it follows that the type of growth response in any specific situation will be a response to the cellular (or extracellular) structures that are in contact with the axon tip. To provide a background of information for attempts to obtain regeneration of cut adult white matter tract axons, therefore, we have studied the organization of the cellular component of adult fiber tracts.

Myelinated adult fiber tracts have a highly conserved and uniform pattern of distribution of oligodendrocytes, astrocytes and microglia (Suzuki, Raisman, 1992). The glial cell bodies are segregated into regularly spaced unicellular rows aligned along the axis of the tract (Figure 1). The oligodendrocytes form contiguous stretches of around 5-15 cell bodies, separated by solitary astrocytes or microglia. Cells of each type give rise to processes which extend across the axis of the tract, permeate the axon fascicles, and in turn generate a large number of longitudinal processes running in parallel with the axons. A major part of the membrane structure of adult fiber tracts consists of a dense carpet of parallel longitudinal-astrocytic processes.

When a tract is damaged, this orderly glial structure is disrupted, and becomes reorganized (e.g. as in an astrocytic scar). The cut axons produce local sprouts at the site of injury (e.g. Cajal, 1928), but the sprouts do not advance through the tract. We have carried out experiments to explore the extent to which this failure can be related to loss of the glial alignment of the fiber tracts.

To minimize the disturbance to the tract glial framework, we devised a micro-lesion approach in which a very fine glass micropipette was passed stereotaxically through the adult cingulum at right angles to its fibers (Davies et al., 1997a). This procedure cuts axons but causes minimal disturbance to the tract structure. We used the proximal accumulation of p75 low affinity neurotrophin receptor to study the responses of individual caudally directed basal forebrain axons. As early as 1 day after operation the cut axon tips produced filopodia-bearing growth cones which in some cases turned back and extended for a distance which (had it been in the forward direction) would have been enough to cross the site of the injury. However, even with this considerably reduced disturbance to the glial tract structure, the new axon sprouts did not cross the injury site, and were unable to enter the distal part of the severed tract.

This prompt post-lesional inhibition of axon advance was associated with a rapid and transient invasion of the lesion site by a linear array of cells which appear to be of monocytic (haematogenous) origin. The invasion of these cells preceded any other obvious anatomical change in the arrangement of the tract glia

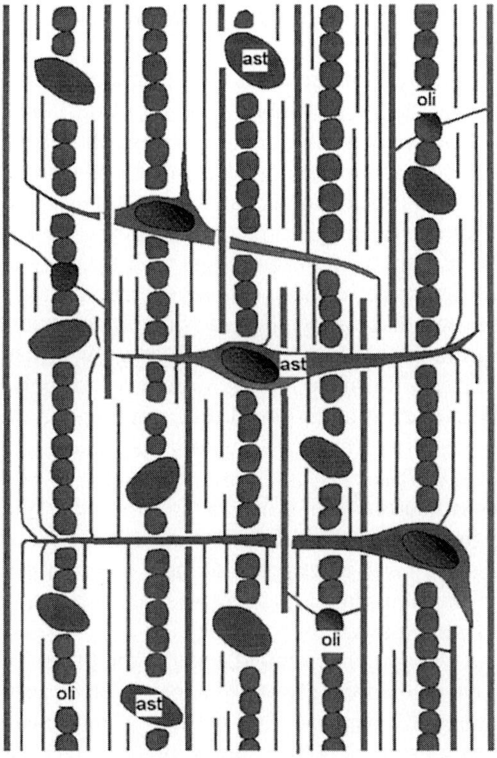

Figure 1 Adult central myelinated fiber tracts have a glial framework consisting of unicellular rows of contiguous oligodendrocytes (blue), solitary astrocytes (green), and microglia (not shown), each of which gives rise to processes running across the axon fascicles, and generating a dense array of parallel, longitudinal processes (myelinating in the case of the oligodendrocytes).

(such as scarring), but was correlated with a marked, highly localized upregulation of molecules such as chondroitin sulphate proteoglycan on the apposed tract astrocytic surfaces (Davies et al.,1997c).

III. DEVELOPMENT AS A MODEL OF ADULT REPAIR

When the first forming embryonic hippocampal axons grow through a tract like the fimbria, the glial framework of the presumptive axon pathway consists of a simple palisade of radial glial processes. During the postnatal period, this is replaced by the dense adult meshwork (Suzuki, Raisman, 1994) containing the three mature glial types (including myelinating oligodendrocytes, which are thought to be inhibitors of axon growth (Schnell, Schwab, 1990). Nonetheless, this transformation of the glial environment does not present an obstacle to the growth of embryonic axons (Wictorin, Björklund, 1992).

Using a minimally traumatic technique (Emmett et al., 1990) for introducing a suspension of embryonic neurons into the adult fimbria (Davies et al.,1993), corpus callosum (Davies et al., 1994) or corticospinal tract (Li, Raisman, 1993), we confirmed that the transplanted embryonic neurons produce axons which can grow as readily in the environment of the adult host myelinated tract as they do in the environment of their normal embryonic radial glial tract. The embryonic axons advanced through, and in alignment with, the adult host glial tract structure at a rate of 1-2 mm per day which is as fast as peripheral nerve regeneration. In the adult spinal cord our observations showed that the myelinated white matter tracts present an environment which is more favorable for embryonic axon growth than that of the adjacent spinal grey matter (Li, Raisman, 1993). Moreover, not only-embryonic neurons but also neonatal and even adult dorsal root ganglionic neurons are able to grow neurites for long distances when micro-transplanted into adult white matter tracts (Davies et al., 1997b).

The observation that embryonic neurons can grow axons in adult white matter tracts that are not permissive for the growth of their own cut (adult) axons suggests that the nerve cells themselves have undergone intrinsic maturational changes as a result of which the adult axons become unresponsive to environments which are favorable for the growth of immature axons.

To characterize the maturational changes which might underlie the failure of axon regeneration in the adult, we have studied the growth of axons in an *in vitro* system. Using organotypic slice cultures of postnatal CNS tissue, we and others (Frotscher, Heimrich, 1993) have demonstrated both anatomically and electrophysiologically that axons grow across the interface between co-cultured hippocampal and entorhinal slices. Retrograde double labelling experiments demonstrate that this is a true regenerating system - i.e. it is the originally cut axons which regenerate. The connections formed by the axons growing in this *in vitro* situation accurately reproduce both the *in vivo* terminal patterns (Li et al., 1993) and the cells of origin (Li et al.,1994) of a number of specific projections. The specificity of the regenerating connectional patterns is robust, and cannot be overridden by selectively altering the availability of the specific targets (Li et al.,1996).

We used a combined retrograde and anterograde labeling paradigm, to follow simultaneously the growth of entorhinal axons into co-cultured hippocampal slices and the growth of hippocampal axons in the opposite direction across the same co-culture interface, into the entorhinal slices. In slices taken at ages up to the 12th postnatal day of life in the rat, entorhinal axons grow into the hippocampal slices, and hippocampal axons grow into the entorhinal slices. However, over the next 24 hour developmental period, both the entorhinal and the hippocampal axons simultaneously lose the ability to regenerate into the co-cultured slice.

To investigate the cause of this failure, younger (P11) slices were confronted with slices from older (P13) tissue. In such pairs of co-cultured slices, the axons of the younger neurons grew into the older slice and formed correct terminal projections there, but the axons of the older neurons did not grow - across the same interface - into the younger slices (Li et al., 1995). The age of failure was the same for both hippocampal and also entorhinal axons. From this we concluded that in this co-culture system, the age related failure of regeneration is correlated with developmental events intrinsic to the neurons, and not to changes in the environment of their pathways.

So how might the clock be turned back so that an adult neuron could be made to behave like an embryonic one? From the experiments quoted so far, it seems that there is nothing present in the lesioned adult CNS environment (or in the slice co-culture environment) that can do this. However, the interventions (below), where regeneration of cut adult axons is stimulated by transplantation of peripheral (Schwann and olfactory ensheathing) cells into the CNS environment, seem, in effect, to be turning back the axotomy responses of the adult nerve cells to a pattern where they are able to express the same regenerative features as they did during their period of development.

IV. THE KEYHOLE APPROACH TO TRACT INJURY AND REPAIR

To analyze the effects of alterations of the cellular environment confronting cut axon tips *in vivo*, we have selected experimental models which maximize the degree of control and the precision of monitoring the tissue rearrangements induced by lesions and transplantation.

We have focused on the spinal cord for two reasons. First, it provides a relatively pure example of axotomy, since the long, white matter fiber tracts can be severed during their course without damage to the cells of origin or to the postsynaptic cells in the terminal fields. Second, it provides the challenge of a human injury which largely affects young, otherwise healthy people, and leads to permanent disabilities which are currently irreparable.

Most laboratory experiments with spinal cord injury have involved large-contusion lesions or surgical transections of the spinal cord. While these compound lesions mimic the situations found in clinical injuries, they cause variable degrees of damage to the surviving tissue, and the tips of the severed axons find themselves confronted with a number of different situations, and considerable misalignment with the distal parts of their original pathways. To complement these 'macro' studies we have devised a 'micro-lesion', or 'keyhole' approach, using much smaller, and precisely controlled electrolytic lesions, placed at a fixed level within the corticospinal tract (CST) on one side (Li, Raisman, 1995).

These lesions provide a window on events occurring in the tract. Within this window, central nervous tissue elements (axons, astrocytes, oligodendrocytes, microglia, and microvessels) are totally destroyed in an area of reproducible size and shape, which is bounded by intact fibers of the adjacent spinal tracts. At the rostral edge of the lesions, the tips of the cut CST axons are swollen, with many fine, local short sprouts.

Such micro-lesions enable us to focus on the responses occurring in individual cut axons in a micro-environment which provides direct access to the glial framework of the distal part of the CST. It is possible to physically bridge the small lesions with microinjection of small numbers of cultured cells (see below), and the micro-approach maximizes the accuracy of assessing the mode of incorporation of transplanted cells and the axonal responses to them.

Disadvantages of the micro-lesion model are that it is difficult to assess the ultimate fate of regenerating axons if they rejoin pathways containing intact axons, and it is difficult to find functional tests sensitive to such small lesions. As a model for clinical spinal cord lesions, the 'keyhole' approach is midway between the more realistic, but complex situation of large compound lesions, and the more controlled, but less realistic situation of tissue culture.

V. INCORPORATION OF TRANSPLANTED CELLS

To try to make the glial framework of damaged tracts more favorable for axon regeneration, we (Li, Raisman, 1997) and others (e.g. Guest et al., 1997; Xu et al., 1995) have studied the effects of transplantation of cultured peripheral nerve Schwann cells (SCs). Micro-transplanted SCs are able to enter the glial environment of CNS tracts, and are incorporated in several specific ways (Brook et al., 1993; Li, Raisman, 1997), leading to the formation of an organized tract glial structure which is composed of a regulated mosaic of both central and peripheral glial elements.

Transplanted SCs exhibit a limited degree of migration in adult white matter tracts. When transplanted into lesions of the corticospinal tract, SCs greatly increase the local axon sprouting. The cut axons grow profusely throughout the transplant, forming a highly tortuous, neuromatous, varicose mass. Some axons form terminal arborizations.

These axogenic effects of transplanted SCs raise some important issues. Spinal tract lesions alone (i.e. without transplants) induce ingrowth of endogenous SCs from the periphery (Bunge et al., 1993; Li, Raisman, 1995). Why do these endogenous SCs not induce comparable axonal growth? Is the timing, distribution, or number of the ingrowing endogenous cells in some way inferior to transplanted (i.e. exogenous) cells?

But even with exogenous SCs, however, we saw little evidence of cut axon sprouts re-entering the distal part of the host tract (Li, Raisman, 1994),and reconnecting with their original targets. The failure of the sprouts to leave the SC environment of the transplant and re-enter the glial tract environment of the distal CST is comparable to the failure of regenerating dorsal root fibers to leave the peripheral nerve/SC environment of the dorsal roots and re-enter the CNS (i.e. glial) environment of the dorsal spinal cord (Stensaas et al., 1979; Bignami et al., 1984).

A factor possibly contributing to the failure of re-entry of regenerating axons could be the limited distance for which the transplanted SCs themselves are able to migrate into the host CNS. One way in which we have tried to make the SCs more able to bridge lesions is to extrude them as a column (Brook et al., 1994). Columns of SCs extruded through the thalamus form aligned cellular structures which induce ingrowth and alignment of CNS astrocytes and microglia, thus effectively forming an organised hybrid PNS/CNS structure (Lawrence, Brook and Raisman, in preparation). The SC columns provoke the ingrowth and extension of adjacent CNS axons, resulting in the formation of new fiber tracts covering distances of several mm. Such axon-bearing SC columns are able to form bridges out of the brain at the dorsal surface of the diencephalon, cross the choroid fissure, and re-enter the ventral surface of the overlying telencephalon. However, there is still no evidence that the axons which enter the columns are able to leave them and re-enter the CNS.

VI. THE USE OF GLIAL CELLS FROM THE ENTRY REGION OF THE OLFACTORY NERVES

To identify a source of cells which might be superior to SCs for promoting axon growth in the CNS, we sought a situation where adult axons are normally able to enter the CNS. The only situation in which this is known to occur is the olfactory system, where the sensory neurons have a limited life, and are replaced throughout adult life, so that their newly formed axons continually re-enter the CNS (Moulton, 1974; Barber, Raisman, 1978a; Wilson, Raisman, 1981; Graziadei, Montigraziadei, 1979; Barber, Raisman, 1978b; Graziadei, Montigraziadei, 1980). The interface at which these entirely unmyelinated olfactory axons enter the olfactory bulb is formed by special types of glia, which have been called olfactory ensheathing glial cells (OECs; Blanes, 1898; Valverde, Lopez-Mascaraque, 1991; Valverde et al., 1992; Doucette, 1990; Doucette, Devon, 1993; Raisman, 1985; Ramón-Cueto, Nieto-Sampedro, 1992; Ramón-Cueto et al., 1993). OECs have been grown in tissue culture (Barnett et al., 1993; Ramón-Cueto, Nieto-Sampedro, 1992; Ramón-Cueto, Valverde, 1995; Doucette, Devon, 1993), where they have been shown to be able to myelinate dorsal root ganglion axons with peripheral-type myelin (Devon, Doucette, 1992). Ramón Cueto and Nieto Sampedro (1994) reported that transplants of cultured OECs can mediate the re-entry of regenerating dorsal root axons into the dorsal spinal grey matter.

We now report some recent findings on the response of cut adult CST axons to transplants of cultured OECs (Li et al., 1997). Precisely localized focal electrolytic lesions were made in the CST on one side at the level of the upper two cervical segments in the adult rat. In contrast to the previous observations with transplanted SCs, we found that after injection of cultured OECs, the cut axons extended as single, fine, tapering, straight, unbranched sprouts. This morphology was not seen in any previous situation. By 3 weeks, the host corticospinal axons and their associated transplanted OECs had accumulated into uniform parallel bundles, and the OECs had formed peripheral-type myelin around the regenerating CS axons.

The regenerating axons extended the full length of the lesioned area and into the caudal part of the host CST, where their re-entry was marked by the resumption of oligodendrocytic myelination (Figure 2). Thus the effect of the transplant was to form a patch of peripheral type tissue across which the cut central axons regenerated. This is the first report of a situation where adult regenerating CNS axons have been seen to re-enter and grow along their original white matter pathway (where we are currently investigating their mode of termination).

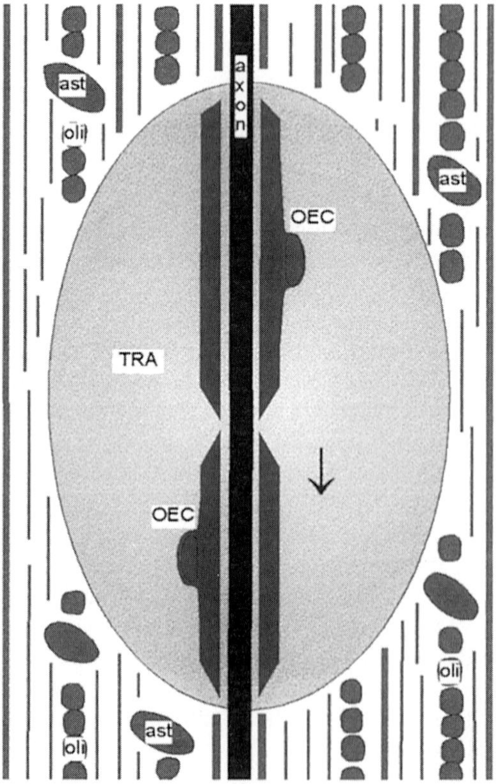

Figure 2 A regenerating axon leaves the glial CNS environment of the proximal tract of the corticospinal tract (containing astrocytes, ast; and myelinating oligodendrocytes, oli). Entering the transplanted lesion area (TRA) from rostrally (above), it passes directly (arrow), without branching, through the lesion area, where it is myelinated by the transplanted olfactory ensheathing cells (OEC), and then re-enters the distal tract caudally (below), where it becomes re-myelinated by oligodendrocytes.

To monitor the return of function, we used a directed forepaw reaching test in which the rat was trained to obtain a food reward by reaching through an aperture (Whishaw et al., 1986). Unilateral CST lesions abolished the acquisition (i.e. in naive animals) of directed forepaw reaching on the operated side for a testing period of 15 days. Transplants completely bridging the defect restored it (Li et al., 1997).

VI. SYNAPTOGENESIS BY ADULT AXONS

So far, this chapter has considered the failure of long fiber regeneration in white matter tracts, and the attempts to overcome it. But what would happen when a regenerating axon reaches its original destination?

One of the first indications that the adult CNS was anything more than passive in the face of injury was the observation that destruction of afferent fibers to the septal nuclei induced short range (1 mm) opportunistic synaptogenesis by terminal sprouting of local surviving axon terminals in the deafferented region (Raisman, 1969; Cotman, Nadler, 1978). Whether or not these new connections are functionally useful, neutral, or even deleterious, is not yet clear, and probably differs in different situations. In considering the long distance regeneration of the original cut axons, this question becomes even more important. By re-occupying deafferented postsynaptic sites, local opportunistic synaptogenesis in the target areas may deny those sites to the original regenerating axons. Hopefully, the sort of activity-dependent plasticity now being shown to be present at the cortical level (Merzenich et al., 1996) may come into operation, and allow the synapses belonging to regenerating axons to be 'preferred' against the adventitious synapses produced by local sprouting, and progressively displace them, so as to re-establish a pattern of connections which, while not necessarily fully normal in distribution or quantity, may yet restore a useful degree of lost functions.

ACKNOWLEDGMENTS

This work was supported by the Medical Research Council (UK), the BritishNeurological Research Trust, the International Spinal Research Trust, the Barnwood House Trust, and Smith's Charity.

REFERENCES

Barber PC, Raisman G (1978a) Cell division in the vomeronasal organ of the adult mouse. Brain Res. 141:57-66.

Barber PC, Raisman G (1978b) Replacement of receptor neurones after section of the vomeronasal nerves in the adult mouse. Brain Res. 147:297-313.

Barnett SC, Hutchins A-M, Noble M (1993) Purification of olfactory nerve ensheathing cells from the olfactory bulb. Dev.Biol. 155:337-350.

Bignami A, Chi NH, Dahl D (1984) Regenerating dorsal roots and the nerve entry zone: an immunofluorescence study with neurofilament and laminin antisera. Exp.Neurol. 85:426-436.

Blanes T (1898) Sobre algunes puntos dudosos de la estructura del bulboolfactorio. Rev Trim.Micro. 3:99-127.

Brook GA, Lawrence JM, Raisman G (1993) Morphology and migration of cultured-Schwann cells transplanted into the fimbria and hippocampus in adult rats. Glia 9:292-304.

Brook GA, Lawrence JM, Shah B, Raisman G (1994) Extrusion transplantation of Schwann cells into the adult rat thalamus induces directional host axon growth. Exp.Neurol. 126:31-43.

Bunge RP, Puckett WR, Becerra JL, Marcillo A, Quencer RM (1993) Observations on the pathology of human spinal cord injury. Adv.Neurol. 59:75-89.

Cajal SR (1928) Degeneration and Regeneration of the Nervous System. New York: Hafner.

Cotman CW, Nadler JV (1978) Reactive synaptogenesis in the hippocampus. In: Neuronal Plasticity (Cotman CW ed), pp 227-271. New York: Raven Press.

Davies SJA, Field PM, Raisman G (1993) Long fiber growth by axons of embryonic mouse hippocampal neurons micro-transplanted into the adult rat fimbria. Eur.J.Neurosci. 5:95-106.

Davies SJA, Field PM, Raisman G (1994) Long interfascicular axon growth from embryonic neurons transplanted into adult myelinated tracts. J.Neurosci. 14:1596-1612.

Davies SJA, Field PM, Raisman G (1997a) Regeneration of cut adult axons fails even in the presence of continuous aligned glial pathways. Exp.Neurol. 142:203-216.

Davies SJA, Fitch MT, Memberg SP, Hall AK, Raisman G, Silver J (1997b) Regeneration of adult axons in white matter tracts of the central nervous system. Nature 390:680-683.

Davies SJA, Fitch MT, Memberg SP, Hall AK, Raisman G, Silver J (1997c) Robust adult axon regeneration in central nervous system white matter tracts. Soc.Neurosci.Abstr. 23:1448

Devon R, Doucette R (1992) Olfactory ensheathing cells myelinate dorsal root ganglion neurites. Brain Res. 589:175-179.

Doucette R (1990) Glial influences on axonal growth in the primary olfactory system. Glia 3:433-449.

Doucette R, Devon R (1993) Olfactory ensheathing cells: factors influencing the phenotype of these glial cells. In: Biology and Pathology of Astrocyte-Neuron Interactions (S.Federoff et al ed), pp 117-124. New York: Plenum Press.

Emmett CJ, Jaques-Berg W, Seeley PJ (1990) Microtransplantation of neural cells into adult rat brain. Neuroscience 38:213-222.

Fan J, Raper JA (1995) Localized collapsing cues can steer growth cones without inducing their full collapse. Neuron 14:263-274.

Frotscher M, Heimrich B (1993) Formation of layer-specific fiber projections to the hippocampus in vitro. Proc.Natl.Acad.Sci.USA 90:10400-10403.

Graziadei PPC, Montigraziadei GA (1979) Neurogenesis and neuron regeneration in the olfactory system of mammals. I. Morphological aspects of differentiation and structural organization of the olfactory sensory neurons. J.Neurocytol. 8:1-18.

Graziadei PPC, Montigraziadei GA (1980) Neurogenesis and neuron regeneration in the olfactory system of mammals. 3. Deafferentation and reinnervation of the olfactory bulb following section of the fila-olfactoria in rat. J.Neurocytol. 9:145-162.

Guest JD, Rao A, Olson L, Bunge MB, Bunge RP (1997) The ability of human Schwann cell grafts to promote regeneration in the transected nude rat spinal cord. Exp.Neurol. 148:502-522.

Li D, Field PM, Raisman G (1995) Failure of axon regeneration in postnatal rat entorhino-hippocampal slice co-culture is due to the age of the axon, not that of the pathway or target. Eur.J.Neurosci. 7:1164-1171.

Li D, Field PM, Raisman G (1996) Connectional specification of regenerating availability in postnatal organotypic slice co-culture. Exp.Neurol. 142:151-160.

Li Y, Field PM, Raisman G (1997) Repair of adult rat corticospinal tract by transplants of olfactory ensheathing cells. Sci 277:2000-2002.

Li D, Field PM, Starega U, Li Y, Raisman G (1993) Entorhinal axons project to dentate gyrus in organotypic slice co-culture. Neuroscience 52:799-813.

Li D, Field PM, Yoshioka N, Raisman G (1994) Axons regenerate with correct specificity in horizontal slice culture of the postnatal rat entorhino-hippocampal system. Eur.J.Neurosci. 6:1026-1037.

Li Y, Raisman G (1993) Long axon growth from embryonic neurons transplanted into myelinated tracts of the adult rat spinal cord. Brain Res.629:115-127.

Li Y, Raisman G (1994) Schwann cells induce sprouting in motor and sensory axons in the adult rat spinal cord. J.Neurosci. 14:4050-4063.

Li Y, Raisman G (1995) Sprouts from cut corticospinal axons persist in the presence of astrocytic scarring in long-term lesions of the adult rat spinal cord. Exp.Neurol. 134:102-111.

Li Y, Raisman G (1997) Integration of transplanted cultured Schwann cells into the long myelinated fibre tracts of the adult spinal cord. Exp.Neurol. 145:397-411.

Mason CA, Wang LC (1997) Growth cone form is behavior-specific and, consequently, position-specific along the retinal axon pathway. J.Neurosci. 17:1086-1100.

Merzenich M, Wright B, Jenkins W, Xerri C, Byl N, Miller S, Tallal P (1996) Cortical plasticity underlying perceptual, motor, and cognitive skill development: implications for neurorehabilitation. Cold Spring Harb.Symp.Quant.Biol. 61:1-8.

Moulton DG (1974) Dynamics of cell populations in the olfactory epithelium. Ann.NY Acad.Sci. 237:52-61.

Raisman G (1969) Neuronal plasticity in the septal nuclei of the adult rat. Brain Res. 14:25-48.

Raisman G (1985) Specialized neuroglial arrangement may explain the capacity of vomeronasal axons to reinnervate central neurons. Neuroscience 14:237-254.

Ramón-Cueto A, Nieto-Sampedro M (1992) Glial cells from adult rat olfactory bulb: immunocytochemical properties of pure cultures of ensheathing cells. Neuroscience 47:213-220.

Ramón-Cueto A, Nieto-Sampedro M (1994) Regeneration into the spinal cord of transected dorsal root axons is promoted by ensheathing glia transplants. Exp.Neurol. 127:232-244.

Ramón-Cueto A, Pérez J, Nieto-Sampedro M (1993) In vitro enfolding of olfactory neurites by p75 NGF receptor positive ensheathing cells from adult rat olfactory bulb. Eur.J.Neurosci. 5:1172-1180.

Ramón-Cueto A, Valverde F (1995) Olfactory bulb ensheathing glia: A unique cell type with axonal growth-promoting properties. Glia 14:163-173.

Schnell L, Schwab ME (1990) Axonal regeneration in the rat spinal cord produced by an antibody against myelin-associated neurite growth inhibitors. Nature 343:269-272.

Stensaas LJ, Burgess PR, Horch KW (1979) Regenerating dorsal root axons are blocked by spinal cord astrocytes. Soc.Neurosci.Abstr. 5:684-684.

Suzuki M, Raisman G (1992) The glial framework of central white matter tracts: Segmented rows of contiguous interfascicular oligodendrocytes and solitary astrocytes give rise to a continuous meshwork of transverse and longitudinal processes in the adult rat fimbria. Glia 6:222-235.

Suzuki M, Raisman G (1994) Multifocal pattern of postnatal development of the macroglial framework of the rat fimbria. Glia 12:294-308.

Tessier-Lavigne M, Goodman CS (1996) The molecular biology of axon guidance. Sci 274:1123-1133.

Valverde F, Lopez-Mascaraque L (1991) Neuroglial arrangements in the olfactory glomeruli of the hedgehog. J.comp.Neurol. 307:658-674.

Valverde F, Santacana M, Heredia M (1992) Formation of an olfactory glomerulus: morphological aspects of development and organization. Neuroscience 49:255-276.

Whishaw IQ, O'Connor RB, Dunnett SB (1986) The contributions of motor cortex, nigrostriatal dopamine and caudate-putamen to skilled forelimb use in the rat. Brain 109:805-843.

Wictorin K, Björklund A (1992) Axon outgrowth from grafts of human embryonicspinal cord in the lesioned adult rat spinal cord. NeuroReport 3:1045-1048.

Wilson KCP, Raisman G (1981) Estimation of numbers of vomeronasal synapses in the glomerular layer of the accessory olfactory bulb of the mouse at different ages. Brain Res. 205:245-253.

Xu XM, Guénard V, Kleitman N, Bunge MB (1995) Axonal regeneration into Schwann cell-seeded guidance channels grafted into transected adult rat spinal cord. J.comp.Neurol. 351:145-160.

18

Cell Surface and Extracellular Molecules That Promote or Inhibit Axonal Growth

M. Grumet

Rutgers State University of New Jersey, Piscataway, New Jersey

I. INTRODUCTION

In this chapter I discuss adhesion molecules and receptors that promote or inhibit axonal growth during development with particular emphasis on recent advances in this field that may be relevant to nerve regeneration. During development, axons are guided to their targets by several different molecular mechanisms that include complex patterns of promoters or inhibitors of axonal growth. Dynamic changes in temporal and spatial expression of sets of these molecules are believed to be important for determining patterns of axonal growth during development. Many of these same molecules have lower levels or different patterns of expression in the mature animal. There is little growth in the mature mammalian nervous system and while nerves can regrow in the peripheral nervous system following injury, they do so abortively in the central nervous system (CNS). Recent progress in understanding molecular mechanisms of axonal growth and guidance and in particular in identifying inhibitors in the CNS, provides a hope for significant improvements in promoting CNS nerve regeneration in the future. Other articles in this volume by (this volume, chapters by Schwab; David and McKerracher) focus in detail on inhibitors in myelin.

Towards the end of the 19th century, Ramon y Cajal discovered the growth cone and predicted its role as a key structure for guiding growing axons along circuitous routes to their targets (Cajal, 1995). Based on the specificity of regenerating retinal axons, Sperry proposed a chemoaffinity hypothesis suggesting the existence of specific molecules used by growth cones for pathway and target recognition. Evidence for labeled pathways was provided in several systems, most elegantly in invertebrates, where the pathfinding of pioneer axonal growth cones was demonstrated to be influenced by guidepost cells expressing certain cell surface molecules (Goodman and Tessier-Lavigne, 1997). Studies in vertebrates verified that cell adhesion molecules (CAMs) and extracellular matrix molecules (ECMs) promote cell adhesion and axonal growth. Only in the last decade has it been recognized that inhibitors of axonal growth play a major role by limiting growth into certain regions.

It is now clear that there are at least four types of interactions that govern axonal growth; these are either attractive or repulsive forces acting either locally or at a distance. Many CAMs and ECM proteins act locally as attractive molecules for axonal growth, while growth factors and other soluble proteins such as netrins can be chemoattractive providing long-range guidance cues. Cells also release proteins such as semaphorins that are chemorepulsive, and certain cell surface and ECM proteins mediate contact repulsion locally. Axonal growth cone receptors are believed to mediate responses to each of these molecules. The receptors can include CAMs and integrins, as well as signaling molecules such as receptor kinases and phosphatases. Particular molecules can serve both as ligand and receptor, and responses to molecules can be attractive or repulsive depending on the state of the cell and its receptors. The following discussion has been organized according to different families of molecules that have been studied for their roles during neural development.

II. CAMS CAN ACT AS BOTH LIGANDS AND RECEPTORS

Most CAMs can bind to themselves, thus they are termed homophilic binders. In that sense, they can serve as both ligand and receptor on adjacent cells. Many CAMs have cytoplasmic domains that can transmit signals across the plasma membrane and therefore behave as signal transducing receptors. Cadherins are a family of CAMs that exhibit primarily homophilic binding and are thought to be involved in neurite outgrowth and synapse formation in the nervous system (Colman, 1997). A number of CAMs have been found to bind heterophilically to other proteins in opposing cells and in the extracellular matrix. The integrins are a family of heterodimeric CAMs that serve as receptors for extracellular matrix proteins (Faissner, 1997). CAM-CAM interactions can also occur within the same plasma membrane as complexes that are thought to confer specificity, or to function as co-receptors, in transmembrane signalling. The Ig superfamily of molecules includes CAMs and other receptors that modulate axonal growth and are discussed below. The Immunoglobulin (Ig) Superfamily of CAMs represents one of the largest and most diverse families of CAMs whose members are characterized by the presence of one or more Ig domains (Fig. 1). It has been subdivided into groups of more closely related molecules based on further similarities in their structures. Several of these subfamilies are characterized by inclusion of another domain found in fibronectin (Fn), the FnIII repeat. It is interesting that there are similarities in polypeptide folding patterns between Ig domains and FnIII repeats.

A. N-CAM

The neural CAM (N-CAM, Fig. 1A) was the first member of this family to be discovered and it consists of five Ig domains and two FnIII repeats (Edelman, 1984). Three major forms of the molecule (~180, 140 and 120 kD) result from alternative splicing at the carboxyterminus of the protein. The largest form has an extended cytoplasmic region that is missing from the 140 kD form and this region can bind to spectrin, a cytoskeletal protein. The shortest form is linked to the membrane via a phosphatidylinositol (GPI) and lacks a cytoplasmic region. Neurons express mainly the two larger forms, astrocytes the two smaller forms, and oligodendrocytes the smallest form (Carbonetto, 1993).

Embryonic forms of N-CAM have a high content of an unusual form of polysialic acid (PSA) on its fifth Ig domain with up to 100 sialic acid residues per chain (Rutishauser and Landmesser, 1996). The addition of PSA to N-CAM is developmentally regulated by two polysialyltransferases that are expressed in the nervous system (Walsh and Doherty, 1997). PSA negatively regulates binding mediated by N-CAM, slowing the rate and extent of binding dramatically by comparison to N-CAM that is deficient in PSA. As development proceeds, N-CAMs are found with decreasing proportions of PSA and therefore abundant expression of PSA is correlated with axon pathfinding and targeting. Manipulations to remove PSA enzymatically indicate that it affects axon pathfinding not only by modifying the function of N-CAM but also by modifying other CAMs such as L1, a CAM that mediates axon fasciculation (see below). This may be due, at least in part, to the negative charge on PSA or to steric hindrance that alters N-CAM homophilic binding and interactions of other CAMs in the plasma membrane. Given that PSA expression on N-CAM can be regulated by electrical activity, it is important to consider the state of N-CAM glycosylation on cells during nerve regeneration. Interestingly, regenerating axons in the adult hippocampal formation were observed in association with PSA and astrocytes (Aubert et al., 1998).

N-CAM is expressed widely on neurons during development and levels of the protein are generally lower in the mature nervous system. It has been implicated in histogenesis in various neural regions during development. N-CAM can promote neurite growth *in vitro* and its expression on neurons and glia suggests that it functions *in vivo* as well. A 10-amino acid variable alternatively spliced exon (VASE) in N-CAM that alters the structure of the fourth Ig domain inhibits the axonal growth response mediated by N-CAM. About half of the N-CAM transcripts in the adult contain VASE and these are commonly found in regions that do not exhibit synaptic plasticity (Walsh and Doherty, 1997). Therefore, N-CAM

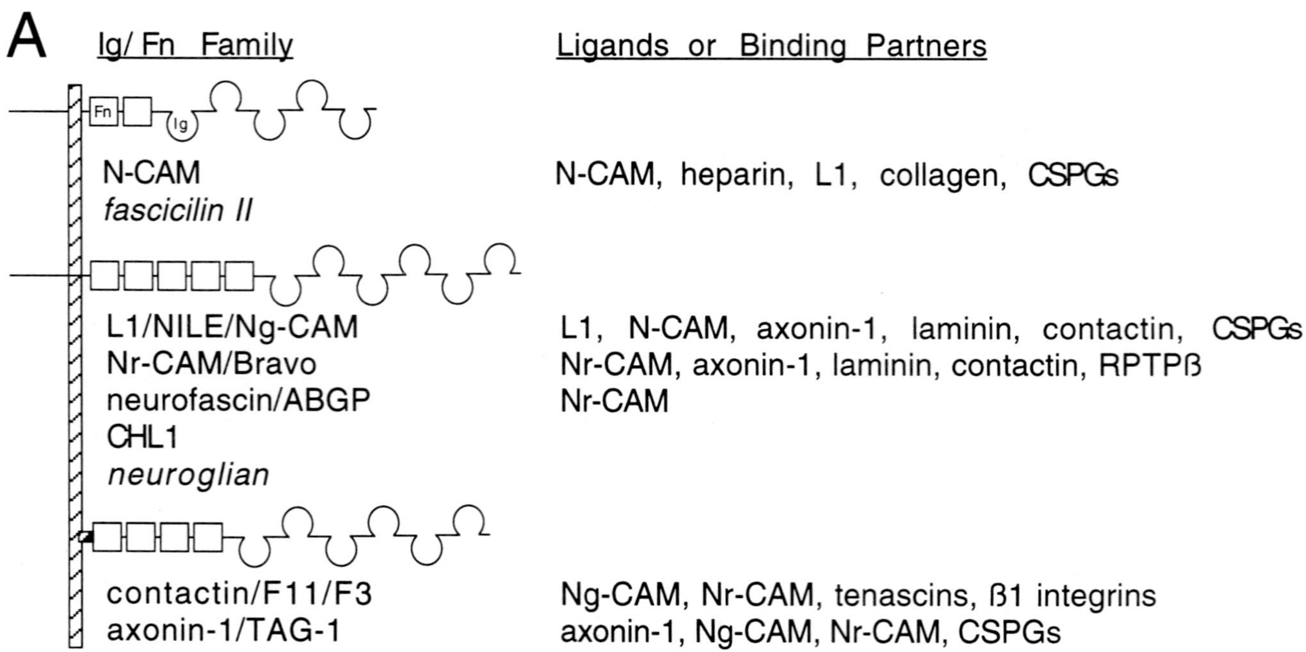
A
Ig/ Fn Family
Ligands or Binding Partners
Fn
Ig
N-CAM
fascicilin II
N-CAM, heparin, L1, collagen, CSPGs
L1/NILE/Ng-CAM
Nr-CAM/Bravo
neurofascin/ABGP
CHL1
neuroglian
L1, N-CAM, axonin-1, laminin, contactin, CSPGs
Nr-CAM, axonin-1, laminin, contactin, RPTPß
Nr-CAM
contactin/F11/F3
axonin-1/TAG-1
Ng-CAM, Nr-CAM, tenascins, ß1 integrins
axonin-1, Ng-CAM, Nr-CAM, CSPGs

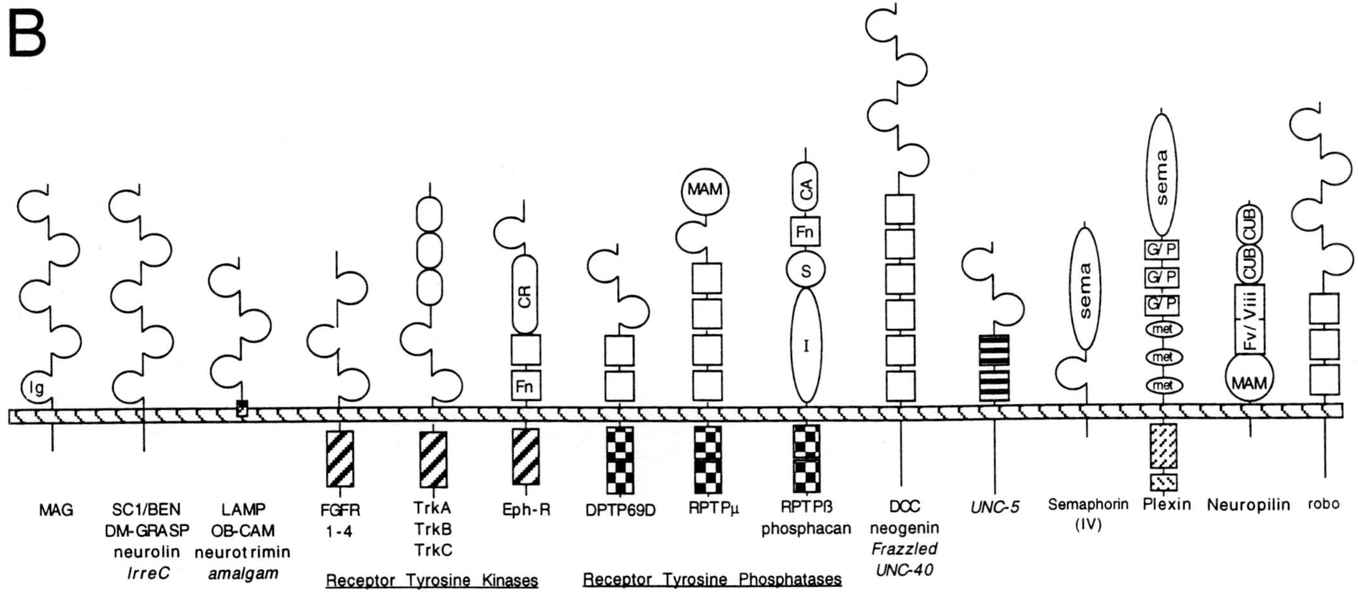

Figure 1 Neural Ig cell adhesion molecules and receptors that mediate axonal growth. A) Three subfamilies of Ig/FnIII cell adhesion molecules (CAMs) and their binding partners on cells or in the extracellular matrix are shown under schematic models of each subgroup. Ig domains (Ig) are denoted by open loops and fibronectin type III repeats (Fn) by squares. Homologues in different species are separated by slashes and related invertebrate proteins are indicated in italics. CSPGs are chondroitin sulfate proteoglycans including neurocan and phosphacan/RPTPß. B) Additional members of the Ig superfamily and receptors that mediate axonal growth. These include receptors for netrins (DCC and *UNC-5*), and representatives of receptor tyrosine kinases and phosphatases. Neuropilins and plexins serve as receptors for some semaphorins (e.g. sema III) and there are also membrane-associated semaphorins (e.g. sema IV). CR, cysteine-rich domain; MAM, MAM domain; CA, carbonic anhydrase domain; S and I are novel domains in RPTPß; Fv/Viii, regions of homology to factors V and Viii, CUB, CUB domain; sema, semaphorin domain; G/P, glycine and proline-rich repeat; met, related to MET receptor repeats. See text for additional details.

may represent an inhibitor of nerve regeneration when regions expressing VASE are considered.

In the PNS, the levels of N-CAM rise dramatically following nerve injury (Daniloff et al., 1986; Martini, 1994). N-CAM is observed at sites of nerve-Schwann cell contact suggesting that it might play a role in axonal regeneration. However, antibody perturbation studies suggest that it may only play a minor role in this process (Carbonetto, 1993). Injury in the CNS is associated with reactive astrocytes that can modulate axonal growth. Therefore, it is interesting that exogenous N-CAM has been found to reduce glial proliferation by binding to N-CAM on astrocytes (Krushel et al., 1998).

B. L1 Subfamily (L1/Ng-CAM, Nr-CAM, Neurofascin and CHL1)

This group represents a subfamily of CAMs with members containing 6 Ig and 4-5 FnIII repeats and a highly conserved cytoplasmic region (Grumet, 1991, Brummendorf, 1995). It is called the L1 subgroup because mouse L1 was the first CAM of this type to be cloned. L1 is homologous to rat NILE (NGF inducible large external glycoprotein) and similar to chick Ng-CAM. Although the extracellular regions of L1 and Ng-CAM are only ~50% identical in amino acid sequence, there is very high conservation in the cytoplasmic region with a 50 amino acid stretch that is identical, suggesting that these are homologous proteins. Nr-CAM is related to L1/Ng-CAM (~40% identity) and conservation among Nr-CAMs from chick to human is fairly high (>80% identity) (Grumet, 1997). Neurofascin is another member of this family that was also identified as an ankyrin binding glycoprotein (ABGP) and it shows a striking resemblance to Nr-CAM particularly in its cytoplasmic region (>70% identity) (Davis et al., 1996). CHL1 (close homology of L1) is the most recent member of this group to be identified and it shows most striking homology to Nr-CAM in its cytoplasmic region (64% identity) (Holm et al., 1996).

Multiple forms of these proteins are generated from several alternative spliced regions that range in size from 3 amino acids to an entire FnIII repeat (~100 amino acids). L1 is the only mammalian CAM that has been found, so far, to be expressed with an alternatively spliced RSLE sequence in the cytoplasmic region that follows a tyrosine residue. This sequence has been proposed to be a signal for sorting of L1 to the axonal growth cone; RSLE-minus forms of L1 are expressed exclusively in non-neuronal cells (Kamiguchi and Lemmon, 1998). This suggests that among these CAMs, L1 may be the only one that is specifically targeted to the growth cone. Another cytoplasmic sequence (FIGQY) that is highly conserved in the L1 subgroup is involved in binding to ankyrin, a cytoskeletal protein, and this interaction is inhibited by phosphorylation on the tyrosine residue (Zhang et al., 1998). Full length L1-subfamily proteins migrate at ~200 kD on denaturing gels and several members, including L1/Ng-CAM and Nr-CAM, are proteolytically cleaved at a furin-like site in the third FnIII repeat to yield amino- and carboxy-terminal fragments of ~140 and 60-80 kD, respectively

(Grumet and Sakurai, 1996). Interestingly, these two fragments appear to be stably associated on the cell surface. Although the function of this cleavage is unclear, it may be an important factor to consider in designing exogenous forms of CAMs for introduction *in vivo* to promote nerve regeneration.

L1/Ng-CAM is expressed by most postmitotic neurons and is most prevalent on growth cones and axons during development (Brummendorf and Rathjen, 1995; Grumet, 1992). Migrating neurons such as granule cells express L1 and antibody perturbation indicates a role for L1 in their migration. Antibody perturbation also indicates that L1 plays a major role in axonal fasciculation. L1 exhibits strong homophilic interactions, and like N-CAM, the rate and extent of binding is highly dependent on the surface density of the CAM. While homophilic L1 binding is believed to be a major function of L1, it has numerous heterophilic-binding partners including other CAMs and extracellular matrix proteins. For example, Ng-CAM interacts with another CAM, axonin-1, in the same plasma membrane and this complex is thought to be important for promoting axonal growth (Kunz et al., 1998). L1 can also bind to laminin and to two major brain chondroitin sulfate proteoglycans, neurocan and phosphacan, that can modulate axonal growth *in vitro* (Grumet and Sakurai, 1996). Some of these interactions may be implicated in the L1-mediated response of neurons to non-neuronal cells expressing these heterophilic ligands including astrocytes and Muller cells that do not express L1, as well as with Schwann cells that do. Antibodies to L1 have also been found to inhibit ensheathment of axons by Schwann cells and subsequent differentiation in these co-cultures (Carbonetto, 1993). Interestingly, there are striking similarities between defects in humans with mutation in L1 and L1-deficient mice that confirm roles for L1 in axonal fasciculation and growth in the CNS (Brummendorf et al., 1998).

In contrast to L1 that is widely expressed on most neurons, the other members of this subgroup are more restricted in their patterns of expression. Nr-CAM is expressed on subsets of neurons in the CNS and is prevalent on peripheral ganglia including dorsal root ganglia and sympathetic ganglia (Krushel et al., 1993, Brummendorf, 1995). It has been found to promote neurite outgrowth in these ganglionic neurons (but not in most CNS neurons) by a heterophilic mechanism involving axonin-1 as a neuronal receptor (Lustig, 1999; Suter et al., 1995). Interestingly, it is transiently expressed in the floorplate where it is involved in guidance of commissural axons across the ventral midline. Nr-CAM is also expressed on many cells in the retina during development including the Muller glia. Neurofascin is expressed on a subset of mammalian neurons during spinal cord development in a pattern that differs from that of Nr-CAM (Moscoso and Sanes, 1995). It is also expressed in oligodendrocytes postnatally. *In vitro* experiments suggest a role for neurofascin in tectal neurite outgrowth by a mechanism involving Nr-CAM as a receptor (Volkmer et al., 1996). In contrast to L1 that shows highest levels of expression during development, neurofascin and Nr-CAM are expressed at highest levels in adult brain (Davis et al., 1993). Both of these CAMs are co-localized with sodium channels and ankyrin to nodes of Ranvier at early stages of node formation and therefore may play a role in this process (Lambert et al., 1997). Given their high levels of expression in the adult, additional studies are needed to study the pattern of expression and functions of these CAMs in the adult nervous system.

Several members of this subgroup of CAMs have been found to promote neurite outgrowth in culture using purified native proteins or recombinant chimeric proteins as dimers with the Fc region of Ig. The use of such dimers may be important for maximal activity insofar as the dimers may serve to increase the stability of the CAM and its binding avidity. In addition, the CAM-Fc chimeras may act to stimulate axonal growth responses in neurons by clustering CAMs as well as co-receptors that may include the FGF receptor (Walsh and Doherty, 1997). Moreover, signalling to CAMs as receptors in neurons may promote neuronal survival (Hulley et al., 1998). Among the Ig-CAMs, L1 is the most potent promoter of neurite growth in culture and it is one of the most widely expressed on neurons. L1 has been found to be expressed on regenerating axons in mammals (Aubert et al., 1998) and L1 expression was found to be increased moderately following spinal cord injury in the adult (Roonprapunt et al., 1996). Therefore, L1-Fc was tested by intrathecal infusion in an adult rat model for spinal cord injury and it was found to promote locomotor recovery (Basso et al., 1996; Roonprapunt, 1998). This result provides strong impetus to test CAMs in combinations with other agents (e.g. growth factors) to promote recovery following CNS injury, but at the same time it is important to clarify the mechanism of L1 action *in vivo.* As we learn more about other CAMs they may be considered for testing *in vivo,* but most other CAMs have restricted distributions that may limit their efficacy to certain populations of neurons. This may be advantageous for targeting responses of certain types of neurons and will depend on the patterns of CAM expression in the adult and how they change following injury.

C. Contactin/F3/F11 and Tag-1/Axonin-1

This group of Ig/FnIII CAMs has a GPI linkage at their carboxyterminus that serves as an anchor to the plasma membrane. Chick contactin/F11, human contactin and mouse F3 are highly conserved representing homologues in different species (Brummendorf and Rathjen, 1995). Contactin is expressed on a subset of neuronal processes including on the axons of granule cells in the cerebellum as well as on certain glial cells (Willbold et al., 1997). It binds heterophilically to tenascins, a receptor protein tyrosine phosphatase (RPTPß), and to other CAMs, and thereby may have multiple functions in cell-cell interaction and signalling (Brummendorf and Rathjen, 1995; Grumet, 1997; Peles et al., 1998). These interactions include both promotion and inhibition of neurite outgrowth, depending on the circumstances.

Chick axonin-1, rodent TAG-1 and human Tax-1 are highly conserved homologues in different species (Brummendorf and Rathjen, 1995). A significant portion of axonin-1 has been found in a soluble form *in vivo* and recent work suggests that it is specifically released by endogenous GPI-specific phospholipases (Lierheimer et al., 1997). *In vitro* studies demonstrated that the soluble form inhibits neurite fasciculation and pathfinding in the developing chick embryo. Axonin-1 is expressed by neurons but not by glia, and is prevalent in motor and sensory systems. The protein is expressed transiently at high levels during development but only at low levels in adult brain (Wolfer et al., 1998). Axonin-1 can bind by a homophilic mechanism but its primary mode of action on cells appears to be by interacting heterophilically for example with Ng-CAM (L1) and Nr-CAM to promote axonal growth. The binding of axonin-1 to other proteins and its release from cells as a soluble form suggests that it modulates axonal growth in vivo (Sonderegger, 1997). Although additional studies are needed to evaluate the potential role of axonin-1/TAG-1 following nerve injury, it was not found to be expressed in regenerating retinal ganglion cells in the rat (Jung et al., 1997), suggesting that it may not play a major role in regeneration.

D. Other Ig CAMs and Subfamilies

The myelin associated glycoprotein MAG (Fig. 1B) is expressed on oligodendrocytes and myelinating Schwann cells and can modulate axonal growth in a complex manner (this volume, Chapter by David and McKerracher). An unrelated CAM also consisting of five Ig domains is called SC1/BEN/DM-GRASP/neurolin. This CAM binds by a homophilic mechanism but has also been reported to bind to Ng-CAM (DeBrenardo and Chang, 1996). It is expressed transiently at high levels during development in axonal pathways for instance in the spinal cord and retinal axons, and is re-expressed at least in goldfish (i.e. neurolin) during retinal axonal regeneration (Paschke et al., 1992). BEN/SC1/DM-GRASP expression is also found in human spinal cord and it is regulated during neuromuscular development suggesting a potential role in muscle re-innervation (Fournier-Thibault et al., 1999; Karagogeos et al., 1997).

LAMP, OB-CAM, neurotrimin, and CEPU-1 constitute a subfamily of CAMs containing three Ig domains that have a GPI link to the plasma membrane. They are expressed in different patterns on subsets of neurons, for example LAMP is a limbic system-associated membrane protein and neurotrimin is expressed on thalamocortical and pontocerebellar projections. LAMP and neurotrimin each bind by a homophilic mechanism and possibly by a heterophilic mechanisms as well (Gil et al., 1998; Pimenta et al., 1995). It is likely that members of this subfamily regulate development of subsets of neuronal projections via attractive and repulsive mechanisms that are mediated by homophilic and heterophilic interaction, respectively.

E. Receptor Protein Tyrosine Kinases and Phosphatase and Their Ligands

In view of the importance of Ig domains and FnIII repeats for interactions mediated by CAMs, it is interesting that various neural receptors that are involved in signalling also express some of these domains. FGF receptors have Ig domains in their extracellular ligand-binding region. In addition to a role of FGF in promoting nerve growth, there is evidence that interactions of FGF receptors with CAMs including N-CAM, L1, and N-cadherin mediate neurite outgrowth promoting signals (Walsh and Doherty, 1997). The trk receptors for neurotrophins also have Ig domains. The largest subfamily of tyrosine kinase receptors is the Eph family of receptors that contain an Ig domain, a cysteine-rich domain and two FnIII repeats. The ligands for these receptors fall into two classes based on the presence of GPI-linkages or transmembrane domains. Their actions are complex insofar as the ephrins must be membrane bound in order to activate the receptors, and there may be bi-directional signalling between cells expressing transmembrane ephrins and Eph receptors. Most interactions mediated by these proteins are repulsive and they act during development in axonal growth, fasciculation and topographic guidance (Flanagan and Vanderhaeghen, 1998). For example, opposing gradients of ephrins and Eph receptors play critical roles in axon pathfinding and retinotectal topographic mapping during development (O'Leary and Wilkinson, 1999). While much has been learned recently about the functions of these molecules during development, little is known of their roles in the adult.

Dynamic regulation of tyrosine phosphorylation in the nervous system also requires protein tyrosine phosphatases (PTP). Several receptor PTPs (RPTP), some containing multiple Ig and FnIII repeats, have been implicated in axonal guidance and target recognition during development in *Drosophila* such as DPTP69D (Stoker and Dutta, 1998). Another subgroup of RPTP contains an amino terminal MAM domain and functions as homophilic adhesion molecules. While little is known about the ligands for RPTPs, evidence that dimerization inactivates phosphatase function suggests that clustering of RPTPs may be functionally important (Majeti et al., 1998). Regulation of RPTPs could also be achieved by heterophilic interactions such as between RPTPß and tenascin in the ECM or contactin on neurons. Changes in tyrosine phosphorylation can ultimately affect several cytoplasmic targets including the growth cone cytoskeleton.

III. EXTRACELLULAR MATRIX MOLECULES CAN MODULATE AXONAL GROWTH AND THEIR RECEPTORS

Extracellular matrix (ECM) molecules including laminins, tenascins, fibronectins, collagens, thrombospondins, and proteoglycans can either act to promote or inhibit neurite outgrowth. Many of these molecules are synthesized by astrocytes in the CNS and Schwann cells in the PNS, and have multiple interactions with other ECM proteins to form an extracellular network that can interact with various cell surface receptors. Laminins are among the most potent promoters of neurite outgrowth while tenascins and proteoglycans can be potent inhibitors. Major receptors for ECM molecules include the integrins, a large family of heterodimeric proteins, and members of the Ig superfamily. Two more recently discovered families of ECM molecules, the netrins and the semaphorins, have chemoattractive and chemorepulsive effects that provide long-range guidance cues. The present discussion will focus on recent progress given that the roles of ECM molecules in neuronal development and regeneration have been reviewed extensively (Aubert et al., 1995; Carbonetto, 1993; Faissner, 1997; Goodman and Tessier-Lavigne, 1997; Martini, 1994; Venstrom and Reichardt, 1993).

The netrins are a family of secreted proteins that were identified in the floor plate of the spinal cord as long range guidance cues for commissural axons (Goodman and Tessier-Lavigne, 1997). Two netrins have been identified in vertebrates, so far. They consist of a ~600 amino acid segment that is structurally related to the short arm of the γ chain of laminin at the amino terminus, followed by three EGF-like repeats, and a highly basic domain at their carboxyterminus that is unrelated to laminin. Members of the Ig superfamily in vertebrates called DCC (deleted in colon cancer; Fig. 1B) act as receptors for netrins that mediate their attractive effects. Evidence from *C. elegans* indicates that in certain situations netrins can be repulsive and utilize a different receptor that is also a member of the Ig Superfamily, the product of the UNC-5 gene. While netrins clearly play a role in axon guidance during development, their patterns of expression and potential functions in the adult remains to be explored.

The semaphorins are a family of secreted and cell surface proteins that were initially named collapsin, by virtue of their ability to collapse growth cones and inhibit axonal growth (Goodman and Tessier-Lavigne, 1997). Like netrins, some semaphorins have a highly basic region at their carboxyterminus that is likely to be important for its distribution in tissues, but they are a much larger family with several vertebrate semaphorins having transmembrane spanning regions. This family of molecules is characterized by a conserved extracellular sema domain of ~500 amino acids that contains 14-16 cysteines. Two groups of receptors have recently been identified for the semaphorins - neuropilins and plexins (Yu and Kolodkin, 1999). Neuropilins 1 and 2 are expressed on sympathetic axons and are believed to be involved in repulsion by certain soluble semaphorins (e.g. sema III). Neuropilins can form homo and heterodimers on cells and thereby may act as receptors for semaphorins. However, neuropilins have very short cytoplasmic regions in contrast to the plexins that are also thought to act as receptors for semaphorins. Interestingly, plexins have structural homology with the MET oncogene, a receptor tyrosine kinase, and contain a semaphorin domain as well (Winberg et al., 1998). Sema III acts as a chemorepellent during spinal cord development for axons of sensory and motor neurons, and decreases in sema III expression following nerve injury are correlated with regeneration (Pasterkamp et al., 1998 a,b). Sema III also appears to act as a chemorepellent for neuropillin-1 in the regeneration of primary olfactory axons (Pasterkamp et al., 1998 a).

In the developing spinal cord, axonal guidace of commissural cells towards the ventral midline floor plate is driven by netrins as chemoattractants, whereas interactions between Nr-CAM and axonin-1 are involved in crossing the floor plate. It is striking that once crossed, these axons do not re-cross the floor plate and genetic studies have revealed proteins that are involved in this process. Slit is an extracellular matrix protein containing leucine-rich regions and EGF repeats that acts as a midline repellent for an axonal receptor called robo (Brose et al., 1999; Li et al., 1999). Mutants in robo (*roundabout*) cross and re-cross the floor plate numerous times, hence its name. Robo consists of five Ig domains and three fibronectin type III repeats with a large cytoplasmic region (Kidd et al., 1998). Slit is also a positive regulator of sensory axon elongation and branching (Wang et al., 1999). It will be important to determine the expression patterns of these proteins in the adult nervous system and in response to injury as a basis to analyze their potential roles in regeneration.

IV. FUTURE DIRECTIONS

There is increasing evidence for roles of various CAMs, ECM molecules and receptors, in axonal growth and guidance during development. Much needs to be learned about the expression and functions of these molecules in the mature nervous system. Many of these molecules are expressed at low levels in the mature nervous system and their dramatic upregulation following injury to the PNS is probably critical for peripheral nerve regeneration. It is likely that upregulating or re-introducing key molecules that promote neurite growth will lead to improvement in CNS regeneration. It will be important to identify axonal growth receptors that are expressed in adult neurons that can be activated by exogenously supplied ligands. Then, it may be possible to design treatments (e.g. with specific growth factors) to activate these systems or to genetically modify cells to express receptors and other factors that promote nerve regrowth *in vivo*. Moreover, it is critical to overcome growth inhibitors that are present in adult brain or upregulated after CNS injury. In view of this consideration, it is exciting that growth cone responses can be converted from repulsive to attractive by mechanisms involving cyclic nucleotides. These effects may be mediated by at least two signal transduction mechanisms involving either cAMP or cGMP that receive inputs from diverse systems involving neurotrophins, netrins, semaphorins, and MAG, as well as additional inhibitors present in myelin (Cai et al., 1999; Song et al., 1998). Therefore, it may also be possible to identify new drugs that activate intracellular signalling downstream of CAMs and other receptors to modulate axonal growth. It is likely that a combination of methods to neutralize growth inhibitors, and promote neuronal survival and axonal growth, will make it possible to achieve substantial regeneration in the CNS and improve functional recovery.

ACKNOWLEDGMENTS

I thank Drs. Takeshi Sakurai, David Friedlander and Jeff Haspel for helpful discussions and critically reading the manuscript. Supported by grants from NIH, American Paralysis Association, Spinal Cord Research Foundation and Acorda Therapeutics Inc.

REFERENCES

Aubert, I., Ridet, J. L., and Gage, F. H. (1995). Regeneration in the adult mammalian CNS: guided by development. Curr Opin Neurobiol *5*, 625-35.

Aubert, I., Ridet, J. L., Schachner, M., Rougon, G., and Gage, F. H. (1998). Expression of L1 and PSA during sprouting and regeneration in the adult hippocampal formation. J Comp Neurol *399*, 1-19.

Basso, D. M., Beattie, M. S., and Bresnahan, J. C. (1996). Graded histological and locomotor outcomes after spinal cord contusion using the NYU weight-drop device versus transection. Exp Neurol *139*, 244-56.

Brose, K., Bland, K. S., Wang, K. H., Arnott, D., Henzel, W., Goodman, C. S., Tessier-Lavigne, M., and Kidd, T. (1999). Slit proteins bind Robo receptors and have an evolutionarily conserved role in repulsive axon guidance. Cell *96*, 795-806.

Brummendorf, T., Kenwrick, S., and Rathjen, F. G. (1998). Neural cell recognition molecule L1: from cell biology to human hereditary brain malformations. Curr Opin Neurobiol *8*, 87-97.

Brummendorf, T., and Rathjen, F. G. (1995). Cell adhesion molecules 1: immunoglobulin superfamily, Volume 2 (London: Academic Press).

Cai, D., Shen, Y., De Bellard, M., Tang, S., and Filbin, M. T. (1999). Prior exposure to neurotrophins blocks inhibition of axonal regeneration by MAG and myelin via a cAMP-dependent mechanism. Neuron *22*, 89-101.

Cajal, R. S. (1995). Histology of the nervous system of man and vertebrates (New York: Oxford University Press).

Carbonetto, S. a. d., S. (1993). Adhesive Molecules of the Cell Surface and Extracellular Matrix in Neural Regeneration. In Neuroregeneration, A. Gorio, ed. (New York: Raven Press), pp. 77-100.

Colman, D. R. (1997). Neurites, Synapses, and Cadherins Reconciled. Mol Cell Neurosci *10*, 1-6.

Daniloff, J. K., Levi, G., Grumet, M., Rieger, F., and Edelman, G. M. (1986). Altered expression of neuronal cell adhesion molecules induced by nerve injury and repair. Journal of Cell Biology *103*, 929-945.

Davis, J. Q., Lambert, S., and Bennett, V. (1996). Molecular composition of the node of Ranvier: Identification of ankyrin-binding cell adhesion molecules neurofascin (mucin+/third FnIII domain-) and Nr-CAM at nodal axon segments. Journal of Cell Biology *135*, 1355-1367.

Davis, J. Q., McLaughlin, T., and Bennett, V. (1993). Ankyrin-binding proteins related to nervous system cell adhesion molecules: Candidates to provide transmembrane and intercellular connections in adult brain. Journal of Cell Biology *121*, 121-133.

DeBrenardo, A. P., and Chang, S. (1996). Heterophilic interactions of DM-GRASP: GRASP-Ng-CAM interactions involved in neurite extension. Journal of Cell Biology *133*, 657-666.

Edelman, G. M. (1984). Modulation of cell adhesion during induction, histogenesis, and perinatal development of the nervous system. Annual Review of Neuroscience *7*, 339-377.

Faissner, A. (1997). Glial derived extracellular matrix compoenents: Important roles in axon growth and guidance. The Neuroscientist *3*, 371-380.

Flanagan, J. G., and Vanderhaeghen, P. (1998). The ephrins and Eph receptors in neural development. Annu Rev Neurosci *21*, 309-45.

Fournier-Thibault, C., Pourquie, O., Rouaud, T., and Le Douarin, N. M. (1999). BEN/SC1/DM-GRASP expression during neuromuscular development: a cell adhesion molecule regulated by innervation. J Neurosci *19*, 1382-92.

Gil, O. D., Zanazzi, G., Struyk, A. F., and Salzer, J. L. (1998). Neurotrimin mediates bifunctional effects on neurite outgrowth via homophilic and heterophilic interactions. J Neurosci *18*, 9312-25.

Goodman, C. S., and Tessier-Lavigne, M. (1997). Molecular mechanisms of axon guidance and target recognition. In Molecular and Cellular Approaches to Neural Development, W. M. Cowan, Jessel, T.M., and Zipursky, S.L., ed. (New York: Oxford UNIVERSITY PRESS), pp. 108-178.

Grumet, M. (1991). Cell adhesion molecules and their subgroups in the nervous system. Curr.Opin.Neurobiol. *1*, 370-376.

Grumet, M. (1992). Structure, expression, and function of Ng-CAM, a member of the immunoglobulin superfamily involved in neuron-neuron and neuron-glia adhesion. Journal of Neuroscience Research *31*, 1-13.

Grumet, M. (1997). Nr-CAM: A cell adhesion molecule with ligand and receptor functions. Cell Tissue Research.

Grumet, M., and Sakurai, T. (1996). Heterophilic interactions of the cell adhesion molecules Ng-CAM and Nr-CAM with neural receptors and extracellular matrix proteins. Semin.Neurosci. *8*, 379-389.

Holm, J., Hillenbrand, R., Steuber, V., Bartsch, U., Moos, M., Lubbert, H., Montag, D., and Schachner, M. (1996). Structural features of a close homologue of L1 (CHL1) in the mouse: a new member of the L1 family of neural recognition molecules. Eur J Neurosci *8*, 1613-29.

Hulley, P., Schachner, M., and Lubbert, H. (1998). L1 neural cell adhesion molecule is a survival factor for fetal dopaminergic neurons. J Neurosci Res *53*, 129-34.

Jung, M., Petrausch, B., and Stuermer, C. A. (1997). Axon-regenerating retinal ganglion cells in adult rats synthesize the cell adhesion molecule L1 but not TAG-1 or SC-1. Mol Cell Neurosci *9*, 116-31.

Kamiguchi, H., and Lemmon, V. (1998). A neuronal form of the cell adhesion molecule L1 contains a tyrosine- based signal required for sorting to the axonal growth cone. J Neurosci *18*, 3749-56.

Karagogeos, D., Pourquie, C., Kyriakopoulou, K., Tavian, M., Stallcup, W., Peault, B., and Pourquie, O. (1997). Expression of the cell adhesion proteins BEN/SC1/DM-GRASP and TAG-1 defines early steps of axonogenesis in the human spinal cord. J Comp Neurol *379*, 415-27.

Kidd, T., Brose, K., Mitchell, K. J., Fetter, R. D., Tessier-Lavigne, M., Goodman, C. S., and Tear, G. (1998). Roundabout controls axon crossing of the CNS midline and defines a novel subfamily of evolutionarily conserved guidance receptors. Cell *92*, 205-15.

Krushel, L. A., Prieto, A. L., Cunningham, B. A., and Edelman, G. M. (1993). Expression patterns of the cell adhesion molecules Nr-CAM during histogenesis of the chick nervous system. Neuroscience *53*, 797-812.

Krushel, L. A., Tai, M. H., Cunningham, B. A., Edelman, G. M., and Crossin, K. L. (1998). Neural cell adhesion molecule (N-CAM) domains and intracellular signaling pathways involved in the inhibition of astrocyte proliferation. Proc Natl Acad Sci U S A *95*, 2592-6.

Kunz, S., Spirig, M., Ginsburg, C., Buchstaller, A., Berger, P., Lanz, R., Rader, C., Vogt, L., Kunz, B., and Sonderegger, P. (1998). Neurite fasciculation mediated by complexes of axonin-1 and Ng cell adhesion molecule. J Cell Biol *143*, 1673-90.

Lambert, S., Davis, J. Q., and Bennett, V. (1997). Morphogenesis of the node of Ranvier: co-clusters of ankyrin and ankyrin-binding integral proteins define early developmental intermediates. J Neurosci *17*, 7025-36.

Li, H. S., Chen, J. H., Wu, W., Fagaly, T., Zhou, L., Yuan, W., Dupuis, S., Jiang, Z. H., Nash, W., Gick, C., Ornitz, D. M., Wu, J. Y., and Rao, Y. (1999). Vertebrate slit, a secreted ligand for the transmembrane protein roundabout, is a repellent for olfactory bulb axons. Cell *96*, 807-18.

Lierheimer, R., Kunz, B., Vogt, L., Savoca, R., Brodbeck, U., and Sonderegger, P. (1997). The neuronal cell-adhesion molecule axonin-1 is specifically released by an endogenous glycosylphosphatidylinositol-specific phospholipase. Eur J Biochem *243*, 502-10.

Lustig, M., Sakurai, T., and Grumet, M. (1999). Nr-CAM Promotes Neurite Outgrowth from Peripheral Ganglia by a Mechanism Involving Axonin-1 as a Receptor. Devel. Bio (in press).

Majeti, R., Bilwes, A. M., Noel, J. P., Hunter, T., and Weiss, A. (1998). Dimerization-induced inhibition of receptor protein tyrosine phosphatase function through an inhibitory wedge. Science *279*, 88-91.

Martini, R. (1994). Expression and functional roles of neural cell surface molecules and extracellular matrix components during development and regeneration of peripheral nerves. J Neurocytol *23*, 1-28.

Moscoso, L. M., and Sanes, J. R. (1995). Expression of four immunoglobulin superfamily adhesion molecules (L1, Nr-CAM/Bravo, neurofascin/ABGP, and N-CAM) in the developing mouse spinal cord. Journal of Comparative Neurology *352*, 321-334.

O'Leary, D. D., and Wilkinson, D. G. (1999). Eph receptors and ephrins in neural development. Curr Opin Neurobiol *9*, 65-73.

Paschke, K. A., Lottspeich, F., and Stuermer, C. A. (1992). Neurolin, a cell surface glycoprotein on growing retinal axons in the goldfish visual system, is reexpressed during retinal axonal regeneration. J Cell Biol *117*, 863-75.

Pasterkamp, R. J., De Winter, F., Holtmaat, A. J., and Verhaagen, J. (1998). Evidence for a role of the chemorepellent semaphorin III and its receptor neuropilin-1 in the regeneration of primary olfactory axons. J Neurosci *18*, 9962-76.

Pasterkamp, R. J., Giger, R. J., and Verhaagen, J. (1998). Regulation of semaphorin III/collapsin-1 gene expression during peripheral nerve regeneration. Exp Neurol *153*, 313-27.

Peles, E., Schlessinger, J., and Grumet, M. (1998). Multi-ligand interactions with receptor-like protein tyrosine phosphatase beta: implications for intercellular signaling. Trends Biochem Sci *23*, 121-4.

Pimenta, A. F., Zhukareva, V., Barbe, M. F., Reinoso, B. S., Grimley, C., Henzel, W., Fischer, I., and Levitt, P. (1995). The limbic system-associated membrane protein is an Ig superfamily member that mediates selective neuronal growth and axon targeting. Neuron *15*, 287-97.

Roonprapunt, C. (1998). The role of the cell adhesion molecule L1 in spinal cord injury and regeneration. In Physiology and Neuroscience (New York: NYU Medical Center), pp. 154.

Roonprapunt, C., Hooper, A., Huang, W., Friedlander, D. R., Grumet, M., and Young, W. (1996). Elevated levels of the cell adhesion molecule, L1, following spinal cord injury in the adult rat. Society for Neuroscience Abstracts *22*, 1018.

Rutishauser, U., and Landmesser, L. (1996). Polysialic acid in the vertebrate nervous system: a promoter of plasticity in cell-cell interactions. Trends in Neuroscience *19*, 422-427.

Sonderegger, P. (1997). Axonin-1 and NgCAM as "recognition" components of the pathway sensor apparatus of growth cones: a synopsis. Cell Tissue Res *290*, 429-39.

Song, H., Ming, G., He, Z., Lehmann, M., Tessier-Lavigne, M., and Poo, M. (1998). Conversion of neuronal growth cone responses from repulsion to attraction by cyclic nucleotides. Science *281*, 1515-8.

Stoker, A., and Dutta, R. (1998). Protein tyrosine phosphatases and neural development. Bioessays *20*, 463-72.

Suter, D. M., Pollerberg, G. E., Buchstaller, A., Giger, R. J., Dreyer, W. J., and Sonderegger, P. (1995). Binding between the neural cell adhesion molecules axonin-1 and Nr-CAM/Bravo is involved in neuron-glia interaction. Journal of Cell Biology *131*, 1067-1081.

Venstrom, K. A., and Reichardt, L. F. (1993). Extracellular matrix 2: Role of extracellular matrix molecules and their receptors in the nervous system. FASEB Journal *7*, 996-1003.

Volkmer, H., Leuschner, R., Zacharias, U., and Rathjen, F. G. (1996). Neurofascin induces neurites by heterophilic interactions with axonal NrCAM while NrCAM requires F11 on the axonal surface to extend neurites. Journal of Cell Biology *135*, 1059-1069.

Walsh, F. S., and Doherty, P. (1997). Neural cell adhesion molecules of the immunoglobulin superfamily: role in axon growth and guidance. Annu Rev Cell Dev Biol *13*, 425-56.

Wang, K. H., Brose, K., Arnott, D., Kidd, T., Goodman, C. S., Henzel, W., and Tessier-Lavigne, M. (1999). Biochemical purification of a mammalian slit protein as a positive regulator of sensory axon elongation and branching. Cell *96*, 771-84.

Willbold, E., Brummendorf, T., Rathjen, F. G., Schwarz, H., and Weiss, B. (1997). The neural cell recognition molecule F11 is expressed on Muller cells and Schwann cells in vitro. J Hirnforsch *38*, 71-80.

Winberg, M. L., Noordermeer, J. N., Tamagnone, L., Comoglio, P. M., Spriggs, M. K., Tessier-Lavigne, M., and Goodman, C. S. (1998). Plexin A is a neuronal semaphorin receptor that controls axon guidance. Cell *95*, 903-16.

Wolfer, D. P., Giger, R. J., Stagliar, M., Sonderegger, P., and Lipp, H. P. (1998). Expression of the axon growth-related neural adhesion molecule TAG-1/axonin-1 in the adult mouse brain. Anat Embryol (Berl) *197*, 177-85.

Yu, H. H., and Kolodkin, A. L. (1999). Semaphorin signaling: a little less per-plexin [In Process Citation]. Neuron *22*, 11-4.

Zhang, X., Davis, J. Q., Carpenter, S., and Bennett, V. (1998). Structural requirements for association of neurofascin with ankyrin. J Biol Chem *273*, 30785-94.

19

Neuroprotection from Cell Death Following Axotomy

B. Timothy Himes and Alan Tessler
MCP Hahnemann University and Department of Veterans Affairs Medical Center, Philadelphia, Pennsylvania

I. INTRODUCTION - REGENERATION IS IMPOSSIBLE WITHOUT NEURONAL SURVIVAL

Failure to recover after central nervous system (CNS) injury is in large part due to the death of damaged neurons, which do not replicate, and inability of the surviving neurons to regenerate their axons. The concept that axons that regenerate and reestablish contact with their normal targets will assist recovery is axiomatic. Even in the absence of regeneration, however, neurons that survive axotomy may contribute to recovery. Surviving neurons might maintain a collateral or principal axon that contributes to a functionally important circuit that would be lost if the neuron died. Lesion induced sprouting (reactive synaptogenesis) could strengthen the contribution of spared axons to such a circuit. Neuron survival is also a prerequisite for strategies designed to increase recovery by encouraging axon sprouting or regeneration, and treatments that increase survival have been shown to enhance recovery due to regeneration (Tuszynski and Gage, 1995).

Treatments that maximize neuron survival are likely to assume increasing importance now that protocols are being designed to use transplants to treat patients in the clinic. To avoid worsening the deficits of evolving spinal cord injuries, the initial recipients of transplants are likely to be patients with chronic injuries and stable deficits. Regeneration of chronically injured axons can only occur if the neurons have survived. The importance of neuron survival for functional recovery has encouraged efforts to understand the requirements of mature and developing neurons for survival and stimulated attempts to increase survival of axotomized neurons. Knowledge about the trophic requirements of normal and axotomized neurons has expanded prodigiously in the past 10-15 years. In this review we consider the interventions that have been employed to increase survival of axotomized neurons. Although most studies of neuron survival after axotomy have focused on well circumscribed nuclei where neurons can readily be counted, retrograde neuron death is likely to be more widespread (Katoh et al., 1996; Bradbury et al., 1998; Yong et al., 1998). We do not discuss attempts to increase survival of neurons whose cell bodies have been damaged directly by processes such as trauma or ischemia, although the similarities in mechanisms by which neurons die suggest that the same treatments will rescue neurons injured by diverse pathologies (for reviews, see Budd, 1998; Martin et al., 1998). We also do not consider chronic neuronal degeneration. Although there may also be similarities between the death of acutely axotomized neurons and those that die due to processes such as Alzheimer's disease and amyotrophic lateral sclerosis, even less is known about the mechanisms that account for indolent degeneration than for acute retrograde neuronal death, and the treatment of these degenerative diseases poses additional complexities (reviewed in Martin et al., 1998).

II. CLASSIFICATION OF NEURON DEATH

For at least two decades cell death has been classified into two distinct processes, necrosis and apoptosis, based primarily on morphological and biochemical criteria (reviewed by Wyllie et al., 1980). Death resulting from insults external to the cell, including trauma and ischemia, has been considered to be necrotic, characterized by swelling of mitochondria and endoplasmic reticulum, membrane rupture and phagocytosis by invading scavengers. Cell death occurring in response to the physiological processes of normal development, including programmed cell death (PCD) in the nervous system, has been considered to be apoptotic. Apoptosis results from the activation of an intrinsic cell suicide program and is characterized by condensation of the nucleus and cytoplasm, intranucleosomal cleavage, and rapid removal of the stricken cell by resident phagocytes or adjacent cells.

A considerable amount of recent evidence has demonstrated points of convergence between necrosis and apoptosis and emphasized instances in which features of both processes coexist (reviewed in Martin et al., 1998). The particular characteristics of cell death in response to trauma, ischemia or axotomy are likely to be influenced by a number of variables, including the type of neuron and its stage of development, but similarities between the morphological and molecular features of neuron death presumably reflect similarities in the underlying pathological mechanisms. The importance of the accumulation of large concentrations of excitatory amino acids, especially glutamate, has received increasing attention as a crucial contributor to cell death after various insults (Lindholm, 1994; Sei et al., 1998; Stout et al., 1998). In those cases in which it has been examined, retrograde neuron death in response to axotomy has shown the morphological and biochemical features of apoptosis (Garcia-Valenzuela et al., 1993; Rossiter et al., 1996; Groves et al., 1997). Only a few of these studies have been based on electron microscopic analyses that are proposed to be the most reliable method for distinguishing apoptosis from necrosis (Martin et al., 1998), and only selected systems of neurons have been examined for evidence of apoptosis. Whether or not retrograde neuron death after axotomy fulfills the most rigorous criteria of apoptosis and whether apoptosis is an entirely distinct process from necrosis, however, are secondary issues. Increased understanding of the importance of excitotoxicity and of the molecular events leading to cell death has resulted in effective interventions for rescuing axotomized neurons. Consistent with the idea that similar mechanisms contribute to the retrograde death of neurons after axotomy and neurons injured directly by, for example, ischemia or trauma, are reports that the same treatments rescue neurons injured by diverse types of insults (Davis and Antonawich, 1997; Antonawich et al., 1998; Hayashi et al., 1998; McConkey, 1998; Parsadanian et al., 1998; Wen et al., 1998; Antonawich et al., 1999).

A. Treatment strategies are being developed for apoptosis

Increased understanding of the mechanisms of the cell suicide program has generated new approaches to treatment (reviewed by Raff et al., 1993; Haanen and Vermes, 1996; Wong et al., 1997; Adams and Cory, 1998; Kinloch et al., 1999). Cell death is often mediated by the activation of a family of at least 10 cytoplasmic cysteine proteases, the caspases, which function both to initiate and to carry out the execution phase of apoptosis by cleaving crucial proteins in the nucleus and cytoplasm (reviewed in Villa et al., 1997; McConkey, 1998; Peter and Krammer, 1998). Caspases are constitutively expressed as inactive precursors that are proteolytically processed to an active form in response to a pro-apoptotic signal and then cleave other caspases that are downstream in a rapid cascade. The target substrates of caspases include cytoskeletal proteins, nuclear proteins such as laminin and poly (ADP-ribose) polymerase and the inhibitor (ICAD) of the caspase-activated deoxyribonuclease (CAD), which causes nuclear DNA fragmentation (Enari et al., 1998). Activation of these proteins accounts for cell disassembly and the morphological features of apoptosis. One strategy for preventing neuron death has been to block the execution phase of apoptosis with agents that specifically inhibit a single caspase or that function as general inhibitors of caspases. For example, both YVAD, a peptide inhibitor of caspase-1 (Milligan et al., 1995), and DEVD-CHO, an inhibitor of caspase-3 (CPP32) (Li et al., 1998), protect motoneurons from naturally occurring cell death in vivo, and inhibitors of the interleukin 1β converting enzyme (ICE) family significantly reduce infarct volume in cortex and striatum after transient focal ischemia (Hara et al., 1997). Caspase inhibitors may be useful in the treatment of neurodegenerative diseases (Holtzman and Deshmukh, 1997), and, as discussed below, caspase inhibitors have been used in several systems to maintain neurons that would otherwise die after axotomy.

Intervention may also be effective in the period between the onset of an apoptotic stimulus and the activation of caspases and other proteases that accomplish the execution phase. According to the model developed by Johnson and coworkers, these stages include a latent period and sequential stages of activation and propagation of the apoptotic signal (Deckwerth and Johnson, 1993; Deshmukh et al., 1996).The appearance and increase in reactive oxygen species (ROS), for example, has been postulated to contribute to the triggering and propagation of apoptosis (Dugan et al., 1998), and inhibition of lipid peroxidation has been reported to decrease axotomy-induced apoptotic degeneration following facial nerve section in neonatal rats (Hall et al., 1996).

The family of peptides related to the proto-oncogene Bcl-2, which are thought to function just proximal to caspase activation (Holtzman and Deshmukh, 1997), offers another potentially useful point of intervention. Some members of this family, such as Bcl-2 and Bcl-xL have anti-apoptotic functions, and others, such as Bax, Bak and Bok, are pro-apoptotic. Bax has been reported to be essential for sympathetic neuron death due to NGF deprivation (Deckwerth et al., 1996). The mechanisms by which these peptides integrate extracellular signals, mitochondrial physiology and caspase/protease activity are not fully known. Bcl-2 is located on the cytoplasmic face of the mitochondria outer membrane and other intracellular membranes (Zamzami et al., 1997; Adams and Cory, 1998; Green and Reed, 1998), and is thought to preserve the integrity of these organelles (Polyak et al., 1997; Zamzami et al., 1997; Pettman and Henderson, 1998). It inhibits the release from mitochondria of cytochrome c, which, in combination with ATP, coactivates the autocatalysis of pro-caspase 9 into caspase 9, enabling it to participate in the execution phase of apoptosis (Thornberry and Lazebnik, 1998). Bcl-2 also suppresses the release of Ca^{++} from mitochondria which is induced by uncouplers of respiration (Green and Reed, 1998) and can prevent alteration of the mitochondrial permeability transition pore complex, which helps to maintain the inner transmembrane potential (Zamzami et al., 1997). It also protects cells from the generation of ROS and from lipid peroxidation (Hockenbery et al., 1993; Davies, 1995; Krajewski et al., 1995). The neurons of transgenic mice that overexpress Bcl-2 show less programmed cell death than wild-type littermates (Martinou et al., 1994), and axotomized neurons show better survival (Farlie et al., 1995; Alberi et al., 1996; Cenni et al., 1996; Coulpier et al., 1996; Zhou et al., 1999). In contrast, Bcl-2 null mutant mice show reduced numbers of peripheral (Michaelidis et al., 1996) and RGC (Cellerino et al., 1999) neurons. Reducing concentrations of pro-apoptotic members of the Bcl-2 family may also be effective. For example, inhibiting expression of the p53 tumor suppresser has been proposed to limit death of cultured sympathetic neurons in response to either NGF withdrawal or p75NTR activation by reducing p53-dependent transcription of the pro-apoptotic protein Bax (Aloyz et al., 1998). Intervention at intermediate stages in the evolution of apoptosis by shifting the balance between pro- and anti-apoptotic members of the Bcl-2 family of proto-oncogenes appears to be an extremely promising approach to the treatment of post-axotomy neuron death, and other strategies that target these stages may also be effective.

The interval for effective treatment between the onset of an apoptotic stimulus and the time when cell death becomes inevitable may vary for different types of neurons and has been defined only in a few cases. For example, fetal spinal cord transplants can keep axotomized Clarke's nucleus neurons alive if provided at the time of injury, but are completely ineffective if transplantation is delayed for more than one week (Shibayama et al., 1998b). In contrast, exogenously supplied NGF reverses atrophy of axotomized DRG neurons for at least 3 weeks following sciatic nerve injury (Verge et al., 1989), and BDNF infusion reverses atrophy of axotomized red nucleus (RN) neurons as long as 12-18 weeks after cervical hemisection (Kobayashi et al., 1995). Exogenous neurotrophic factor treatment also increases the number of RN neurons whose axons regenerate into a peripheral nerve graft four weeks after cervical hemisection (Ye and Houle, 1997).

B. Trophic factors can prevent apoptosis

The most frequently reported strategy for rescuing axotomized neurons is the exogenous administration of neurotrophic factors, particularly the specific ligands of receptors expressed by the injured neurons. Whether the success of this treatment means that the survival of adult neurons, like that of immature neurons, depends on a supply of target-derived neurotrophic factors or whether the neurotrophic factor acts pharmacologically is unknown. One rationale for this treatment is based on an analogy between retrograde neuron death and programmed cell death (PCD). PCD refers to the process in which large numbers of neurons in most areas of the developing nervous system die by apoptosis. PCD can be enhanced by target removal and decreased by provision of supernumerary targets (reviewed by Burek and Oppenheim, 1996). In at least one system in which the question has been studied, however, adult medial septal neurons have been reported not to die when their targets in the hippocampus were ablated (Sofroniew et al., 1993), suggesting that their survival is independent of support from the target. It has become clear that additional sources of trophic support are available to neurons besides those that originate in the target, including support from glia, extracellular matrix, afferent neurons and the neurons themselves (reviewed by Burek and Oppenheim, 1996). Given the multiplicity of potential sources of trophic support that are available to mature neurons, it has been difficult to determine whether the survival of mature neurons continues to depend on neurotrophic support and, if so, to identify the sources of this support. It has also been difficult to account for the lesser dependence for survival of mature neurons than immature neurons on target-derived neurotrophic support. One possibility is that mature neurons become more dependent on other sources of trophic support than the target, another is that mature neurons become better able than developing neurons to buffer changes in intracellular calcium or other intracellular challenges induced by axotomy (reviewed by Burek and Oppenheim, 1996). Other mechanisms besides inadequate trophic support from the target also contribute to PCD. For example, death of developing sympathetic neurons appears to be initiated by signals mediated by the p75 neurotrophin receptor (p75NTR), since BDNF can cause apoptosis via this receptor even in the presence of small quantities of NGF (Bamji et al., 1998). These authors point out that one implication of their findings is that survival at the time of target innervation depends on a complex interaction among the neurotrophins that neurons encounter. Exogenously administered neurotrophic factors may therefore rescue axotomized neurons by adding to the sum of survival-promoting factors available to the neuron through its collateral axons, the axons afferent to it, and those available by an autocrine mechanism.

C. Delivery of Trophic Factors

A number of constraints limit the routes by which trophic factors can be administered. Systemic administration is limited by the short half-lives of trophic factors in the general circulation and by the development of antibodies, by the inability of relatively large peptides to pass through the blood brain barrier, and by the systemic side effects of the large amounts of trophic factors necessary to attain therapeutic concentrations in the CNS (Penn et al., 1997). Intraventricular infusion delivers effective amounts of neurotrophic factors only to neurons with perikarya or processes close to the ventricles or subarachnoid space. Administration of BDNF by this route is particularly ineffective because it is bound by trkB receptors present in ependymal cells and brain parenchyma and therapeutic levels are unavailable to target neurons (Yan et al., 1994). The amounts of neurotrophic factors that can be administered intraventricularly are also limited by a major weight loss that is thought to be caused by actions within the hypothalamus (Pelleymounter et al., 1995; Giehl et al., 1997). Intracisternal administration of neurotrophic factors may avoid weight loss, but also is likely to supply adequate levels of factor only to neurons close to the ventricles or subarachnoid space (Giehl et al., 1997; Giehl et al., 1998a). The rescue of most axotomized neurons will therefore require that factors be delivered close to their perikarya or cut axons. Intraparenchymal diffusion of neurotrophic factors is limited to 1.5 to 3 mm around an infusion cannula (Giehl and Tetzlaff, 1996).

Local delivery of trophic factors is also problematic. (1) As a component of their response to injury, astrocytes upregulate the expression of truncated trkB receptors, a form of the high affinity receptor for BDNF and NT4/5 (Frisen et al., 1993). These receptors can compete with axotomized axons for BDNF delivered exogenously and account for the failure of BDNF delivered to the spinal cord to be as effective as BDNF delivered close to the perikarya in preventing atrophy of RN neurons (Kobayashi et al., 1997). (2) Trophic factors administered by gelfoam are only transiently available. Gelfoam pledgets soaked in NT-3 removed from the spinal cord 1 week after insertion, for example, retained bioactivity whereas activity was lost at 2 weeks (Shibayama et al., 1998a). Degradation or washout may account for instances in which neurotrophic factors administered by gelfoam have rescued axotomized neurons only temporarily (Schmalbruch and Rosenthal, 1995). Osmotic minipumps can deliver neurotrophic factors continuously into the parenchyma and prevent degenerative changes in septal neurons (Fischer and Bjorklund, 1991), but this method of administration does not invariably rescue axotomized neurons more effectively than a single application (Shibayama et al., 1998a). (3) Rescue from retrograde neuron death depends on achieving optimal concentrations of trophic factors, and concentrations that were too low or too high have been ineffective. The failure of excessive concentrations of neurotrophic factors to rescue axotomized neurons has been attributed to a toxic effect (von Bartheld et al., 1994), to desensitization or decrease of receptor protein (Frank et al., 1997) and to cross-reactivity with a receptor that interferes with binding its physiologic ligand (reviewed in Pinon et al., 1995). Gene therapy techniques are a newly developed method for providing axotomized neurons with a continuous supply of neurotrophic factors at nearly physiological concentrations (see below).

II. MODEL SYSTEMS FOR THE STUDY OF RETROGRADE NEURON DEATH AND RESCUE

A. Retinal ganglion cells (RGC) are particularly vulnerable to axotomy

RGCs provide one of the most thoroughly studied models of retrograde death following axotomy, in which various treatments based on an understanding of the mechanisms of apoptosis have been used for rescue (this volume, Chapter by Chaudary and Sharma). In addition to their accessibility for surgery and labeling, RGCs offer the advantage of serving as a model for CNS injury because their axons are surrounded by CNS glia and do not spontaneously regenerate. They appear to be particularly vulnerable to axotomy. Following intracranial crush (8 or 10 mm from the eye) or intraorbital cut (0.5 or 3 mm), approximately 95% of injured RGCs eventually die in adult rats (Villegas-Perez et al., 1992). Death after both types of injury proceeds rapidly for the first 2 weeks and then more slowly, suggesting that different processes are responsible for the two phases. Death after intraorbital transection is complete by approximately 6 months; after intracranial crush, death continues over a 20-month survival period. When the optic nerve of adult rats is sectioned within the orbit (0.5 mm from the eye), RGC do not die for the first 5 days, but death by apoptosis (Isenmann et al., 1997) is rapid and virtually complete thereafter; 50% survive at day 7 and less than 10% at 14 days (Berkelaar et al., 1994). This is the baseline against which most rescue strategies are measured.

The explanation for the vulnerability of RGCs is uncertain, but it may be related not only to the short distance between the cell body and the site of injury, but also to a paucity of neurotrophic support derived from sources other than their targets. RGCs give off no recurrent collaterals within the retina (Shepherd, 1979), they receive relatively few synapses, and the spread of their dendrites is limited compared to other types of output neuron (reviewed by Sterling, 1990). They are also particularly difficult to rescue; several sources of trophic support, including target-derived fragments (Huxlin et al., 1995a; Huxlin et al., 1995b) and Schwann cells (Maffei et al., 1990), allowed limited long-term survival after intraorbital transection, which at best was 22% at 14 weeks with Schwann cell grafts (Maffei et al., 1990).

Specific neurotrophic factors have been used to promote RGC survival. Intravitreal injections of glial-derived neurotrophic factor (GDNF), which is retrogradely transported from targets in the superior colliculus (Yan et al., 1999), allowed 35-50% of RGC neurons to survive to 14 days after injury, the longest time studied (Klocker et al., 1997; Yan et al., 1999). Ciliary neurotrophic factor (Mey and Thanos, 1993) as well as members of the fibroblast growth factor family (Sievers et al., 1987) also promote RGC survival in vivo. RGCs express trkB, the high-affinity receptor for BDNF and NT4/5, and retrogradely transport BDNF when it is applied to the cut end of the optic nerve, making BDNF and NT-4/5 promising agents for rescue (Sawai et al., 1996). A single intravitreous injection of BDNF delayed the onset of RGC death beyond 1 week and increased survival significantly, although to a diminishing extent, at both 2 and 4 weeks; by 6 and 8 weeks, however, even multiple injections of BDNF failed to increase survival over control injections (Mansour-Robaey et al., 1994). A single intravitreous injection of NT4/5 also delayed the onset of RGC death after axotomy and protected RGCs up to 14 days, the longest time studied, although to a lesser extent than BDNF (Peinado-Ramon et al., 1996). One injection of NT-3 was ineffective (Peinado-Ramon et al., 1996), but the combination of BDNF and GDNF produced survival at 14 days that was slightly better than that achieved with either factor alone (Yan et al., 1999).

To avoid the repeated injections required by the short half-life of BDNF and to obtain a longer-lasting exposure, recombinant adenovirus genetically modified to express BDNF (Ad.BDNF) was administered by a single intravitreal injection. In a study in which this injection led to AD.BDNF infection of Muller glia cells rather than RGC, the Muller cells expressed the c-myc tagged BDNF for about 10 days and appeared to secrete it in the vicinity of RGC perikarya (Di Polo et al., 1998). Ad.BDNF increased RGC survival more than four-fold over that seen following control injections of adenovirus containing only the lacZ gene at 16 days and continued to have a beneficial, although sharply diminishing, effect on survival at 28 days. The maximum ~35% survival seen at 16 days did not exceed that observed following a single intravitreous injection of BDNF, however, and was not increased by immunosuppression with FK-506, even though immunosuppression prolonged high-level expression of transgene to 30 days. Administration of a different Ad.BDNF vector by a single intravitreal injection infected several different types of cells, including Muller glia cells and RGC (Isenmann et al., 1998). Expression of the lacZ marker gene continued for ~10 days, decreased during the second and third weeks and persisted only weakly after 4 weeks. About 40% of axotomized RGC that otherwise would have died survived at 14 days, which was less than that found with repeated injections of BDNF.

Several different mechanisms could account for the failure of BDNF to obtain permanent survival of RGC. Axotomy has been found to down-regulate levels of expression of mRNA for the full length trkB receptor by 3 days after injury and to cause an up-regulation of truncated trkB receptor levels in astrocytes in the optic nerve stump at ~1 week (Di Polo et al., 1998). These changes could desensitize RGCs to the effects of BDNF and limit its availability to the injured axons. Another possibility is that BDNF limits its own neuroprotective capacity by inducing free radical formation, particularly nitric oxide (NO) (Klocker et al., 1998). Consistent with this notion, systemic administration of either an unspecified free radical scavenger (S-PBN) or a specific inhibitor of NO synthase (L-NAME) together with intraocularly administered BDNF produced a significantly greater survival of axotomized RGC at 14 days than BDNF alone. Neither scavenger increased survival without BDNF (Klocker et al., 1998).

The incomplete and transient rescue of axotomized RGCs by grafts and neurotrophic factors is consistent with the idea that their survival depends on more than one neurotrophic factor and that multiple pathways can lead to delayed death of axotomized neurons. This realization has prompted attempts to increase survival by intervening at steps along apoptotic pathways that may be common to several different pathologic processes. To examine the neuroprotective potential of the antiapoptotic gene Bcl-2, RGC survival in transgenic mice that overexpress Bcl-2 has been compared to that found in wild-type mice after optic nerve section in newborns (Bonfanti et al., 1996) and adults (Cenni et al., 1996). Many more RGC of wild-type than transgenic mice show pyknotic nuclei and fragmented DNA at 24 and 30 hours, and nearly 50% of RGC have degenerated by 24 hours, whereas no degeneration appeared in transgenic mice. Following optic nerve section in adults, only 5% of RGCs survived axotomy in wild-type mice at 3.5 months, whereas 63% survived in transgenic mice. The perikarya of surviving RGC neurons were atrophied, but electrophysiological recordings indicated that, in contrast to those that survived in wild-type mice, they remained functional.

Because caspases play a critical role as effectors of apoptosis, the protective effect of caspase inhibitors has been examined (Kermer et al., 1998). Intraocular injections of an irreversible wide-range protease inhibitor (ZVAD-fmk) rescued 22% of RGC neurons that would otherwise have died 14 days after optic nerve section, and injections of an irreversible inhibitor of CPP-32-like caspases (ADEVD-cmk) yielded a significantly greater rescue of 34%. CPP-32-like inhibitors also increase short-term RGC survival if administered 3 days after injury, but not if administration is delayed until 7 days (Chaudhary et al., 1999). Whether inhibitors of caspases can produce long-term survival and whether these agents act synergistically with neurotrophic factors in this system remain to be determined.

B. Corticospinal tract (CST) neurons die after injury very close to the cell body

In contrast to the vulnerability of RGCs, corticospinal tract (CST) neurons do not die after axotomy at the spinal level in adult animals, although their perikarya are slightly atrophied (Pruitt et al., 1988; Merline and Kalil, 1990). Axotomy within the internal capsule causes the death of 40% of injured CST neurons by 5 days, ~50% by 7 days, and only a small additional cell loss at 28 days (Giehl and Tetzlaff, 1996). The properties of neurons that allow some members of a nucleus to survive while others die are unknown, but a similar observation of differential vulnerability has been reported for neurons in other systems, including those of Clarke's Nucleus (Himes et al., 1994), RN (Mori et al., 1997) and dorsal root ganglion (Himes and Tessler, 1989). Studies of CST neurons have provided some insight into the mechanisms of trophic support that might allow axotomized neurons to survive (discussed in Giehl and Tetzlaff, 1996). Very few CST neurons have supraspinal collateral axons that could provide trophic support, but NT-3 produced at the lesion site could exert an effect mediated by trkC receptors present on CST neurons. Intracortical collaterals could also contribute; virtually all (90%) CST neurons express trkB (Giehl and Tetzlaff, 1996), and BDNF mRNA and protein are expressed throughout the cerebral cortex (Kokaia et al., 1993). Additional trophic support may derive from paracrine or autocrine effects. *In situ* hybridization analysis reveals that ~50% of CST neurons express mRNA for BDNF (Giehl et al., 1998b). Axotomized CST neurons, however, upregulate expression of mRNA for BDNF only slightly and decrease their expression of mRNA for trkB (Giehl et al., 1998b). Whether CST neurons increase retrograde transport of neurotrophic factors after injury has not been studied. DRG neurons and spinal cord motor neurons increase retrograde transport of neurotrophins by a receptor-mediated process that may contribute to their survival after sciatic nerve injury (Curtis et al., 1998). Intracortical infusion of either NT-3 or BDNF enables all CST neurons axotomized in the internal capsule to survive for 1 week (Giehl & Tetzlaff, '96), and BDNF has long-term effects that promote survival for at least 42 days (Hammond et al., '99). GDNF also insures both short- and long-term survival (Giehl et al., '97) through mechanisms that depend on endogenous BDNF (Hammond et al., '99).

C. Medial Septal Nucleus neurons are rescued by exogenous neurotrophic factor

Transection of the fimbria-fornix provides a well defined central system in which to study retrograde degeneration since it interrupts axons of the medial septal (MS) nucleus that project to the hippocampus and efferent axons of hippocampal pyramidal cells. The appearance of few degenerative changes in the hippocampal neurons has been attributed to the presence of numerous local collaterals that escape axotomy (reviewed in Naumann et al., 1992). In contrast, the absence of locally arborizing collateral axons may account for many of the pronounced physiological changes seen in the MS after axotomy. Transection of the fimbria-fornix produces prominent degenerative changes in MS neurons. Large MS neurons disappear, staining for the cholinergic marker enzymes choline acetyltransferase (ChAT) and acetylcholinesterase (AChE) is almost completely lost by 2 weeks (Hefti, 1986; Williams et al., 1986; Kromer, 1987), and immunoreactivity for glutamate decarboxylase (GAD) is greatly diminished by 6 weeks (Peterson et al., 1987). These changes suggest that interruption of a supply of neurotrophic factors from target neurons in the hippocampus leads to degenerative changes in MS neurons.

The extent of neuron death after fimbria-fornix transection has been disputed. Counts of neurons retrogradely labeled by tracers injected into the hippocampus indicated that most MS neurons died after fimbria-fornix transection (O'Brien and Oppenheim, 1990; Tuszynski et al., 1990). Other evidence suggests, however, that fewer MS neurons die than counts based on transmitter-related enzymes would suggest (reviewed in Naumann et al., 1992). Some investigations using electron microscopy (Naumann et al., 1992; Ginsberg and Martin, 1998) and the TUNEL technique (Haas et al., 1996) have failed to provide evidence for apoptosis.

A number of studies have demonstrated that the exogenous administration of trophic factors can attenuate changes in MS phenotype and reduce neuron death after axotomy. Continuous intraventricular infusion of NGF for 2 or 4 weeks significantly reduced or prevented the decline in ChAT or AChE-positive cell bodies that follows axotomy of MS neurons (Hefti, 1986; Williams et al., 1986; Kromer, 1987), but only partially prevented their atrophy (Hefti, 1986). Infusion of BDNF also rescued markers of cholinergic neuron phenotype (Knusel et al., 1992; Morse et al., 1993). Intraventricular administration of NGF for 3 weeks did not prevent a decline in staining for the calcium-binding protein parvalbumin (PARV), a marker for axotomized GABAergic septohippocampal neurons, and did not increase the spontaneous recovery in ChAT or PARV immunoreactivity that occurs by 6 months in operated rats that have not received NGF (Naumann et al., 1994). trkA activation accounts for the rescue observed with NGF because intraventricular infusion of polyclonal antibodies that act as specific agonists of trkA in combination with an antibody that blocks the low affinity NGF receptor (p75 NGF) prevented short-term decline in the number of axotomized MS neurons that were immunoreactive for p75NGF, another marker of cholinergic neurons (Lucidi-Phillipi et al., 1996). Injection of a lentiviral vector expressing human NGF into the septum 3 weeks prior to transection of the fimbria fornix also acted prophylactically to prevent a decline of ChAT-stained septal neurons 3 weeks after axotomy (Blomer et al., 1998). Recombinant adeno-associated virus may provide another vector for the long-term delivery to medial septal neurons of high levels of neurotrophic factors (Klein et al., 1999). Overexpression of the anti-apoptotic peptide Bcl-xL in the same model of injury also reduced the loss of ChAT-immunoreactive septal neurons, although the rescue was smaller than that observed with NGF. This result suggested that, although both NGF and Bcl-xL prevented apoptosis, the effect of NGF was in part mediated through a paracrine mechanism.

Very few mature MS neurons die when their target is ablated without damaging the axon (Sofroniew et al., 1990). Excitotoxic ablation of target neurons in the hippocampus did not cause a significant decline in immunocytochemically detected cholinergic neurons in the MS although the surviving neurons were shrunken and their cholinergic staining was reduced. These observations suggested that several aspects of neuron phenotype depended on target-derived neurotrophic support but that death was due to changes induced by axotomy (Sofroniew et al., 1990; Sofroniew et al., 1993). If this is so for other populations of neurons, then it suggests that death or survival of injured neurons reflects a balance between the changes induced by axotomy and the capacity of the neuron to adapt to these changes. Whatever the explanation, neurons differ greatly in their vulnerability after axotomy.

D. Clarke's Nucleus neurons atrophy even when cell death is prevented

CN has provided another useful model system for developing strategies to rescue neurons from retrograde cell death. These neurons provide an exception to the general observations that newborn neurons are more dependent on target-derived neurotrophic support than adult neurons and that newborn neurons are more likely than mature neurons to die after axotomy. Axotomy by unilateral hemisection at the T8 segment in newborn rats causes 40% of CN neurons at L1 to die, and the same lesion in adults kills 30% (Himes et al., 1994). Several different types of intervention have successfully rescued virtually all of these neurons. Transplants of embryonic spinal cord, cerebellum, and neocortex enable the axotomized neurons to survive in both newborns and adults, whereas transplants of embryonic striatum are ineffective (Himes et al., 1994). Several lines of evidence suggest that one mechanism by which transplants enable injured CN neurons to survive is by acting as a source of diffusible neurotrophic factors. Although not directly tested, it is unlikely that axotomized CN neurons send axons into transplants because regeneration into fetal transplants from neurons with perikarya as distant as these is distinctly uncommon (Jakeman and Reier,

1991). Therefore rescue is likely to depend on diffusion of trophic factors rather than on synapse formation with neurons in the grafts or with the normal targets of CN neurons in rostral spinal cord or cerebellum. The three types of tissues that rescue CN neurons express high levels of NT-3 mRNA at the time of transplantation (Maisonpierre et al., 1990), but embryonic striatum does not. In one test of the notion that NT-3 was responsible for the rescue, NT-3 was administered by gelfoam pledget or continuously for a 2-month survival period by Alzet minipump (Shibayama et al., 1998a). Exogenous administration by either route of NT-3, but not other neurotrophins, prevented at least 50% of the cell death observed in CN following axotomy. This result made it likely, therefore, that NT-3 is responsible for the CN neuron rescue. In addition, because bioactive NT-3 is only available from gelfoam pledgets for at most 2 weeks but administration by gelfoam is as effective as continuous administration by mini-pump, it appears that many axotomized CN neurons are only transiently vulnerable to the effects of axotomy (Shibayama et al., 1998a). If enabled to survive through this vulnerable period, the neurons appear to be able to survive permanently. Grafts of embryonic CNS are more effective than NT-3 administered exogenously; this could be because cell grafts produce more NT-3, because the supply of neurotrophic factors is more continuous or because the CNS transplants produce other factors that are also beneficial to the injured neurons. When, however, NT-3 is provided by grafts of fibroblasts or the C17 immortalized stem-like cell line genetically modified to express NT-3, rescue is as effective as with embryonic CNS transplants and virtually all of the axotomized CN neurons survive (Himes et al., 1999). Whether CN neurons express trkC, the specific receptor for NT-3, remains to be determined.

Whether the survival of mature uninjured CN neurons depends on target-derived neurotrophic factors is unknown, but axotomy appears to make these injured neurons more vulnerable to excitotoxic input from afferent axons. Deafferentation of CN by dorsal rhizotomy at the time of axotomy (Sanner et al., 1993) or blocking NMDA receptors by administration of the NMDA receptor antagonist MK-801 prevents CN cell death (Sanner et al., 1994). These results suggest that axotomized neurons are susceptible to excitotoxic cell death even when the CNS injury is well removed from the region of the cell body.

The apoptotic mechanisms which lead to cell death require the active synthesis of new proteins and the activation of a cascade of specific proteases (caspases) that participate in the execution phase of apoptosis (Thornberry and Lazebnik, 1998). Blocking synthetic pathways that are stimulated by axotomy can prevent or at least delay apoptotic cell death (Maas et al., 1998), but in most cases surviving neurons are atrophied. For example, neurotrophins (Sendtner et al., 1992) and GDNF (Matheson et al., 1997) have been found to increase short term survival of axotomized facial neurons when applied to the cut nerves of newborn rats, but only GDNF prevented atrophy. The virtually complete rescue of axotomized CN neurons found with transplants of fetal CNS tissue or of genetically engineered cells and the partial rescue found with exogenous administration of NT-3 alone also failed to maintain perikaryal area. These observations suggest that larger amounts of NT-3 are necessary to maintain neuron size after axotomy than to ensure neuron survival. Decreases in cytoskeletal elements that could account for atrophy have been reported in the proximal dendrites and cell bodies of axotomized CN neurons (Brook et al., 1998); caspases hydrolyze proteins involved in cytoskeleton regulation (reviewed by Pettman and Henderson, 1998; Thornberry and Lazebnik, 1998). To determine whether a strategy designed to intervene at a point at which several different survival signals converge, we examined whether supplying axotomized CN neurons with the antiapoptotic gene Bcl-2 would prevent loss and atrophy of the injured neurons. We have found that human Bcl-2 delivered by intraspinal injection of a DNA/lipid plasmid to axotomized CN neurons prevented retrograde neuron loss and significantly attenuated atrophy (Takahashi et al., 1999). Figure 1a and b summarizes the effects of several interventions on CN neurons.

E. Red nucleus neurons can be rescued with BDNF and can be induced to regenerate

Several strategies have been used to treat the retrograde neuron loss and atrophy that follow transection of RN axons (Figure 1). Neurons located in the magnocellular portion of the RN are the source of axons that cross in the midbrain and descend to the spinal cord via the contralateral lateral funiculus. When axotomized at the C3 level in adult rats, these neurons initially increase their synthesis of regeneration associated genes, including tubulins, actin and GAP-43, but during the second week expression of these genes decreases and the neurons atrophy (Tetzlaff et al., 1991). By 2 months following axotomy at this level 35% of the RN neurons are lost (Mori et al., 1997). Axotomy at the midthoracic level produces a neuron loss that is considerably more massive in newborn than in adult rats (Prendergast and Stelzner, 1976), consistent with the generalization that newborn neurons are more vulnerable to axotomy than adult neurons. Transplants of embryonic spinal cord placed into the midthoracic hemisection site in newborns completely prevent the extensive loss of RN neurons that follows this lesion (Bregman and Reier, 1986). The effect is specific for the normal target of rubrospinal axons because transplants of other regions of the embryonic CNS or sciatic nerves keep RN neurons alive only transiently (Bregman and Kunkel-Bagden, 1988). Transplants of embryonic spinal cord prevent about 50% of the RN neuron loss otherwise observed after C3 axotomy in adults (Mori et al., 1997) but do not prevent the axotomized neurons from atrophying. Delivery of the human Bcl-2 gene rescues RN neurons as effectively as transplants and in addition attenuates atrophy (Shibata et al., 2000) (Figure 2).

The rescue effects of transplants in both newborns and adults are likely to be due at least in part to the transplant acting as a surrogate source of neurotrophic factors. In adult operates axotomized RN neurons remain close to the margins of the transplants but do not enter or traverse them (Mori et al., 1997).

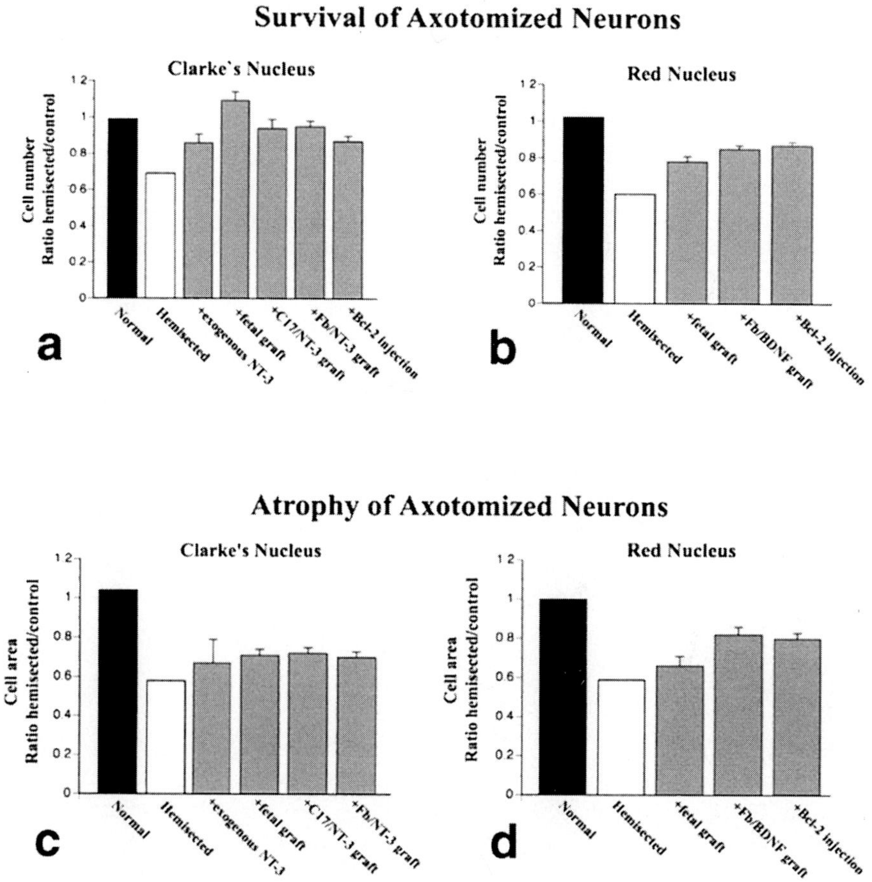

Figure 1 Bar graphs summarizing the effects of several different treatments on loss and atrophy of axotomized Clarke's nucleus and Red Nucleus neurons. All treatments were administered at the time of unilateral spinal cord hemisection. For the studies of Red Nucleus neurons, the hemisection was performed at C3/4. The hemisection was at T8 for the Clarke's nucleus studies. Fb/NT-3 grafts are fibroblasts that have been genetically modified to express NT-3; C17/NT-3 grafts are immortalized stem-like cells isolated from newborn mouse cerebellum.

In newborn operates regenerated axons establish synaptic contacts with neurons within the transplants (Bregman et al., 1991; Bregman, 1994), and many regenerated rubrospinal axons grow into spinal cord caudal to the grafts (Bregman and Bernstein-Goral, 1991; Bernstein-Goral and Bregman, 1993). Successful regeneration presumably ensures permanent survival by providing trophic support from the transplants and from the normal targets of RN neurons, although additional support to regenerated newborn RN neurons may derive from collateral axons that are maintained in cervical spinal cord (Bernstein-Goral and Bregman, 1997).

Exogenous administration of specific neurotrophic factors has also prevented or reversed the retrograde effects of RN neuron axotomy. RN neurons

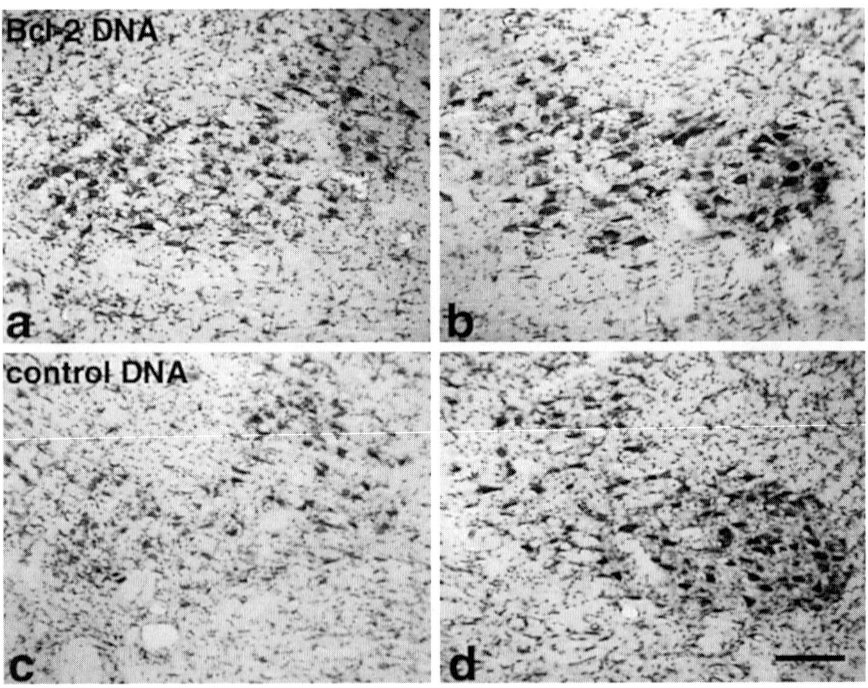

Figure 2 Photomicrographs through the magnocellular Red Nucleus 2 months following unilateral cervical lateral funiculus injury and injection of human Bcl-2 DNA (a, b) or control DNA (c, d). Left RN (a, c) is contralateral to the lesion and right RN (b, d) is ipsilateral. A single injection of Bcl-2 DNA prevents much of the cell loss and atrophy in RN (a), while an injection of DNA that does not contain the Bcl-2 gene is ineffective (c). Scale bar = 100 μm.

express trkB and trkC receptors but not trkA (Kobayashi et al., 1997). Within 7 days following a cervical hemisection expression of full length trkB receptors on RN neurons dramatically declines (Kobayashi et al., 1997). Infusion of BDNF or NT-4/5 into the midbrain close to the perikarya of RN neurons from 7-14 days after axotomy nevertheless causes an increase in the expression of regeneration associated proteins GAP-43 and $t\alpha 1$-tubulin mRNA and prevents cell atrophy for at least two weeks following the termination of the treatment (Kobayashi et al., 1997). Administration of BDNF by gelfoam pledget into the midthoracic hemisection site of newborn rats kept alive significantly larger numbers of RN neurons than gelfoam soaked in saline; NT-3 and NGF rescued these neurons only temporarily (Diener and Bregman, 1994). Although RN neurons did not die after midthoracic hemisection in adult rats, the axotomized neurons were considerably atrophied; BDNF or NT-3 alone or transplants of fetal spinal cord alone partially prevented this decrease in mean soma size whereas mean soma size was indistinguishable from normal at 28 days after injury when either BDNF or NT-3 was administered by gelfoam pledget in combination with a transplant (Bregman et al., 1998). We have observed that, when adult RN neurons axotomized by a partial unilateral hemisection at C3 are provided with a transplant of fibroblasts genetically modified to express BDNF, the axons regenerate through and around the transplants and into host spinal cord as far caudal as T8 (Liu et al., 1999b). The RN neurons of these rats do not die and atrophy is largely prevented (Liu et al., 1999a) (Figure 3).

III. FUTURE DIRECTIONS

Increased understanding of the mechanisms by which a neuron dies of apoptosis is leading to new treatments. The strategies of inhibiting the actions of the caspases, which carry out the execution phase of apoptosis, and influencing the balance toward the antiapoptotic members of the Bcl-2 family of proto-oncogenes, have built directly on this knowledge. Administration of neurotrophic factors, the most commonly used treatment, has allowed various types of neuron to survive axotomy even if the method of delivery made the factor available only transiently and the mechanisms by which the factors act are unknown. Gene therapy techniques have the potential to make neurotrophic factors available for longer times and at concentrations that are more physiological. The most effective strategies for increasing the survival of injured neurons may be those that also increase regeneration and functional recovery, and these strategies are coming closer to application in the clinic. Once neuronal death can be reliably prevented following injury the critical issue of how these cells can reintegrate into the CNS and restore function can be addressed.

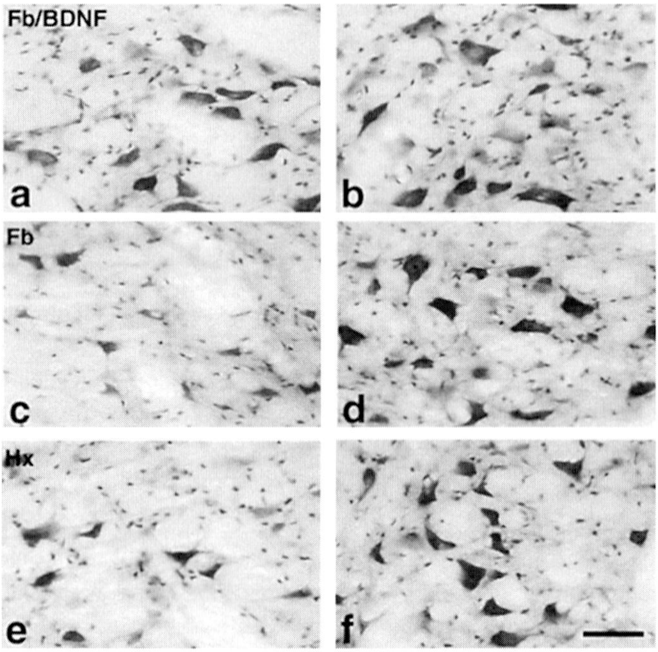

Figure 3 Photomicrographs through the magnocellular Red Nucleus 2 months following unilateral cervical lateral funiculus injury and transplantation of BDNF-secreting fibroblasts (a, b) or unmodified fibroblasts (c, d) or injury alone (e, f). Large neurons are present on control sides (b, d, f) and contralateral to BDNF-fibroblast transplant (a). Fewer neurons are present contralateral to the transplant of unmodified fibroblasts (c) or injury alone (e) and no large neurons are present. Scale bar = 50 μm.

ACKNOWLEDGMENTS

We are grateful for support from the Research Service of the Department of Veterans Affairs, NIH (NS24707), American Paralysis Association, Eastern Paralyzed Veterans Association, International Research for Paraplegia, International Spinal Research Trust and Paralyzed Veterans of America.

REFERENCES

Adams JM, Cory S (1998) The Bcl-2 protein family: arbiters of cell survival. Science 281:1322-1326.

Alberi S, Raggenbass M, de Bilbao F, Dubois-Dauphin M (1996) Axotomized neonatal motoneurons overexpressing the bcl2 proto-oncogene retain functional electrophysiological properties. Proc. Natl. Acad. Sci. USA 93:3978-3983.

Aloyz RS, Bamji SX, Pozniak CD, Toma JG, Atwal J, Kaplan DR, Miller FD (1998) P53 is essential for developmental neuron death as regulated by the trkA and p75 neurotrophin receptors. J. Cell Biol. 143:1691-1703.

Antonawich FJ, Federoff HJ, Davis JN (1999) BCL-2 transduction, using a herpes simplex virus amplicon, protects hippocampal neurons from transient global ischemia. Exp. Neurol. 156:130-137.

Antonawich FJ, Krajewski S, Reed JC, Davis JN (1998) Bcl-x(l) Bax interaction after transient global ischemia. J. Cereb. Blood Flow Metab. 18:882-886.

Bamji SX, Majdan M, Pozniak CD, Belliveau DJ, Aloyz R, Kohn J, Causing CG, Miller FD (1998) The p75 neurotrophin receptor mediates neuronal apoptosis and is essential for naturally occurring sympathetic neuron death. J. Cell Biol. 140:911-923.

Berkelaar M, Clarke DB, Wang YC, Bray GM, Aguayo AJ (1994) Axotomy results in delayed death and apoptosis of retinal ganglion cells in adult rats. J. Neurosci. 14:4368-4374.

Bernstein-Goral H, Bregman BS (1993) Spinal cord transplants support the regeneration of axotomized neurons after spinal cord lesions at birth: a quantitative double-labeling study. Exp. Neurol. 123:118-132.

Bernstein-Goral H, Bregman BS (1997) Axotomized rubrospinal neurons rescued by fetal spinal cord transplants maintain axon collaterals to rostral CNS targets. Exp. Neurol. 148:13-25.

Blomer U, Kafri T, Randolph-Moore L, Verma IM, Gage FH (1998) Bcl-xL protects adult septal cholinergic neurons from axotomized cell death. Proc. Natl. Acad. Sci. USA 95:2603-2608.

Bonfanti L, Strettoi E, Chierzi S, Cenni MC, Liu X-H, Martinou J-C, Maffei L, Rabacchi SA (1996) Protection of retinal ganglion cells from natural and axotomy-induced cell death in neonatal transgenic mice overexpressing bcl-2. J. Neurosci. 16:4186-4194.

Bradbury EJ, King VR, Simmons LJ, Priestley JV, McMahon SB (1998) NT-3, but not BDNF, prevents atrophy and death of axotomized spinal cord projection neurons. Eur. J. Neurosci. 10:3058-3068.

Bregman BS (1994) Recovery of function after spinal cord injury: transplantation strategies. In: Functional Neural Transplantation (Dunnett SB, Bjorklund A, eds.), pp. 489-529. New York: Raven Press.

Bregman BS, Bernstein-Goral H (1991) Both regenerating and late-developing pathways contribute to transplant-induced anatomical plasticity after spinal cord lesion at birth. Exp. Neurol. 112:49-63.

Bregman BS, Bernstein-Goral H, Kunkel-Bagden E (1991) CNS transplants promote anatomical plasticity and recovery of function after spinal cord injury. Restorative Neurol. Neurosci. 2:327-338.

Bregman BS, Broude E, McAtee M, Kelley MS (1998) Transplants and neurotrophic factors prevent atrophy of mature CNS neurons after spinal cord injury. Exp. Neurol. 149:13-27.

Bregman BS, Kunkel-Bagden E (1988) Effect of target and non-target transplants on neuronal survival and axonal elongation after injury to the developing spinal cord. Prog. Brain Res. 78:205-211.

Bregman BS, Reier PJ (1986) Neural tissue transplants rescue axotomized rubrospinal cells from retrograde death. J. Comp. Neurol. 244:86-95.

Brook GA, Spitzer C, Nacimiento W, Woodhams PL, Noth J (1998) A novel early component of the cell body response in axotomized Clarke's nucleus neurons revealed by monoclonal antibody Py. Exp. Neurol. 149:64-72.

Budd SL (1998) Mechanisms of neuronal damage in brain hypoxia/ischemia: Focus on the role of mitochondrial calcium accumulation. Pharmacol. ther. 80:203-229.

Burek MJ, Oppenheim RW (1996) Programmed cell death in the nervous system. Brain Pathol. 6:427-446.

Cellerino A, Michaelidis T, Barski J, Bahr M, Thoenen H, Meyer M (1999) Retinal ganglion cell loss after the period of naturally occurring cell death in bcl-2(-/-) mice. Neuroreport 10:1091-1095.

Cenni MC, Bonfanti L, Martinou JC, Ratto GM, Strettoi E, Maffei L (1996) Long-term survival of retinal ganglion cells following optic nerve section in adult bcl-2 transgenic mice. Eur. J. Neurosci. 8:1735-1745.

Chaudhary P, Ahmed F, Quebada P, Sharma SC (1999) Caspase inhibitors block retinal ganglion cell death following optic nerve transection. Mol. Brain Res. 67:36-45.

Coulpier M, Junier M-P, Peschanski M, Dreyfus PA (1996) Bcl-2 sensitivity differentiates two pathways for motoneuronal death in the wobbler mutant mouse. J. Neurosci. 16:5897-5904.

Curtis R, Tonra JR, Stark JL, Adryan KM, Park JS, Cliffer KD, Lindsay RM, DiStefano PS (1998) Neuronal injury increases retrograde axonal transport of the neurotrophins to spinal sensory neurons and motor neurons via multiple receptor mechanisms. Mol. Cell. Neurosci. 12:105-118.

Davies AM (1995) The Bcl-2 family of proteins, and the regulation of neuronal survival. Trends Neurosci. 18:355-358.

Davis JN, Antonawich FJ (1997) Role of apoptotic proteins in ischemic hippocampal damage. Annals of the New York Academy of Sciences 835:309-320.

Deckwerth TL, Elliott JL, Knudson CM, Johnson EM, Jr., Snider WD, Korsmeyer SJ (1996) BAX is required for neuronal death after trophic factor deprivation and during development. Neuron 17:401-411.

Deckwerth TL, Johnson EM, Jr. (1993) Temporal analysis of events associated with programmed cell death (apoptosis) of sympathetic neurons deprived of nerve growth factor. J. Cell Biol. 123:1207-1222.

Deshmukh M, Vasilakos J, Deckwerth TL, Lampe PA, Shivers BD, Johnson J, E. M. (1996) Genetic and metabolic status of NGF-deprived sympathetic neurons saved by an inhibitor of ICE family proteases. J. Cell Biol. 135:1341-1354.

Di Polo A, Aigner LJ, Dunn RJ, Bray GM, Aguayo AG (1998) Prolonged delivery of brain-derived neurotrophic factor by adenovirus-infected Muller cells temporarily rescues injured retinal ganglion cells. Proc. Natl. Acad. Sci. USA 95:3978-3983.

Diener PS, Bregman BS (1994) Neurotrophic factors prevent the death of CNS neurons after spinal cord lesions in newborn rats. Neuroreport 5:1913-1917.

Dugan LL, Creedon DJ, Johnson J, E. M., Holtzman DM (1998) Rapid suppression of free radical formation by nerve growth factor involves the mitogen-activated protein kinase pathway. Proc. Natl. Acad. Sci. USA 94:4086-4091.

Enari M, Sakahira H, Yokoyama H, Okawa K, Iwamatsu A, Nagata S (1998) A caspase-activated DNase that degrades DNA during apoptosis, and its inhibitor ICAD. Nature 391:43-50.

Farlie PG, Dringen R, Rees SM, Kannourakis G, Bernard O (1995) bcl-2 transgene expression can protect neurons against developmental and induced cell death. Proc. Natl. Acad. Sci. USA 92:4397-4401.

Fischer W, Bjorklund A (1991) Loss of AchE- and NGFr-labeling precedes neuronal death of axotomized septal-diagonal band neurons: reversal by intraventricular NGF infusion. Exp. Neurol. 113:93-108.

Frank L, Wiegand SJ, Siuciak JA, Lindsay RM, Rudge JS (1997) Effects of BDNF on the regulation of TrkB protein and message in adult rat brain. Exp. Neurol. 145:62-70.

Frisen J, Verge VM, Fried K, Risling M, Persson H, Trotter J, Hokfelt T, Lindholm D (1993) Characterization of glial trkB receptors: differential response to injury in the central and peripheral nervous systems. Proc. Natl. Acad. Sci. USA 90:4971-4975.

Garcia-Valenzuela E, Gorczyca W, Darzynkiewicz Z, Sharma SC (1993) Apoptosis in adult retinal ganglion cells after axotomy. J. Neurobiol. 25:431-438.

Giehl KM, Schacht CM, Yan Q, Mestres P (1997) GDNF is a trophic factor for adult rat corticospinal neurons and promotes their long-term survival after axotomy in vivo. Eur. J. Neurosci. 9:2479-2488.

Giehl KM, Schacht CM, Yan Q, Mestres P (1998a) Infusion of GDNF into the cerebral spinal fluid through two different routes: effects on body weight and corticospinal neuron survival. Neuroreport 9:2809-2813.

Giehl KM, Schutte A, Mestres P, Yan Q (1998b) The survival-promoting effect of glial cell line-derived neurotrophic factor on axotomized corticospinal neurons in vivo is mediated by an endogenous brain-derived neurotrophic factor mechanism. J. Neurosci. 18:7351-7360.

Giehl KM, Tetzlaff W (1996) BDNF and NT-3, but not NGF, prevent axotomy-induced death of rat corticospinal neurons in vivo. Eur. J. Neurosci. 8:1167-1175.

Ginsberg SD, Martin LJ (1998) Ultrastructural analysis of the progression of neurodegeneration in the septum following fimbria-fornix transection. Neuroscience 86:1259-1272.

Green DR, Reed JC (1998) Mitochondria and apoptosis. Science 281:1309-1312.

Groves MJ, Christopherson T, Giometto B, Scaravilli F (1997) Axotomy-induced apoptosis in adult rat primary sensory neurons. J. Neurocytol. 26:615-624.

Haanen C, Vermes I (1996) Apoptosis: programmed cell death in fetal development. Eur. J. Obstet. Gynecol. Reprod. Biol. 64:129-133.

Haas CA, Deller T, Naumann T, Frotscher M (1996) Selective expression of the immediate early gene c-jun in axotomized rat medial septal neurons is not related to neuronal degeneration. J. Neurosci. 16:1894-1903.

Hall ED, Smith SL, Oostveen JA (1996) Inhibition of lipid peroxidation attenuates axotomy-induced apoptotic degeneration of facial motor neurons in neonatal rats. J. Neurosci. Res. 44:293-299.

Hammond ENL, Tetzlaff W, Mestres P, Giehl KM (1999) BDNF, but not NT-3, promotes long-term survival of axotomized adult rat corticospinal neurons in vivo. NeuroReport 10:2671-2675.

Hara H, Friedlander RM, Gagliardini V, Ayata C, Fink K, Huang Z, Shimizu-Sasamata M, Yuan J, Moskowitz MA (1997) Inhibition of interleukin 1b converting enzyme family proteases reduces ischemic and excitotoxic neuronal damage. Proc. Natl. Acad. Sci. USA 94:2007-2012.

Hayashi T, Sakurai M, Abe K, Sadahiro M, Tabayashi K, Itoyama Y (1998) Apoptosis of motor neurons with induction of caspases in the spinal cord after ischemia. Stroke 29:1007-1012.

Hefti F (1986) Nerve growth factor promotes survival of septal cholinergic neurons after fimbrial transections. J. Neurosci. 6:2155-2162.

Himes BT, Goldberger ME, Tessler A (1994) Grafts of fetal central nervous system tissue rescue axotomized Clarke's nucleus neurons in adult and neonatal operates. J. Comp. Neurol. 339:117-131.

Himes BT, Liu Y, Solowska JM, Snyder EY, Fischer I, Tessler A (1999) Transplants of cells genetically modified to express neurotrophin-3 rescue axotomized Clarke's nucleus neurons after spinal cord injury. Exp. Neurol. Submitted.

Himes BT, Tessler A (1989) Death of some dorsal root ganglion neurons and plasticity of others following sciatic nerve section in adult and neonatal rats. J. Comp. Neurol. 284:215-230.

Hockenbery DM, Oltvai ZN, Yin XM, Milliman CL, Korsmeyer SJ (1993) Bcl-2 functions in an antioxidant pathway to prevent apoptosis. Cell 75:241-251.

Holtzman DM, Deshmukh M (1997) Caspases: a treatment target for neurodegenerative disease? Nature Med. 3:954-955.

Huxlin KR, Carr R, Schulz M, Sefton AJ, Bennett MR (1995a) Trophic effect of collicular proteoglycan on neonatal rat retinal ganglion cells in situ. Brain Res. Dev. Brain Res. 84:77-88.

Huxlin KR, Dreher B, Schulz M, Sefton AJ, Bennett MR (1995b) Effect of collicular proteoglycan on the survival of adult rat retinal ganglion cells following axotomy. Eur. J. Neurosci. 7:96-107.

Isenmann S, Klocker N, Gravel C, Bahr M (1998) Protection of axotomized retinal ganglion cells by adenovirally delivered BDNF in vivo. Eur. J. Neurosci. 10:2751-2756.

Isenmann S, Wahl C, Krajewski S, Reed JC, Bahr M (1997) Up-regulation of bax protein in degenerating retinal ganglion cells precedes apoptotic cell death after optic nerve lesion in the rat. Eur. J. Neurosci. 9:1763-1772.

Jakeman LB, Reier PJ (1991) Axonal projections between fetal spinal cord transplants and the adult rat spinal cord: a neuroanatomical tracing study of local interactions. J. Comp. Neurol. 307:311-334.

Katoh K, Ikata T, Katoh S, Hamada Y, Nakauchi K, Sano T, Niwa M (1996) Induction and its spread of apoptosis in rat spinal cord after mechanical trauma. Neuroscience Lett. 216:9-12.

Kermer P, Klocker N, Labes M, Bahr M (1998) Inhibition of CPP32-like proteases rescues axotomized retinal ganglion cells from secondary cell death in vivo. J. Neurosci. 18:4656-4662.

Kinloch RA, Treherne JM, Furness LM, Hajimohamadreza I (1999) The pharmacology of apoptosis. Trends Pharmacol. Sci. 20:35-42.

Klein RL, Muir D, King MA, Peel AL, Zolotukhin S, Moller JC, Kruttgen A, Heymach Jr. JV, Muzyczka N, Meyer EM (1999) Long-term actions of vector-derived nerve growth factor or brain-derived neurotrophic factor on choline acetyltransferase and trk receptor levels in the adult rat basal forebrain. Neuroscience 90:815-821.

Klocker N, Braunling F, Isenmann S, Bahr M (1997) In vivo neurotrophic effects of GDNF on axotomized retinal ganglion cells. Neuroreport 8:3439-3442.

Klocker N, Cellerino A, Bahr M (1998) Free radical scavenging and inhibition of nitric oxide synthase potentiates the neurotrophic effects of brain-derived neurotrophic factor on axotomized retinal ganglion cells In vivo. J. Neurosci. 18:1038-1046.

Knusel B, Beck KD, Winslow JW, Rosenthal A, Burton LE, Widmer HR, Nikolics K, Hefti F (1992) Brain-derived neurotrophic factor administration protects basal forebrain cholinergic but not nigral dopaminergic neurons from degenerative changes after axotomy in the adult rat brain. J. Neurosci. 12:4391-4402.

Kobayashi NR, Bedared AM, Tetzlaff W (1995) BDNF reverses the atrophy of chronically injured rat rubrospinal neurons after cervical (C3) axotomy. Soc. Neurosci. Abst. 21 (2):1056.

Kobayashi NR, Fan D-P, Giehl KM, Bedard AM, Wiegand SJ, Tetzlaff W (1997) BDNF and NT-4/5 prevent atrophy of rat rubrospinal neurons after cervical axotomy, stimulate GAP-43 and Tα1-tubulin mRNA expression, and promote axonal regeneration. J. Neurosci. 17:9583-9595.

Kokaia Z, Bengzon J, Metsis M, Kokaia M, Persson H, Lindvall O (1993) Coexpression of neurotrophins and their receptors in neurons of the CNS. Proc. Natl. Acad. Sci. USA 90:6711-6715.

Krajewski S, Mai JK, Krajewska M, Sikorska M, Mossakowski MJ, Reed JC (1995) Upregulation of bax protein levels in neurons following cerebral ischemia. J. Neurosci. 15:6364-6376.

Kromer L (1987) Nerve growth factor treatment after brain injury prevents neuronal death. Science 235:214-216.

Li L, Prevette D, Oppenheim RW, Milligan CE (1998) Involvement of specific caspases in motoneuron cell death in vivo and in vitro following trophic factor deprivation. Mol. Cell. Neurosci. 12:157-167.

Lindholm D (1994) Role of neurotrophins in preventing glutamate induced neuronal cell death. J. Neurol. 242:S16-18.

Liu Y, Himes BT, Murray M, Tessler A, Fischer I (1999a) Grafts of BDNF-producing fibroblasts that promote regeneration of axotomized rubrospinal neurons also rescue most neurons from retrograde death and prevent their atrophy. J. Comp. Neurol. submitted.

Liu Y, Kim D, Himes BT, Chow S, Murray M, Tessler A, Fischer I (1999b) Transplants of fibroblasts genetically modified to express BDNF promote regeneration of adult rat rubrospinal axons. J. Neurosci. 19:4370-4387.

Lucidi-Phillipi CA, Clary DO, Reichardt LF, Gage FH (1996) TrkA activation is sufficient to rescue axotomized cholinergic neurons. Neuron 16:653-663.

Maas JW, Horstmann S, Borasio GD, Anneser JMH, Shooter EM, Kahle PJ (1998) Apoptosis of central and peripheral neurons can be prevented with cyclin-dependent kinase mitogen-activated protein kinase inhibitors. J. Neurochem. 70:1401-1410.

Maffei L, Carmignoto G, Perry VH, Candec P, Ferrari G (1990) Schwann cells promote the survival of rat retinal ganglion cells after optic nerve section. Proc. Natl. Acad. Sci. USA 87:1855-1859.

Maisonpierre PC, Belluscio L, Friedman B, Alderson RF, Wiegand SJ, Furth ME, Lindsay RM, Yancopoulos GD (1990) NT-3, BDNF, and NGF in the developing rat nervous system: Parallel as well as reciprocal patterns of expression. Neuron 5:501-509.

Mansour-Robaey S, Clarke DB, Wang Y-C, Bray GM, Aguayo AJ (1994) Effects of ocular injury and administration of brain-derived neurotrophic factor on survival and regrowth of axotomized retinal ganglion cells. Proc. Natl. Acad. Sci. USA 91:1632-1636.

Martin LJ, Al-Abdulla NA, Brambrink AM, Kirsch JR, Sieber FE, Portera-Cailliau C (1998) Neurodegeneration in excitotoxicity, global cerebral ischemia, and target deprivation: A perspective on the contributions of apoptosis and necrosis. Brain Res. Bull. 46:281-309.

Martinou JC, Dubois-Dauphin M, Staple JK, Rodriguez I, Frankowski H, Missotten M, Albertini P, Talabot D, Catsicas S, Pietra C, et al. (1994) Overexpression of BCL-2 in transgenic mice protects neurons from naturally occurring cell death and experimental ischemia. Neuron 13:1017-1030.

Matheson CR, Wang J, Collins FD, Yan Q (1997) Long-term survival effects of GDNF on neonatal rat facial motoneurons after axotomy. Neuroreport 8:1739-1742.

McConkey DJ (1998) Biochemical determinants of apoptosis and necrosis. Toxicol. Lett. 99:157-168.

Merline M, Kalil K (1990) Cell death of corticospinal neurons is induced by axotomy before but not after innervation of spinal targets. J. Comp. Neurol. 296:506-516.

Mey J, Thanos S (1993) Intravitreal injections of neurotrophic factors support the survival of axotomized retinal ganglion cells in adult rats in vivo. Brain Res. 602:304-317.

Michaelidis TM, Sendtner M, Cooper JD, Airaksinen MS, Holtmann B, Meyer M, Thoenen H (1996) Inactivation of bcl-2 results in progressive degeneration of motoneurons, sympathetic and sensory neurons during early postnatal development. Neuron 17:75-89.

Milligan CE, Prevette D, Yaginuma H, Homma S, Cardwell C, Fritz LC, Tomaselli KJ, Oppenheim RW, Schwartz LM (1995) Peptide inhibitors of the ICE protease family arrest programmed cell death of motoneurons in vivo and in vitro. Neuron 15:385-393.

Mori F, Himes BT, Kowada M, Murray M, Tessler A (1997) Fetal spinal cord transplants rescue some axotomized rubrospinal neurons from retrograde cell death in adult rats. Exp. Neurol. 143:45-60.

Morse JK, Wiegand SJ, Anderson K, You Y, Cai N, Carnahan J, Miller J, DiStefano PS, Altar CA, Lindsay RM, Alderson RF (1993) Brain-derived neurotrophic factor (BDNF) prevents the degeneration of medial septal cholinergic neurons following fimbria transection. J. Neurosci. 13:4146-4156.

Naumann T, Kermer P, Seydewitz V, Ortmann R, D'Amato F, Frotscher M (1994) Is there a long-lasting effect of a short-term nerve growth factor application on axotomized rat septohippocampal neurons? Neurosci. Letts. 173:213-215.

Naumann T, Peterson GM, Frotscher M (1992) Fine structure of rat septohippocampal neurons: II. A time course analysis following axotomy. J. Comp. Neurol. 325:219-242.

O'Brien MK, Oppenheim RW (1990) Development and survival of thoracic motorneurons and hindlimb musculature following transplantation of the thoracic neural tube to the lumbar region in the chick embryo: Anatomical aspects. J. Neurobiol. 21(2):313-340.

Parsadanian AS, Cheng Y, Keller-Peck CR, Holtzman DM, Snider WD (1998) Bcl-x(L) is an antiapoptotic regulator for postnatal CNS neurons. J. Neurosci. 18:1009-1019.

Peinado-Ramon P, Salvador M, Villegas-Perez MP, Vidal-Sanz M (1996) Effects of axotomy and intraocular administration of NT-4, NT-3, and brain-derived neurotrophic factor on the survival of adult rat retinal ganglion cells. Invest. Ophthalmol. Vis. Sci. 37:489-500.

Pelleymounter MA, Cullen MJ, Wellman CL (1995) Characteristics of BDNF-induced weight loss. Exp. Neurol. 131:229-238.

Penn RD, Kroin JS, York MM, Cedarbaum JM (1997) Intrathecal ciliary neurotrophic factor delivery for treatment of amyotrophic lateral sclerosis (phase I trial). Neurosurgery 40:94-100.

Peter ME, Krammer PH (1998) Mechanisms of CD95 (APO-1/Fas)-mediated apoptosis. Curr. Opin. Immunol. 10:545-551.

Peterson GM, Williams LR, Varon S, Gage FH (1987) Loss of GABAergic neurons in medial septum after fimbria-fornix transection. Neurosci. Lett. 76:140-144.

Pettman B, Henderson CE (1998) Neuronal cell death. Neuron 20:633-647.

Pinon LGP, Robinson M, Davies AM (1995) High specificity of neurotrophins in the embryonic chicken trigeminal system. Eur. J. Neurosci. 7:2397-2402.

Polyak K, Xia Y, Zweier JL, Kinzler KW, Vogelstein B (1997) A model for p53-induced apoptosis. Nature 389:300-305.

Prendergast J, Stelzner DJ (1976) Changes in the magnocellular portion of the red nucleus following thoracic hemisection in the neonatal and adult rat. J. Comp. Neurol. 166:163-172.

Pruitt JN, 2nd, Feringa ER, McBride RL (1988) Corticospinal axons persist in cervical and high thoracic regions 10 weeks after a T-9 spinal cord transection. Neurology 38:946-950.

Raff MC, Barres BA, Burne JF, Coles HS, Ishizaki Y, Jacobson MD (1993) Programmed cell death and the control of cell survival: lessons from the nervous system. Science 262:695-700.

Rossiter JP, Riopelle RJ, Bisby MA (1996) Axotomy-induced apoptotic cell death of neonatal rat facial motoneurons: time course analysis and relation to NADPH-diaphorase activity. Exp. Neurol. 138:33-44.

Sanner CA, Cunningham TJ, Goldberger ME (1994) NMDA receptor blockade rescues Clarke's and red nucleus neurons after spinal hemisection. J. Neurosci. 14:6472-6480.

Sanner CA, Murray M, Goldberger ME (1993) Removal of dorsal root afferents prevents retrograde death of Clarke's nucleus neurons in the cat. Exp. Neurol. 123:81-90.

Sawai H, Clarke DB, Kittlerova P, Bray GM, Aguayo AJ (1996) Brain-derived neurotrophic factor and neurotrophin-4/5 stimulate growth of axonal branches from regenerating retinal ganglion cells. J. Neurosci. 16:3887-3894.

Schmalbruch H, Rosenthal A (1995) Neurotrophin 4/5 postpones the death of injured spinal motoneurons in newborn rats. Brain Res. 700:254-260.

Sei Y, Fossom L, Goping G, Skolnick P, Basile AS (1998) Quinolinic acid protects rat cerebellar granule cells from glutamate-induced apoptosis. Neurosci. Lett. 241:180-184.

Sendtner M, Holtmann B, Kolbeck R, Thoenen H, Barde Y-A (1992) Brain-derived neurotrophic factor prevents the death of motoneurons in newborn rats after nerve section. Nature 360:757-759.

Shepherd GM (1979) In: The synaptic organization of the brain, 2 Edition, p 188. New York: Oxford University Press.

Shibata M, Murray M, Tessler A, Ljubetic C, Saavedra RA. 2000. Single injections of a DNA plasmid that contains the human bcl-2 gene prevent loss and atrophy of distinct neuronal populations after spinal cord injury in adult rats. Exp. Neurol. (submitted).

Shibayama M, Hattori S, Himes BT, Murray M, Tessler A (1998a) Neurotrophin-3 prevents death of axotomized Clarke's nucleus neurons in adult rat. J. Comp. Neurol. 390:102-111.

Shibayama M, Matsui N, Himes BT, Murray M, Tessler A (1998b) Critical interval for rescue of axotomized neurons by transplants. Neuroreport 9:11-14.

Sievers J, Hausmann B, Unsicker K, Berry M (1987) Fibroblast growth factors promote the survival of adult rat retinal ganglion cells after transection of the optic nerve. Neurosci. Letts. 76:157-162.

Sofroniew MV, Cooper JD, Svendsen CN, Crossman P, Ip NY, Lindsay RM, Zafra F, Lindholm D (1993) Atrophy but not death of adult septal cholinergic neurons after ablation of target capacity to produce mRNAs for NGF, BDNF, and NT3. J. Neurosci. 13:5263-5276.

Sofroniew MV, Galletly NP, Isacson O, Svendsen CN (1990) Survival of adult basal forebrain cholinergic neurons after loss of target neurons. Science 247:338-342.

Sterling P (1990) Retina. In: The synaptic organization of the brain, 3 Edition (Shepherd GM, ed.), pp. 170-188. New York: Oxford University Press.

Stout AK, Raphael HM, Kanterewicz BI, Klann E, Reynolds IJ (1998) Glutamate-induced neuron death requires mitochondrial calcium uptake. Nat. Neurosci. 1:366-373.

Takahashi K, Schwarz E, Ljubetic C, Murray M, Tessler A, Saavedra R (1999) DNA plasmid that codes for human Bcl-2 gene preserves axotomized Clarke's nucleus neurons and reduces atrophy after spinal cord hemisection in adult rats. J. Comp. Neurol. 404:159-171.

Tetzlaff W, Alexander SW, Miller FD, Bisby MA (1991) Response of facial and rubrospinal neurons to axotomy: changes in mRNA expression for cytoskeletal proteins and GAP-43. J. Neurosci. 11:2528-2544.

Thornberry NA, Lazebnik Y (1998) Caspases: enemies within. Science 281:1312-1316.

Tuszynski MH, Gage FH (1995) Bridging grafts and transient nerve growth factor infusions promote long-term central nervous system neuronal rescue and partial functional recovery. Proc. Natl. Acad. Sci. USA 92:4621-4625.

Tuszynski MH, U HS, Amaral DG, Gage FH (1990) Nerve growth factor infusion in the primate brain reduces lesion-induced cholinergic neuronal degeneration. J. Neurosci. 10:3604-3514.

Verge VMK, Riopelle RJ, Richardson PM (1989) Nerve growth factor receptors on normal and injured sensory neurons. J. Neurosci. 9:914-922.

Villa P, Kaufmann SH, Earnshaw WC (1997) Caspases and caspase inhibitors. Trends Biochem. Sci. 22:388-393.

Villegas-Perez M-P, Vidal-Sanz M, Rasminsky M, Bray GM, Aguayo AG (1992) Rapid and protracted phases of retinal ganglion cell loss follow axotomy in the optic nerve of adult rats. J. Neurobiol. 24:23-36.

von Bartheld CS, Kinoshita Y, Prevette D, Yin Q-W, Oppenheim RW, Bothwell M (1994) Positive and negative effects of neurotrophins on the isthmo-optic nucleus in chick embryos. Neuron 12:639-654.

Wen TC, Tanaka J, Peng H, Desaki J, Matsuda S, Maeda N, Fujita H, Sato K, Sakanaka M (1998) Interleukin 3 prevents delayed neuronal death in the hippocampal CA1 field. J. Exp. Med. 188:635-649.

Williams LR, Varon S, Peterson GM, Wictorin K, Fischer W, Bjorklund A, Gage FH (1986) Continuous infusion of nerve growth factor prevents basal forebrain neuronal death after fimbria fornix transection. Proc. Natl. Acad. Sci. USA 83:9231-9235.

Wong B, Park CG, Choi Y (1997) Identifying the molecular control of T-cell death; on the hunt for killer genes. Semin. Immunol. 9:7-16.

Wyllie AH, Kerr JFR, Currie AR (1980) Cell death: the significance of apoptosis. Int. Rev. Cytol. 68:251-306.

Yan Q, Matheson C, Sun J, Radeke MJ, Feinstein SC, Miller JA (1994) Distribution of intracerebral ventricularly administered neurotrophins in rat brain and its correlation with trk receptor expression. Exp. Neurol. 127:23-36.

Yan Q, Wang J, Matheson CR, Urich JL (1999) Glial cell line-derived neurotrophic factor (GDNF) promotes the survival of axotomized retinal ganglion cells in adult rats: comparison to and combination with brain-derived neurotrophic factor (BDNF). J. Neurobiol. 38:382-390.

Ye JH, Houle JD (1997) Treatment of the chronically injured spinal cord with neurotrophic factors can promote axonal regeneration from supraspinal neurons. Exp. Neurol. 143:70-81.

Yong C, Arnold AM, Zoubine MN, Citron BA, Watanabe I, Berman NEJ, Festoff BW (1998) Apoptosis in cell compartments of rat spinal cord after severe contusion injury. J. Neurotrauma 15:459-472.

Zamzami N, Hirsch T, Dallaporta B, Petit PX, Kroemer G (1997) Mitochondrial implication in accidental and programmed cell death: apoptosis and necrosis. J. Bioenerg. Biomembr. 29:185-193.

Zhou L, Connors T, Chen DF, Murray M, Tessler A, Kambin P, Saavedra RA (1999) Red nucleus neurons of Bcl-2 over-expressing mice are protected from cell death induced by axotomy. NeuroReport 10:3417-3421.

20

The Use of Peripheral Nerve Transplants to Enhance Axonal Regeneration in CNS Neurons

Kwok-Fai So and Henry K. Yip
The University of Hong Kong, Hong Kong, China

I. INTRODUCTION

The marked difference between the regenerative ability of neurons in the mammalian peripheral and central nervous systems has fascinated neuroscientists for many years. The Nobel Laureate, Ramon y Cajal, has beautifully summarized this aspect of the work in his monumental book on Degeneration and Regeneration of the Nervous System (DeFelipe and Jones, 1991). In fact, Cajal and his student, Tello, recognized that this critical difference in axonal regeneration is due to the physical or chemical environment in which the axon is located and they attempted to use a peripheral nerve to enhance regeneration of the optic nerves in adult rabbits (DeFelipe and Jones, 1991). Cajal wrote "*This is a new indication of what we have repeatedly stated, namely, that the irregularity of the central paths is not a fatal result of the imminent organization of the axonic protoplasm, but an accidental condition, due to the conditions of the neuroglial environment, in which, since the embryonic period, all excitatory activity of neuronal trophism and neurocladism has definitely ceased.*" (DeFelipe and Jones, 1991, p. 589). In spite of this insightful observation, the use of peripheral nerve transplants to enhance axonal regeneration of CNS neurons did not take off until the publication of a series of elegant studies conducted by Aguayo and his colleagues in the '80s (Richardson et al., 1980; David and Aguayo, 1981; Benfey and Aguayo, 1982; So and Aguayo, 1985). Using the most modern axonal tracing technique available at that time, Aguayo and colleagues were able to convince the scientific community that many types of CNS neurons can indeed regenerate their axons if a favorable environment (peripheral nerve) is provided.

Many research groups have since used the peripheral nerve transplantation paradigm to enhance axonal regeneration of CNS neurons from the spinal cord and brainstem (Richardson et al., 1980; David and Aguayo, 1981; Wu et al., 1994; Houle et al., 1994; Cheng et al., 1996; Jin, 1998), thalamus and cortex (Benfey and Aguayo, 1982; Xiao et al., 1989; Morrow et al., 1993), and retina or optic nerve (So and Aguayo 1985; Berry et al., 1986; Politis and Spencer, 1986; Vidal-Sanz et al., 1987; Thanos, 1988; Watanabe et al., 1991; Bähr et al., 1992; Lau et al., 1994; Robinson, 1994; Carter and Jhaveri, 1997). Many regeneration studies have been carried out using the retina and optic nerve as a model system because the somata and myelinated axons of retinal ganglion cells (RGCs) can be manipulated separately and the retina can be studied as a flat-mounted preparation which facilitates the analysis of the RGCs in the entire retina. Thus, in this chapter, we will concentrate on reviewing experiments that have used peripheral nerve transplants to enhance axonal regeneration of RGCs.

We will focus on how peripheral nerve is used: 1) to overcome the unfavorable extrinsic CNS environment, 2) as a source of trophic factors, 3) to upregulate the intrinsic growth potential of the axotomized neurons (since recent studies suggest that the lack of intrinsic growth potential in neurons is also an important factor contributing to the failure of CNS regeneration Chen et al., 1995; So and Yip, 1998) and 4) to enhance neuronal survival. The chapter is divided into three main sections. First, we will describe experiments using peripheral nerve transplants, second, studies using Schwann cells or fibroblast isolated from peripheral nerve, and third the work on using trophic factors which are known to be present in the peripheral nerve graft. In each case we will discuss how these manipulations effect the survival and axonal regeneration of RGCs.

II. THE USE OF PERIPHERAL NERVE TO ENHANCE THE SURVIVAL AND REGENERATION OF RGCS

The peripheral nerve used for transplantation experiments is normally taken from the peroneal or tibial branch of the sciatic nerve in the hind limb. The entire sciatic nerve is used in some studies. Up to 3 cm of the peroneal branch of the sciatic nerve can be dissected from rodents for transplantation. To provide a favorable environment for axonal regeneration of RGCs, the peripheral nerve can be attached to the retina (So and Aguayo, 1985) or to the transected optic nerve (Berry et al., 1986; Politis and Spencer, 1986; Vidal-Sanz et al., 1987; Watanabe et al., 1991). The growth potential of RGCs is enhanced by transplanting a short segment (2 mm) of peripheral nerve into the vitreous of the eye (Cho and So, 1992). The peripheral nerve is a good conduit for regeneration of axons from CNS neurons for the following reasons: 1) The degenerating myelin is removed rapidly so the inhibitory molecules presented on the peripheral myelin such as myelin associated glycoprotein (MAG) (McKerracher et al., 1994; Mukhopadhyay et al., 1994; this volume, Chapter by David and McKerracher) is also removed. 2) The inhibitory molecules found in CNS myelin (this volume, Chapter by Schwab) are not present in the peripheral nerve. 3) Schwann cells have been shown to divide (Bradley and Asbury, 1970) and form columns of cells within the basal lamina tubes (Bungner bands) following injury of the nerve. Schwann cells and fibroblasts are known to secrete various types of trophic factors and some of them may be important for enhancing the survival or axonal regeneration of RGCs. 4) Basement membranes of the Schwann cell tubes are known to possess many adhesion molecules such as L1, J1, intergins and laminin which enhance axonal growth (Daniloff et al., 1986; Kuffler, 1986; Martini et al., 1990; Mirsky and Jessen, 1990; Guénard et al., 1993).

A. Transplantation of a peripheral nerve to the optic nerve can promote survival

Transplanting a peripheral nerve to the optic nerve can promote the survival of axotomized RGCs and prevent axonal degeneration of the optic fibers inside the retina for 6 and 9 months after optic nerve injury (Villegas-Perez et al., 1988). A precrushed graft will further enhance the survival of RGCs (Bähr et al., 1992). Since Schwann cells divide in the distal portion of the peripheral nerve following injury, the enhancement of the precrushed graft may be due to an increase in the number of Schwann cells which can secrete more trophic factors to influence the survival of RGCs.

Transplants of the peripheral nerve into the retina (Turner et al., 1987) can also delay the death of axotomized RGCs. However, our recent study using a retrograde labeling technique by applying FluoroGold in the optic nerve showed that transplantation of a 2 mm segment of peripheral nerve into the vitreous does not prevent the death of axotomized RGCs (Cho et al., 1997), but can induce sprouting of some of the damaged RGCs (Cho and So, 1992; Lei et al., 1995). Interestingly, intravitreal transplant of a short segment of optic nerve is able to reduce the death of RGCs up to 1 week after axotomy and transplantation (Cho et al., 1997).

B. Transplantation of a peripheral nerve to the optic nerve can promote regeneration

After demonstrating the ability of CNS neurons in adult rats to regenerate axons into peripheral nerve graft, Richardson was not able to show the similar ability in RGCs by transplanting peripheral nerve to the intracranial portion of the optic nerve (Richardson et al., 1982). The result was puzzling at that time but we now have good reason to suspect that this is because the peripheral nerve was transplanted too far away from the optic disc. Distance of grafting in the optic nerve is an important factor in controlling the number of RGCs that regenerate axons into the graft although the reason for this is still not completely clear (see below).

The first convincing study to show that axotomized RGCs in adult rats can regenerate axons into a peripheral nerve was conducted by So and Aguayo (1985). Inspired by the findings that most of the neurons regenerating axons into the peripheral nerve were concentrated around the transplantation site (David and Aguayo, 1981), the desheathed end of the peripheral nerve graft was inserted directly into the retina so that the peripheral nerve contacted the damaged axons of RGCs (Fig. 1A). The distal end of the graft was blind-ended and laid subcutaneously over the skull. One month later, different sizes of RGCs were labeled with horseradish peroxidase applied to the stump of the graft (So and Aguayo, 1985). The RGCs were distributed within pie-shaped areas peripheral to the sites of grafting and their number was greater for grafts near the optic disc than for those in the outer portions of the retina. Axotomy appears to be a prerequisite to induce RGCs to regrow axons into the graft since axonal growth does not occur from uninjured RGCs which still retain their axons in the optic nerve (So and Aguayo, 1985, So et al., 1986).

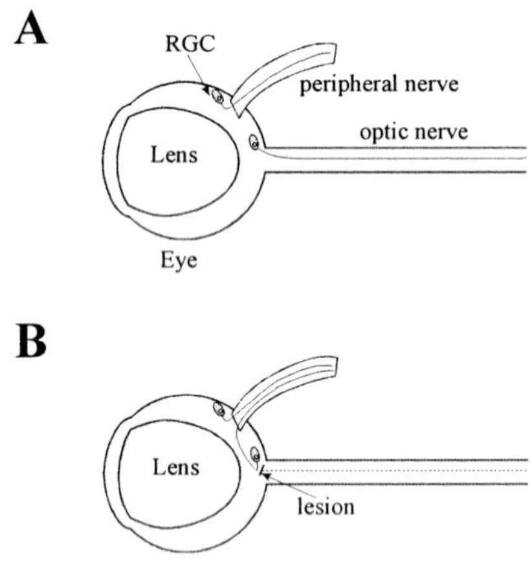

Figure 1 A. Schematic diagram illustrating the growth of an axon from a representative axotomized RGC (retinal ganglion cell) into the peripheral nerve transplanted into the eye. Note that the undamaged RGC with an axon in the optic nerve does not send an axon into the graft. Only one RGC is drawn to made the point. B. In addition to the transplantation of a peripheral nerve into the eye, a lesion made between the peripheral nerve graft and the optic disc transects the axons of another population of RGCs which will also send an axon into the graft (see text for details).

The graft in the retina seems to be able to actively attract damaged axons to grow into the graft. By studying the responses of RGCs with axons transected at locations of 1.5 or 3 mm from the peripheral nerve transplantation site (So et al., 1986), we have shown that a population of RGCs situated between the graft and the optic disc can also send axons into the graft if the lesion is placed at 1.5 mm from the site of grafting. No effect is shown if the lesion is placed 3 mm away suggesting that this is a distance-dependent phenomenon (Fig. 1B). It is likely that Schwann cells and fibroblasts in the peripheral nerve graft secrete diffusible factors to attract sprouts from the damaged axons. This interpretation is supported by our results of co-culturing a segment of peripheral nerve and a strip of retina from adult hamsters. The direction of growth of the regenerating axons from the RGCs is affected by the location of the peripheral nerve suggesting a tropic effect of the nerve (Liu and So, 1990).

The number of regenerating RGCs is greatly increased if the peripheral nerve is transplanted to the orbital portion of the optic nerve because more damaged axons are in contact with the peripheral nerve graft (Fig. 2A). This has been shown in the rat (Berry et al., 1986, Politis and Spencer, 1986; Vidal-Sanz et al., 1987; Thanos et al., 1993), hamster (Cho and So, 1992; Ng et al., 1995), and cat (Watanabe et al., 1991). The percentage of regenerating RGCs is normally not more than 10% of the total population of RGCs and their numbers decrease over time.

Different types of RGCs can regenerate axons along the peripheral nerve graft (So and Aguayo, 1985; Watanada et al., 1993; Thanos and Mey, 1995). Using the peripheral nerve to connect the optic nerve with target cells in the pretectum or the superior colliculus results in a preferential survival of different groups of regenerating RGCs (Thanos and Mey, 1995). Implantation of the distal stump into the pretectum leads to selective survival of large RGCs whereas implantation into the superior colliculus results in survival of many small RGCs. It has been shown that retinal axons enter the peripheral nerve graft at about 4 days after transplantation (Cho and So, 1987; Berry et al., 1988) and the axons regenerate along the basement membrane of the Schwann cells (Berry et al., 1988) at a maximal rate of 1 to 2 mm/day (Trecarten et al., 1986; Cho and So, 1987). Tight junctions have been observed between regenerating RGC axons and Schwann cells (Dezawa and Nagano, 1993). Peripheral nerve grafts with intact basement membrane but lacking viable Schwann cells do not support axonal regeneration (Berry et al., 1988). Using the electron microscope to examine the interface between the proximal stump of the transected optic nerve and a peripheral nerve graft with or without viable Schwann cells, RGC axons growing out from the proximal optic nerve stump are shown to be accompanied by processes of astrocytes, only in grafts containing viable Schwann cell (Hall and Berry, 1989; Dewaza et al., 1998). In those experiments using viable peripheral nerve grafts Schwann cells are identified in the junctional zone suggesting that they might play an active role in guiding the RGC axons into the peripheral nerve graft (Hall and Berry, 1989). Using morphometric technique at the electron microscopic level

(Chau et al., 1992) we have shown that there is an active interaction of the regenerated RGC axons and Schwann cells which provide the new growth environment for the optic fibers. Thus, the mean myelinated axon diameter of regenerated RGC axons is significantly greater than that of retinal axons in the intact optic nerve. In addition, the myelination behavior of Schwann cells is shown to be influenced by the regenerating RGC axons.

During normal development in hamsters, RGCs exhibit spines on their dendrites (Lau et al., 1992) which are retracted in adults. A similar phenomenon is observed in some of the RGCs regenerating axons into a peripheral nerve graft (Lau et al., 1991). The dendrites of these cells retract over time (Thanos, 1988; Lau et al., 1991) and administration of macrophage inhibitory factor (MIF) is able to prevent some of the retraction (Thanos and Mey, 1995) so that the dendrites of the small cells (RII-like RGCs) overlap uniformly and completely cover the retinal surface. MIF seems to be able to decrease the microglial reaction in the retina after axotomy of the optic nerve and with the transplantation of a peripheral nerve is able to enhance the number of RGCs regeneratinng axons into the graft. Irradiation of the eye with a low level laser following axotomy also can delay RGC death and promote the axonal regeneration of RGCs (Leung et al., 1996; Yip et al., 1999). The laser effect may also be related to a decrease in microglial reaction. (Leung et al., 1997).

Aguayo and colleagues (Vidal-Sanz et al., 1987; Carter et al., 1989) have demonstrated normal appearing synaptic contacts made by retinal axons growing in peripheral nerve implants, into the superior colliculus. These synapses remain in the superior colliculus for a long period of time (Vidal-Sanz et al., 1991) and the number of synaptic contacts per axon seems to be preserved although the terminal field is compressed (Carter et al., 1991). Recording from the axons that had regenerated in the peripheral nerve showed nearly normal receptive visual fields (Keirstead et al., 1985; Diao et al., 1987). Also, after inserting the peripheral nerve into the superior colliculus, postsynaptic potentials with normal visual fields could be recorded from neurons in the superior colliculus (Keirstead et al., 1989; Sauve et al., 1995). Similar experiment in the cat further illustrated that the number of regenerating ON-center cells dominates over those of OFF-center cells (Watanabe and Fukuda, 1997). Normal appearing synaptic contacts have also been observed in the dorsal lateral geniculate nucleus after connecting the optic nerve to the thalamus with a peripheral nerve (Carter and Jhaveri, 1997). Whether normal postsynaptic potentials can be recorded in the reconstructed retinogeniculate connections remains to be investigated.

Behavioral recovery of some visual functions has been shown in several studies. The pupillary light reflex is restored in animals with RGC axons connected to the pretectum (Thanos, 1992; Whiteley et al., 1998). Connecting the RGC axons to the superior colliculus in rats can restore the light-dark discrimination behavior (Sasaki et al., 1993) and behavioral arousal (Sasaki et al., 1996). Simple pattern discrimination behavior seems to be restored if RGCs are guided into the optic tract with a peripheral nerve graft (Thanos, 1997). These studies provide a good basis for further functional studies of regenerated RGC axons.

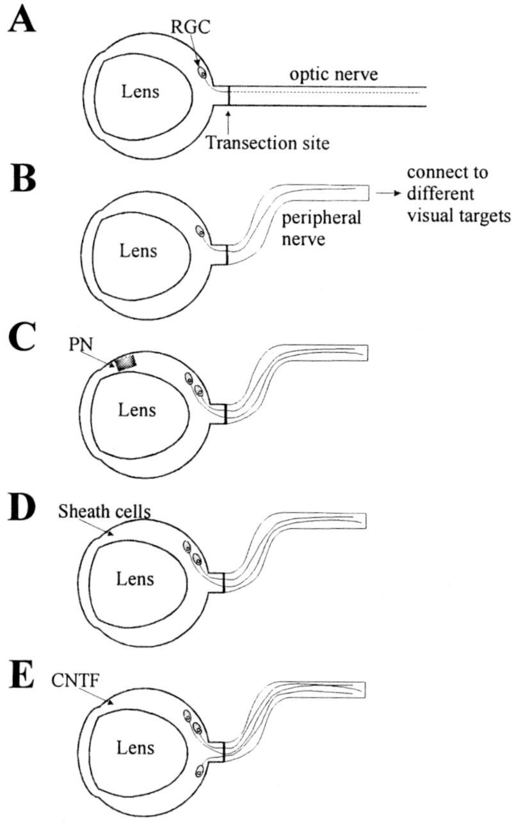

Figure 2 A. Transection of the optic nerve will lead to degeneration of the portion of the axon distal to the site of damage. No regeneration of axons from the RGCs is observed. Only one RGC is drawn to illustrate the point.
B. Axotomized RGCs will regenerate axons into a peripheral nerve graft attached to the ocular stump of the transected optic nerve. The distal end of the peripheral nerve can be connected to different visual targets in the brain.
C. The additional transplantation of a small segment of peripheral nerve into the eye will double the number of RGCs to regenerate axons into the attached peripheral nerve graft.
D. Injection of sheath cells into the vitreous will result in the same enhancement of regeneration of RGC axons into the attached peripheral nerve graft.
E. Intravitreal injection of CNTF (ciliary neurotrophic factor) but not other trophic factors will markedly increase the number of RGCs to regenerate axons into the attached peripheral nerve graft.

Unlike lower vertebrates (Grafstein, 1991; this volume, Foreword by Grafstein and Part I), a prior lesion (conditioning lesion) of the optic nerve in rats cannot induce regeneration of the RGC axons in the optic nerve (Kiernam, 1985) nor does it enhance the number of RGC axons regenerating into a peripheral nerve graft (You et al., 1996) or increase the maximal rate of axonal regeneration (Cho and So, 1987) in hamsters, although it can shorten the delay time for growth into a peripheral nerve graft in hamsters and rats (Cho and So, 1987; Thanos and Vanselow, 1989). A peripheral nerve which has been damaged about 1 week before grafting (predegenerated graft) has been shown to increase the number of regenerating RGCs in some (Bähr et al., 1992; You et al.,1998) but not other studies (Thanos and Mey, 1995; You et al., 1996).

Distance of axotomy from RGC soma plays an important role in determining the ability of RGCs to regenerate axons into the peripheral nerve graft. Grafting of the peripheral nerve into the eye (So and Aguayo, 1985) or about 2 mm from the optic disc (Berry et al., 1986; Vidal-Sanz et al., 1987) leads to regeneration of RGC axons. But grafting to the optic nerve intracranially (about 7 mm from the optic disc) (Richarson et al., 1982; Lau et al., 1994) or to the cut optic tract (Stevenson et al., 1985) results in little, if any, regeneration of RGC axons into the graft. Our recent study shows that the maximal number of regenerating RGCs is obtained if the peripheral nerve is grafted 0.5 mm from the optic disc (You et al., 1997). This approach does not damage the vascular supply to the eye since the central retinal artery enters the optic nerve at about 0.2 mm from the optic disc. Grafting the peripheral nerve to the optic nerve intraorbitally at 0.5, 1, 1.5, 2, 2.5 and 3 mm from the optic disc results in a proportional and dramatic drop of the ability of the RGCs to regenerate axons into the graft (You et al., 1997). The reason for this is not clear but it might be related to the accumulative inhibitory effect of the non-neuronal cells in the optic nerve including astrocytes (Bähr et al., 1995), oligodendrocytes and CNS myelin (Schwab et al., 1993). The variation in the number of regenerating RGCs reported in different studies may partly be due to the attachment of the peripheral nerve graft to different sites of the optic nerve. Interestingly, bridging the superior colliculus and the transected optic fibers at the brachium of the superior colliculus with a segment of peripheral nerve results in regeneration of RGC axons into the superior colliculus (Sawai et al., 1996a; So et al., 1996a). The presence of collateral projections of the retinocollicular projections to the thalamus may be one of the reasons why some of the inhibitory effect can be overcome.

III. TRANSPLANTATION OF A PERIPHERAL NERVE INTO THE VITREOUS CAN ACTIVATE THE INTRINSIC GROWTH POTENTIAL OF RGCS

Transplantation of a short segment of peripheral nerve into the vitreous (Fig. 2B) is one way to upregulate the intrinsic growth potential of the RGCs probably because the Schwann cells and fibroblasts in the nerve can secrete different types of tropic factors and adhesion molecules (see below).

Following axotomy of RGCs and transplantation of an intravitreal peripheral nerve, the expression of GAP-43 (Ng et al., 1995) and c-Jun (Cho et al., 1994) of the RGCs is upregulated. A small number of the RGCs also display morphological plasticity by exhibiting axon-like and spine-like processes (Lau et al., 1991; Cho and So, 1992; Lei et al., 1995). The number of axon-like processes presented on each RGC decreases with time and the processes most likely arise from dendrites, then the intraretinal portion of the axons, and lastly from the somata suggesting a hierarchy of sprouting sites (Cho and So, 1992). No axon-like processes are detected in the regenerating RGCs when they are allowed to grow axons into a peripheral nerve graft suggesting that the axon tip is the most favoured site for regenerative sprouting if the environment is appropriate.

A segment of peripheral nerve transplanted into the vitreous can greatly increase the number of RGCs regenerating axons into a peripheral nerve graft (Fig. 2B) following both a proximal (Ng et al., 1995; Lu et al., 1998) or distal axotomy (Lau et al., 1994; So et al., 1996b; Cui et al., 1999). This may be related to the upregulation of the intrinsic growth potential of the RGCs since the expression of growth associated genes including GAP-43 (protein: Ng et al., 1995, mRNA: Chan et al., 1997) and c-jun (Lu et al., 1998) are upregulated in such cells. An intravitreal peripheral nerve graft has also been shown to be able to induce damaged RGC axons to regenerate across a lesion site of a crushed optic nerve (Fig. 3B) and to grow along the optic nerve (Berry et al., 1996; Zeng et al., 1998).

IV. INTRAVITREAL IMPLANTATION OF SHEATH CELLS FROM PERIPHERAL NERVE CAN PROMOTE SURVIVAL AND GROWTH

The effectiveness of the intravitreal peripheral graft in eliciting growth responses and guiding growing axons can be explained by its constituent cells. Attempts to repair the damaged visual pathways may also include the promotion of survival of injured RGCs by grafting with sheath cells.

A. Survival Studies

Schwann cells secrete neurotrophic factors and therefore can enhance the ability of injured RGCs to survive (Maffei et al., 1990). Recently, it was demonstrated that the enhancement of RGC survival by intravitreal implantation of Schwann cells is dose-dependent (Li et al., 1997a). Intravitreally implanted fibroblasts isolated from peripheral nerve could also promote RGC survival after intraorbital transection of the optic nerve (Li et al., 1997a). These results suggest that the effects of peripheral nerve on the survival of axotomized RGCs could be attributed to both Schwann cells and fibroblasts. Both Schwann cells and fibroblasts can produce BDNF, NT-3, NGF, and IL-6 (Acheson et al., 1991; Hayashi 1996; Ohnishi et al., 1996; Reichert et al., 1996). In addition, Schwann cells can also produce CNTF,

GDNF and FGF (Neuberger and De Vires, 1993; Henderson et al., 1994; MacLennan et al., 1994; Watabe et al., 1995; Meisinger et al., 1996) and fibroblasts are known to synthesize cytokine colony stimulating factor (Maysinger et al., 1996). Exogenous administration of growth factors, including BDNF, CNTF, GDNF and FGF promote the survival of axotomized RGCs (Sievers et al., 1987; Mey and Thanos, 1993; Mansour-Robaey et al., 1994; Sawai et al., 1996b). IL-6 and cytokine colony stimulating factor (CSF) could play an important role in the survival and neurite outgrowth of CNS neurons (McCaffery et al., 1984; Maysinger et al., 1996). Although Schwann cells have been suggested to be the main source of trophic support from the peripheral nerve in promoting the survival and regeneration of injured neurons (Berry et al., 1988; Smith and Stevenson, 1988; Maffei et al., 1990; Dezawa and Nagano, 1993), fibroblasts secrete many of these trophic factors, and may contribute to enhancing the survival of axotomized RGCs. Intravitreal implantation of Schwann cells and/or fibroblasts may then provide a better sourve of neurotrophic factors to the eye and thus enhance RGC survival and regeneration. This technique could offer axotomized RGCs with a variety of neurotrophic factors. Evidence shows that neurons may need combinations of growth factors to maintain their physiological functions and to prevent cell death (Nishi, 1994). In this regard, it is interesting that multiple trophic factors promote RGC survival *in vitro* (Meyer-Franke et al., 1995). Furthermore, these injected cells could provide a continuous supply of neurotrophic factors negating concerns about the long-term stability of the desired proteins and the need for repeated injections.

B. Regeneration Studies

The importance of peripheral nerve-derived trophic factors in promoting RGC regeneration is demonstrated by work in which an intravitreal peripheral nerve graft enhances the expression of GAP-43 (Ng et al., 1995; So et al., 1996a) and regeneration of RGCs into a peripheral nerve graft (Lau et al., 1994; Ng et al., 1995). Furthermore, Berry et al. (1996) show that by implanting a piece of predegenerated peripheral nerve in the vitreous, large numbers of optic axons can regenerate several millimeters beyond the crush site. These results indicate that graft-derived trophic factors can act directly on the axotomized RGC bodies to change the intrinsic properties of the cells, including their ability to upregulate the expression of growth-related genes and overcome the inhibitory environment. In agreement with the effect of intravitreal peripheral nerve grafts on RGC regeneration, Schwann cells implanted in the vitreous body of the eye (Fig. 2D) also enhance regeneration of the optic axons either into the distal segment of peripheral nerve graft or directly across a crush site (Fig. 3C) of the optic nerve (Li et al., 1997b). In addition, in Schwann cell-treated retinas, a profusion of RT-97 positive axonal processes is found near the optic disc and at the same time fewer beaded-degenerating axons are detected. These results suggest that intravitreally transplanted Schwann cells could promote axonal regeneration and intraretinal sprouting, and decrease axonal degeneration of injured RGCs. In addition, neurotrophic molecules secreted by peripheral nerve grafts also exert tropic effects on axonal outgrowth both *in vivo* and *in vitro* (Conner and Varon, 1995; Malgrange et al., 1996). Thus it is possible that regenerating axons in the peripheral nerve graft respond to such molecules derived from the graft.

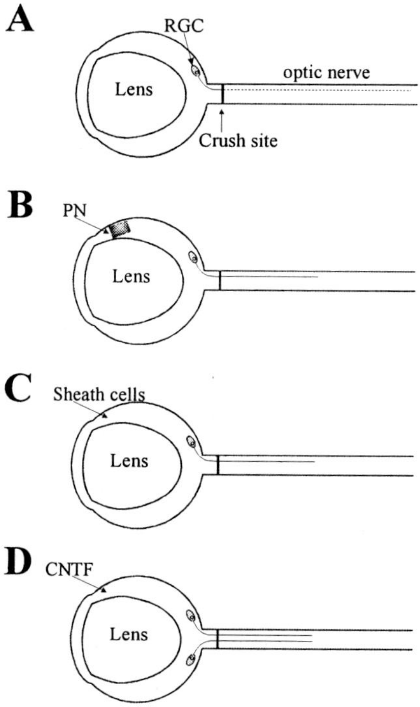

Figure 3 A. A crush of the optic nerve damages all axons of RGCs. No regeneration of axons beyond the crush site is observed. Only one RGC is illustrated.
B. Following transplanation of a small segment of peripheral nerve into the vitreous, a small number of axotomized RGCs can regrow their axons beyond the damage site.
C. Intravitreal transplantation of sheath cells into the vitreous results in the same enhancement of axonal regeneration beyond the crush site.
D. Intravitreal injection of CNTF (ciliary neurotrophic factor) results in additonal enhancement of number of RGCs to regenerate axons beyond the crush site.

V. PERINEURONAL APPLICATION OF NEUROTROPHIC FACTORS CAN HELP RGCS REGENERATE

Given the fact that neurotrophic support from the intravitreal graft arises from the trophic factors synthesized by the cellular constituents (Schwann cells and fibroblasts) of the peripheral nerve, direct delivery of a trophic factor near the cell bodies can increase the availability of neurotrophic support to the axotomized neurons. Increased neurotrophic influence at the cell body may induce an intrinsic, genetic program (Chen et al., 1995; Bonfanti et al., 1996; Cenni et al., 1996; Chen et al., 1997; this volume, chapter by Fernandes) and new protein synthesis (Grafstein and McQuarrie, 1978), resulting in enhanced neuronal survival and axonal elongation, or down-regulation of proteins that are normally expressed on the membrane of CNS axons and respond to the surrounding inhibitory environment.

A. Survival Studies

The use of neurotrophins to prevent or reduce RGC loss after injury has been a subject of intense study. BDNF (Johnson et al., 1986; Rodrigeuz-Tebar et al., 1989; Mey and Thanos, 1993; Cohen et al., 1994; Mansour-Robaey, 1994; Cui et al., 1995; Ma et al., 1998) and NT-4/5 (Cohen et al., 1994; Cui et al., 1995) have been consistently shown to rescue developing and mature RGCs both *in vivo* and *in vitro*. These results are compatible with the localization of trkB, the specific high affinity receptor for BDNF and NT-4/5, in the retina (Berkemeier et al., 1991; Klein et al., 1991). Although the high affinity NGF receptor trkA (Carmingnoto et al., 1991; Ernfors et al., 1992; Zanellato et al., 1993) and high affinity NT-3 receptor trkC (Carmingnoto et al., 1991; Allendoerfer et al., 1994) are expressed in the retina, the effect of NGF and NT-3 on RGC survival is still controversial (Carmingnoto et al., 1989; Lehwalder et al., 1989; Cohen et al., 1994; de la Rossa et al., 1994; Rabacchi et al., 1994; Cui et al., 1995). Recently, we have found that trkA is not expressed in the normal retina but low levels of trkB and trkC can be detected (Cui, et al., 1999). The optic fiber layer in the retina is intensely labeled with trkB, suggesting that trkB is axonally transported (Hendry and Crouch, 1993; Bhattacharyya et al., 1997; Fournier et al., 1997; Herzog and Bartheld, 1997; Altar and DiStefano, 1998). BDNF is present in the superior colliculus of adult rats (Hofer et al., 1990; Wetmore et al., 1990; Ma et al., 1997) and levels of BDNF in the hamster superior colliculus correlate well with the developmental events of RGC axons in the target (Ma et al., 1997). Furthermore, BDNF injected into the superior colliculus reduces developmental RGC death (Ma et al., 1998). All these results indicate that BDNF is a target-derived survival factor for developing RGCs.

The binding of the different neurotrophins to their relative high-affinity trk receptors is modulated by the low-affinity receptor, $p75^{NTR}$. The low-affinity receptor binds all members of the family of neurotrophin with similar affinity. The precise role of $p75^{NTR}$ has not been fully characterized and its role in the neurotrophic effects in axotomized and regenerating mammalian retina is still unknown. Alternative functions have been proposed for $p75^{NTR}$, such as buffering the concentration of available extracellular neurotrophins and maintaining a high concentration of neurotrophins near the site of release, or allowing neurotrophins bound to $p75^{NTR}$ on one cell and to be presented to trk receptors on other cells (Taniuchi et al., 1988; Barbacid, 1995). It has been suggested that $p75^{NTR}$ acts as an accessory subunit of trk receptors and facilitates trk signaling (Bothwell, 1996). New evidences demonstrate that $p75^{NTR}$ can trigger cellular responses without the participation of trk receptors and $p75^{NTR}$ signaling is of biological relevance *in vivo* (Frade et al., 1996; Carter and Lewin, 1997; Dechant and Barde, 1997). $p75^{NTR}$ has been reported to be involved in regulating apoptosis (Rabizadeh et al., 1993; Dobrowsky et al., 1994; Frade et al., 1996; Frade and Barde, 1998; Frade and Barde, 1999). It has also been shown that injured RGCs undergo apoptotic cell death in the adult mammalian retina (Berkelaar et al., 1994 and our unpublished observation). Thus $p75^{NTR}$ is proposed to play a pro-apoptotic role in RGC death after optic nerve injury in rat retina (Suzuki et al., 1998). Although, $p75^{NTR}$ mRNA is localized in the RGC layer of both developing (Koide et al., 1995) and adult rat retina (Suzuki et al., 1998), our recent investigation failed to detect $p75^{NTR}$ expression on retrogradely-labeled RGCs in the axotomized and regenerating adult retinas. The low affinity $p75^{NTR}$ is instead, primarily localized on Müller cell processes, identified with vimentin antibody (Hu et al., 1998,1999). Our results indicate that the previously reported light microscopic localization of $p75^{NTR}$ on RGCs might belong to the surrounding Müller cell processes. Thus, the pathway of neurotrophic effects on RGCs might be, at least partially, through a glial-neuronal pathway rather than on RGCs directly. Since $p75^{NTR}$ is not present in RGCs, the proposed pro-apoptotic role of $p75^{NTR}$ involved in RGC death after optic nerve injury is unlikely to occur in rats.

B. Regeneration Studies

Because most of the studies of neurotrophic factors have been directed towards neuronal viability, less information is available on their role in axonal regeneration (Cui et al., 1998). For example, BDNF, NT-4/5, and bFGF have all been shown to promote the survival of developing or adult RGCs (Sievers et al., 1987; Mey and Thanos, 1993; Cohen et al., 1994; Mansour-Robaey et al., 1994; Cui et al., 1995). Their effects on axonal regeneration are limited to enhancing neurite outgrowth *in vitro* (Cohen et al., 1994) and axonal branching and sprouting *in vivo* (Mansour-Robaey et al., 1994; Sawai et al., 1996), but they are reported to have no effect on long distance axonal regeneration (Mansour-Robaey et al., 1994; Chen et al., 1997). Studies on NGF, NT-3, and CNTF reveal no significant effects on RGC neurite outgrowth (Cohen et al., 1994; Sawai et al., 1996; Chen et al., 1997). Our recent investigation is the first to demonstrate that CNTF (Fig. 2E), and not neurotrophins (NGF, BDNF, NT-3, NT-4/5) and bFGF, substantially enhances the regeneration of injured optic axons (about 25% of RGCs) into a sciatic nerve graft but does not increase the survival of distally axotomized RGCs (Cui et al., 1999). In addition, CNTF significantly increases a very small number of RGCs (about 0.5%) to cross the lesion site (Fig. 3D) to the distal stump of the optic nerve (So et al., 1999). The fewer regenerating axons detected in the latter model may be due to lack of a peripheral nerve graft and possibly, the formation of an inhibitory scar environment after optic nerve crush. The level of CNTF expression has previously been shown to change significantly after injury in both the central and peripheral nervous systems (Ip et al., 1993). Changes of CNTF expression are also a marker of neuronal injury in the retina (LeVail et al., 1992; Ip and Yancopoulos, 1996). Both CNTFRα and its mRNA are expressed at high levels in developing retinas (Kirsch et al., 1997), indicating a role during the developing of the visual system and suggesting a possible role in the injury response in the retina.

VI. OTHER FACTORS IN THE PERIPHERAL NERVE GRAFT THAT PROMOTE AXONAL REGENERATION

The outgrowth of a regenerating RGC axon into peripheral nerve grafts and its final termination in the appropriate target tissue requires interaction between the axon and its environment involving a full array of chemical constituents of cell membranes and signaling molecules. Developmental studies have generated insights into some of the underlying molecular mechanisms that underlie promotion or inhibition of neurite growth. For example, several recognition molecules have been identified (Martini, 1994; Schachner et al., 1994). Schwann cells express integrins and cell adhesion molecules on their surfaces (Daniloff et al., 1986; Mirsky and Jessen, 1990; Schachner, 1990). The neural adhesion molecules L1 is one of several recognition molecules which could enhance neurite elongation (Schachner, 1990). L1-dependent neurite outgrowth is mediated by a number of homophilic and heterophilic receptor ligand interactions with molecules on axonal surfaces which not only results in promotion of neurite outgrowth but also acts as a signal transducer leading to changes in intracellular messengers (Atashi, et al., 1992; Doherty and Walsh, 1992; Saffell et al., 1997). The highly sialylated form of N-CAM present in the embryo axons is re-expressed in regenerating nerves (Rutishauser and Landmesser, 1996) and is necessary for the extension of RGC neurite on cell membranes *in vitro* (Zhang et al., 1992). The direct interaction between the regenerating axons and Schwann cell surfaces, mediated by N-CAM, can strongly promote axonal elongation after axons enter the graft. Schwann cells also produce ECM molecules such as laminin and collagens (Bunge, 1993). The upregulation of $\beta1$ integrin in RGCs is observed when they regenerate their axons through the peripheral nerve graft (Knoops et al., 1993), lending support to the concept that ECM could influence CNS regeneration.

VII. FUTURE DIRECTIONS

The use of peripheral nerve to enhance axonal regeneration of CNS neurons has played an important role in convincing the scientific community that adult CNS neurons have the capacity to regenerate. It will continue to be a useful model to study the molecular mechanisms of axonal regeneration including the molecular interaction between CNS axons and PNS or CNS environments. The comparison of these two types of interactions will generate insights into understanding CNS regeneration leading to possible future manipulation of axonal regeneration with modern molecular techniques.

Bridging the transected site and target area with a segment of peripheral nerve will continue to be exploited as a possible strategy of clinical treatment. However, more basic research is required including more works on the behavioral recovery of function.

It is now clear that in order for maximum axonal regeneration to occur, changing the environment and upregulation of the growth potential of axotomized neurons are both important. The use of peripheral nerve transplant, neutralization of inhibitory molecules or addition of growth promoting molecules in the CNS are ways to change the CNS environment. Administration of Schwann cells or the appropriate type of trophic factors close to the cell bodies of the axotomized neurons are alternate ways to upregulate the growth potential of the axotomized neurons. For example, future work involving RGCs may be directed at understanding how perineuronal application of Schwann cells or CNTF so markedly enhances axonal regeneration into a peripheral nerve graft (Fig. 2D and E) or along the optic nerve (Fig. 3C and D). It would be pertinent to establish whether the expression of particular growth-associated genes is the limiting factor for those CNS neurons that do not regenerate. If that is the case, then inserting genes into these neurons or applying appropriate trophic factor directly to the cell bodies or the injured axons to increase the expression of these genes, should enable them to mount an adequate regenerative response after injury. The use of CNTF to promote axonal regeneration of RGC axons in the optic nerve following a crush lesion (Fig. 3D) is particularly exciting as it can be easily applied in a clinical setting. However, it is necessary to find ways (e.g. decrease scar formation) to markedly increase the number of regenerating axons and to show that they can reach the targets and mediate meaningful behavioral functions before this technique can be applied in humans.

ACKNOWLEDGEMENTS

The research from the authors' laboratories that is described herein was supported by research grants from the University of Hong Kong, the Research Grant Council of Hong Kong and from the Croucher Foundation of Hong Kong.

REFERENCES

Acheson A, Barker PA, Alderson RF, Miller FD, Murphy RA (1991) Detection of brain-derived neurotrophic factor-like activity in fibroblasts and Schwann cells: inhibition by antibodies to NGF. Neuron 7:265-275.

Allendoerfer KL, Cabelli RJ, Escandon E, Kaplan DR, Nikolics K, Shatz CJ (1994) Regulation of neurotrophin receptors during the maturation of the mammalian visual system. J Neurosci 14:1795-1811.

Altar CA, DiStefano PS (1998) Neurotrophin trafficking by anterograde transport. Trends Neurosci 21:433-437.

Atashi JR, Klinz SG, Ingraham CA, Matten WT, Schachner M, Maness PF (1992) Neural cell adhesion molecules modulate tyrosine phosphorylation of tubulin in nerve growth cone membranes. Neuron 8:831-842.

Bähr M, Eschweiler GW, Wolburg H (1992) Precrushed sciatic nerve grafts enhance the survival and axonal regrowth of retinal ganglion cells in adult rats. Exp Neurol 116:13-22.

Bähr M, Przyrembel C, Bastmeyer M (1995) Astrocytes from adult rat optic nerve are non-permissive for regenerating retinal ganglion cell axons. Exp Neurol 131:211-220.

Barbacid M (1995) Neurotrophic factors and their receptors. Curr Opin Cell Biol 7:148-155.

Benfey M, Aguayo AJ (1982) Extensive elongation of axons from rat brain into peripheral nerve grafts. Nature 296:150-152.

Berkelaar M, Clarke DB, Wang YC, Bray GM, Aguayo AJ (1994) Axotomy results in delayed death and apoptosis of retinal ganglion cells in adult rats. J Neurosci 14:4368-4374.

Berkemeier LR, Winslow JW, Kaplan DR, Nikolics K, Goeddel DV, Rosenthal A (1991) Neurotrophin-5: A novel neurotrophic factor that activates trk and trkB. Neuron 7:857-866.

Berry M, Carlile J, Hunter A (1996) Peripheral nerve explants grafted into the vitreous body of the eye promote the regeneration of retinal ganglion cell axons severed in the optic nerve. J Neurocytol 25:147-170.

Berry M, Rees L, Hall S, Yiu P, Sievers J (1988) Optic axons regenerate into sciatic nerve isografts only in the presence of Schwann cells. Brain Res Bull 20:223-231.

Berry M, Rees L, Sievers J (1986) Unequivocal regeneration of rat optic nerve axons into sciatic nerve isografts. In: Neural Transplantation and Regeneration (Das GD, Wallace RB, eds) pp 63-79. New York: Springer.

Bhattacharyya A, Watson FL, Bradlee TA, Pomeroy SL, Stiles CD, Segal RA (1997) Trk receptors function as rapid retrograde signal carriers in the adult nervous system. J Neurosci 17:7007-7016.

Bonfanti L, Strettoi E, Chierzi S, Cenni MC, Liu XH, Martinou JC, Maffei L, Rabacchi SA (1996) Protection of retinal ganglion cells form natural and axotomy-induced cell death in the neonatal transgenic mice overexpressiong bcl-2. J Neurosci 16:4186-4194.

Bothwell M (1996) p75NTR: A receptor after all. Science 272:506-507.

Bradley WG, Asbury AK (1970) Duration of synthesis phase in neuilemma cells in mouse sciatic nerve during degeneration. Exp Neurol 26:275-282.

Bunge MB (1993) Schwann cell regulation of extracellular matrix biosynthesis and assembley. In: Peripheral Neuropathy, 3rd edn (Dyck PJ, Thomas PK, Griffin JW, Low PA, Poduslo JF, eds) pp 299-316. Philadelphia: WB Saunders.

Carmignoto, G, Comelli MC, Candeo P, Cavicchioli L, Yan Q, Merighi A, Maffei L (1991) Expression of NGF receptor and NGF receptor mRNA in the developing and adult rat retina. Exp Neurol 111:302-311.

Carmignoto G, Maffei L, Candeo P, Canella R, Comelli C (1989) Effect of NGF on the survival of rat retinal ganglion cells following optic nerve section. J Neurosci 9:1263-1272.

Carter BD, Lewin GR (1997) Neurotrophins live or let die: Does p75NTR decide? Neuron 18:187-190.

Carter DA, Bray GM, Aguayo AJ (1989) Regenerated retinal ganglion cell axons can form well-differentiated synapses in the superior colliculus of adult hamsters. J Neurosci 9:4042-4050.

Carter DA, Bray GM, Aguayo AJ (1991) Patterns of the arborization made by retinal ganglion cell axons regenerating into the superior colliculus of adult hamsters. Soc Neurosci Abstr 17:568.

Carter DA, Jhaveri S (1997) Retino-geniculate axons regenerating in adult hamsters are able to form morphologically distinct terminals. Exp Neurol 146:315-322.

Cenni MC, Bonfanti L, Martinou JC, Ratto GM, Strettoi E, Maffei L (1996) Long-term survival of retinal ganglion cells following optic nerve section in adult bcl-2 transgenic mice. Eur J Neurosci 8:1735-1745.

Chan PM, Chung SK, So KF (1997) Regulation of GAP-43 mRNA in retinal ganglion cells following axotomy and intravitreal peripheral nerve transplantation. Soc Neurosci Abstr 23:1449.

Chau WK, Dockery P, So KF, Lau KC (1992) Interaction of central axons with Schwann cells of peripheral nervous tissue. Soc Neurosci Abstr 18:964.

Chen DF, Jhaveri S, Schneider GE (1995) Intrinsic changes in developing retinal neurons result in regenerative failure of their axons. Proc Natl Acad Sci USA 92:7287-7291.

Chen DF, Schneider GE, Martinou JC, Tonegawa S (1997) Bcl-2 promotes regeneration of severed axons in mammalian CNS. Nature 385:434-439.

Cheng H, Cao Y, Olson L (1996) Spinal cord repair in adult paraplegic rats: partial restoration of hind limb function. Science 273:510-513.

Cho EY, So KF (1987) Rate of regrowth of damaged retinal ganglion cell axons regenerating in a peripheral nerve graft in adult hamsters. Brain Res 419:369-374.

Cho EY, So KF (1992) Characterization of the sprouting response of axon-like processes from retinal ganglion cells after axotomy in adult hamsters: a model using intravitreal implantation of a peripheral nerve. J Neurocytol 21:589-603.

Cho KS, Shen L, So KF, Chung SK (1994) Intravitreal transplantation of a peripheral nerve enhances c-Jun expression in a subpopulation of axotomized retinal ganglion cells in hamsters. Proceeding of the 5th International Symposium on Neural Transplantation, Chatenay-Malabry, Paris, France. p O56.

Cho KS, So KF, Chung SK (1997) Intravitreal optic nerve graft retards death and enhances axonal regeneration of retinal ganglion cells in adult hamster. Soc Neurosci Abstr 23:1449.

Cohen A, Bray GM, Aguayo AJ (1994) Neurotrophin-4/5 (NT-4/5) increases adult rat retinal ganglion cell survival and neurite outgrowth in vitro. J Neurobiol 25:953-959.

Conner JM, Varon S (1995) Effects of exogenous nerve growth factor upon sympathetic sprouting into the hippocampal formation. Exp Neurol 136:123-135.

Cui Q, Harvey AR (1995) At least two mechanisms are involved in the death of retinal ganglion cells following target ablation in neonatal rats. J Neurosci 15:8143-8155.

Cui Q, Lu Q, So KF, Yip HK (1999) CNTF, not other trophic factors, promotes axonal regeneration of axotomized retinal ganglion cells in adult hamsters. Invest Ophthalmol Vis Sci 40:760-766.

Cui Q, So KF, Yip HK (1998) Major biological effects of neurotrophic factors on retinal ganglion cells in mammals. Biol Signals Recept 7:220-226.

Daniloff JK, Levi G, Grumet M, Rieger F, Edelman GM (1986) Altered expression of neuronal cell adhesion molecules induced by nerve injury and repair. J Cell Biol 103:929-945.

David S, Aguayo AJ (1981) Axonal elongation into peripheral nervous system 'bridges' after central nervous system injury in adult rats. Science 214:931-933.

Dechant G, Barde YA (1997) Signalling through the neurotrophin receptor p75NTR. Curr Opin Neurobiol 7:413-418.

DeFelipe J, Jones EG (1991) In Cajal's Degeneration and Regeneration of the Nervous System. New York: Oxford University Press.

de la Rossa EJ, Arribas A, Frade JM, Rodriguez-Tebar A (1994) Role of neurotrophins in the control of neural development: Neurotrophin-3 promotes both neuron differentiation and survival of cultured chick retinal cells. Neurosci 58:347-352.

Dezawa M, Nagano T (1993) Contacts between regenerating axons and the Schwann cells of sciatic nerve segments grafted to the optic nerve of adult rats. J Neurocytol 22:1103-1112.

Dezawa M, Negishi H, Kawana K, Adachi-Usami E (1998) Response of glial population during adult rat optic nerve regeneration into a peripheral nerve graft. Invest Ophthalmol Vis Sci 39:S807.

Diao YC, Xiao YM, So KF (1987) Retinal ganglion cell regeneration axons into peripheral nerve graft in adult hamster can respond to light. Sci Bull 32:369-374.

Dobrowsky RT, Werner MH, Castellino AM, Chao MV, Hannun YA (1994) Activation of the sphingomyelin cycle through the low-affinity neurotrophin receptor. Science 265:1596-1599.

Doherty P, Walsh FS (1992) Cell adhesion molecules, second messengers and axonal growth. Curr Opin Neurobiol 2:595-601.

Ernfors P, Merlio JP, Persson H (1992) Cells expressing mRNA for neurotrophins and their receptors during embryonic rat development. Eur J Neurosci 4:1140-1158.

Fournier AE, Beer J, Arregui CO, Essagian C, Aguayo AJ, McKerracher L (1997) Brain-derived neurotrophic factor modulates GAP-43 but not Ta1 expression in injured retinal ganglion cells of adult rats. J Neurosci Res 47:561-572.

Frade JM, Barde YA (1998) Nerve growth factor: two receptors, multiple functions. Bioessays 20:137-145.

Frade JM, Barde YA (1999) Genetic evidence for cell death mediated by nerve growth factor and the neurotrophin receptor p75 in the developing mouse retina and spinal cord. Development 126:683-690.

Frade JM, Rodriguez-Tebar A, Barde YA (1996) Induction of cell death by endogenous nerve growth factor through its p75 receptor. Nature 383:166-168.

Grafstein B (1991) The goldfish visual system as a model for the study of regeneration in the central nervous system. In: Development and plasticity of the visual system. (Cronly-Dillon J, ed) pp 190-200. London: Macmillan Press.

Grafstein B, McQuarrie IG (1978) Role of the nerve cell body in axonal regeneration. In: Neuronal Plasticity (Cotman CT, ed) pp 155-195. New York: Raven.

Guénard V, Xu X, Bunge M (1993) The use of Schwann cell transplantation to foster central nervous system repair. The Neurosci 5:401-411.

Hall S, Berry M (1989) Electron microscopic study of the interaction of axons and glia at the site of anastomosis between the optic nerve and cellular or acellular sciatic nerve grafts. J Neurocytol 18:171-184.

Hayashi K (1996) Biochemical studies on functional proteins in the brain nervous system. Neurobiochemical studies on nerve growth factor. Yakugaku-Zasshi 116:286-308.

Henderson CE, Philips HS, Pollock RA (1994) GDNF: a potent survival factor for motoneurons present in peripheral nerve and muscle. Science 266:1062-1064.

Hendry IA, Crouch M (1993) Synergy, retrograde transport, and cell death. In: Neurotrophic factors (Loughlin S, Fallon J, eds) pp 51-88. Boston: Academic Press.

Herzog KH, von Bartheld CS (1997) Contributions of the optic tectum and the retina as sources of BDNF for retinal ganglion cells in the chick embryo. Sco Neurosci Abstr 23:2244.

Hofer M, Pagliusi SR, Hohn A, Leibrock J, Barde YA (1990) Regional distribution of brain-derived neurotrophic factor mRNA in the adult mouse brain. Eur Mol Biol Org J 9:2459-2464.

Houle JD, Wright JW, Ziegler MK (1994) After spinal cord injury, chronically injured neurons retain the potential for axonal regeneration. In: Neuronal Transplantation, CNS Neuronal Injury and Regeneration. (Marwah J, Teitelbaum H, Prasad KN, eds) pp 103-118.

Hu B, Yip HK, So KF (1998) Localization of p75 neurotrophin receptor in the retina of the adult SD rat: An immunocytochemical study at light and electron microscopic levels. Glia 24:187-197.

Hu B, Yip HK, So KF (1999) Expression of p75 neurotrophin receptor in the injured and regenerating rat retina. NeuroReport, 10:1293-1297.

Ip NY, Wiegand SJ, Morse J, Rudge JS (1993) Injury-induced regulation of ciliary neurotrophic factor mRNA in the adult rat brain. Eur J Neurosci 5:25-33.

Ip NY, Yancopoulos GD (1996) The neurotrophins and CNTF: two families of collaborative neurotrophic factors. Annu Rev Neurosci 19:491-515.

Jin Y (1998) Neuronal survival and axonal regeneration of the lateral vestibular nucleus in rats after spinal cord injury. Ph.D thesis. The University of Hong Kong.

Johnson JE, Barde YA, Schwab M, Thoenen H (1986) Brain-derived neurotrophic factor supports the survival of cultured rat retinal ganglion cells. J Neurosci 6:3031-3038.

Keirstead SA, Rasminsky M, Fukuda Y, Carter DA, Aguayo AJ, Vidal Sanz M (1989) Electrophysiologic responses in hamster superior colliculus evoked by regenerating retinal axons. Science 246:255-257.

Keirstead SA, Vidal-Sanz M, Rasminsky M, Aguayo AJ, Levesque M, So KF (1985) Responses to light of retinal neurons regenerating axons into peripheral nerve grafts in the rat. Brain Res 359:402-406.

Kiernan JA (1985) A conditioning lesion does not induce axonal regeneration in the optic nerve of the rat. Exp Neurol 87:181-184.

Kirsch M, Lee MY, Meyer V, Wiese A, Hofmann HD (1997) Evidence for multiple, local functions of ciliary neurotrophic factor (CNTF) in retinal development: expression of CNTF and its receptors and in vitro effects on target cells. J Neurochem 68:979-990.

Klein R, Nanduri V, Jing SA, Lamballe F, Tapley P, Bryant S, Cordon-Cardo C, Jones KR, Reichardt LF, Barbacid M (1991) The trkB tyrosine protein kinase is a receptor for brain-derived neurotrophic factor and neurotrophin-3. Cell 66:395-403.

Knoops B, Carbonetto S, Aguayo AJ (1993) β1 intergrin subunit expression by central nervous system neurons is regulated following contact with the environment of the peripheral nervous system. Soc Neurosci Abstr 19:679.

Koide T, Takahashi JB, Hoshimaru M, Kojima M, Otsuka T, Asahi M, Kikuchi H (1995) Localization of trkB and low-affinity nerve growth factor receptor mRNA in the developing rat retina. Neurosci Lett 185:183-186.

Kuffler DP (1986) Isolated satellite cells of a peripheral nerve direct the growth of regenerating frog axons. J Comp Neurol 249:57-64.

Lau KC, So KF, Cho EY (1991) Morphological changes of retinal ganglion cells regenerating axons along peripheral nerve grafts: a Lucifer Yellow and silver staining study. Restor Neurol Neurosci 3:235-246.

Lau KC, So KF, Tay D (1992) Postnatal development of type I retinal ganglion cells in hamsters: a lucifer yellow study. J Comp Neurol 315:375-381.

Lau KC, So KF, Tay D (1994) Intravitreal transplantation of a segment of peripheral nerve enhances axonal regeneration of retinal ganglion cells following distal axotomy. Exp Neurol 128:211-215.

Lehwalder D, Jefferey PL, Unsicker K (1989) Survival of purified embryonic chick retinal ganglion cells in the presence of neurotrophic factors. J Neurosci Res 24:329-337.

Lei JL, Lau KC, So KF, Cho EY, Tay D (1995) Morphological plasticity of axotomized retinal ganglion cells following intravitreal transplantation of a peripheral nerve segment. J Neurocytol 24:497-506.

Leung MCP, So KF, Tay DKC (1996) Low level laser irradiation rescues axotomized retinal ganglion cells in adult hamsters. Neurosci Lett Suppl 47:S17.

Leung MCP, So KF, Tay DKC, Cho EYP, Kong WC (1997) The effect of laser irradiation of microglial responses in the retina of adult hamster after optic nerve axotomy. Neurosci Lett Suppl 47:S17.

LeVail MM, Unoki K, Yasumura D, Matthes MT, Yancopoulos GD, Steinberg RH (1992) Multiple growth factors, cytokines, and neurotrophins rescue photoreceptors from the damaging effects of constant light. Proc Natl Acad Sci USA 89:11249-11253.

Li SX, Yip HK, Hu B, So KF (1997a) The role of fibroblasts and Schwann cells in promoting the survival of axotomized retinal ganglion cells. Soc Neurosci Abstr 23:1992.

Li SX, Yip HK, So KF (1997b) The role of transplanted Schwann cells in promoting regeneration of rat optic nerve. Neurosci Lett 49:S12.

Liu L, So KF (1990) Effect of peripheral nerve on the neurite growth from retinal explants in culture. Cell Res 1:77-87.

Lu Q, So KF, Yip HK (1998) The effect of an intravitreal peripheral nerve graft on c-jun expression in regenerating retinal ganglion cells in hamsters. Soc Neurosci Abstr 24:2007.

Ma YT, Hsieh T, Forbes ME, Johnson JE, Frost DO (1997) BDNF protein levels in developing hamster visual system. Soc Neurosci Abstr 23:329.

Ma YT, Hsieh T, Forbes ME, Johnson JE, Frost DO (1998) BDNF injected into the superior colliculus reduces developmental retinal ganglion cell death. J Neurosci 18:2097-2107.

MacLennan AJ, Gaskin AA, Lado DC (1994) CNTF receptor alpha mRNA expression in rodent cell lines and developing rat. Brain Res Mol Brain Res 25:251-256.

Maffei L, Carmignoto G, Perry VH, Candeo P, Ferrari G (1990) Schwann cells promote the survival of rat retinal ganglion cells after optic nerve section. Proc Natl Acad Sci USA 87:1855-1859.

Malgrange B, Lefebvre PP, Martin D, Staecker H, Van de Water TR, Moonen G (1996) NT-3 has a tropic effect on process outgrowth by postnatal auditory neurones in vitro. NeuroReport 7:2495-2499.

Mansour-Robaey S, Clarke DB, Wang YC, Bray GM, Aguayo AJ (1994) Effects of ocular injury and administration of brain-derived neurotrophic factor on survival and regrowth of axotomized retinal ganglion cells. Proc Natl Acad Sci USA 91:1632-1636.

Martini R, Schachner M, Faissner A (1990) Enhanced expression of extracellar matrix molecules J1/tenascin in the regenerating adult mouse sciatic nerve. J Neurocytol 19:601-616.

Martini R (1994) Expression and functional roles of neural cell surface molecules and extracellular matrix components during development and regeneration of peripheral nerves. J Neurocytol 23:1-28.

Maysinger D, Berezovskaya O, Fedoroff S (1996) The hematopoietic cytokine colony stimulating factor 1 is also a growth factor in the CNS: (II). Microencapsulated CSF-1 and LM-10 cells as delivery systems. Exp Neurol 141:47-56.

McCaffery CA, Raju TR, Bennett MR (1984) Effects of cultured astroglia on the survival of neonatal rat retinal ganglion cells in vitro. Dev Biol 104:441-448.

McKerracher L, David S, Jackson DL, Kottis V, Dunn RJ, Braun PE (1994) Identification of myelin-associated glycoprotein as a major myelin-derived inhibitor of neurite growth. Neuron 13:805-811.

Meisinger C, Zeschnigk C, Grothe C (1996) In vivo and in vitro effect of glucocorticoids on fibroblast growth factor (FGF)-2 and FGF receptor 1 expression. J Biol Chem 271:16520-16525.

Mey J, Thanos S (1993) Intravitreal injections of neurotrophic factors support the survival of axotomized retinal ganglion cells in adult rats in vivo. Brain Res 602:304-317.

Meyer-Franke A, Kaplan MR, Pfrieger FW, Barres BA (1995) Characterization of the signaling interactions that promote the survival and growth of developing retinal ganglion cells in culture. Neuron 15:805-819.

Mirsky R, Jessen KR (1990) Schwann cell development and regulation of myelination. Semin Neurosci 2:423-435.

Morrow DR, Campbell G, Lieberman AR, Anderson PN (1993) Differential regenerative growth of CNS axons into tibial and peroneal nerve grafts in the thalamus of adult rats. Exp Neurol 120:60-69.

Mukhopadhyay G, Doherty P, Walsh FS, Crocker PR, Filbin MT (1994) A novel role for myelin-associated glycoprotein as an inhibitor of axonal regeneration. Neuron 13:757-767.

Neuberger TJ, De Vires GH (1993) Distribution of fibroblast growth factor in cultured dorsal root ganglion neurons and Schwann cells. J Neurocytol 22:436-448.

Nishi R (1994) Neurotrophic factors: Two are better than one. Science 265:1052-1053.

Ng TF, So KF, Chung SK (1995) Influence of peripheral nerve grafts on the expression of GAP-43 in regenerating retinal ganglion cells in adult hamsters. J Neurocytol 24:487-496.

Ohnishi A, Yamamoto T, Her Q, Han M, Murai Y, Ikeda M (1996) The effect of brain-derived neurotrophic factor on regeneration of nerve fibers after crush injury–morphometric evaluation. Sangyo Ika Daigaku Zasshi 18:261-271.

Politis MJ, Spencer PS (1986) Regeneration of rat optic axons into peripheral nerve grafts. Exp Neurol 91:52-59.

Rabacchi SA, Ensini M, Bonfanti L, Gravina A, Maffei L (1994) Nerve growth factor reduces apoptosis of axotomized retinal ganglion cells in the neonatal rat. Neurosci 63:969-973.

Rabizadeh S, Oh J, Zhong LT, Yang J, Bitler CM, Butcher LL, Bredesen DE (1993) Induction of apoptosis by the low-affinity NGF receptor. Science 261:345-348.

Reichert F, Levitzky R, Rotshenker S (1996) Interleukin 6 in intact and injured mouse peripheral nerves. Eur J Neurosci 8:530-535.
Richardson PM, Issa VM, Shemie S (1982) Regeneration and Retrograde degeneration of axons in the rat optic nerve. J Neurocytol 11:949-966.
Richardson PM, McGuinness UM, Aguayo AJ (1980) Axons from CNS neurons regenerate into PNS grafts. Nature 284:264-265.
Robinson GA (1994) Immediate early gene expression in axotomized and regenerating retinal ganglion cells of the adult rat. Brain Res Mol Brain Res 24:43-54.
Rodriguez-Tebar A, Jeffrey PL, Thoenen H, Barde YA (1989) The survival of chick retinal ganglion cells in response to brain-derived neurotrophic factor depends on their embryonic age. Dev Biol 136:296-303.
Rutishauser U, Landmesser L (1996) Polysialic acid in the vertebrate nervous system: A promoter of plasticity in cell-cell interactions. Trends Neurosci 19:422-427.
Saffell JL, Williams EJ, Mason IJ, Walsh FS, Doherty P (1997) Expression of a dominant negative FGF receptor inhibits axonal growth and FGF receptor phosphorylation stimulated by CAMs. Neuron 18:231-242.
Sasaki H, Coffey P, Villegas-Perez MP, Vidal-Sanz M, Young MJ, Lund RD, Fukuda Y (1996) Light induced EEG desynchronization and behavioral arousal in rats with restored retinocollicular projection by peripheral nerve graft. Neurosci Lett 218:45-48.
Sasaki H, Inoue T, Iso H, Fukuda Y, Hayashi Y (1993) Light-dark discrimination after sciatic nerve transplantation to the sectioned optic nerve in adult hamsters. Vis Res 33:877-880.
Sauve Y, Sawai H, Rasminsky M (1995) Functional synaptic connections made by regenerated retinal ganglion cell axons in the superior colliculus of adult hamsters. J Neurosci 15:665-675.
Sawai H, Clarke DB, Kittlerova P, Bray GM, Aguayo AJ (1996b) Brain-derived neurotrophic factor and neurotrophin-4/5 stimulate growth of axonal branches from regenerating retinal ganglion cells. J Neurosci 16:3887-3894.
Sawai H, Sugioka M, Morigiwa K, Sasaki H, So KF, Fukuda Y (1996a) Functional and morphological restoration of intracranial brachial lesion of the retinocollicular pathway by peripheral nerve autografts in adult hamsters. Exp Neurol 137:94-104.
Schachner M (1990) Function implications of glial cell recognition molecules. Semin Neurosci 2:492-507.
Schachner M (1994) Neural recognition molecules in disease and regeneration. Curr Opin Neurobiol 4:726-734.
Schwab ME, Kapfhammer JP, Bandtlow CE (1993) Inhibitors of neurite growth. Annu Rev Neurosci 16:565-595.
Sievers J, Hausmann B, Unsicker K, Berry M (1987) Fibroblast growth factors promote the survival of adult rat retinal ganglion cells after transection of the optic nerve. Neurosci Lett 76:157-162.
Smith GV, Stevenson JA (1988) Peripheral nerve grafts lacking viable Schwann cells fail to support central nervous system axonal regeneration. Exp Brain Res 69:299-306.
So KF, Aguayo AJ (1985) Lengthy regrowth of cut axons from ganglion cells after peripheral nerve transplantation into the retina of adult rats. Brain Res 328:349-354.
So KF, Ng TF, Chung SK (1996b) The Relationship of the Expression of GAP-43 and the Axonal Regeneration of Retinal Ganglion Cells in Adult Mammals. In: Perspectives in Neuroscience Research (Tan CK, Ling EA, Tan CBC, eds) pp 137-152.

So KF, Sawai H, Ireland S, Tay D, Fukuda Y (1996a) The effect of damage of the brachium of the superior colliculus in neonatal and adult hamsters and the use of peripheral nerve to restore retinocollicular projections. Prog Brain Res 112:363-372.

So KF, Xiao YM, Diao YC (1986) Effects on the growth of damaged ganglion cell axons after peripheral nerve transplantation in adult hamsters. Brain Res 377:168-172.

So KF, Yip HK (1998) Regenerative capacity of retinal ganglion cells in mammals. Vis Res 38:1525-1535.

So KF, Zeng QR, Yip HK, Cho KS (1999) CNTF induced axonal re-growth across the crush site of the optic nerve. ARVO Abstr, 40:S267.

Stevenson JA (1985) Growth of optic tract axons in nerve grafts in hamsters. Exp Neurol 87:446-457.

Suzuki A, Nomura S, Morii E, Fukuda Y, Kosaka J (1998) Localization of mRNAs for trkB isoforms and p75 in rat retinal ganglion cells. J Neurosci Res 54:27-37.

Taniuchi M, Clark HB, Schweitzer JB, Johnson EM Jr (1988) Expression of nerve growth factor receptors by Schwann cells of axotomized peripheral nerves: Ultrastructural location, suppression by axonal contact, and binding properties. J Neurosci 8:664-681.

Thanos S (1988) Alterations in the morphology of ganglion cell dendrites in the adult rat retina after optic nerve transection and grafting of peripheral nerve segments. Cell Tissue Res 254:599-609.

Thanos S (1992) Adult retinofugal axons regenerating through peripheral nerve grafts can restore the light-induced pupilloconstriction reflex. Eur J Neurosci 4:691-699.

Thanos S (1997) Neurobiology of the regenerating retina and its functional reconnection with the brain by means of peripheral nerve transplants in adult rats. Survey Ophthalmol 42 [Suppl] 1:5-26.

Thanos S, Mey J (1995) Type-specific stabilization and target-dependent survival of regenerating ganglion cells in the retina of adult rats. J Neurosci 15:1057-1079.

Thanos S, Mey J, Wild M (1993) Treatment of the adult retina with microglia-suppressing factors retards axotomy-induced neuronal degradation and enhances axonal regeneration in vivo and in vitro. J Neurosci 13:455-466.

Thanos S, Vanselow J (1989) Adult retinal ganglion cells retain the ability to regenerate their axons up to several weeks after axotomy. J Neurosci Res 22:144-149.

Trecarten MJ, Villegas-Perez MP, Vidal-Sanz M, Thanos S, Aguayo AJ (1986) Growth of retinal axons along peripheral nerve system grafts inserted into retina of adult rats. Soc Neurosci Abstr 12:701.

Turner JE, Blair JR, Chappel ET (1987) Peripheral nerve implant effects on survival of retinal ganglion layer cells after axotomy initiated by a penetrating lesion. Brain Res 419:46-54.

Vidal-Sanz M, Bray GM, Aguayo AJ (1991) Regenerated synapses persist in the superior colliculus after the regrowth of retinal ganglion cell axons. J Neurocytol 20:940-952.

Vidal-Sanz M, Bray GM, Villegas-Perez MP, Thanos S, Aguayo AJ (1987) Axonal regeneration and synapse formation in the superior colliculus by retinal ganglion cells in the adult rat. J Neurosci 7:2894-2909.

Villegas-Perez MP, Vidal-Sanz M, Bray GM, Aguayo AJ (1988) Influences of peripheral nerve grafts on the survival and regrowth of axotomized retinal ganglion cells in adult rats. J Neurosci 8:265-280.

Watanabe M, Fukuda Y (1997) Proportions of ON-center versus OFF-center cells in retinal ganglion cells with regenerated axons of adult cats. Exp Neurol 143:117-123.

Watabe K, Fukuda T, Tanaka J, Honda H, Toyohara K, Sakai O (1995) Spontaneously immortalized adult mouse Schwann cells secrete autocrine and paracrine growth-promoting activities. J Neurosci Res 41:279-290.

Watanabe M, Sawai H, Fukuda Y (1991) Axonal regeneration of retinal ganglion cells in the cat geniculocortical pathway. Brain Res 560:330-333.

Watanabe M, Sawai H, Fukuda Y (1993) Number, distribution, and morphology of retinal ganglion cells with axons regenerated into peripheral nerve graft in adult cats. J Neurosci 13:2105-2117.

Wetmore C, Ernfors P, Persson H, Olson L (1990) Localization of brain-derived neurotrophic factor mRNA to neurons in the brain by in situ hybridization. Exp Neurol 109:141-152.

Whiteley SJO, Sauve Y, Aviles-Trigueros M, Vidal-Sanz M, Lund RD (1998) Extent and duration of recovered pupillary light reflex following retinal ganglion cell axon regeneration through peripheral nerve grafts directed to the pretectum in adult rats. Exp Neurol 154:560-572.

Wu W, Han K, Li L, Schinco FP (1994) Implantation of PNS graft inhibits the induction of neuronal nitric oxide synthase and enhances the survival of spinal motoneurons following root avulsion. Exp Neurol 129:335-339.

Xiao YM, So KF, Diao YC, Wang LH (1989) The axonal regeneration of visual cortical neurons in golden hamsters. Acta Anatomica Sinica 20:306-313.

Yip HK, Lam LW, So KF (1999) Short period of low level laser enhances retinal ganglion cell (RGC) survival after optic nerve axotomy in adult SD rats. ARVO 40:S132.

You SW (1998) Neuronal survival and axonal regeneration of retinal ganglion cells in adult hamsters. Ph.D thesis. The University of Hong Kong.

You SW, So KF, Yip HK (1997) Effects of distance of axotomy on axonal regeneration of retinal ganglion cells into a peripheral nerve graft. Soc Neurosci Abstr 23:1449.

You SW, So KF, Yip HK, Bedi KS (1996) Effect of a pre-degenerated peripheral nerve graft and a conditioning lesion of optic nerve on axonal regeneration of retinal ganglion cells. Soc Neurosci Abstr 22:1230.

Zanaletto A, Comelli MC, Dal Toso R, Carmignoto G (1993) Developing rat retinal ganglion cells express the functional NGF receptor p140trkA. Dev Biol 159:105-113.

Zeng QR, So KF, Yip HK (1998) The effect of intravitreal peripheral nerve on axonal regeneration following the crush injury of the optic nerve. Proc Aust Neurosci Soc 9:8.

Zhang H, Miller RH, Rutishauser U (1992) Polysialic acid is required for optimal growth of axons on a neuronal substrate. J Neurosci 12:3107-3114.

21

Transplantation of Schwann Cells and Ensheathing Glia to Improve Regeneration in Adult Spinal Cord

Giles W. Plant[1], Almudena Ramón-Cueto[2] and Mary Bartlett Bunge[1]

[1]The Miami Project to Cure Paralysis, & the Departments of Anatomy, Cell Biology and Neurological Surgery, University of Miami School of Medicine, Miami, Florida

[2]Centro de Biologia Molecular "Severo Ochoa" (Consejo Superior de Investigaciones Cientificas), Facultad de Ciencias, Universidad Autonoma de Madrid, Cantoblanco, Madrid, Spain

I. INTRODUCTION

Spinal cord injury is a devastating injury that interrupts the communication of information from the brain to the spinal cord. Injuries to the spinal cord can vary from a small compression to a complete disruption of the entire width of the cord caused by bone shards cutting through the cord, gun shot wounds or knife attacks. One suggested way of repairing this injury is to use tissue bridges to span the lesion and reconnect both ascending and descending spinal tracts involved in sensory and motor function, respectively.

After an extensive spinal cord lesion, the necrotic tissue of the injury region should be removed by the neurosurgeon before application of any further treatment. This will create a gap at the injury site that cannot be crossed by regenerating axons unless a bridge between both cord stumps is provided. Therefore, the use of bridges containing supportive substrates for axonal elongation in combination with other successful repair strategies seems necessary. These bridges could be tubes containing either molecules (e.g., extracellular matrix molecules, neurotrophins) or cells (e.g., Schwann cells, olfactory ensheathing glia, fibroblasts genetically modified to produce neurotrophins) proven to be promoters of axonal regeneration (Bunge, 1999). Much attention on spinal cord bridging transplantation has been focused on the use of peripheral nerves.

In this chapter, we compare the use of peripheral nerve and Schwann cells as appropriate candidates for bridging areas of injury. Because large numbers of Schwann cells are needed for transplantation, we next outline methods of Schwann cell preparation. Following that, there is a discussion on improving outcome when additional strategies are used in combination with Schwann cell transplantation. One of the additional strategies is the transplantation of ensheathing glia to modify the inhibitory barrier that forms between the Schwann cell transplant and host spinal cord. The promise of ensheathing glia in spinal cord repair, methods of preparation, generation of cell lines, and results of their transplantation into the spinal cord to promote remyelination as well as regeneration are discussed. Future directions are also considered.

II. PERIPHERAL NERVE TRANSPLANTATION INTO THE SPINAL CORD

In contrast to the central nervous system (CNS), the peripheral nervous system (PNS) has the ability to regenerate axons without intervention, leading to some sensory and motor improvement (Ramon y Cajal, 1928; Fawcett and Keynes, 1990; Son and Thompson., 1996a, b). CNS regeneration is very limited but axons can regenerate under the right conditions and providing the distance from the injury site is not too far from the soma. The earliest results obtained by Ramon y Cajal and his fellow researchers (1928) suggested that CNS nerve cells can regenerate in an environment in which appropriate nutrients and guidance molecules are provided. In the early 1980s, Richardson and colleagues (1980,1984) proved that spinal cord axonal populations regenerate when a peripheral nerve is placed into a surgical gap created in the rat spinal cord.

Recently a group in Sweden (Cheng et al., 1996) developed a multiple peripheral nerve approach in combination with other strategies to enhance regeneration in the completely transected spinal cord of the adult rat. They used 18 pieces of small diameter peripheral nerve to span a 3-5 mm gap in the cord. The peripheral nerve segments were carefully placed within the intraspinal gap and directed from white to gray matter to stimulate axonal growth into a more growth permissive area. These segments (derived from intercostal nerves of the same animal) were stabilized within the lesion site by fibrin glue. The fibrin glue contained a growth factor called acidic fibroblast growth factor (FGF-1). This growth factor has also been reported to prevent die-back of the corticospinal tract after complete transection of the spinal cord (Guest et al., 1997b). In addition to this, the spinal column was stabilized using a wiring system. The authors reported an improvement in hind limb locomotion in the rats, and anatomical WGA/HRP tracing in the sensory/motor cortex indicated growth of corticospinal tract axons into and out of the peripheral nerve grafts.

This multifaceted-approach using peripheral nerves may be limited, however, by the difficulty in obtaining the amount of peripheral nerve needed in a large injury and the lesion may not have appropriate edges for positioning the nerves within the lesion. To enable the nerves to be positioned correctly, the injury site would have to be debrided and in so doing re-injury would occur, with additional functional loss. A number of spinal cord injured patients may have a gap larger than that used in the rat model (4-5mm). One example of a large spinal cord lesion is the ongoing clinical condition of syringomyelia that can lead to functional deterioration over time (Fox et al., 1988; MacDonald et al., 1988; Caplan et al., 1990; William, 1990). Thus, not dissimilar to inducing successful regeneration in large peripheral nerve injury gaps, the availability and feasibility of spanning large injury gaps with peripheral nerve transplants has its limitations. The ethical considerations to use cadaver peripheral nerve and the possibility of immune rejection have led to the development of other strategies to bridge spinal cord injuries. One such strategy is the use of Schwann cells isolated from the peripheral nerves (Bunge, 1975).

III. REASONS FOR USING SCHWANN CELLS TO PROMOTE AXONAL REGENERATION

Storage of peripheral nerves diminishes their ability to support regeneration (Levi et al., 1994). Levi and colleagues (1994) studied the viability of both rat and human peripheral nerves after various time periods at 4°C. After 3 weeks, there were no viable Schwann cells or fibroblasts. Schwann cells survived up to a week; numbers and purity obtained were similar to fresh nerves and the Schwann cells were able to myelinate DRG axons. It appears that a period of axon/myelin breakdown permits Schwann cells to detach from the degenerating axons, thereby possibly making them easier to dissociate and improving their survival. Successful freezing and thawing of nerves to produce viable nerve for transplantation has not been elucidated; in fact, repeated freeze/thawing of peripheral nerves provides a non-conducive regenerative graft (Berry et al., 1988; Hall and Berry, 1989; Hall, 1989).

In response to the considerations outlined above, research groups have investigated the proliferation of Schwann cells extracted from adult peripheral nerve tissue and tested their ability to promote CNS regeneration. The eventual aim is to find ways to isolate Schwann cells from adult peripheral nerves (from sensory nerves of a spinal cord injured patient, for example), and purify and expand them substantially in tissue culture before using them as transplants. In addition, it will be important to be able to freeze and store Schwann cells for future use and to perhaps match donors, not unlike the matching procedures in use for organ donors today. The ability to expand Schwann cell numbers from pieces of isolated peripheral nerve is important because the expansion treatment does not alter markedly the ability of Schwann cells to express important growth-promoting molecules and phenotypic markers normally expressed (Morrissey et al., 1991; Casella et al., 1996; Levi, 1996; Li et al., 1996).

Schwann cells play a major role in the regenerative capacity of peripheral nerve (Fawcett and Keynes, 1990). If frozen and thawed, the ability of the nerve to stimulate axonal regeneration is lost, mainly due to the loss of Schwann cells (see above). Schwann cells form a continuous basal lamina along the entire length of the axon/Schwann cell unit. After injury the Schwann cells and the basal lamina persist; these structures in which the Schwann cells are housed are called bands of Büngner. Schwann cells have a number of attributes that make them suitable for axonal growth. They synthesize neurotrophic factors, release chemoattractant molecules, express on their surfaces a number of integrins, and cell surface adhesion molecules (Bandtlow et al., 1987; Acheson et al., 1991; Rende et al., 1992), and produce extracellular matrix molecules such as laminin and collagens (Daniloff et al., 1986; Kuffler, 1986; Mirsky and Jessen, 1990; Schachner, 1990; Bunge, 1993) known to promote axonal growth. A large body of literature supports the idea that Schwann cells promote the regeneration of CNS axons both *in vitro* and *in vivo* (reviewed in Bunge and Hopkins, 1990, and Guenard et al., 1993; also Montgomery and Robson, 1993; Harvey et al., 1994; Plant et al., 1995, 1998a; Xu et al., 1995a, 1997). In this review, however, we will concentrate on Schwann cells transplanted to the injured spinal cord of the rodent and the possibility in the future to autotransplant human Schwann cells into the spinal cord injured patient.

A major advantage of using Schwann cells derived from peripheral nerve is that large numbers of Schwann cells can be produced *in vitro* in a short period of time. Schwann cells, because of the ease of culturing them, were for a long time derived from prenatal or postnatal but not adult PNS tissues (Wood, 1976; Brockes et al., 1979). In a clinically relevant paradigm, availability of donor tissue becomes a central issue and dependence upon perinatal tissue is problematic due to ethical reasons. Autologous grafting of Schwann cells would enable surgeons to circumvent the problem of finding suitable donors and rejection problems often associated with transplantation. In most cases, autotransplantation would require the production of Schwann cells from adult peripheral nerve. After isolation from peripheral nerve, Schwann cells need to be expanded in number and care taken to ensure that the cells have growth control and functional capacity matching the Schwann cells in their normal milieu.

IV. GENERATION OF RAT AND HUMAN SCHWANN CELLS

In order to use Schwann cells as bridges or transplants it is necessary to produce not only high numbers but also to obtain purified populations from adult nerves

(Morrissey et al., 1991) for subsequent expansion *in vitro*. In the mid to late-1970s, Wood (1976) and Brockes and colleagues (1979) described procedures to purify and culture rodent Schwann cells. Since that time, the procedures have been steadily improving so that now greater numbers and higher purity of cells can be obtained. Morrissey and colleagues (1991) developed a technique which utilized the natural axonal and myelin breakdown of the peripheral nerve *in vitro*. This breakdown (Wallerian degeneration) led to a mitogenic response of the Schwann cells (Abercrombie et al., 1946; Bradley and Asbury, 1970), thereby enabling an increase in Schwann cell number. After several explant transfers in culture during which fibroblasts emigrated from the piece of peripheral nerve, the nerve no longer contained fibroblasts (Morrissey et al., 1991). Yields greater than $2x10^4$ cells/mg of starting weight were obtained after growing cells in the presence of 20μg/ml glial growth factor (GGF) and 2μM forskolin with Schwann cell purity as high as 98%. These cells were then shown to behave normally by their ability to myelinate dorsal root ganglion cell axons. The same methodology applied to human phrenic nerve yielded similar results except that the time course was slower (Morrissey et al., 1991).

Since the development of this technique, there have been substantial advances for potential autologous human Schwann cell transplantation. Some of these advances (see Askansas et al., 1980; Morrissey et al., 1991; Rutkowski et al., 1992) were combined in a study by Levi and Bunge (1994) who obtained sufficient human Schwann cell numbers and purity to perform transplantation studies in rodents. An important part of the study was the use of Schwann cell mitogens, such as heregulin, forskolin and cholera toxin. The method described by Levi and Bunge (1994), however, had a few disadvantages. The initial period for maintaining and transferring the nerve explants (for fibroblast exclusion) was long and labor intensive with a high possibility of contamination. Division of Schwann cells following dissociation was relatively slow and the amount of expansion limited. The fourth passage of these cells also caused detachment of the cells, with subsequent aggregation. Increased fibroblast contamination was also seen. Casella and colleagues (1996) described an improvement of the above described technique for human Schwann cell generation. The authors utilized a combination of known Schwann cell mitogens, heregulin and forskolin, in medium in which the peripheral nerve fragments were kept before harvest and dissociation. This modification allowed dissociation of the fragments at two weeks rather than four, thus eliminating the need to transfer explants, which increased cell yield and purity. Laminin or collagen were also used instead of the normal tissue culture coating of poly-L-Lysine. This change allowed multiple passages in medium containing heregulin and forskolin and solved the problem of cell aggregation and detachment. Cholera toxin use was also eliminated. Higher cell yields were also observed compared with previous studies (Morrissey et al., 1991; Rutkowski et al., 1992) and phenotypic characteristics were maintained (Fig. 1).

Another important observation was the dramatic difference in proliferation, migratory behavior, and morphology of human Schwann cells on different sub-

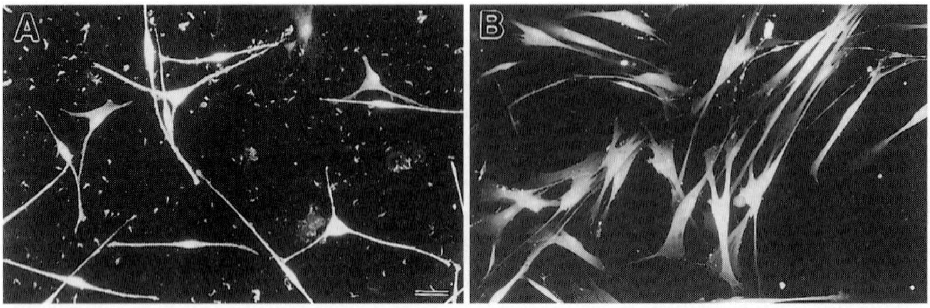

Figure 1 In vitro immunostaining for S100 in human SCs. (**A**) Schwann cells at first passage and (**B**) after six passages. Note the more flattened morphology in (**B**) compared with the typical elongated bipolar morphology at the earlier passage (**A**). S100 immunostaining was not diminished after six passages. Bar: 50μm

strates (Casella et al., 1996). With regard to substrate, the function of integrins on the cell surface and the interaction with ligands on the extracellular matrix must be kept in mind, particularly when discussing cell death by apoptosis (Boudreau et al., 1995). The addition of laminin or collagen as a growth substratum may partly explain the increased expansion as well as resolution of the problem of aggregation and detachment. Casella et al. (1996) also noted that their method increased the cell number from nerves by 3,000 times after dissociation. This number was obtained after 10 weeks including the two weeks pre-incubation in mitogens prior to dissociation. The final purities obtained were also very high, between 90-95 percent. One centimeter of intercostal peripheral nerve (9.9±1.6 mg of dry fascicles) provides approximately 10^6 cells at the time of the dissociation and has a potential to generate 3x 10^9 cells after expansion. This number of cells could fill a 5 meter long guidance channel of 2.6 mm inner diameter at a concentration of 120 X 10^6 Schwann cells/ml (see below). Schwann cells are known to be effective in promoting axonal regeneration at this concentration (Xu et al., 1997). More recent work has further improved the yield by growing Schwann cells at lower density. This modification allows up to a 17,000-fold increase in Schwann cell number, yielding a transplant nearly 30 meters long in 30-35 days (GTB Casella and PM Wood, unpublished observations). Age of the Schwann cell donor does not affect the isolation, number or purity of the Schwann cells generated (Levi, 1996).

A recent paper by Li and colleagues (1996) explored another avenue to provide pure cultures of human Schwann cells. They described the use of a serum-free medium that contained Gas6. Gas6 was originally cloned as a growth arrest-specific protein from fibroblasts (Manfioletti et al., 1993). Cultures of human

Schwann cells grown with Gas6 contained only low numbers of contaminating fibroblasts and showed an increase in proliferation and incorporation of thymidine (Li et al., 1996). Gas6 also had synergistic effects with the other known human Schwann cell mitogens, heregulin, glial growth factor and forskolin. The combination of Gas6, heregulin and forskolin supports maximal cell proliferation, while importantly preserving typical Schwann cell morphology and expression of Schwann cell markers (GFAP, S100 and p75). This ability to maintain the normal Schwann cell phenotype while expanding numbers quickly gives more support for their possible use in human spinal cord injuries.

V. SCHWANN CELL TRANSPLANTATION INTO THE SPINAL CORD

The spinal cord is a prime candidate for axonal tract repair; the serious and currently irreparable functional effects are due to disconnection of neurons from their targets by lesions of long spinal fiber tracts. The spinal cord has long ascending and descending tracts which contain axons recruited from many different sites at all levels of the brain and spinal cord and deliver them to targets no less dispersed. To use multiple peripheral nerves to reconnect them to specific sites is problematic. One method to try to circumvent this problem, pioneered by Raisman's group (this volume, chapter by Raisman), was to design a micro-transplantation technique to reduce trauma at the site of injection. Following their success in delivering embryonic neurons to the CNS in this manner (Davies et al., 1994), Schwann cells were injected by means of an air pressure delivery system (Emmett et al., 1990) and a glass micro-pipette (Brook et al., 1993) into a circumscribed location in the corticospinal tract and ascending dorsal column tracts in rat cord. The results indicated that Schwann cells were able, unlike peripheral nerves, to induce local sprouting of the corticospinal tract fibers. Ascending dorsal column axons also sprouted into the area of Schwann cells (Li and Raisman, 1994). In a later paper, Li and Raisman (1997) described the injection of a suspension of 10,000 Schwann cells into a discrete site in the upper cervical level of the corticospinal tract. From 4 days after transplantation, a central mass of p75 positive Schwann cells and cuffs of Schwann cells along the perivascular space of blood vessels could be seen. After 6 weeks, p75 immunoreactivity of the interfascicular Schwann cells had become down-regulated, but P_0 immunostaining revealed that the Schwann cells were still present and, moreover, had myelinated segments of the host corticospinal tract in the region of the transplant. In conclusion, the authors showed that Schwann cells can be intimately integrated into the cytoarchitecture of the myelinated adult host corticospinal tract. Moreover, this integration was not random in damaged areas, but it involved direct interaction with the host cells .

The surface area available for axonal ingrowth may be greater when a suspension of Schwann cells is used compared with peripheral nerve and, additionally, the inhibitory peripheral myelin molecules are lacking (Bedi et al., 1994).

Also, the further damage due to insertion of peripheral nerves is avoided. On the other hand, the longitudinally aligned substrates found in damaged peripheral nerve (Bands of Büngner) are lost, and the cells also lack contact with a stable matrix. This could induce anoikis (Frisch and Ruoslahti, 1997) or may make the cells more vulnerable to attack from debris-clearing cells such as macrophages or microglia.

A rat model which leads to cyst formation closely mirrors many human injuries. This type of model is currently being investigated for the feasibility of cellular transplantation by a number of groups. Martin and colleagues (1996) used Schwann cell suspensions in the lesion site, not principally to induce axons to regenerate, but to prevent further axonal or cellular loss. Their results showed that survival of Schwann cells varied depending upon the time of injection; cell survival was better if cells were injected immediately or 10 days after injury than at 3 days after lesioning. Possible interaction with toxic metabolites and the presence or absence of appropriate neurotrophins or cytokines were suggested as reasons for cell loss. Another advantage of the immediate injection of Schwann cells was to decrease the astrogliotic scar; later transplants did not reduce this scar (Martin et al., 1996). The grafts at 0 and 10 days injection were invaded by numerous axons, with most originating from the nearby dorsal roots; no regeneration of corticospinal or monoaminergic tracts was seen. Schwann cell transplantation into a cavity resulting from a photochemical lesion is discussed below.

VI. SCHWANN CELL/MATRIX TRANSPLANTATION INTO THE SPINAL CORD

In the spinal cord, limited work has been done on the transplantation of Schwann cells in suspension, in contrast to transplantation in association with matrices. Strategies to promote axonal regeneration across spinal cord transections have involved grafting a number of scaffolds, including highly orientated growth promoting substrates such as matrix bridges, carbon filaments (Khan et al., 1991; Onifer et al., 1997), collagen (Kuhlengel et al., 1990; Paino and Bunge, 1991, Paino et al., 1994), and Matrigel (Xu et al., 1995a,b, 1997; Chen et al., 1996; Oudega et al., 1997).

Bridges of cultured Schwann cells have been used successfully to join two completely separated spinal cord stumps (Xu et al., 1997; see also Xu et al., 1995a). These grafts were comprised of a mixture of Matrigel (which contains extracellular matrix molecules such as laminin, collagen IV, entactin and heparan sulphate proteoglycan) and cultured Schwann cells derived from adult rat peripheral nerve (see above); 1990±594 myelinated axons and eight times more nonmyelinated axons were found inside these grafts (Xu et al., 1997). Control grafts containing no Schwann cells contained very few myelinated and unmyelinated axons. Limited growth of brainstem neurons (serotonergic and noradrenergic) into the Schwann cell grafts was observed by immunostaining. The Schwann cell grafts did support regeneration of descending and ascending axons (from spinal and sensory neurons), but no corticospinal fibers were seen. This result was similar to that seen by Martin and colleagues (1991).

In addition to the complete transection model, further studies using matrices made of Matrigel or fibrin glue have been explored in a lateral hemisection model of spinal cord injury (Xu et al., 1999; Bamber et al., 1998). The hemisection was at T8 and the right half of the spinal cord was removed for 2.5 mm. A 1 mm diameter tube containing Schwann cells was implanted into the lesion area and the dura was closed. A mean axonal count of 1,000 fibers was found with approximately 9 times more unmyelinated axons. Propriospinal, sensory and some brainstem neurons had projected into the graft and, significantly, some axons had reentered the distal spinal cord for distances up to 3.5 mm. One notable difference from the complete transection model was the return of cerebrospinal fluid circulation due to the repair of the dural covering. Also, there was less damage to the vertebral column in the hemisection model.

Recently, Bamber and colleagues (1998) have used fibrin instead of Matrigel in the same hemisection/tube model. Fibrin has the advantage in that the content is known, compared with the complexity of the Matrigel mixture. The amount of astrocytic gliosis appeared attenuated at the host-graft interfaces after one month and neurofilament positive axons were present in the graft; whether axonal growth is increased through these interfaces remains to be determined. Fibrin may be used as a delivery system for neurotrophic factors; NT-3 mixed into the fibrin appeared to stabilize the grafts, promoting increased axonal ingrowth. Further exploration of the application of fibrin needs to be done because the grafts did not appear to be as stable as the Matrigel (Bamber et al., 1998; NI Bamber and XM Xu, personal communication).

Previous studies of similar lesions to the spinal cord have also utilized Schwann cells in either a polycarbonate tube (Montgomery et al., 1996) or associated with the collagen matrix used as a growth substratum for the cultured cells (Kuhlengel., 1990; Paino and Bunge, 1991, Paino et al., 1994). The polycarbonate tube used by Montgomery and colleagues (1996) to house cultured Schwann cells was transplanted into the dorsal half of the spinal cord. Axons were seen at all time points studied (1 week – 2 months), grew in a longitudinal direction, and were ensheathed and myelinated by the transplanted Schwann cells. Cultured Schwann cells accompanying cultured sensory neurons were placed into lesioned neonatal spinal cord (Kuhlengel et al., 1990). The collagen coated Nitex filters carrying the DRG/SC implants were placed into the aspirated dorsal columns of the spinal cord immediately or 5 days after injury. DRG/SC implants became well vascularized, and implant survival was better at immediate implantation than 5 days later. Electron microscopy revealed astrocytes populating the implant/cord junction zone and some had migrated into the implant. Schwann cells were associated with non-myelinated and myelinated axons in the implants. Neuronatomical tracing for CST neurons using WGA/HRP revealed that labeled fibers were not present in the implant but were present and well fasciculated just beneath in the gray matter.

Paino and colleagues (1994) also used Schwann cells derived from cultured dorsal root ganglion preparations. Instead of Nitex filters, the Schwann cells, implanted either elongated and associated with their extracellular matrix, or dissociated and without matrix, were rolled in polymerized collagen to form an implant 4-6mm long. This was grafted into a photochemical lesion of the dorsal columns (Bunge et al., 1994) at 5 or 28 days after lesioning. At 14, 28, and 90 days and 4 and 6 months after grafting, animals were analyzed histologically with silver and toluidine blue stains and electron microscopy. Numerous unmyelinated and myelinated axons were seen at 28 days in most grafts; the number of myelinated axons ranged from 517-3,214. Typical Schwann cell ensheathment and myelination were present in the grafts. Dissociated Schwann cell grafts performed as well as the Schwann cell + extracellular matrix grafts. The grafts that were implanted later (28 days) seemed to be as successful if not more so than those grafted at 5 days postlesion. No axons were seen in collagen grafts lacking Schwann cells.

VII. HUMAN SCHWANN CELL TRANSPLANTATION INTO THE SPINAL CORD

In addition to transplantation of rat Schwann cells purified from adult nerves, Schwann cells dissociated, expanded and purified from adult human donors have been transplanted into the injured spinal cord of an immunodeficient rat (Nude rat) (Guest et al., 1997a,b). These Schwann cells were grafted with Matrigel inside a PAN/PVC polymer channel or without the channel. The human Schwann cells were found to be as effective as rat Schwann cells. The improved regenerative response found was related to the use of the nude rat rather than to the Fischer rat strain previously used. (This also raises the possibility of better regeneration when the inflammatory response is delayed or minimized.) Schwann cell survival, as demonstrated by Hoechst dye labeling, was good (40-45 days). The number of axons found in the graft was 1442±514 myelinated axons (Guest et al., 1997a). Serotonergic and noradrenergic axons were seen within the grafts but not reentering the distal spinal cord, although tracing revealed fiber growth into the distal cord. Behavioral tests, the inclined plane and open field locomotion tests (Basso et al., 1995), were also carried out; there was a modest but statistically significant improvement in both when Schwann cells were present in the grafts. In a few animals there was evidence of some form of contact placing response but due to the lack of tracing evidence of corticospinal tract regrowth the authors proposed that local neuronal circuitry was involved (Guest et al., 1997a). In summary, the human Schwann cell/nude rat model was more effective than the Fischer rat model in stimulating fiber growth into the distal cord and eliciting a response from brainstem neurons, particularly raphe and coeruleus, despite the distant thoracic placement of the graft.

VIII. COMBINATION OF SCHWANN CELL TRANSPLANTS WITH OTHER STRATEGIES

Schwann cell grafts placed into thoracic injuries of the Fischer rat spinal cord, as evident from the results above, do not elicit a regenerative axonal response from brainstem or cortical neurons, and do not promote axonal growth out of the graft. Additional strategies, therefore, will be required to achieve these goals. Chen et al. (1996) combined the administratioan of the steroid drug, methylprednisolone, with Schwann cell transplantation into the thoracic cord. With intravenous methylprednisolone, the Schwann cell bridge contained an average of 3,237 myelinated axons plus more numerous unmyelinated axons. Brainstem neurons were observed to respond to this treatment paradigm with a mean of 57 neurons that extended axons into the grafts and serotonergic and noradrenergic axons were found 2-2.5 mm into the graft. Also, a modest number of axons were found to have grown through the graft and into the host distal cord only when methylprednisolone had been administered. Methylprednisolone appeared to have reduced secondary tissue loss after the initial injury.

A second therapeutic treatment added to Schwann cell grafts was the addition of neurotrophic factors (Xu et al.,1995b). Neurotrophins have a multitude of functions, among them supporting neuronal survival and axonal extension (Lindsay et al., 1994). Xu and colleagues (1995b) used two neurotrophins, brain-derived neurotrophic factor (BDNF) and neurotrophin –3 (NT-3), delivered via an Alzet pump attached to the distal end of a capped PAN/PVC channel housing the Schwann cell graft. The neurotrophins were delivered for 14 days and the rats were maintained for an additional 14 days. A mean of 1,523±292 myelinated axons was present in the Schwann cell/neurotrophin grafts and retrogradely labeled neurons were present throughout the proximal cord (967±104). Retrograde tracing from the Schwann cell/neurotrophin grafts in the thoracic cord also labeled neurons in a number of brainstem nuclei, with 67% of these being in vestibular nuclei. The mean number of labeled brainstem neurons in the Schwann cell/neurotrophin group (92) contrasted with the control Schwann cell/vehicle group (6). The results showed that administration of neurotrophins in combination with Schwann cell/Matrigel grafts increased propriospinal axon regeneration and also, more significantly, elicited growth from distant supraspinal neuronal populations.

Two further neurotrophic factors were analyzed for their ability to enhance regeneration in the PAN/PVC channel/Schwann cell-Matrigel grafts/complete transection paradigm (Oudega et al., 1997). Insulin-like growth factor-I (IGF-I) and platelet derived growth factor (PDGF) together have been shown to promote axonal regeneration in the PNS (Wells et al., 1994). *In vitro* data have also shown recently that IGF-I is a survival factor for Schwann cells (Syroid et al., 1999). Four weeks after implantation, electron microscopic analysis showed that the addition of IGF-I and PDGF resulted in an increase in the myelinated:unmyelinated fiber ratio from 1:7 to 1:3 in the Schwann cell graft and, additionally, in the myelin thickness (2-fold). Importantly, overall fiber regeneration was diminished by 63%

by the addition of IGF-I and PDGF. The authors postulated that this reduction may have been caused by the increase of tissue cavitation in the proximal spinal cord stumps. These results indicate that careful choice of growth factor administration is needed to avoid deleterious effects on fiber regeneration and the integrity of host spinal cord tissue.

Further exploration of neurotrophin administration has involved altering the Schwann cell itself by viral vectors to deliver a gene to encode BDNF (Menei et al., 1998) and nerve growth factor (NGF) (Tuszynski et al., 1998) and then transplanting these genetically altered cells into the injured rat spinal cord. Menei and colleagues (1998) used a retroviral vector carrying the sequence for human pre-proBDNF cDNA to infect primary Schwann cells derived from adult rat peripheral nerve. These cells after infection and appropriate selection for the gene produced 23ng/24 hours/million cells BDNF *in vitro* as tested by ELISA. The infected Schwann cells were transplanted into the completely transected rat spinal cord (T8) at the lesion site and as a 5 mm long trail in the cord distal to the transection. More serotonergic and noradrenergic positive fibers were seen beyond the transection site in the infected Schwann cell transplanted cords compared with the normal non-infected Schwann cell transplants. Fast blue, injected 5 mm below the lesion (at the distal end of the trail), labeled as many as 135 neurons in the brainstem (mostly in reticular and raphe nuclei); normal Schwann cell transplants traced in the same way revealed a maximum of 22 labeled neurons mostly in vestibular nuclei. These results indicated increased supraspinal axonal growth across a spinal cord transection site and into the distal cord when BDNF was administered via Schwann cells. There was a lack of Po staining around the axons associated with the BDNF-secreting Schwann cells. The authors proposed that the BDNF may have maintained the Schwann cells in a less differentiated state, one that promotes axonal regeneration rather than myelination. One could speculate that delay in myelination may be a welcome defect if the cell is producing regenerative molecules instead of inhibitory myelin.

Tuszynski and colleagues (1998) have produced Schwann cells secreting the human form of NGF; the NGF levels as measured by ELISA were 1.5±0.1ng NGF/ml/24 hours/million cells. After grafting the NGF-producing Schwann cells into the intact spinal cord, they were penetrated by numerous sensory axons originating primarily from the dorsolateral fasciculus, whereas non-infected Schwann cell grafts did not elicit this effect. Over time, the Schwann cell grafts secreting NGF supported growth of tyrosine hydroxylase and dopamine-β-hydroxylase immunostained labeled axons of putative coerulospinal origin, unlike control grafts. Myelination was present in either non-modified or modified NGF-secreting Schwann cell grafts.

Clearly, these new methods to increase the potency of Schwann cell grafts by either genetically modifying them with viral vectors or adding other therapeutic agents, for example, have proved to be important in stimulating more axons to regenerate, including those from distant supraspinal neurons. One should consider altering the host spinal cord terrain after injury as well so as to improve regeneration and eventually function. Studies in our laboratory have shown the presence of proteoglycans at the interfaces of Schwann cell grafts placed into a complete transection of the spinal cord (Fig. 2) (Plant et al., 1998b). Interestingly, the level of CSPG expression as visualized by use of the antibody, CS56, is increased more at the distal host/Schwann cell interface than at the proximal interface. The Schwann cells at the proximal interface show little or no expression whereas, in the distal-most portion of the grafts and at the distal interface, they show substantial expression of this molecule. One can speculate that this may be a contributing factor to axon failure to exit from the Schwann cell grafts into the host distal cord as shown in previous Schwann cell graft models (Xu et al., 1997). We have attempted to overcome this inhibitory barrier to axonal growth by transplantating ensheathing glia into areas near the Schwann cell/host interfaces (Ramón-Cueto et al., 1998). The results of this work will be discussed in the latter part of this chapter.

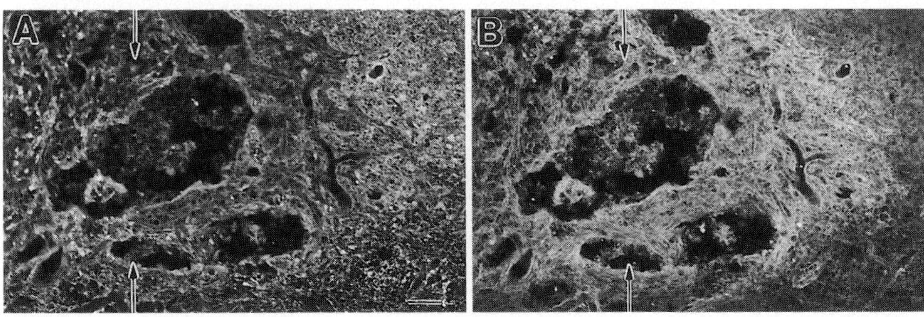

Figure 2 Immunostaining for chondroitin sulfate proteoglycan (CSPG) at the distal Schwann cell graft - host spinal cord interface. A, GFAP staining of astrocytes at the interface (arrows) and (B) the high expression of CSPG in the same section. Bar: 100μm.

IX. OLFACTORY ENSHEATHING GLIA

Olfactory neurons have the unique property of extending their axons into the olfactory bulb to properly connect with CNS target neurons in adult mammals (Graziadei and Monti Graziadei, 1978, 1979, 1980, 1986; Monti Graziadei and Graziadei, 1979, 1992; Monti Graziadei et al., 1980; Barber, 1982; Doucette et al., 1983; Cancalon, 1987; Costanzo and Graziadei, 1987; Doucette, 1990; Wellis and Scott, 1991; Oakley and Riddle, 1992; Gong et al., 1994; Roskams et al., 1996; Munirathinam et al., 1997). The ability of these axons to elongate through the CNS milieu appears related to the presence of olfactory ensheathing glia (OEG) which enfold growing axons, perhaps isolating them from the nonpermissive CNS environment (Barber and Lindsay, 1982; Doucette, 1984, 1986, 1990, 1991, 1993a; Raisman, 1985; Valverde and Lopez-Mascaraque, 1991; Pixley, 1992a; Ramón-Cueto and Valverde, 1995; Ramón-Cueto and Avila, 1998). During the past years, several groups have focused their attention on OEG because they are located in a region of the mammalian CNS where axonal growth occurs throughout life, and also because these cells appear responsible for the growth-promoting properties of the olfactory bulb. Moreover, OEG are present where axons leave the PNS to enter central nervous tissue. In this section, we present an overview of OEG features related to axonal regeneration, the methods used to obtain this unique glial type, and the repair properties that OEG have promoted in different spinal cord injury models.

A. OEG properties related to promotion of axonal regeneration

In order to regenerate, injured neurons need to be supplied with the appropriate combination of survival and growth-promoting factors, as well as with blockers of environmental inhibitory molecules (Fawcett and Keynes, 1990; Bovolenta et al., 1992; Schwab et al., 1993; Silver, 1994; Olson, 1997; Bregman, 1998). OEG seem to be a source of trophic factors, express adhesion molecules on their plasma membranes, and possess the ability to promote neuronal survival and ensheath and myelinate axons after their purification from olfactory structures (reviewed in Ramón-Cueto and Valverde, 1995; Ramón-Cueto and Avila, 1998). OEG produce platelet-derived growth factor (Kott et al., 1994), neuropeptide Y (Ubink et al., 1994), and S100 (Barnett et al., 1993; Gong et al., 1994, 1996; Cummings and Brunjes, 1995; Doucette and Devon, 1995; Franceschini and Barnett, 1996) which are known growth and survival factors. Furthermore, evidence suggests that these cells might secrete nerve growth factor (NGF), brain-derived neurotrophic factor (BDNF), neurotrophin-3 (NT-3), and neurotrophin-4 (NT-4) (discussed in Ramon-Cueto and Avila, 1998). These cells also contain the low affinity p75 NGF receptor (NGFR) in their plasma membranes (Vickland et al., 1991; Ramón-Cueto and Nieto-Sampedro, 1992; Ramón-Cueto et al., 1993; Doucette, 1993b; Barnett et al., 1993; Goodman et al., 1993; Turner and Perez-Polo, 1993, 1994; Miwa et al., 1993; Gong et al., 1994, 1996; Franceschini and Barnett, 1996; Sonigra et al.,

1996) that might favor the action of secreted neurotrophins on neurons. In addition to neurotrophins, OEG express L1, N-CAM, PSA-N-CAM, laminin, fibronectin, and glia-derived nexin (Liesi, 1985; ; Reinhardt et al., 1988; Key and Akeson, 1990; Pixley, 1992, 1996; Ramón-Cueto and Nieto-Sampedro, 1992 Barnett et al., 1993; Goodman et al., 1993; Chuah and Au, 1993; Franceschini and Barnett, 1996; Doucette, 1996; Kafitz et al., 1997; Miragell et al., 1998) which are adhesion- and neurite-promoting molecules known to be involved in axonal elongation (Bixby et al., 1988; Kleitman et al., 1988; Luckenbill-Edds, 1997). These factors are likely related to the ability of OEG to support neuronal survival and neurite elongation in culture (Goodman et al., 1993; Ramón-Cueto et al., 1993; Kafitz and Greer, 1999; Sonigra et al., 1999) and axonal regeneration within the CNS after transplantation (see below). OEG retain the ability to enfold neurites when they are cocultured with olfactory neurons (Ramon-Cueto et al., 1993).

OEG are unique cells in many ways. In addition to the survival, growth, and neurite-promoting properties, they present features not exhibited by other glial types (reviewed in Ramón-Cueto and Valverde, 1995; Ramón-Cueto and Avila, 1998). Furthermore, the monoclonal antibody, 1.9.E., which reacts with an as yet unidentified protein of the OEG cytoskeleton, does not recognize any molecule of adult CNS and PNS glial cells (Fig. 3; Heredia et al., 1998). All available data, therefore, strongly support the idea that OEG belong to a different class of glia and cannot be included within one of the known glial groups.

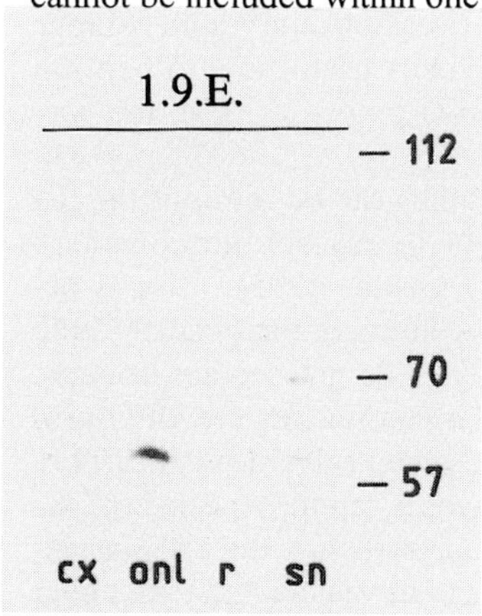

Figure 3 Western blot showing electrophoretic bands recognized by antibody 1.9E. in tissue samples from different adult rat nervous tissue regions. OEG are exclusively localized in the olfactory nerve and glomerular layers (onl). This monoclonal antibody immunoreacted with one band of an apparent molecular weight of 60 KDa in the lane containing these two olfactory bulb layers. Immunohistochemistry revealed that this is a molecule contained in the cytoskeleton of OEG. 1.9.E. did not recognize any band in neural tissue containing other glial types or neurons, such as cortex (cx), remaining layers of the olfactory bulb (r), and sciatic nerves (sn) (from the work of Heredia et al., 1998).

B. Methods to obtain and culture OEG

The extraordinary features exhibited by OEG make these cells very attractive candidates to repair CNS injuries. Hence, the development of a reliable and easy method to obtain large amounts of pure OEG appears necessary to generate adequate cell numbers for transplantation into the injured CNS. Different techniques are used to culture OEG from embryonic, neonatal, and adult rodent olfactory tissue. The morphological and immunocytochemical features exhibited by OEG *in vitro* are very variable depending upon the age of tissue donor, culture conditions (culture medium, purity of the cultures, etc.), and time in culture. Because we have recently reviewed the phenotypic properties displayed by OEG under different experimental conditions (Ramón-Cueto and Avila, 1998), we will not discuss them in this chapter, but we will outline the different methods used to obtain OEG, emphasizing those more suitable to provide cells for CNS transplantation.

1. OEG cultured from embryonic rodent olfactory tissue

Dissociated OEG cultures may be obtained from the olfactory bulbs of E14-E16 mouse and E18 rat embryos (Doucette, 1993b: Fracek et al., 1994; Doucette and Devon, 1995). When cultures are gotten from whole olfactory bulbs, however, they contain a mixed population of cells which includes neurons, astroglia and OEG (Fracek et al., 1994). The cultures can be maintained for up to 120 days in serum-containing medium, and synapse formation between olfactory bulb neurons can be observed. These olfactory bulb cultures provide a useful tool to perform longevity studies which could include changes in OEG properties or in the way that OEG associate with axons over time in culture.

Pure OEG cultures from embryonic olfactory bulbs can be set up if the tissue is obtained from the olfactory nerve layers of 14-16 day-old mouse and 18 day-old rat embryos (Doucette, 1993b; Doucette and Devon, 1995). This is because OEG are exclusively localized in the nerve fiber layers of the olfactory bulb and, moreover, at this developmental stage, these layers do not contain neurons, are almost devoid of astrocytes, and the main cellular constituents are OEG progenitors (Doucette, 1989; Marin-Padilla and Amieva, 1989; Valverde et al., 1992). To prepare pure OEG cultures, the olfactory nerve layer is carefully peeled off the bulb primordium and, after mechanical dissociation of the tissue, the cell suspension is plated onto glass coverslips. These cultures can be maintained with either serum-containing or chemically defined medium for four weeks. Preparation of pure OEG embryonic cultures appears very useful to study the normal developmental changes and differentiation of OEG, either in culture or after transplantation, as well as to repair specific CNS lesions (see below).

For those *in vitro* studies in which the integrity of the olfactory tissue is required, either organotypic slice cultures (Gong et al., 1996) or explant cultures (Chuah and Au, 1991) from embryonic olfactory epithelium may be prepared. Both of these groups used Sprague-Dawley rat embryos at a similar developmental stage (E13 and E14, respectively). To obtain organotypic cultures, the rostral portion of the embryonic head was embedded in agarose, 400um sections cut, the olfactory epithelium dissected, and the slices placed on Millicell-CM membranes (Millipore) coated with type I collagen, laminin, or fibronectin. They used serum-containing and serum-free culture medium; healthier slices with robust neurite outgrowth were obtained when chemically-defined medium was supplied (Gong et al., 1996). The olfactory epithelium was obtained by dissecting the olfactory mucosa, treating it with trypsin and pancreatin solutions, and then removing the olfactory epithelium from the underlying connective tissue. Olfactory explants were placed onto poly-L-lysine-coated coverslips and grown in serum-containing medium supplemented with a vitamin solution. Under the experimental conditions described above, OEG migrated out of the slices and explants and associated with growing axons. All these culture methods are very useful to study the cellular and molecular bases of OEG migration, neuron-glia interactions, and ensheathment of growing axons.

2. OEG cultures from neonatal rodent olfactory tissue

OEG cultures from neonates can be set up from either olfactory epithelium (Barber and Lindsay, 1982; Chuah and Au, 1991; Pixley, 1992, 1996 or bulb (Barber and Lindsay, 1982; Barnett et al,., 1993; Chuah and Au, 1993; Goodman et al., 1993; Franceschini and Barnett, 1996). From olfactory epithelium, cells can be grown as dissociated neonatal cultures (Barber and Lindsay, 1982; Pixley, 1992, 1996) or explants from juvenile rats (Chuah and Au, 1991). Although the latter protocol was the same as that used to prepare explants from embryos, the extent of survival, neurite outgrowth, OEG migration, and ensheathment of axons was less compared with that of embryonic explants. Dissociated OEG cultures from neonatal olfactory epithelium (Pixley, 1992 1996) and mucosa (Barber and Lindsay, 1982) contain a mixed population of cell types, including olfactory receptor neurons, fibroblasts, chondrocytes and myoepithelial cells as well as OEG. Therefore, these "micro-nose" cultures constitute a better system for the study of cellular interactions during development and maturation than as a source of OEG for transplantation.

Olfactory bulbs from neonates are also a source of OEG (Barber and Lindsay, 1982; Barnett et al., 1993; Chuah and Au, 1993; Goodman et al., 1993; Franceschini and Barnett, 1996). When whole olfactory bulbs are dissociated and placed onto a dish, a culture containing not only OEG but also neurons, astroyctes, oligodendrocytes, and microglia is obtained (Barber and Lindsay, 1982; Goodman et al., 1993). When the olfactory nerve fiber layer of 1-3 day-old rats is dissected and plated, the cultures contain, in addition to OEG, some astrocytes that may proliferate and contaminate the cultures (Chuah and Au, 1991); after birth astrocytes arising from the olfactory ventricle have already started to populate this layer (Doucette, 1989; Marin-Padilla and Amieva, 1989; Valverde et al., 1992).

Barnett et al. (1993) have developed a method to obtain pure OEG cultures from neonatal olfactory bulbs. These authors dissected olfactory bulbs from 7 day-old Sprague-Dawley rats, dissociated the tissue, and incubated the resulting cell suspension with a mixture of 04 and anti-fluorescent secondary antibodies. Immunolabeled cells were purified using a FACStar fluorescence-activated cell sorter and grown in the appropriate medium. Because OEG are 04 positive and GalC negative, sorted cells correspond to OEG. Pure OEG cultures for either *in vitro* or transplantation studies can be set up from neonatal rat olfactory bulbs using this procedure.

3. OEG cultures from adult rat olfactory tissue

Although it is complicated to set up cultures from adult olfactory mucosa, some viable cells can be obtained and their number increased if the cultures are prepared one week after lesioning the olfactory bulb (lesion-induced priming procedure; Barber and Lindsay, 1982). On the other hand, OEG can be cultured easily from adult rat olfactory bulbs (Goodman et al., 1993; Ramón-Cueto et al., 1993; Sonigra et al., 1996). Three different cell types are obtained from adult bulbs: endothelial-like cells, microglia, and OEG (Ramón-Cueto et al., 1993). The olfactory nerve fiber layer is dissected from the rest of the bulb, the pia mater completely removed, and the tissue obtained dissociated and seeded onto poly-L-lysine-coated flasks as a cell suspension. Dissection of the nerve fiber layer and removal of meninges are important steps because the former diminishes the number of microglial cells that would come from the other bulb layers, and the latter avoids fibroblast contamination from the pia mater. These non-pure OEG cultures can be maintained for several weeks *in vitro.* However, the rate of division of endothelial cells is higher than that of OEG, and the former cell type very rapidly overruns the cultures.

OEG purification is an important step, especially if the final aim is to use OEG for transplantation studies. OEG can be separated from the other cell types and grown in pure populations in culture (Fig. 4; Ramón-Cueto and Nieto-Sampedro, 1994; Ramón-Cueto et al., 1998).

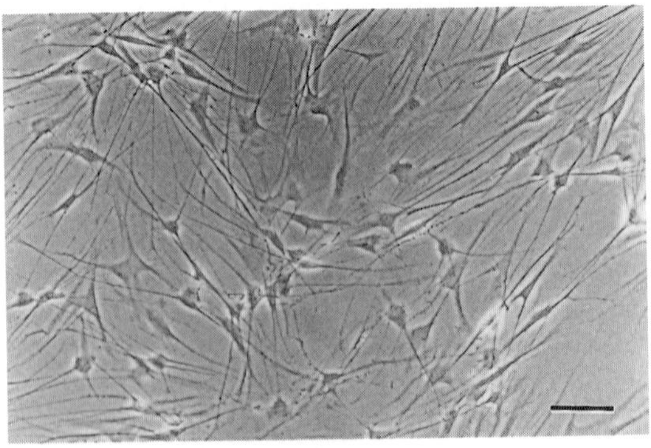

Figure 4 Phase contrast micrograph of a pure OEG culture from adult rat olfactory bulb. Bar: 50μm.

Purification from adult rat olfactory bulb cultures can be achieved by immunoaffinity, using an antibody against p75 NGFR. Seven to ten days after plating the primary cultures, cells are detached from the flasks and resuspended in serum-containing medium. They are plated next onto petri dishes, pretreated first with biotinylated anti-mouse IgG antibody and then with supernatants of cultured 192 hybridoma cells containing anti-p75 NGFR antibody. Because OEG are the only cell type in the primary cultures expressing p75 NGFR in their plasma membranes, all cells attached to the surface are OEG. Accordingly, cells unbound to the antibody-treated surface are discarded and bound OEG are detached with a cell scraper. Purified OEG are replated onto poly-L-lysine-treated flasks and grown in serum-containing medium supplemented with forskolin and pituitary extract. This protocol leads to 98% pure OEG cultures after 15 days *in vitro*, when the cells can be used for transplantation into the injured spinal cord (see below).

4. Generation of OEG cell lines

OEG immortalization provides a useful technique to obtain, in a short period of time, large numbers of OEG for either *in vitro* studies or CNS transplantation. OEG from either neonatal or adult olfactory bulbs have been immortalized following different procedures (Goodman et al., 1993; Franceschini and Barnett, 1996; Sonigra et al., 1996). Retroviral infection of neonatal and adult olfactory bulb cultures, using defective retroviruses encoding wild type (pZIPTEX) or mutant (U19) SV40 large T-antigens, led to several astrocyte lines and one neonatal and three adult OEG lines (Goodman et al., 1993). OEG lines exhibited similar morphological and immunocytochemical features as OEG and were able to support neurite outgrowth when cocultured with neurons. Franceschini and Barnett (1996) used the retrovirus containing the temperature-sensitive mutant genes of the SV40 large T-antigen to infect and immortalize pure OEG 04 positive FACS-sorted cultures from neonatal bulbs. The advantage of this immortalization procedure is that the gene product functions at the permissive temperature (33°C) and it is inactive at 39°C; large numbers of OEG can be obtained in culture at 33°C and cell division stopped at the nonpermissive temperature. Furthermore, these OEG lines can be used for transplantation because the higher body temperature curbs cell division. With this procedure, the authors constructed a clonal OEG line which shared growth, survival, morphological and antigenic phenotypes with sorted OEG. In addition, they have transplanted this OEG line to repair demyelinating CNS lesions (Franklin et al., 1996).

OEG immortalization also can be achieved spontaneously without retroviral infection (Sonigra et al., 1996). The cell line of Rolf B1.T was obtained from primary cultures of the intracranial portion of the olfactory nerve. After 19 passages of the primary cultures, clones were obtained by limiting dilution of the cells. Rolf B1.T was grown in serum-containing medium for 18 months. During this period, the growth rate was maintained and the cells did not change their phenotypic features. The properties of this line, as well as their ability to support neurite outgrowth, closely resemble those of OEG. Interestingly, the Rolf B1.T line does not grow in semi-solid agar, indicating that the cells did not transform and that they can be safely used for CNS transplantation.

C. OEG transplantation into the adult rat spinal cord

Although all the procedures outlined above provide useful methods to obtain OEG, the most suitable techniques to obtain OEG for transplantation into the CNS should be those yielding pure OEG cultures. There are three methods yielding pure OEG cultures from embryonic (Doucette, 1993b; Doucette and Devon, 1995), neonatal (Barnett et al., 1993), and adult (Ramón-Cueto and Nieto-Sampedro, 1994; Ramón-Cueto et al., 1998) rat olfactory bulbs, respectively. All of these were used successfully to repair specific lesions of the adult CNS in which promotion of axonal regeneration or myelination was the goal (Ramón-Cueto and Nieto-Sampedro, 1994; Franklin et al., 1996; Smale et al., 1996; Ramón-Cueto et al., 1998). In this section, we describe the repair properties of transplanted OEG in the damaged spinal cord, when different lesion models are used.

1. Promotion of axonal regeneration

a. After specific tract lesions. Two lesion models have been used to test the ability of OEG from adult rats to promote the regeneration of selectively injured fibers in the adult rat spinal cord (Ramón-Cueto and Nieto-Sampedro, 1994; Li et al., 1997, 1998; Navarro et al., 1999). In one of the models, either a rhizotomy of one thoracic root (Ramón-Cueto and Nietro-Sampedro, 1994) or multiple lumbar rhizotomies (Navarro et al., 1999) were performed, and pure OEG were transplanted at the dorsal root entry zone where the roots had entered before transection. Roots were anastomosed to the cord. After OEG transplantation, regrowing dorsal root axons were able to cross the root-cord transitional zone, enter and regenerate within an otherwise inhibitory environment of the spinal cord. Regenerating sensory axons elongated through the spinal cord gray matter, reaching the ipsilateral and contralateral laminae that they innervate under normal conditions but not the ventral horn and the dorsal columns (Ramón-Cueto and Nieto-Sampedro, 1994). OEG appeared to migrate from the injection site and associate with the growing axons, possibly providing the appropriate conditions for their regeneration (Ramón-Cueto and Nieto-Sampedro, 1994; Navarro et al., 1999). In addition, recent experiments revealed that regenerated dorsal root axons were functionally active because specific lost bladder reflexes were restored (Navarro et al., 1999).

In a different injury model (Li et al., 1997, 1998), focal stereotaxic electrolytic lesions were performed in the corticospinal tract on one side and between cervical segments 1 and 2. Cells from cultures of adult rat olfactory nerve and glomerular layers, containing OEG, endothelial cells, and microglia (Ramón-Cueto et al., 1993), were transplanted into the lesioned area (Li et al., 1997, 1998). Using this experimental paradigm, injured corticospinal axons regenerated and crossed the lesioned area after transplantation. Cells migrated from the transplantation site and were found aligned along the tract axis, making direct contact with the membrane of growing axons. As in the other model, the authors reported a recovery of lost function after OEG transplantation (Li et al., 1997). These results indicate that OEG transplants not only provide axons with the conditions needed for regeneration, but they also may allow axons to find and synapse with appropriate target neurons and thus restore function.

b. After complete spinal cord transection. A complete spinal cord thoracic segment (T9) was removed and the gap was bridged with a Schwann cell-filled polymer guidance channel (Xu et al., 1995a, 1997). Although this type of graft successfully joins both cord stumps, sustaining axonal growth through it, axons fail to exit and do not invade more distal or rostral cord locations (see above). A suspension of pure OEG cells from adult olfactory bulb cultures (Ramón-Cueto et al., 1993) was transplanted into both spinal cord stumps near the ends of the channel with two main purposes; first, to determine if regenerating axons inside the channels were able to cross the interface and regenerate through the CNS environment of the spinal cord stumps; and second, to determine whether more axons and other axonal types regenerate across the bridge. Six weeks after OEG transplantation, profuse axonal growth of axons inside the channels was observed. Strikingly, OEG promoted long distance axonal regeneration of ascending fibers (2.5 cm) and descending fibers (1.5 cm, serotonergic, Fig. 5) in both spinal cord stumps, respectively. Regenerating axons and transplanted OEG were found in both the Schwann cell graft inside the channel and the connective tissue surrounding the channel. Fibers invaded the glial scars formed at the transection site and elongated within the white and grey matter of the spinal cord stumps. OEG migrated from the transplantation sites through the inhibitory CNS environment and appeared to accompany the growing axons. Thus, transplants of pure OEG enabled regenerating axons to exit the Schwann cell grafts and enter the spinal cord and promoted long distance axonal regeneration in the completely transected adult rat spinal cord (Ramón-Cueto et al., 1998).

2. Repair of demyelinated spinal cord lesions

During the past years, two groups have transplanted OEG into the demyelinated spinal cord with the goal of myelinating denuded axons (Franklin et al., 1996; Imaizumi et al., 1998). The rationale was that *in vitro* experiments had shown that OEG were capable of myelinating axons when cocultured with dorsal root ganglia neurons (Devon and Doucette, 1992, 1995). In both studies, the dorsal columns of adult rats were demyelinated by X-irradiation followed by focal ethidium bromide injections into the irradiated zone. In the first study, Franklin et al. (1996) transplanted a clonal OEG cell line obtained from pure OEG cultures from neonatal olfactory bulbs (Franceschini and Barnett, 1996; see above). These authors observed that the transplanted OEG line remyelinated dorsal column axons and that the cells exhibited many of the features of Schwann cells myelinating CNS axons. In the second and more recent study (Imaizumi et al., 1998), the authors transplanted OEG obtained from the olfactory fiber layer of neonatal rat olfactory bulbs

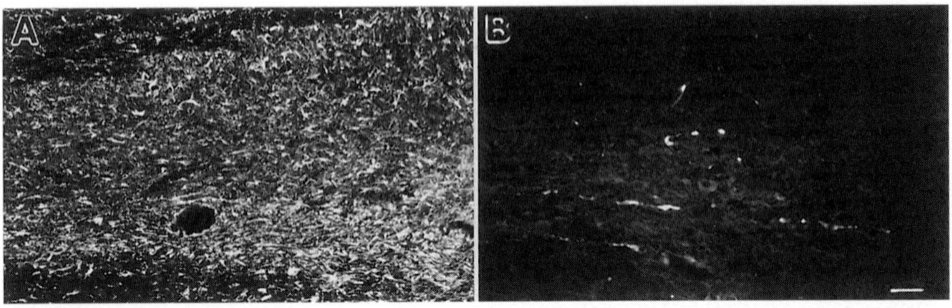

Figure 5 Long distance axonal regeneration of descending serotonergic fibers in the transected adult rat spinal cord in the presence of OEG transplants. A, B. Adjacent sections (saggital of the distal spinal cord stump immunolabeled with anti-glial fibrillary acidic protein (GFAP) (A) and serotonin (B). A, GFAP immunoreactive astrocytes in the same spinal cord region as in B. B, Serotonergic fibers regenerating through the lateral region of the gray commisure (lamina X) in the distal cord stump, at 1 cm from the transection site. Bar: 100μm.

(Chuah and Au, 1993). Similar to the previous study, Schwann cell-like remyelination of dorsal column axons was observed. In addition, OEG migrated from the injection site and enhanced conduction velocity and frequency-response properties of the axons they myelinated. Transplants obtained from adult rat olfactory bulbs, not purified for OEG, also led to myelination of regenerated corticospinal axons (Li et al., 1998). The type of myelin illustrated in the Li et al. (1998) experimental paradigm was of the peripheral type. In none of these studies were the OEG labeled before transplantation to demonstrate conclusively that the transplanted OEG were the myelin-forming cells.

X. FUTURE DIRECTIONS

How can the transplantation of Schwann cells be improved to provide a better environment for CNS axons to grow in the spinal cord, reconnect to correct target sites, and lead to improved sensory and motor function for the recipient? One improvement in the transplantation of Schwann cells may include provision of an environment for their optimal integration into the CNS and improvement in their growth promoting phenotype. In accordance with this the host CNS needs to be more permissive for the implant to adhere, or to prevent or reduce any subsequent inflammatory and rejection reactions. A field of study, relatively new to the CNS, is the use of biomaterials or biomolecules to enhance regeneration. The use of polymer tubes such as the PAN/PVC tube (Xu et al., 1995a; Chen et al., 1996; Xu et al., 1997) to deliver Schwann cells to a lesion in the spinal cord has some difficulties, particularly when kept in the animal for extended periods of time such as 3 months. The ends of the tubes can repeatedly irritate the host cord tissue and potentially cause increased gliosis, inflammation, cavitation, and even disruption of the host-graft junction, thereby diminishing growth (Guest et al., 1997a). Because the Schwann cell/Matrigel graft constricts over time, its surface area becomes smaller than that of the inner diameter of the tube (2.6 mm). This reduces the size of the area for axons to enter and grow along the entire length of the implant.

Another biopolymer recently tried in our laboratory, in collaboration with Dr. Jean Marie-Parel's group at the Bascom Palmer Eye Institute, University of Miami, has utilized a mixture of two polymers, polylactic and polyglycolic acids, to form a tube which can disappear over time. Gautier and colleagues (1998) studied their *in vitro* and *in vivo* degradability as well as their effects on rat Schwann cells *in vitro* and in spinal cord tissue *in vivo.* The aim was to ascertain the feasibility of producing biocompatible implants containing Schwann cells that could be resorbed by the body over time, leaving only the Schwann cells behind. These polymers could lead also to lessened scarring by way of their eventual resorption. This study provided the first evidence that this technique could be used in the mammalian spinal cord and be well tolerated.

Hydrogel based, three-dimensional matrices in neural tissue repair and regeneration is another avenue of research currently being studied. Hydrogels can provide multiple shapes and the appropriate physical and elastic requirements that can mimic those found in CNS tissue. When produced with a highly porous structure and after collagen I (Woerly and Marchand 1990; Plant et al., 1995) or collagen IV (Plant et al., 1998a) infiltration, they are capable of supporting and orientating new tissue growth, thereby facilitating tissue reconstruction and regeneration. Additionally, these compounds can be prepared with incorporated sequences found in extracellular matrix macromolecules such as the RGD sequence (Plant et al., 1997). When transplanted into the CNS, these hydrogels initiated axonal regeneration and continued to support host glial survival.

A recent paper by Woerly and colleagues (1996) went one step further in this biotechnology by producing a type of biohybrid polymer incorporating hydrogel mechanical characteristics with the growth promoting ability of Schwann cells; Schwann cells were able to survive, although in small numbers. This technology could lead to organized channel microstructures containing matrix, integrins, growth factors and cells for reconstruction after spinal cord injury. More recent compelling evidence for the use of hydrogels in spinal cord injury has been obtained in the cat (Woerly et al, 1998). The authors describe a new hydrogel based on the polymer, poly[N-(2-hydroxypropyl) methacrylamide] (PHPMA). After 3 months, the hydrogel appropriately bridged the tissue defect and provided a permissive interface with the host tissue which favored host glial cell ingrowth, angiogenesis, and axonal growth within the microstructure of the network. The gels also showed physiological parameters that closely resembled extracellular space characteristics *in vivo*.

We have discussed above the improvement in axonal regeneration when OEG are transplanted into the adult mammalian spinal cord. These cells offer advantages compared with other repair strategies. OEG migrate from the injection sites, associate with growing axons, and accompany them through the inhibitory environment of the glial scar and the white matter (Ramón-Cueto and Nieto-Sampedro, 1994; Li et al., 1997, 1998; Ramón-Cueto et al., 1998). These cells likely provide regenerating axons with an appropriate cocktail of neurite growth-promoting factors for their regeneration and, moreover, may ensheath regenerating axons, isolating them from the non-permissive CNS environment. In addition, transplanted OEG integrate successfully within the host CNS, and neither inflammatory reaction nor a disruption of the spinal cord cytoarchitecture is observed. By comparison, in other repair paradigms, the permissive environment remains at the grafting or injection sites (David and Aguayo, 1981; Kromer and Cornbrooks, 1985; Xu et al., 1995a, 1997; Cheng et al., 1996; Nakahara et al., 1996; Olson, 1997; Menei et al., 1998; Bregman, 1998; Fawcett, 1998). Axons are sequestered within this suportive milieu, cannot exit it, and are thus impeded in reinnervating denervated targets.

Thus, OEG open up the prospect of new therapeutic approaches to treat spinal cord injuries and CNS trauma. These cells may be particularly valuable in combination with other promising repair strategies described elsewhere in this volume, such as blockade of myelin inhibitory molecules (Schwab et al., 1993; Bregman et al., 1995; Dyer et al., 1998; Thallmair et al., 1998), macrophage manipulation (Rapalino et al., 1998), or neurotrophic factor administration (Schnell et al., 1994; Xu et al., 1995b; Grill et al., 1998; Menei et al., 1998). The addition of OEG to Schwann cell bridges placed to span a complete transection gap improved the regenerative response (Ramón-Cueto et al., 1998). In the regeneration studies performed so far in the spinal cord, OEG were obtained from adult donors (Ramón-Cueto and Nieto-Sampedro, 1994; Li et al., 1997, 1998; Ramón-Cueto et al., 1998), suggesting that these cells, as well as Schwann cells, may be candidates for autologous transplantation in the future. More extensive combination strategies need to be devised to achieve better functional recovery, both in acute and chronic injury. It is a time of great promise for spinal cord injury repair. The results of applying advanced tissue culture techniques, developing new biomaterials and anti-rejection drugs, creating new vectors for gene delivery, better understanding the expression of guidance molecules, and exploration of improved neuroprotective compounds will aid in the creation of new and more effective combination strategies to improve the quality of life for spinal cord injured persons.

ACKNOWLEDGMENTS

We thank Charlaine Rowlette for word processing and R Camerena, M Bautista J Belio, and JA Perez for photographic assistance. GWP and MBB are currently funded by American Paralysis Association, NIH NS 09923-28, the Miami Project, NHMRC #9935975 (Australia), the NRP (Western Australia). AR-C is presently supported by CICYT, an institutional grant from Fundacion Ramon Aveces and by Levantina del Calzado s.h.

REFERENCES

Abercrombie M, Johnson ML (1946) Quantitative histology of Wallerian degeneration; Nuclear population in rabbit sciatic nerve. J. Anat 80:37-50.

Acheson A, Barker PA, Alderson RF, Miller FD, Murphy RA (1991) Detection of brain-derived neurotrophic factor-like activity in fibroblasts and Schwann cells: inhibtion by antibodies to NGF. Neuron 7:265-275.

Askansas V, King E, Dalakas, MC, Lawrence JV, Carter LS (1980) Human Schwann cells in tissue culture, histochemical and ultrastructural studies. Arch Neurol 37:329-337

Bamber NI, Li H, Lu X, Aebischer P, Xu XM (1998) Fibrin "Glue" as an alternative matrix for implanting Schwann cells into partially injured adult rat spinal cords. Soc Neurosci Abstr 24:69.

Bandtlow CE, Heumann R, Schwab ME, Thoenen H (1987) Cellular localization of nerve growth factor synthesis by in situ hybridization. EMBO J 6:891-899.

Barber PC (1982) Neurogenesis and regeneration in the primary olfactory pathway of mammals. Bibl. Anat 23:12-25.

Barber PC, Lindsay RM (1982) Schwann cells of the olfactory nerves contain glial fibrillary acidic protein and resemble astrocytes. Neurosci 7:3077-3090.

Barnett SC, Hutchins AM, Noble M (1993) Purification of olfactory nerve ensheathing cells from the olfactory bulb. Dev Biol 155:337-350.

Basso DM, Beattie MS, Bresnahan JC (1995) A sensitive and reliable locomotor rating scale for open field testing in rats. J Neurotrauma 12:1-21.

Bedi KS, Winter J, Berry M, Cohen J (1994) Adult rat dorsal root ganglion neurons extend neurites on predegenerated but not on normal peripheral nerves in vitro. Eur J Neurosci 4: 193-200.

Berry M, Hall SM, Rees L, Gregson N, Sievers J (1988) Response of axons and glia at the site of anastomosis between the optic nerve and cellular or acellular sciatic nerve grafts. J Neurocytol 17: 727-744.

Bixby JL, Lilien J, Reichardt LF (1988) Identification of the major proteins that promote neuronal process outgrowth on Schwann cells in vitro. J Cell Biol 107:352-361.

Boudreau N, Sympson CJ, Werb Z, Bissel MJ (1995) Suppression of ICE and apoptosis in mammary cells by extracellular matrix. Science 267:891-893.

Bovolenta P, Wandosell F, Nieto-Sampedro M (1992) CNS glial scar tissue: a source of molecules which inhibit central neurite outgrowth. Prog Brain Res 94:367-379.

Bradley WG, Asbury AK (1970) Duration of synthesis phase in neurilemma cells in mouse sciatic nerve during degeneration. Exp Neurol 26:275-282.

Bregman BS, Kunkel-Baden E, Schnell L, Dai HN, Gao D, Schwab ME (1995) Recovery from spinal cord injury mediated by antibodies to neurite growth inhibitors. Nature 378:498-501.

Bregman BS (1998) Regeneration in the spinal cord. Curr Opin Neurobiol 8:800-807.

Brockes JP, Fields KP, Raff MC (1979) Studies on cultured rat Schwnn cells. I. Establishment of purified populations from cultures of peripheral nerve. Brain Res 165:105-108.

Brook GA, Lawrence JM, Raisman, G (1993) Morphology and migration of cultured Schwann cells transplanted into the fimbria and hippocampus in adult rats. Glia 9:292-304.

Bunge MB (1993) Schwann cell regulation of exracellular matrix biosynthesis and assembly, In Peripheral Neuropathy, 3rd Edn (Dyck PJ, Thomas PK, Griffin JW, Low PA, Poduslo JF, eds), pp 299-316, WB Saunders, Philadelphia.

Bunge MB (1999) What type of bridges will best promote axonal regeneration across an area of injury in the adult mammalian spinal cord? In: Degeneration and Regeneration in the Nervous System. Saunders N (ed) Harwood Academic Publishers, Berkshire, UK (in press).

Bunge MB, Holets VR, Bates ML, Clarke T, Watson BD (1994) Characterization of photochemically induced spinal cord injury in the rat by light and electron microscopy. Exp Neurol 127: 76-93.

Bunge RP (1975) Changing uses of nerve tissue culture 1950-1975, In The Nervous System vol 1: The Basic Neurosciences (Tower DB, ed), pp 31-42, Raven Press, New York.

Bunge RP, Hopkins JM (1990) The role of peripheral and central neuroglia in neural regeneration in vertebrates. Sem Neurosci 2:509-518.

Cancalon PF (1987) Survival and subsequent regeneration of olfactory neurons after a distal axonal lesion. J Neurocytol 16:829-841.

Caplan LR, Norohna AB, Amico LL, (1990) Syringomyelia and arachnoiditis. J Neurol Neurosurg Psychiat 53:106-113.

Casella GTB, Bunge RP, Wood PM (1996) Improved method for harvesting Human Schwann cells from mature peripheral nerve and expansion in vitro. Glia 17:327-338.

Chen A, Xu XM, Kleitman N, Bunge MB (1996) Methylprednisolone administration improves axonal regeneration into Schwann cell grafts in transected adult rat thoracic spinal cord. Exp Neurol 138:261-276.

Cheng H, Cao Y, Olson L (1996) Spinal cord repair in adult paraplegic rats: Partial restoration of hind limb function. Science 273:510-513.

Chuah MI, Au C (1991) Olfactory Schwann cells are derived from precursor cells in the olfactory epithelium. J Neurosci Res 29:172-180.

Chuah MI, Au C (1993) Cultures of ensheathing cells from neonatal rat olfactory bulbs. Brain Res 601:213-220.

Costanzo RM, Graziadei PPC (1987) Development and plasticity of the olfactory system. In: Finger TE, Silver WL eds. Neurobiology of Taste and Smell. New York: John Wiley and Sons; 233-250.

Cummings DM, Brunjes PC (1995) Migrating luteinizing hormone-releasing hormone (LHEH) neurons and processes are associated with a substrate that express S 100. Dev Brain Res 88:148-157.

Daniloff JK, Levi G, Grumet M, Rieger F, Edelman GM (1986) altered expression of neuronal cell adhesion molecules induced by nerve injury and repair. J Cell Biol 103:929-945.

David S, Aguayo AJ (1981) Axonal elongation into peripheral nervous system bridges after central nervous system injury in adult rats. Science 214:931-933.

Davies SJA, Field PM, Raisman G (1994) Long interfascicular axon grwoth from embryonic neurons transplanted into adult myelinated tracts. J Neurosci 14:1596 1612.

Devon R, Doucette R (1992) Olfactory ensheathing cells myelinate dorsal root ganglion neurites. Brain Res 589:175-179.

Devon R, Doucette R (1995) Olfactory ensheathing cells do not require L-ascorbic acid in vitro to assemble a basal lamina or to myelinate dorsal root ganglion neurites. Brain Res 688:223-229.

Doucette JR (1984) The glial cells in the nerve fiber layer of the rat olfactory bulb. Anat Rec 210:385-391.

Doucette JR (1986) Astrocytes in the olfactory bulb. In: Fedoroff S, Vernadakis A, eds. Astrocytes. New York, Academic Press. 293-310.

Doucette JR (1989) Development of the nerve fiber layer in the olfactory bulb of mouse embryos. J Comp Neurol 285:514-527.

Doucette JR (1990) Glial influences on axonal growth in the primary olfactory system. Glia 3:433-449.

Doucette JR (1991) PNS-CNS transitional zone of the first cranial nerve. J Comp Neurol 312:451-466.

Doucette JR (1993) Glial cells in the nerve fiber layer of the main olfactory bulb of embryonic and adult mammals. Microsc Res Tech 24:113-130.

Doucette JR (1993) Glial progenitor cells of the nerve fiber layer of the olfactory bulb. Effect of astrocyte growth media. J Neurosci Res 35:274-287.

Doucette JR (1996) Immunocytochemical localization of laminin, fibronectin and collagen type IV in the nerve fiber layer of the olfactory bulb. Int J Devl Neurosci 14:945-959.

Doucette JR, Devon R (1995) Elevated intracellular levels of cAMP induce olfactory ensheathing cells to express GAL-C and GFAP but not MBP. Glia 13:130-140.

Doucette JR, Kiernan JA, Flumerfelt BA (1983) The re-innervation of olfactory glomeruli following transection of primary olfactory axons in the central or prepheral nervous system. J Anat 137:1-19.

Dyer JK, Bourque JA, Steeves JD (1998) Regeneration of brainstem-spinal axons after lesion and immunological disruption of myelin in adult rat. Exp Neurol 154:12-22.

Emmett CJ, Jaques-Berg W, Seeley PJ (1990) Microtransplantation of neural cells into adult rat brain. Neurosci 38:213-222.

Fawcett JW, Keynes RJ (1990) Peripheral nerve regeneration. Annu Rev Neurosci 13:43-60.

Fawcett JW (1998) Spinal cord repair: from experimental models to human application. Spinal cord 36:811-817.

Fox JL, Wener L, Drennam DC, Manz HJ, Won DJ, Al-Mefty O (1988) Central spinal cord injury: magnetic resonance imaging confirmation and operative considerations. Neurosurg 22:340-347.

Fracek Jr SP, Guo L, Schafer R (1994) Morphological characteristics of cultured olfactory bulb cells. Exp Brain Res 100:421-436.

Franceschini IA, Barnett SC (1996) Low-affinity NGF-receptor and E-N-CAM expression define two types of olfactory nerve ensheathing cells that share a common lineage. Dev Biol 173:327-343.

Franklin RJM, Gilson JM, Franceschini IA, Barnett SC (1996) Schwann cell-like myelination following transplantation of an olfactory bulb-ensheathing cell line into areas of demyelination in the adult CNS. Glia 17:217-224.

Frisch SM, Ruoslahti E (1997) Integrins and anoikis. Curr Opin Cell Biol 9:701-706.

Gautier SE, Oudega M, Fragoso M, Chapon P, Plant GW, Bunge MB, Parel J-P (1998) Poly(α-hydroxyacids) for application in the spinal cord: resorbability and biocompatibility with adult rat Schwann cells and spinal cord. J. Biomed Mater 42:642-654.

Gong QZ, Bailey MS, Pixley SK, Ennis M, Liu W, Shipley MT (1994) Localization and regulation of the low affinity nerve growth factor receptor expression in the rat olfactory system during development and regeneration. J Comp Neurol 344:336-348.

Gong QZ, Liu W-L, Srodon M, Foster TD, Shipley MT (1996) Olfactory epithelial organotypic slice cultures: A useful tool for investigation olfactory neural development. Int J Devel Neurosci 14:841-852.

Goodman MN, Silver J, Jacobberger JW (1993) Establishment and neurite outgrowth properties of neonatal and adult rat olfactory bulb glial cell lines. Brain Res 619:199-213.

Graziadei P, Monti Graziadei G (1978) The olfactory system: A model for the study of neurogenesis and axon regeneration in mammals. In: Cotman CW (ed). Neuronal Plasticity. New York: Raven Press: 131-153.

Graziadei PPC, Monti Graziadei GA (1979) Neurogenesis and neuron regeneration in the olfactory system of mammals. I. Morphological aspects of differentiation and structual organization of the olfactory sensory neurons. J Neurocytol 8:1-18.

Graziadei PPC, Monti Graziadei GA (1986) Neuronal changes in the forebrain of mice following penetration by regenerating olfactory axons. J Comp Neurol 247:344-356.

Grill R, Murai K, Blesch A, Gage FH, Tuszynski MH (1998) Cellular delivery of Neurotrophin-3 promotes corticospinal axonal growth and partial functional recovery after spinal cord injury. J Neurosci 17:5560-5572.

Guenard V, Xu XM, Bunge MB (1993) The use of Schwann cell transplantation to foster central nervous system repair. Sem Neurosci 5:401-411.

Guest JD, Hesse D, Schnell L, Schwab ME, Bunge MB, Bunge RP (1997b) Influence of IN-1 antibody and acidic FGF-fibrin glue on the response of injured corticospinal tract axons to human Schwann cell grafts. J Neurosci Res 50:888-905.

Guest JD, Rao, A, Olson L, Bunge MB, Bunge RP (1997a) The ability of human Schwann cell grafts to promote regeneration in the transected nude rat spinal cord. Exp Neurol 148:502-522.

Hall SM (1989) Regeneration in the peripheral nervous system. Neuropath Appl Neurobiol 15:513-529.

Hall S, Berry M (1989) Electron microscopic study of the interaction of axons and glia at the site of anastomosis between the optic nerve and cellular and acellular sciatic nerve grafts. J Neurocytol 18:171-184.

Harvey AR, Chen M, Plant GW, Dyson SE (1994) Regrowth of axons within Schwann cell-filled polycarbonate tubes implanted to the damaged rat optic tract and cerebral cortex of rats. Res Neurol Neurosci 6:221-237

Heredia M, Gascuel J, Ram∴n-Cueto A, Santacana M, Avila J, Mason C, Valverde F (1998) Two novel monoclonal antibodies (1.9.E. and 4.11.C.) against olfactory bulb ensheathing glia. Glia 24:352-364.

Imaizumi T, Lankford KL, Waxman SG, Greer CA, Kocsis JD (1998) Tansplanted olfactory ensheathing cells remyelinate and enhance axonal conduction in the demyelinated dorsal columns of the rat spinal cord. J Neurosci 18:6176-6185.

Kafitz KW, Greer CA (1997) Role of laminin in axonal extension from olfactory receptor cells. J Neurobiol 32:298-310.

Kafitz KW, Greer CA (1999) Olfactory ensheathing cells promote neurite extension from embryonic olfactory receptor cells *in vitro.* Glia 25:99-110.

Key B, Akeson RA (1990) Olfactory neurons express a unique glycosylatedform of neural cell adhesion molecule (N-CAM). J Cell Biol 110:1729-1743.

Khan T, Dauzvardis M, Sayers S (1991) Carbon filaments promote axonal growth across the transected rat spinal cord. Brain Res 541:139-145.

Kleitman N, Simon DK, Schachner M, Bunge RP (1988) Growth of embryonic retinal neurites elicited by contact with Schwann cell surfaces is blocked by antibodies to L1. Exp Neurol 102:298-306.

Kott JN, Westrum LE, Raines EW, Sasahara M, Ross R (1994) Olfactory ensheathing glia and platelet-derived growth factor B-chain reactivity in the transplanted rat olfactory bulb. Int Dev Neurosci 12:315-323.

Kromer LF, Cornbrooks CJ (1985) Transplants of Schwann cell cultures promote axonal regeneration in the adult mammalian brain. Proc Natl Acad Sci 82:6330-6334.

Kuffler DP (1986) Isolated satellite cells of a peripheral nerve direct the growth of regenerating frog axons. J Comp Neurol 249:57-64.

Kuhlengel, KR, Bunge MB, Bunge RP, Burton, H (1990) Implantation of cultured sensory neurons and Schwann cells into lesioned neonatal rat spinal cord. II. Implant characteristics and examination of corticospinal tract growth.

Levi ADO (1996) Characterization of the technique involved in isolating Schwaan cells from adult human peripheral nerve. J Neurosci Meths 68:21-26.

Levi ADO, Bunge RP (1994) Studies of myelin formation after transplantation of human Schwann cells into the severe combined immunodeficient mouse. Exp Neurol 130:41-52.

Levi ADO, Evans PJ, Mackinnon SE, Bunge RP (1994) Cold storage of peripheral nerves : An in vitro of cell viability and function. Glia 10:121-131.

Li, RH, Chen, J, Hammonds G, Philips H, Armanini, Wood P, Bunge RP, Godowski PJ, Sliwkowski MX, Mather JP (1996) Identification of Gas6 as a growth factor for human Schwann cells. J Neurosci 16:2012-2019.

Li Y, Field PM, Raisman G (1997) Repair of rat corticospinal tract by transplants of olfactory ensheathing glia. Science 277:2000-2002.

Li Y, Field PM, Raisman G (1998) Regeneration of adult rat corticospinal axons induced by transplanted olfactory ensheathing cells. J Neurosci 19:10514-10524.

Li Y, Raisman G (1994) Schwann cells induce sprouting in motor and sensory axons in the adult rat spinal cord.

Li Y, Raisman G (1997) Integration of transplanted cultured Schwann cells into the long myelinated fiber tracts of the adult spinal cord. Exp Neurol 145:397-411.

Liesi P (1985) Laminin immunoreactive glia distinguish regenerative adult CNS systems from non-regenerative ones. EMBO 4:2505-2511.

Lindsay RM, Wiegand SJ, Altar CA, DiStefano PS (1994) Neurotrophic factors: from molecule to man. Trends Neurosci 17:182-190

Luckenbill-Edds L (1997) Laminin and the mechanism of neuronal outgrowth. Brain Res Rev 23:1-27.

MacDonald RL, Findlay JM, Tator CH (1988) Microcystic spinal cord degeneration causing posttraumatic myelopathy. Report of two cases. J Neurosurg 68:466-471.

Manfioletti G, Brancolini Avanzi G, Schneider C (1993) The protein encoded by a growth arrest-specific gene (gas6) is a new member of the vitamin K-dependent proteins related to protein S, a negative coregulator in the blood coagulation cascade. Moll Cell Biol 13:4976-4985.

Marin-Padilla M, Amieva BMR (1989) Early neurogenesis of the mouse olfactory nerve: Golgi and electron microscopic studies. J comp Neurol 288:339-352.

Martin D, Robe P, Franzen R, Delree P, Schoenen J, Stevenaert A, Moonen G (1996) Effects of Schwann cell transplantation in a contusion model of rat spinal cord injury. J Neurosci Res 45:588-597.

Martin D, Schoenen J, Delree P, Leprince P, Rogister B, Moonen G (1991) Grafts of syngenic cultured, adult dorsal root ganglion-derived Schwann cells to the injured spinal cord of adult rats: preliminary morphological studies. Neurosci Lett 124:44-48.

Menei P, Montero-Menei C, Whittemore SR, Bunge RP, Bunge MB (1998) Schwann cells genetically modified to secrete human BDNF promote enhanced axonal regrowth across transected adult rat spinal cord. Eur J Neurosci 10:607-621.

Miragall F, Kadmon G, Husmann M, Schachner M (1988) Expression of cell adhesion molecules in the olfactory system of the adult mouse: Presence of the embryonic form of N-CAM. Devel Biol 129:516-531.

Mirsky K, Jessen KR (1990) Schwann cell development and the regulation of myelination. Semin Neurosci 2:423-435.

Miwa T, Moriizumi T, Sakashita H, Kimura Y, Donjo T, Furukawa M (1993) Transection of the olfactory nerves induces expression of nerve growth factor receptor in mouse olfactory epithelium. Neurosci Lett 155:96-98.

Montgomery CT, Robson JA (1993) Implants of cultured Schwann cells support axonal growth in the central nervous system of adult rats. Exp Neurol 122:107-124.

Montgomery CT, Tenaglia EA, Robson JA (1996) Axonal growth into tubes implanted within lesions in the spinal cords of adult rats. Exp Neurol 137:277-290.

Monti Graziadei GA, Graziadei PPC (1979) Neurogenesis and neuron regeneration in the olfactory system of mammals. II. Regeneration and reconstitution of the olfactory sensory neurons after axotomy. J Neurocytol 8:197-213.

Monti Graziadei GA, Graziadei PPC (1992) Sensory reinnervation after partial removal of the olfactory bulb. J Comp Neurol 316:32-44.

Monti Graziadei G, Karlan MS, Bernstein JJ, Graziadei P (1980) Reinnervation of the olfactory bulb after section of the olfactory nerve in monkey *(Saimiri sciureus).* Brain Res 189:343-354.

Morrissey TK, Kleitman N, Bunge RP (1991) Isolation and characterization of Schwann cells derived from adult peripheral nerve. J Neurosci 11:2433-2442.

Munirathinam S, Rao MS, Mohan YR, Raju TR (1997) Regeneration of the olfactory tract following neonatal lesions in rat. Exp Neurol 144:174-182.

Nakahara Y, Gage FH, Tuszynski MH (1996) Grafts of fibroblasts genetically modified to secrete NGF, BDNF, NT-3, or basic FGF elicit differential responses in the adult spinal cord. Cell Trans 5:191-204.

Navarro X, Valero A, Gudino G, Fores J, Rodriguez FJ, Verdu E, Pascual R, Cuadras J, Nieto-Sampedro M (1999) Ensheathing glia transplants promote dorsal root regeneration and spinal reflex restitution after multiple lumbar rhizotomy. Ann Neurol 45:207-215.

Oakley B, Riddle DR (1992) Receptor cell regeneation and connectivity in olfaction and taste. Exp Neurol 115:50-54.

Olson L (1997) Regeneration in the adult central nervous system. Experimental repair strategies. Nat Med 3:1329-1335.

Onifer S, Grover VP, Vargas CG, White LA, Gomez AM, Bunge MB, Bunge RP (1997) Schwann cell, carbon filament, and collagen grafts placed in the adult rat cervical spinal cord to promote chronically injured axon regeneration. Soc Neurosci Abstr 676.17.

Oudega M, Xu XM, Guenard V, Kleitman N, Bunge MB (1997) A combination of insulin-like growth factor-I and Platelet-derived growth factor enhances myelination but diminishes axonal regeneration into Schwann cell grafts in the adult rat spinal cord. Glia 19:247-258.

Paino CL, Bunge MB (1991) Induction of axon growth into Schwann cell implants grafted into lesioned adult rat spinal cord. Exp Neurol 114:254-257.

Paino CL, Fernandez-Valle C, Bates ML, Bunge MB (1994) Regrowth of axons in lesioned adult rat spinal cord: promotion by implants of cultured Schwann cells. J Neurocytol 23:433-452.

Pixley SK (1992) The olfactory nerve contains two populations of glia, identified both *in vivo* and *in vitro.* Glia 5:269-284.

Pixley SK (1996) Characteristics of olfactory receptor neurons and other cell types in dissociated rat olfactory cell cultures. Int J Devel Neurosci 14:823-839.

Plant GW, Chirila, TV, Harvey AR (1998a) Transplantation of collagen IV/ poly(2-hydroxyethyl methacrylate) hydrogels containing Schwann cells into the lesioned rat optic tract. Cell Trans 7:381-391.

Plant GW, Dimitropoulou A, Bates ML, Bunge MB (1998b) The expression of inhibitory proteoglycans following transplantation of Schwann cell grafts into a completely transected adult rat spinal cord. Soc Neurosci Abstr 33.8.

Plant GW, Harvey AR, Chirila TV (1995) Axonal regrowth within poly (2-hydroxyethyl methacrylate) sponges infiltrated with Schwann cells and implanted into the lesioned rat optic tract. Brain Res 671:119-130.

Plant GW, Woerly S, Harvey AR (1997) Hydrogels containing peptide or aminosugar sequences implanted into the rat brain: Influence on cellular migration and axonal growth. Exp Neurol 143:287-299.

Raisman G (1985) Specialized neuroglial arrangement may explain the capacity of vomeronasal axons to reinnervate central neurons. Neurosci 14:237-254.

Ramón -Cueto A, Avila J (1998) Olfactory ensheathing glia: Properties and functionl Brain Res Bull 46:175-187.

Ramón -Cueto A, Nieto-Sampedro M (1992) Glial cells from the adult rat olfactory bulb: Immunocytochemical properties of pure cultures of ensheathing cells. Neurosci 47:213-220.

Ramón -Cueto A, Nieto-Sampedro M (1994) Regeneration into the spinal cord of transected dorsal root axons is promoted by ensheathing glia transplants. Exp Neurol 127:232-244.

Ramón -Cueto A, Perez J, Nieto-Sampedro M (1993) *In vitro* enfolding of olfactory neurites by p75 receptor positive ensheathing cells from adult rat olfactory bulb. Eur J Neurosci 5:1172-1180.

Ramón -Cueto A, Plant GW, Avila J, Bunge MB (1998) Long-distance axonal regeneration in the transected adult rat spinal cord is promoted by olfactory ensheathing glia transplants. J Neurosci 18:3803-3815.

Ramón -Cueto A, Valverde F (1995) Olfactory bulb ensheathing glia: A unique cell type with axonal growth-promoting properties. Glia 14:163-173.

Ramón y Cajal (1928) Degeneration and regeneration of the nervous system (May, RM, translator). New York: Oxford UP.

Rapalino O, Lazarov-Spiegler O, Agranov E, Velan GJ, Yoles E, Fraidakas M, Solomon A, Gepstein R, Katz A, Belkin M, Hadani M, Schwartz M (1998) Implantation of stimulated homologous macrophages results in partial recovery of paraplegic rats. Nat Med 4:814-821.

Reinhardt E, Meier R, Halfter W, Rovelli G, Monard D (1988) Detection of glia-derived nexin in the olfactory system of the rat. Neuron 1:387-394.

Rende M, Muir D, Ruoslahti E, Hagg T, Varon S, Manthorpe M (1992) Immunolocalization of ciliary neurotrophic factor in adult rat sciatic nerve. Glia 5:25-32.

Richardson PM, Issa VMK, Aguayo AJ (1984) Regeneration of long spinal axons in the rat. J Neurocytol 13:165-182.

Richardson PM, McGuinness UM, Aguayo AJ (1980) Axons from CNS Neurons regenerate into PNS grafts. Nature 284:264-265

Roskams AJI, Bethel MA, Hurt KJ, Ronett GV (1996) Sequential expression of Trks A, B, and C in the regenerating olfactory neuroepithelium. J Neurosci 16:1294-1307.

Rutkowski JL, Tennekoon GI, McGillicuddy JE (1992) Selective culture of mitotically active human Schwann cells from adult sural nerves. Ann Neurol 31:580-586.

Schachner M (1990) Functional implications of glial cell recognition molecules. Semin Neurosci 2:497-507.

Schnell L, Schneider R, Kolbeck R, Barde Y-A, Schwab, ME (1994) Neurotrophin-3 enhances sprouting of corticospinal tract during development and after adult spinal cord lesion. Nature 367:170-173.

Schwab ME, Kapfhammer JP, Bandtlow CE (1993) Inhibitors of neurite growth. Annu Rev Neurosci 16:565-595.

Silver J (1994) Inhibitory molecules in development and regeneration. J Neurol 242:22-44.

Smale KA, Doucette R, Kawaja MD (1996) Implantation of olfactory ensheathing cells in the adult rat brain following fimbria-formix transection. Exp Neurol 137:225-233.

Son Y-J, Thompson WJ (1996a) Schwann cell processes guide regeneration of peripheral axons. Neuron 14:125-132.

Son Y-J, Thompson WJ (1996b) Nerve sprouting in muscle is induced and guided by processes extended by Schwann cells. Neuron 14:133-141.

Sonigra RJ, Brighton PC, Jacoby J, Hall S, Wigley CB (1999) Adult rat olfactory ensheathing cells are effective promoters of adult central nervous system neurite outgrowth in co-culture. Glia 25:256-269.

Sonigra RJ, Kandiah SS, Wigley CB (1996) Spontaneous immortalisation of ensheathing cells from adult rat olfactory nerve. Glia 16:247-256.

Syroid DE, Zorick TS, Arbet-Engels C, Kilpatrick TJ, Eckhart W,Lemke, G (1999) A role for insulin-Like growth factor in the regulation of Schwann cell survival. J Neurosci 19:2059-2068.

Thallmair M, Metz GAS, Graggen WJZ, Raineteau O, Kartje GL, Schwab ME (1998) Neurite growth inhibitors restrict plasticity and functional recovery following recovery following corticospinal tract lesions. Nat Neurosci 1:124-131.

Turner CP, Perez-Polo JR (1993) Expression of p75 NGFR in the olfactory system following peripheral deafferentation. Neuroreport 4:1023-1026.

Turner CP, Perez-Polo JR (1994) Changes in the expression of the low-affinity receptor for neurotrophins, p75, in the regenerating olfactory system. Int J Devel Neurosci 12:767-773.

Tuszynski MH, Weidner N, McCormack M, Miller I, Powell H, Conner J (1998) grafts of genetically modified Schwann cells to the spinal cord: survival, axon growth and myelination. Cell Trans 7:187-196

Ubink R, Halasz N, Zhang X, Dagerlind A, Hokfelt T (1994) Neuropeptide tyrosine is expressed in ensheathing cells around the olfactory nerves in the rat olfactory bulb. Neurosci 60:709-726.

Valverde F, Lopez-Mascaraque L (1991) Neuroglial arrangements in the olfactory glomeruli of the hedgehog. J Comp Neurol 307:658-674.

Valverde F, Santacana M, Heredia M (1992) Formation of an olfactory glomerulus: Morphological aspects of development and organization. Neurosci 49:255-275.

Vickland H, Westrum LE, Kott JN, Patterson SL, Bothwell MA (1991) Nerve growth factor receptor expression in the young and adult rat olfactory system. Brain Res 565:269-279.

Wells MR, Batter DK, Antoniades HN, Blunt DG, Weremowicz J, Lynch GE, Hansson HA (1994) PDGF-BB and IGF-I in combination enhance axonal regeneration in a gap model of peripheral nerve injury. Soc Neurosci Abstr 20:545.16.

Wellis DP, Scott JW (1991) Localized denervation demonstrates the innervation pattern of olfactory bulb glomeruli and second order cells. J Comp Neurol 304:544-554.

William B (1990) Post-traumatic syringomyelia, an update. Paraplegia 28:296-313.

Woerly S, Marchand R (1990) Brain tissue and neural graft reactivity to the implantation of in situ self assembled collagen matrices. Restor Neurol Neurosci 1:369-385.

Woerly S, Pinet E, De Robertis L, Bousmina M, Laroche G, Roitback T, Vargova L, Sykova E (1998) Heterogeneous PHPMA hydrogels for tissue repair and axonal regeneration in the injured spinal cord. J Biomater Sci Polym Ed 9:681-711.

Woerly S, Plant GW, Harvey AR (1996) Cultured rat neuronal and glial cells entrapped within hydrogel polymer matrices: a potential tool for neural tissue replacement. Neurosci Lett 205: 197-201.

Wood PM (1976) Separation of functional Schwann cells and neurons from normal peripheral nerve tissue. Brain Res 115:361-375

Xu XM, Chen A, Guenard V, Kleitman N, Bunge MB (1997) Bridging Schwann cell transplants promte axonal regeneration from both the rostral and caudal stumps of transected adult rat spinal cord. J Neurocytol 26:1-16.

Xu XM, Guenard V, Kleitman N, Aebischer P, Bunge MB (1995b) A combination of BDNF and NT-3 promotes supraspinal axonal regeneration into Schwann cell grafts in adult rat thoracic spinal cord. Exp Neurol 134:261-272.

Xu XM, Guenard V, Kleitman N, Bunge MB (1995a) Axonal regeneration into Schwann cell-seeded guidance channels grafted into transected adult rat spinal cord. J Comp Neurol 351:145-160.

Xu XM, Zhang S-X, Li H, Aebischer P, Bunge MB (1999) Regrowth of axons into the distal spinal cord through a Schwann cell-seeded mini-channel implanted into hemisected adult rat spinal cord. Eur J Neurosci 11:1723-1740.

22

Gene Therapy Strategies

Itzhak Fischer and Yi Liu
MCP Hahnemann University, Philadelphia, Pennsylvania

I. EXPLORING THE GENE THERAPY SPACE

Gene therapy is a new concept based on the development during the past decade of methods for delivering genetic material into mammalian cells. The rationale for using gene therapy is to treat inherited or acquired disorders by providing deficient genes or by inhibiting detrimental genes (Miller, 1992; Mulligan, 1993; Miller and Vile, 1995; Blomer et al., 1996; Karpati et al., 1996; Tuszynski, 1998). The application of the gene therapy concept can also be extended to include delivery of genes with therapeutic potential to compensate for cellular dysfunction, malignant tumors or injury. Advances in biotechnology and in understanding the molecular basis of human diseases have propelled human gene therapy from theory into a promising clinical application. One of the earliest clinical trials for human gene therapy, begun in the fall of 1990 with an attempt to transfer the adenosine deaminase (ADA) gene into lymphocytes to compensate for a lethal enzyme deficiency, produced encouraging clinical results (Miller, 1992). Since then, gene therapy has been tested on a wide spectrum of human diseases, but the jury is still out on deciding the effectiveness of this genetic approach (Crystal, 1995; Blomer 1996; Verma and Somia, 1997).

Disorders of the central nervous system (CNS) are a formidable challenge for gene therapy. Direct gene transfer or gene transfer in combination with neurotransplantation are powerful therapeutic strategies for repairing damaged CNS tissue. The potential applications include the enhancement of neuronal function by providing exogenous supplies of deficient neurotransmitters; the use of therapeutic molecules (e.g. neurotrophins and anti-apoptotic factors) to prevent neuronal cell loss and to promote axon regeneration; and the replacement of damaged neurons and glial cells to reconstruct the appropriate neural circuitry (Doering, 1994). There are two major therapeutic modalities for somatic gene therapy, the *ex vivo* and the *in vivo* strategies. In the *ex vivo* approach, cultured cells are genetically modified *in vitro* by recombinant vectors and transplanted into the host. The transduced donor cells then release the therapeutic gene products. With the *in vivo* approach, special vectors, such as viruses, that can introduce genes into the organism, directly deliver the genetic material. The therapeutic gene products are therefore produced by the genetically modified host cells, and may act on either the modified cells themselves, other host cells or both.

Gene therapy can be viewed as having three dimensions: 1) the vector system for *in vivo* or *ex vivo* gene transfer, 2) the donor cells that can be genetically modified for *ex vivo* gene therapy, and 3) the therapeutic genes to be delivered (Fig.1). Appropriate decisions in all three dimensions are crucial for effective CNS gene therapy. The constant improvement of the vector systems has allowed convenient and efficient gene delivery into mammalian CNS cells (Neve, 1993; Miller and Vile, 1995; Blomer et al., 1996; Hermens and Verhaagen, 1998). The isolation, characterization and genetic modification of various types of cells have provided diverse donor sources for neurotransplantation (Anton et al., 1994; Luskin; 1994; Gage et al., 1995; Stemple and Mahanthappa, 1997; Weiss et al., 1996; Whittermore and Snyder 1996; Snyder and Wolfe, 1996; McKay, 1997). Finally, the extraordinary progress in cloning and characterizing the mammalian genome has identified numerous genes with therapeutic value, including neurotrophic factors, anti-apoptotic proteins, transcription control elements, cell adhesion, cytoskeleton and extracellular matrix molecules, and genes associated with axon growth and regeneration. Although gene therapy can be applied to a variety of neurodegenerative disorders including Parkinson's and Alzheimer's diseases (see recent review by Tuszynski, 1998), this review is focused on strategies that promote regeneration in the CNS that can be applied to brain trauma and spinal cord injury.

II. FIRST DIMENSION: THERE ARE MANY VECTORS FOR GENE DELIVERY. CHOOSE WISELY!

Successful gene therapy requires an accurate and efficient delivery system that transfers therapeutic genes to desired cell types at appropriate locations. The vector of choice "dimension" (Fig. 1) presents several types of systems, including both viral and non-viral vectors, that have been proven useful for gene delivery with individual strengths and weaknesses as detailed in the following sections (Review by Doering, 1994; Miller and Vile, 1995; Crystal, 1995; Blomer, 1996; Hermens and Verhaagen, 1998). In designing the vector of choice it is also important to consider the promoter that drives the expression of the transgene. For

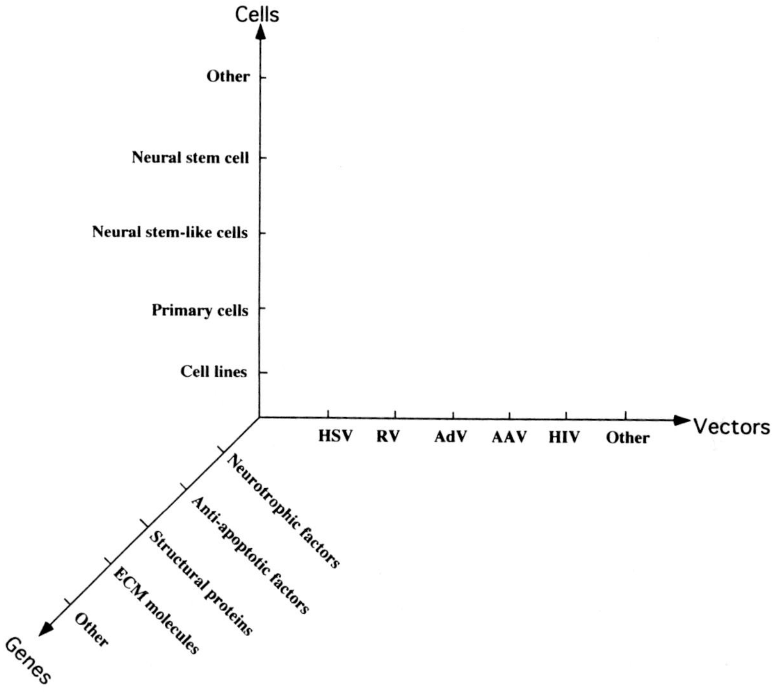

Figure 1 Three dimensions of the gene therapy strategy.

example, is there a need for high level, long term, cell specific or regulated expression of the therapeutic genes? The original promoters used in the recombinant vectors were mostly constitutive viral promoters that in many cases exhibited unpredictable shut off in the nervous system. Currently, it is possible to use a variety of neural promoters, which can be targeted to specific types of cells (GFAP to astrocytes) or a subpopulation of neurons (tyrosine hydroxylase to dopaminergic neurons). There has also been progress in development of inducible promoters such as the glucocorticoid-inducible, the tetracycline-inducible (tet) and the metallothionein-inducible by heavy metal ions. Finally, for many experiments it is very useful to include a reporter gene for easy detection of transduced cells. The most common strategies have been to either use two promoters to drive the expression of the reporter gene and the transgene or to use a single promoter in combination with the IRES sequence (internal ribosome entry site) to direct the expression of two products from a single mRNA (Liu et al., 1999a). The original reporter genes of β-galactosidase and alkaline phosphatase have been replaced by the many variants of the green fluorescent protein (GFP) whose major advantages are a relatively small coding region (to save insert "space") and the ability to observe the expression in live cells without the need for fixation and staining.

A. Viral Vector Systems

Viral vectors exploit the natural abilities of mammalian cell viruses to infect host cells and to utilize the host DNA and protein synthetic machinery. These vectors can be designed to express efficiently a gene of interest, but are made replication-deficient to prevent them from producing infectious particles and gene products that are detrimental to the host cells or induce a strong immune response (Blomer et al., 1996). Differences among the viral vectors include their state in the host nucleus (integration or episomal), the maximal size of the transgene (4 - 35 kb), the type of their genetic material (RNA, and single stranded and double stranded DNA), the titer of purified viruses, requirement for helper virus, host range of infectivity and the risk they pose to host cells. The major viral systems that have been employed for gene therapy include Herpes Simplex virus, retrovirus, adenovirus, adeno-associated virus and lentivirus.

1. Herpes Simplex virus vectors

The Herpes Simplex virus (HSV) vectors are constructed from a large DNA virus of about 150 kb with a carrying capacity for cloning of up to 35 kb of additional DNA. They have a broad range of host cell types, and are capable of infecting both neurons and glial cells, although the infection efficiency is better in neurons (Neve, 1993; Blomer, 1996; Hermens and Verhaagen, 1998). HSV vectors can be used as a replication-deficient construct of the recombinant HSV-1 virus carrying a single copy of the gene of interest. They can also be used as a defective virus amplicon system, which is generated from plasmids containing multiple copies of the gene of interest packaged into HSV virions, but needs a helper virus function. After infecting the host cells and releasing the capsid into the cytoplasm, the viral DNA enters the nucleus through nuclear pores and remains as an epichromosomal entity in a latency stage. HSV vectors can be transported retrogradely or anterogradely along axonal projections. In addition, limited trans-synaptic transfer may also occur.

The major application of HSV vectors is for *in vivo* gene delivery into the CNS. Both reporter genes (e.g., LacZ) and therapeutic genes such as β-glucoridase and glucose transporter genes have been delivered by direct injection of the vector into the CNS parenchyma (Kaplitt et al., 1991; Wolfe et al., 1992; Ho et al., 1993). Transgene expression is usually transient however, and loss of expression occurs as early as 2 weeks following injection of the virus (Chiocca et al., 1990; Andersen et al., 1992). This is probably attributable to promoter down regulation and elimination of virally transduced cells by immunological mechanisms (Blomer et al., 1996). Some other disadvantages of HSV vectors include low viral titer ($<10^7$ TU/ml), a requirement for a helper virus to produce defective amplicons, well documented cytotoxicity and unknown long term safety (Neve, 1993; Hermens and Verhaagen, 1998). The trans-synaptic transfer of the virus is potentially undesirable, because it may compromise the specificity of target gene delivery.

2. Retrovirus vectors

Retroviral vectors are small RNA viruses with a carrying capacity of less than 7 kb. These viruses are characterized by the enzyme reverse transcriptase, which transcribes viral RNA genome into proviral DNA. The cDNA is then randomly integrated into the host genome resulting in a permanently modified host genotype (Crystal, 1995; Mulligan, 1993; Miller, 1992; Temin et al., 1990). The retroviral vectors are prepared by removing the gag, pol and env genes to accommodate the cloning of transgenes and to render the virus replication deficient (but still able to infect cells). The specificity of the retroviral infection depends on the packaging cells that provides the missing viral genes including the envelope gene for either an ecotropic virus limited to mostly rodents or an amphotropic virus with a wide host specificity that includes human. Because the viral genome replicates as the host cell divides, there is no transgene dilution following division. The integration of the retrovirus genomic material into the host genome is both advantageous and problematic. The permanent modification of host cells and the lack of transgene dilution, should ensure stable transgene expression required in chronic disorders such as inherited enzymatic deficiencies. However, prolonged transgene overexpression and accumulation of transgene products may also be toxic to the host cells. More importantly, because the integration of the viral DNA into the host genome is random, insertional mutagenesis by disruption of critical functions such as tumor suppressor genes or by activation of proto-oncogenes is a potential risk factor (Miller, 1992; Crystal, 1995). A major limitation is that the conventional retroviral vectors, such as the Moloney murine leukemia virus vectors, require cell division for infection. As most neuronal cells are postmitotic, they are not susceptible to retroviral infection, and consequently cannot be targeted and modified by these types of vectors. Other disadvantages of retroviral vectors include low titer ($<10^6$ cfu/ml) and low infection efficiency. These disadvantages make retroviral vectors not suitable for *in vivo* gene transfer. They are, however very useful in *ex vivo* applications in which neural and non-neural cell lines, infected with recombinant retrovirus carrying therapeutic genes, are transplanted into the CNS (Blomer et al., 1996; Liu et al., 1999b).

To date, the majority of approved human gene-therapy trials have utilized retroviral vectors. Some of the examples include transfer of genes encoding for adenosine deaminase, low density lipoprotein receptor and tumor necrosis factor. (Reviewed by Miller, 1992). Retrovirus-mediated *ex vivo* gene transfer has also received attention in experimental models of CNS diseases and conditions including Parkinson's disease (Fisher et al., 1991; Horellou et al., 1994; Lundberg et al., 1996b; Anton et al., 1994; Leviver et al., 1995; Horellou et al., 1997; Review by Reymon et al., 1997); Huntington's disease (Emerich et al., 1996); Alzheimer's disease (Rosenberg et al., 1988); Sly disease (Snyder, 1994); Tay-Sachs disease (Lacorazza et al., 1996); aging (Martinez-Serrano et al., 1996a); and spinal cord injury (Tuszynski et al., 1994; 1996; Kim et al., 1996; Grill et al., 1997; Liu et al., 1999b).

Another important application of retroviral vectors for CNS gene therapy is to establish immortalized neural progenitor and stem-like cell lines by transferring oncogenes such as v-myc, neu, Simian Virus 40 large T antigen and adenovirus E1A region (reviewed by Martinez-Serrano and Bjorklund, 1997, Snyder, 1998). The immortalized cells retain the properties of neural cells without becoming tumorigenic, making them an excellent source of cellular grafting (see next section). Numerous studies have demonstrated the therapeutic potential of these cell lines in treatment of CNS disease (Reviewed by Whittermore and Snyder, 1996; Martinez-Serrano and Bjorklund, 1997; Snyder et al., 1997; Snyder 1998).

3. Adenovirus vectors

Adenoviral vectors are double-stranded linear DNA viruses of about 36 kb based on type 2 and type 5 human adenoviruses. Deletion of selective genes creates a carrying capacity of 8 kb (in fourth generation and gutless adenovirus the transgene capacity increased to 25 kb), rendering the virus replication defective (Neve, 1993; Doering, 1994; Crystal, 1995; Miller and Vile, 1995; Hermens and Verhaagen, 1998). The adsorption and penetration of the adenovirus occur by receptor-mediated endocytosis. The virus binds to a cellular receptor with the fiber protein present on the viral capsid, and is then internalized through the interaction of the penton capsid protein with α-type integrins. After internalization and uncoating, the viral DNA enters the host nucleus where it exists as an episome. Since the viral DNA does not integrate into the host genome, the modification of the host cells is not permanent and cell division will result in transgene dilution. This is one of the reasons why transgene expression is usually transient in adenovirus mediated gene transfer experiments (Crystal et al., 1995). Unlike retroviral vectors, however, chronic transgene expression and insertional mutagenesis are not major concerns with adenoviral vectors.

Adenoviral vectors have several major advantages. 1) High titer of viruses (up to 10^{12} pfu/ml) can be prepared in the producer cell line HEK-293 and purified without concerns about helper virus. The high titer also allows convenient adjustment of multiplicity of infection (MOI) for optimal transgene expression and minimal cytopathological effect (Crystal, 1995; Neve, 1993; Liu et al., 1998). 2) Adenoviral vectors have a broad host range, infecting almost any type of mammalian cell, including both neurons and glia (Akli et al., 1993; Bajocchi et al., 1993; Davidson et al., 1993; Le Gal La Salle et al., 1993; Liu et al., 1997). Since adenovirus vectors can modify both dividing and post-mitotic cells, the vector is useful in both *in vivo* and *ex vivo* gene transfer paradigms (Blomer et al., 1996; Davidson and Bohn, 1997; Liu et al., 1997; 1998). 3) Both gene transfer efficiency and levels of transgene expression are high, another consequence of the high titer of this virus. 4) Most adenoviral vectors are constructed based on human type 2 and type 5 adenoviruses, well characterized viruses that cause only mild upper respiratory tract symptoms, and are therefore safe for clinical trials of gene therapy. 5) Adenoviral vectors can be efficiently transported retrogradely along axons, but unlike the HSV vectors are not transported trans-synaptically as HSV vectors. This allows *in vivo* gene delivery to specific areas without the concern of unrestricted spreading of the virus. This feature is especially advantageous for *in vivo* delivery of neurotrophic factors, since the vectors can induce expression of the neurotrophic factors both in the cell bodies and around their axon terminals, therefore providing trophic support to the neurons by target derived and autocrine/paracrine modes (Liu et al., 1997).

Disadvantages of adenoviral vectors include unstable transgene expression due to the episomal location of the viral genome, and host immune response as a result of "leaky viral" replication, the expression of immunogenic late viral proteins and low level viral particle packaging (Yang et al., 1994). There can also be direct toxicity to host cells due to accumulation of the viral proteins (Zhang and Schneider, 1994) and tissue inflammation due to the host immune reaction (Yang et al., 1994; Byrnes et al., 1995). Therefore, an important requirement for an effective recombinant adenovirus vector is the establishment of a strict replication deficiency.

In an attempt to solve these problems, several generations of adenoviral vectors have been designed. The first generation adenovirus vector was generated by deletion of the E-1 region, which encodes several factors important for transactivation of late gene expression and therefore renders the virus replication deficient. This blockage can be overcome if the virus is used at high multiplicity of infection (Wang et al., 1996) or through the expression of host E1-A like gene products. To increase the carrying capacity, the commonly used first generation vectors also had a deletion in the E-3 region. However, the E-3 region encodes several important proteins, including the gp19K protein which helps the virus evade host immune surveillance by binding the major histocompatibility complex I (MHC I) molecules and inhibiting their transport onto the cell surface. This inhibition of MHC I expression on the host cell surface prevents the infected host cells from presenting viral antigens in the context of MHC I molecules which is essential for the immune recognition by cytotoxic T lymphocytes (CTLs). It is therefore possible that the deletion in the E-3 region is responsible for the immune reaction triggered by the first generation vectors (Lee et al., 1995). A modified version of the first generation viral vector was then generated with the gp19k gene constitutively driven by a RSV LTR promoter (Lee et al., 1995). *In vitro* studies have shown that cells infected by this vector were free of CTL mediated cytolysis. The second and third generation adenoviral vectors were designed to minimize the "leaky" replication. The second generation vectors employ a temperature sensitive mutation in E-2A region. E-2A encodes a single-stranded DNA binding protein, which is essential for initiation of DNA replication and chain elongation (Horwitz et al., 1994). The resulting second generation vector is a ΔE-1/ts E-2A vector which has been shown to cause less inflammatory response in liver (Engelhardt et al., 1994) and lung (Goldman et al., 1995). However, there are no reports about its application in CNS. In the third generation vectors, a second deletion in the E-4 region was added to the first generation vector (Wang et al., 1996). This double lethal deletion greatly reduces the possibility of "leaky" replication caused by host E-1A like products or by spontaneous repair through homologous recombination with wild type virus. A fourth generation adenoviral vector with large deletion of the viral genome has been generated using the Cre/lox-P recombinase system, in which the Cre-recombinase is used to remove a 25 kb viral region flanked by the lox-P sequence (Lieber et al., 1996). The resulting vector has a very high transgene capacity and no toxicity, but so far it has proven to be unstable in host cells. The most recent version of the Cre/lox-P system is called the "gutless" vector that has no adenovirus sequences except the packaging sequences and the inverted terminal repeats (Kochanek et al., 1996). In addition to genetic modification of the adenoviral vectors, immune suppression is also an option for reduction of the host immune response. We have reported that the immune response that causes elimination of host spinal cord cells transduced by a recombinant adenoviral vector can be ameliorated by immunosuppression with Cyclosporin A (Liu et al., 1997).

4. Adeno-associated virus vectors

Adeno-associated virus (AAV) vectors are single stranded DNA non-autonomous parvoviruses with a small carrying capacity (4.7 kb). When AAV infects cells it integrates into the genome and remains in a latent state until it is induced by the presence of a helper virus (e.g., adenovirus) to replicate. AAV vectors can be produced at reasonably high titers (10^{10} IU/ml), and gene transfer efficiency is quite high (Xiao et al., 1997; Hermens and Verhaagen, 1998). Like HSV and adenoviral vectors, AAV has a broad host spectrum and is capable of transducing both dividing and non-dividing cells (Flotte et al., 1993; Kaplitt et al., 1994; Podsakoff et al., 1994; Russell et al, 1994; McCown et al, 1996; Mandel et al., 1997; Peel et al., 1997; Xiao et al., 1997). Another major advantage of AAV vectors is that they are nonpathogenic and do not elicit host immune responses. AAV vectors can integrate into the host genome, although the efficiency is low and the vast majority of the vector genome remains episomal. The integration into the human genome is site-specific, and occurs on chromosome 19, in contrast to random integration in retroviral vectors. Also, transduction of host cells following integration is stable for hundreds of passages. These features have drawn attention to AAV vectors in recent years (reviewed in Xiao et al, 1997; Hermens and Verhaagen, 1998). Applications of AAV in CNS have included the use of cell specific promoters to improve the long term expression of the GFP transgene (Peel et al., 1997). The disadvantages of AAV vectors include dependence on adenovirus or HSV as helper virus for transcription and translation, which makes the production of AAV relatively difficult, and the small carrying capacity, which limits the choice of transgenes.

5. Lentivirus vectors

In order to target post-mitotic cells, a new retroviral vector system based on human immune deficiency virus (HIV) has been developed. These vectors infect dividing and post-mitotic cells and integrate into the host genome (Naldini et al., 1996; Reiser et al., 1996; Blomer et al., 1997; Miyoshi et al., 1997). A new series of lentivirus vectors was constructed that can transduce nondividing cells and have the ability to self-inactivate (Miyoshi et al., 1998). Therefore, they combine the merits of conventional retroviral vectors with that of the HSV and adenoviral vectors. Stable integration, long-term transgene expression and lack of expression of viral protein associated with immune response make the HIV-derived vectors attractive in CNS gene therapy (Blomer et al., 1996; Hermens and Verhaagen, 1998), but safety remains the major concern for future applications.

B. Non-viral Vector Systems

Non-viral systems include purified uncomplexed plasmids, DNA-liposome complexes, particle bombardment-mediated gene transfer (gene gun), receptor-mediated endocytosis transfer of genes by linkage with cell surface ligands and adenovirus proteins, mRNA, ribozyme and antisense oligonucleotides. These vectors are safe, easy to synthesize and modify, and impose no limitation on the size of transgenes. There are, however, other disadvantages. The DNA-liposome system has low gene transfer efficiency, cytotoxicity associated with cationic lipid and limited target cell population (Neve, 1993; Crystal, 1995; Miller and Vile, 1995; Scherman et al., 1998). Delivery of genes by conjugating the DNA with a biological ligand unitizes a receptor-mediated pathway and avoids cytotoxicity associated with membrane disruption because endocytosis is a physiological process. The DNA-ligand complex also allows cell targeting by selecting the appropriate receptor and ligand. The initial constructs were not effective because the endocytosed complex was degraded by the lysosomes. To avoid lysosomal delivery, adenoviruses were linked to the conjugated vectors. This startegy added a functional capacity of both binding and endosome disruption and facilitated an efficient gene transfer (Sharon and Curiel, 1994). The main advantages of the linked adenovirus-DNA complex over recombinant viral vectors are that the design and size of the DNA are not constrained by virus packaging and that the gene transfer process is not dependent on the viral genome.

III. SECOND DIMENSION: THERE IS ALSO A WIDE CHOICE OF CELLS FOR *EX VIVO* GENE THERAPY

Advances in neurotransplantation techniques and the refinement of gene delivery vector systems inspired the idea of *ex vivo* CNS gene therapy: transplanting cells that are genetically modified to express exogenous therapeutic gene products. The advantages of *ex vivo* gene transfer include avoiding the problems associated with the use of fetal tissue, unlimited sources of donor cells with homogeneous and well defined characteristics, easy genetic modification using targeted gene delivery vectors, well defined source of exogenous therapeutic substances that can diffuse to appropriate targets, and the ability of neural donor cells to integrate into the host CNS cytoarchitecture and to repair and reconstruct the damaged neuronal connectivity (Gage et al., 1987; Doering et al., 1994; Blomer et al., 1996; Whittermore and Snyder et al., 1996; Snyder and Senut, 1997; Martinez-Serrano and Bjorklund, 1997; Raymon et al., 1997). The choice of cells "dimension" in designing *ex vivo* gene therapy (Fig. 1) presents numerous types of cells that have been genetically modified using various types of vectors and grafted into a variety of CNS structures (reviewed in Whittermore and Snyder, 1996; Snyder et al., 1997; Martinez-Serrano and Bjorklund, 1997; Snyder, 1998). The major challenges of effective and safe *ex vivo* gene therapy in the CNS include avoiding disruptive effects when grafted (non-tumorigenic, minimal immune response), the ability of modifying the cells to express the therapeutic genes at optimal efficacy (high levels, long term, regulatable expression) and the potential for integration and cellular replacement.

Because of the great interest in using multipotential progenitor and stem cells for *ex vivo* gene transfer (for which we will use the general term precursor cells), we have categorized the section on donor cells by their state of differentiation into non-precursor cells (e.g., fibroblasts, astrocytes and Schwann cells, both primary and cell lines) and precursor cells (e.g., neural stem cells and immortalized stem-like cell lines).

A. Non-precursor Cells

1. Primary cells

Primary cells that have been used in CNS gene delivery include primary fibroblasts (Fisher et al., 1991; 1993; Kawaja et al., 1992; Grill et al., 1997; Liu et al., 1999b), Schwann cells (Paino and Bunge, 1991; Xu et al., 1995a,b; Brook et al., 1994), primary astrocytes (Cunninghan et al., 1991a; La Gamma et al., 1993; Lundberg et al., 1996b); and myoblasts (Jiao et al., 1992). A major advantage of primary cells is that they allow autologous or isogenic grafting, therefore reducing the possibility of immune rejection. Primary cells also avoid the problem of tumor formation that is associated with the use of some transformed cell lines (Snyder and Senut, 1997; Blomer, 1996).

Autografts and isografts of primary fibroblasts into adult rat spinal cord integrate well with the host and the graft size remains stable for at least 8 weeks (Kawaja et al., 1991; Tuszynski et al., 1994), while allografts suffer from immune rejection and graft atrophy unless the host has been immunosuppressed (Kawaja et al., 1992; Liu et al., 1998). Recently, primary fibroblasts modified by adenovirus have been successfully allografted into adult Sprague-Dawley rat, immunosuppressed by cyclosporin A, with survival and transgene expression comparable to that observed in isografts or autografts (Liu et al., 1998). Primary fibroblasts, easily prepared from skin biopsy, exhibit contact inhibition that avoids formation of tumors, but allows the growth and storage of large numbers of cells. Primary fibroblasts have been genetically modified, usually by recombinant retroviral vectors, to produce a variety of therapeutic gene products including neurotrophins (Kawaja et al., 1992; Tuszynski et al., 1994; 1996; Grill et al., 1997; Liu et al., 1999b), and enzymes such as tyrosine hydroxylase (Fisher et al., 1991) at high enough levels for physiological effects. A potential problem of both adenoviral and retroviral modified fibroblast grafts is that the highest transgene expression is usually observed within 2 weeks post-transplantation. Down-regulation of the transgene is reflected both in the number of cells expressing the transgene and in the level of expression; only a small number of cells expressed the transgene at 8 weeks post transplantation (Snyder and Senut 1997; Liu et al., 1998). Possible mechanisms for the reduction in transgene expression include promoter down regulation, host immune response and, in the absence of DNA integration, dilution of the transgene due to cell division (Liu et al., 1998). It is, however, important to note that, unlike the life long expression required in therapy of disorders such as Parkinson's disease, it may be enough to express the therapeutic gene (such as a neurotrophin) for only a short time to promote regeneration.

The ability of Schwann cells, associated with peripheral nerve grafts, to promote regeneration in the CNS was initially observed in the pioneering studies of Tello (1911), revisited by Le Gros Clarke (1942), characterized in detail by Aguayo and colleagues (1980) and applied, using cultured Schwann cells, to spinal cord repair by Raisman and colleagues (Li and Raisman, 1994; this volume, Chapter by Raisman), and Bunge and colleagues (Levi et al., 1994; this volume, Chapter by Plant et al.,). Schwann cells provide a favorable environment for regenerating CNS axons (Xu et al., 1995a; Bahr and Bonhoeffer, 1995; Honmou et al., 1996; Guest et al., 1997) by expressing appropriate cell-adhesion molecules such as L1, cadherin and integrin, by providing permissive extracellular matrix components such as collagen and laminin and by secreting neurotrophic factors such as NGF and BDNF (Snyder and Senut et al., 1997). Axonal regeneration through the graft into host is, however, limited. Recently, grafting of olfactory ensheating glial cells has been used successfully to repair adult corticospinal tracts

(Lie et al., 1977; Ramon-Cueto et al., 1998; this volume, Chapter by Plant et al.,). Primary immature astrocytes and microglial cells may also be suitable for *ex vivo* CNS gene therapy because of their capacity to promote regeneration (reviewed by Fawcett, 1997; Stichel and Muller, 1998).

2. Cell lines

Many established cell lines, such as pheochromocytoma, neuroblastoma, glioma, schwannoma, and fibroblastic or astrocytic cell lines have been employed in earlier experimental gene therapy studies (Gage et al., 1987; Rosenberg et al., 1988; Cunningham et al., 1991b; Whittermore et al., 1991; Schinstine et al., 1995; Tornatore et al., 1996). Cell lines have been gradually replaced by primary cells as the graft of choice because of the risk of tumorigenesis. However, some cell lines derived from embryonal carcinoma (such as hNT) that have a potential to differentiate into neurons, and cell lines with properties of radial glia (such as C6-R) that can direct migration of neurons (Friedlander et al., 1998), are still under extensive study as candidates for clinical gene therapy.

B. Multipotential Neural Precursor Cells

1. Immortalized neural progenitor/stem-like cell lines

Using retrovirus mediated gene transfer of oncogenes such as c-myc (Ryder et a., 1990) and SV40 large T-antigen (Renfranz et al., 1991; White and Whittermore, 1992), a spectrum of immortalized neural stem-like cell lines has been isolated from newborn mouse cerebellum, C17.2 (Ryder et al., 1990), embryonic rat hippocampus, HiB5 (Renfranz et al., 1991), embryonic rat striatum, ST14A (Cattaneo et al., 1994) and embryonic rat medullary raphe, RN33B and RN46A (Whittermore and White, 1993; White et al., 1994). Immortalized progenitor cell lines have been prepared from oligodendrocytes (Almazan and McKay, 1992), astrocytes (Radany et al., 1992) and neuroblasts (Giordano et al., 1993). Immortalized neural progenitor/stem-like cells are excellent candidates for *ex vivo* CNS transplantation, to replace fetal transplants, because they are self-renewing, have stable transgene expression, and most importantly, they are multipotent and can differentiate into a variety of phenotypes (Martinez-Serrano and Bjorklund, 1997). The multipotential properties of the progenitor/stem-like cells have been demonstrated *in vitro* by showing that they can be induced to differentiate into neurons and glial cells by extrinsic signals as well as intrinsic programs (Ryder et al., 1990; Mehler et al., 1993; Whittermore and White 1993; Eves et al., 1994; White et al., 1994; Seigel et al 1996; Snyder, 1988). When grafted at an early developmental stage into different CNS regions, stem-like cells can integrate in a cytoarchitecturally appropriate manner and participate in the normal host CNS development (Snyder et al., 1992; 1998). When grafted into different adult CNS regions, in response to the local host cues, these cells can differentiate into neurons and glia, assuming appropriate cytoarchitecture without tumor formation (Renfranz et al., 1991; Snyder et al., 1992; Onifer et al., 1993; Shihabuddin et al., 1995).

In recent years, many studies have demonstrated the therapeutic potential of genetically modified immortalized neural progenitor/stem-like cells in a variety of brain diseases or conditions (Anton et al., 1994; Micklis et al., 1994; Snyder et al., 1995; Lacorazza et al., 1996; Martinez-Serrano et al., 1995 a, b; Martinez-Serrano et al., 1996 a, b; Martinez-Serrano and Bjorkland, 1996). For example, the NGF-producing HiB5 cells grafted into various degeneration models (fimbria-fornix transection, quinolinic acid lesion to nucleus basalis) prevented atrophy of cholinergic neurons (Martinez-Serrano et al., 1995a, b), the BDNF-producing RN46A cells grafted into the brain had positive effects on survival and differentiation of the graft (Eaton and Whittemore, 1996), the NT-3-producing C17.2 cells grafted into hemisected spinal cord rescued Clarke's nucleus neurons that would otherwise die (Himes et al., 1995, 1999b). The same NT-3 producing C17.2 cells grafted into a model of hypoxia-ischemia differentiated into neurons and ameliorated the excitotoxic damage (Park et al., 1998). In addition the C17-2 cell line has been shown to be effective for *ex vivo* gene therapy treatment of various metabolic disorders including Sly disease deficient in β-glucuronidase (Snyder et al., 1995) and Tay-Sachs disease deficient in the α-subunit of hexosaminidase A (Lacorazza, 1996). Their potential in treating spinal cord injury is only beginning to be examined.

2. Neural stem cells

Stem cells are defined operationally by their multipotency and their ability of self-renewal and self-maintenance, but the understanding of neural stem cells is still incomplete and open to much debate (Weiss et al., 1996; Snyder, 1998). The isolation and characterization of neural stem cells initially focused on studies that explored their properties *in vitro* to determine the factors that guide phenotypic choices of the cells. More recently, the emphasis has shifted to studies where the cells are implanted into the CNS and where the properties of the stem cells can be exploited for repair of damaged CNS (Fisher, 1997; Martinez-Serrano and Bjorklund, 1997; Snyder, 1998). There are two potential outcomes for the progeny of a stem cell. If the stem cell follows a symmetric mitotic pathway, both daughter cells will be stem cells. If the stem cells follow an asymmetric pathway, it will produce a stem cell and a progenitor cell (Gage et al., 1995; Weiss et al., 1996). A neural stem cell has the potential to generate all cell types in the CNS, including neurons astrocytes and oligodendrocytes (McKay, 1997). A progenitor cell, in contrast, follows a pathway leading towards terminal differentiation, and thus, has limited capacity for self-renewal and gives rise to limited types of terminally differentiated cells, for instance (Gage et al., 1995; Weiss et al., 1996; McKay, 1997;

Martinez-Serrano and Bjorklund, 1997). The "Precursor cell" term has been used here to refer in general to both stem cells and progenitor cells.

The advantages of neural stem cells over neural progenitor cells for *ex vivo* gene therapy lies in the fact that neural stem cells have unlimited ability for self-renewal and a wider repertoire of phenotypic choices. Consequently, it is possible to prepare and store large numbers of stem cells and avoid the need for immortalization techniques. Because neural stem cells can give rise to many types of neuronal and glial cells, compared to the restricted potential of progenitor cells which produce only limited cell types, they can be used for cell replacement and repair in a large variety of diseases or conditions throughout the CNS as well as a combination therapy with gene transfer in *ex vivo* CNS gene therapy. However, research on-going in our laboratory has shown promising results. Chow has isolated neural stem cells from embryonic rat spinal cord, which have demonstrated proliferation, self-renewal, multipotentiality over a period of at least a year. These cells are readily modified by recombinant adenoviral vectors. When transplanted into intact or lesioned spinal cord, the genetically modified neural stem cells expressed transgenes for at least 4 months (Fig. 2). They also migrated for long distances, differentiated into both neuronal and glial phenotypes and integrated into the host cytoarchitecture (Chow et al., 1997 a-c, 1998).

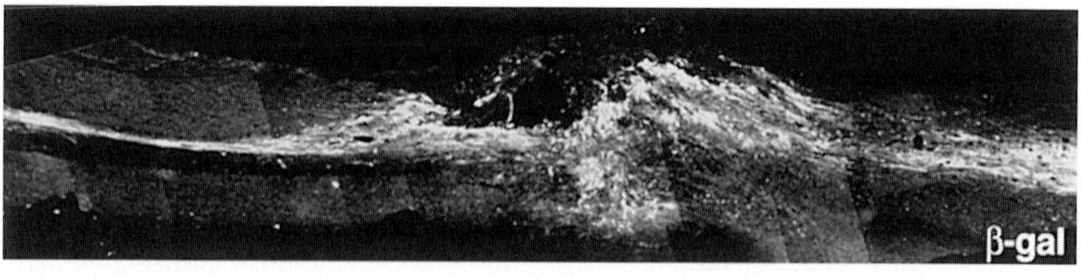

Figure 2 Spinal cord stem cells from Fischer 344 rats, infected with the recombinant adenovirus AD.CMV.lacZ (Liu et al., 1997), were grafted into a partial T8 hemisected spinal cord of Fischer 344 rats with no immunosuppression. Sections were fluorescently immunostained for β-galactosidase 4 months following surgery showing excellent survival of the stem cells, their migration and the continued expression of the transgene.

C. Other Precursor Cells

1. Bone marrow stromal cells

Bone marrow contains, in addition to hematopoietic cells, stem-like cells for nonhematopoietic tissue that are referred to as mesenchymal stem cells or marrow stromal cells (MSCs). Although it has been difficult to generate clones of MSCs, the protocols for isolation of MSCs are relatively simple and based on their ability to adhere tightly to the culture dishes. The resulting stromal cells represent heterogeneous populations that are multipotential and can differentiate into a variety of phenotypes. The full potential of these cells to differentiate and the molecular events involved in their differentiation are not well understood. The MSCs are, however, relatively easy to obtain from a patient under local anesthesia using small aspirates of bone marrow. The cells can be expanded in culture and stored. The ability to genetically modify MSCs with recombinant viral vectors makes them suitable candidates for delivery of therapeutic genes to correct a variety of genetic disorders. When human MSCs are grafted into rat brain without immune suppression they survive for several months with no evidence of an inflammatory response or rejection (Azizi et al., 1998). We have shown that MSCs grafted into spinal cord lesions survive, integrate well and appear to be permissive for axonal growth (Fig. 3). In addition, we have shown that MSCs can be genetically modified with recombinant adenovirus and retrovirus vectors (Himes et al., 1999a). These properties make MSCs an attractive candidate for the delivery of therapeutic genes to injured spinal cord.

IV. THIRD DIMENSION: DELIVERY OF THERAPEUTIC GENES BY *EX VIVO* AND *IN VIVO* GENE THERAPY CAN PROMOTE CNS REGENERATION

The development of *in vivo* and *ex vivo* gene transfer techniques in mammalian CNS, has stimulated great hope that gene therapy strategies might be able to promote CNS repair and regeneration. The third "dimension" of gene therapy (Fig. 1), the choice of therapeutic genes, includes genes encoding neurotrophic/neurotropic factors and their receptors, growth associated proteins, anti-apoptotic factors, extracellular matrix molecules, cell adhesion molecules and proteases that may promote axon growth. These genes have been tested in both *in vivo* and *ex vivo* systems. Recent studies have reported very encouraging results demonstrating successful regeneration in several CNS pathways. In the following section we will focus on studies that have demonstrated the feasibility of gene therapy to promote axon regeneration in mammalian CNS.

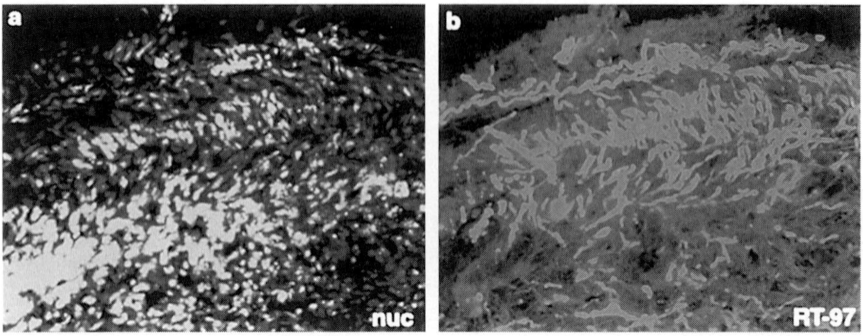

Figure 3 Human marrow stromal cells were labeled with 1 mg/ml bis-benzamide, a fluorescent nuclear dye, for 24 hr before transplantation. The cells were grafted into a partial hemisectioned spinal cord of Sprague Dawley rats. The marrow stromal cells, identified by their nuclear staining (A) filled the lesion cavity and survived for 2 months. Staining with a neurofilament antibody (B) showed numerous axons within the graft and indicated that the cells provide a permissive environment for growing axons.

A. Application of *ex vivo* Gene Therapy

Until recently, gene therapy strategies used to repair CNS injury employed the *ex vivo* paradigm. In most of these reports, retroviral vectors encoding therapeutic factors were used to engineer a variety of types of cells in culture including immortalized cell lines, primary cells and neural precursor cells. The engineered cells are then grafted into brain or spinal cord as the vehicle of the therapeutic gene product. Neuroanatomical studies demonstrated cell survival, axon sprouting, growth and regeneration; behavioral and physiological tests evaluated functional recovery. Several studies also have employed adenoviral vectors for *ex vivo* gene transfer into the CNS (Ridoux et al., 1994; Sabate et al., 1995; Van Esseveldt et al., 1997; Barkats et al., 1997; Boer et al., 1997; Liu et al., 1998). Some of these studies used only reporter genes (lacZ or GFP) to demonstrate the feasibility of adenoviral mediated *ex vivo* gene transfer. Others have demonstrated adenovirus-mediated delivery of therapeutic genes such as the human Cu/Zn superoxide dismutase gene for Parkinson's disease (Barkats et al., 1997) and neurotrophic factors for protection from injury-induced cell death (Baumgartner et al., 1997). The following sections, therefore, focus on retroviral mediated *ex vivo* gene delivery and are organized according to the types of cells engineered as transplants.

1. Fibroblasts

The study of genetically engineered fibroblasts for *ex vivo* gene therapy of CNS lesions was pioneered by Gage, Tuszynski and colleagues a decade ago (reviewed by Gage et al., 1987; Snyder and Senut, 1997; Tuszynski, 1998). Both immortalized and primary fibroblasts were initially studied, but primary fibroblasts were favored because they do not pose the risk of tumorigenesis (Kawaja et al., 1991). Among the therapeutic genes that have been transferred into CNS tissues of experimental animals, neurotrophic factors, (NGF, NT-3 and BDNF) have received the most attention (Rosenberg et al., 1988; Kawaja et al., 1992; Tuszynski et al., 1994, 1996; Senut et al., 1995; Chen and Gage, 1995; Nakahara et al., 1996; Grill et al., 1997; McTigue et al., 1998; Liu et al., 1999b; for a more comprehensive list of references see Hermens and Verhaagen, 1998). In general, these experiments demonstrated three levels of therapeutic potential of genetically engineered fibroblasts expressing neurotrophic factors.

[1] Neuroprotection. While 92% of septal cholinergic neurons axotomized by a fimbra-formix lesion survive in rats receiving NGF-producing fibroblast grafts, only 49% survive in animals receiving unmodified control grafts (Rosenberg et al., 1988). In spinal cords following a mid-thoracic hemisection, NT-3 producing fibroblasts completely rescue the 30% of neurons which would otherwise die (Himes et al., 1995; Tessler et al., 1997).

[2] Axon growth and sprouting. In a series of experiments, Gage, Tuszynski and colleagues have demonstrated that fibroblasts expressing NGF, NT-3 or BDNF grafted into normal or injured spinal cord and a variety of brain regions, including hippocampus and locus coeruleus, induce robust axon growth and sprouting into the transplants (Tuszynski et al., 1994, 1996; Senut et al., 1995; Nakahara et al., 1996). Different neurotrophins elicited different effects (Nakahara et al., 1996); also different CNS regions responded differently (Senut et al., 1995), indicating the specificity of neurotrophins.

[3] Regeneration and functional recovery. Genetically engineered fibroblasts expressing NGF, NT-3 and BDNF have proven effective in promoting regeneration from several CNS pathways, including the fimbria-fornix pathway, corticospinal tract (CST) and rubrospinal tract (RST).

Unilateral ablation of projections from septal cholinergic neurons, resulting in denervation of the ipsilateral hippocampus is demonstrated by the lack of histochemical staining for AchE. Grafts of NGF-secreting fibroblasts induced axon regeneration from the axotomized septal cholinergic neurons and resulted in re-innervation of hippocampus demonstrated by AchE staining (Kawaja et al., 1992).

Primary fibroblasts engineered to produce NT-3 were grafted into the lesion cavities of a dorsal spinal cord hemisection which bilaterally disrupted corticospinal, rubrospinal and cerulospinal projections. The transgenic cellular delivery of NT-3 induced robust axon regrowth from the CST which was demonstrated by anterograde tracing with WGA-HRP injected into the sensorimotor cortex representing the hindlimbs (Grill et al., 1997). When locomotion was assessed, animals with the therapeutic grafts showed significant recovery compared to rats receiving control grafts in a test (the grid task) that requires sensorimotor integration. However, the CST axon regrowth was limited to 12 mm caudal to the NT-3 producing grafts. Also, the CST axons failed to enter the grafts and the regrowth was restricted to the gray matter (Grill et al., 1997).

Using a similar experimental paradigm, the regenerative capacity of RST axons was tested with BDNF-producing grafts (Liu et al., 1999b). Animals were subjected to a partial spinal cord hemisection at C3-4 levels, which removed the right lateral funiculus containing the entire right RST (Fig 4a). Primary skin fibroblasts were engineered with a retroviral construct encoding the human-BDNF gene linked with a fusion reporter gene of β-galactosidase and neomycin resistance (Liu et al., 1999b). The graft of the genetically modified fibroblasts showed excellent survival and integration into the hemisection with no invasion of immune-related cells. RST axon regeneration was analyzed using both anterograde and retrograde tracing techniques (Fig. 4b).

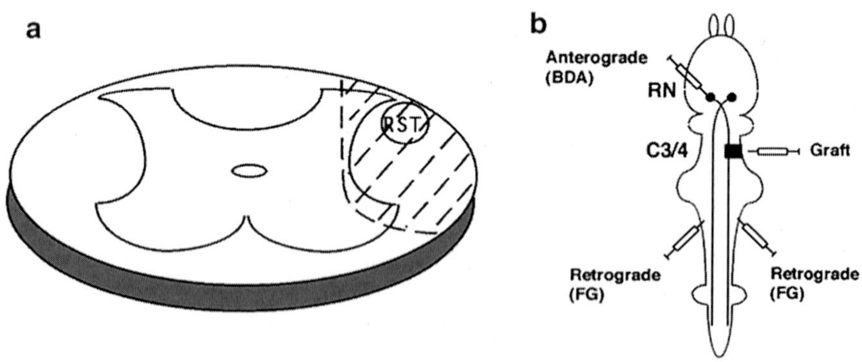

Figure 4 A schematic diagram of the experimental paradigm (From Liu et al., 1999b). Animals received a right C3-4 partial hemisection that disrupted the axons from the left RN. Panel A shows a spinal cord cross section, the shaded area represents the lesion and transplant.. Immediately following the spinal cord lesion, gelfoam, Fibroblasts or BDNF-producing fibroblasts cells were grafted into the lesion cavity. RST axon regeneration was studied using either BDA anterograde tracing or FG retrograde tracing (B).

Based on the retrograde tracing with fluorogold caudal to the lesion, it was estimated that 7-10% of RST axons regenerated up to10 segments (Fig. 6). Anterograde labeling by BDA injection into the Red Nucleus traced the regenerating axons through and around the transplants and into the caudal white matter (Fig. 5). Animals were also tested for functional recovery that assessed limb usage. There was significant recovery of function in animals receiving the therapeutic transplants within the first month of treatment. The functional recovery was abolished by a second hemisection just rostral to the transplants, which indicated that the functional recovery was, at least in part, mediated by the presence in the graft. The BDNF-producing fibroblasts that promote regeneration of axotomized rubrospinal neurons also rescue most neurons from retrograde death and prevent their atrophy (Liu et al., 1999c).

RST regeneration had several striking features that appear different from CST: robust growth through and around the transplants, long distance growth in the white matter (up to several centimeters caudal to the lesions transplant), fast growth rate (1-1.5 mm/day) and formation of projections bearing terminal bouton-like structures in the appropriate laminae of the gray matter (Fig. 5). These differences may reflect intrinsic differences between two major supraspinal motor control systems including the ability to regenerate, the interaction between regenerating axons with the environment in the transplants and in the white matter; and the effects of NT-3 and BDNF on CST and RST axons, respectively.

The effects of NGF and BDNF, delivered by genetically modified cells, on functional recovery following spinal cord injury were also tested in a contusion model (Kim et al., 1996). Fibroblasts modified to produce NGF or BDNF or unmodified fibroblasts were grafted into the mid-thoracic contusion site. Both NGF and BDNF producing fibroblasts significantly accelerated recovery in locomotor performance during the test period, whereas unmodified control fibroblast failed to do so. Histological analysis of the cross-section area at the injury site demonstrated significant neuroprotective effects by the neurotrophin-secreting fibroblasts.

Besides genes encoding neurotrophic factors, fibroblasts have also been engineered to express the neural cell adhesion molecule L1 (Kobayashi et al., 1995). The L1-secreting fibroblasts transplanted into hemisection or extensive dorsal funiculotomy lesions elicited axon ingrowth into the producing grafts or control unmodified grafts.

2. Schwann cells

Schwann cells are known to support axonal growth. Channels seeded with Schwann cells, grafted into a mid-thoracic spinal cord transection site, elicited regeneration only from dorsal root ganglia (DRG) and propriospinal axons (Xu et al., 1995a). When BDNF and NT-3 were infused into such transplants, sig

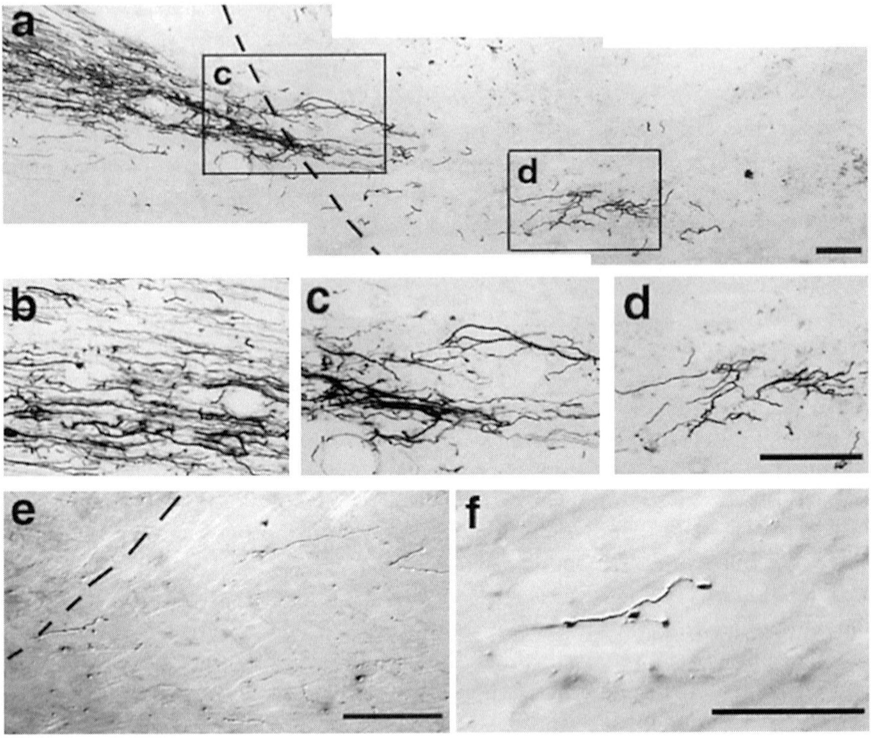

Figure 5 Photomicrographs of cervical spinal cord sections showing regeneration of RST axons through the BDNF-producing fibroblast transplants one month after transplantation. Animals received a right cervical hemisection and a transplant. The left Red Nucleus was anterogradely traced with BDA and the spinal cord tissue was cut into sagittal sections. For all sections left is rostral and right is caudal. A. The BDA labeled RST axons enter the transplant, where the dashed line indicates the rostral graft-host interface. B. In the region rostral to the transplant, numerous axon branches are evident, suggesting sprouting induced by the transplant. C. The BDA labeled axons penetrate the rostral graft-host interface. D. The RST axons deep in the transplant. E. A region in the host white matter immediately caudal to the transplant. The dashed line indicates the caudal graft-host interface. BDA labeled axons exit the transplant and elongate caudally. Some axons bear varicosities resembling terminal boutons (From Liu et al., 1999b).

nificantly more axon ingrowth was induced, including brain stem neurons (Xu et al.,1995b). These findings inspired Bunge and colleagues to engineer Schwann cells to produce human-BDNF using a retroviral vector. The genetically modified Schwann cells were then grafted into a T8 transection site. The unique feature of this study is that the cells were also injected into the caudal spinal cord as a 5 mm trail. This procedure was designed to guide regenerating axons into caudal spinal cord stump (Menei et al., 1998). Axon regeneration from brainstem, DRG and propriospinal neurons was studied by tracing with Fast Blue and by immunocytochemical staining with 5-HT, DβH and CGRP antibodies 1 month post-operatively. The BDNF-producing Schwann cell transplants promoted reticular, vestibular and raphe nucleus neurons to regenerate axons across the transection site. Such a procedure also induced more DRG and propriospinal neurons to regenerate for significantly longer distance (Menei et al., 1998). The response from CST and RST neurons was as robust. These findings again suggest that different supraspinal structures may be amenable to different interventions and therefore, that the choice of donor cells and therapeutic factors will need to be tailored to the type of injury to be repaired.

3. Astrocytes

Several studies with genetically modified astrocytes demonstrated the feasibility of using these cells for *ex vivo* gene transfer to promote CNS regeneration. Primary type I rat astrocytes modified with a retroviral vector encoding a mouse β-NGF cDNA and co-grafted with adrenal chromaffin cells into rat striatum enhanced the survival and neurite outgrowth of chromaffin cells (Cunningham et al., 1991a, 1994). Primary astrocytes were also engineered by adenoviral vectors containing genes of CNTF or NT-3. The modified astrocytes secreted high levels of bioactive CNTF or NT-3 and supported the survival of motor neurons *in vitro* (Smith et al., 1996). Furthermore, an astrocyte cell line, Neu7 transfected with a plasmid expressing urokinase, a major enzyme controlling the extracellular proteolytic cas-

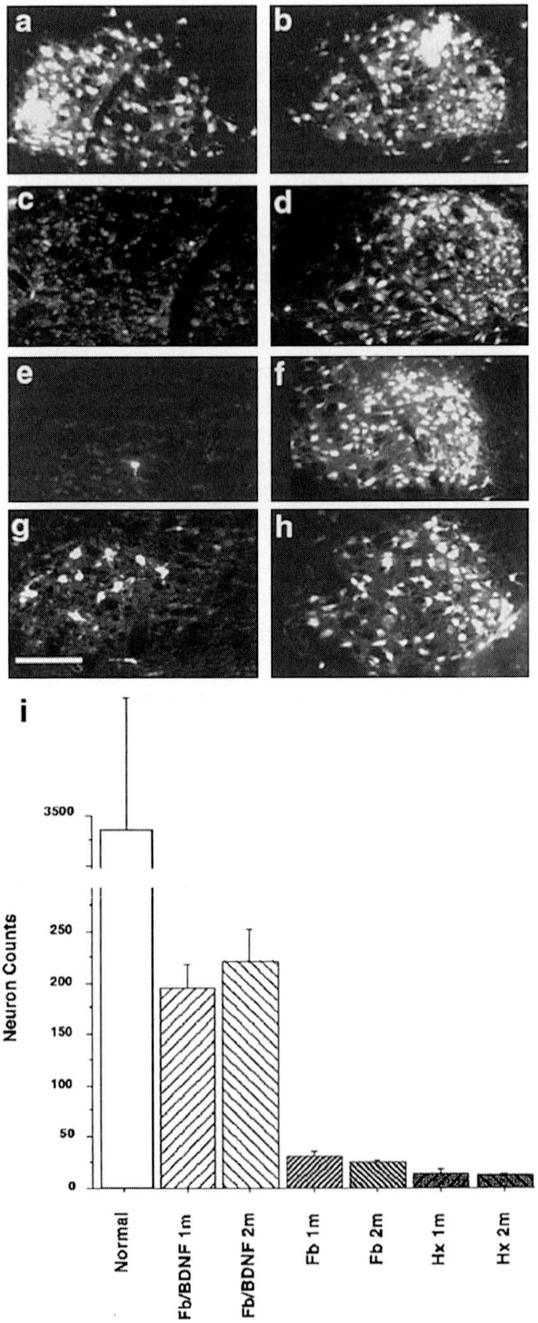
a
b
c
d
e
f
g
h
i
Neuron Counts
3500
250
200
150
100
50
0
Normal
Fb/BDNF 1m
Fb/BDNF 2m
Fb 1m
Fb 2m
Hx 1m
Hx 2m

cade, promoted axon regeneration from DRG neurons in monolayer and three-dimensional cultures (Muir et al., 1998). Even though these studies do not provide direct evidence that genetically modified astrocytes are suitable for *ex vivo* gene therapy to promote CNS regeneration, they do support this possibility.

4. Immortalized neural progenitor/stem-like cells

A great many immortalized neural progenitor cell lines have been used for *ex vivo* gene transfer into the CNS (reviewed by Martinez-Serrano and Bjorklund, 1997). Genes that have been transferred include reporter genes (lacZ and luciferase) and therapeutic genes (neurotrophins, β-Glucoronidase, β-Hexosaminidase, tyrosine hydroxylase, etc.). CNS regions targeted have included cortex (Snyder, 1994; Snyder and Macklis, 1995; Eaton and Whittemore, 1996), cerebellum (Renfranz et al., 1991; Snyder et al., 1992), hippocampus (Renfranz et al., 1991; Onifer et al., 1993; Shihabuddin et al., 1995, 1996; Eaton and Whittemore, 1996), striatum (Lundberg et al., 1996 a, b, 1997; Lundberg and Bjorklund et al., 1996), septum (Martinez-Serrano et al., 1995 a), ventricles (Lacorazza et al., 1996; Snyder and Macklis, 1995), raphe nuclei (Onifer et al., 1993) and spinal cord (Onifer et al., 1993; Himes et al., 1995; Eaton et al., 1997; Liu et al., 1999b). The therapeutic potential of genetically modified immortalized neural progenitor cells was evaluated in several animal models of disease and injury including Parkinson's disease (Anton et al., 1994), Huntington's disease (Martinez-Serrano and Bjorklund, 1996), Alzheimer's disease (Martinez-Serrano et al., 1995b), stroke (Martinez-Serrano and Bjorklund, 1997; Park et al., 1999), mucopolysaccharidosis type VII (Snyder et al., 1995), Tay-Sachs disease (Lacorazza et al., 1996), aging (Martinez-Serrano et al., 1996a) and spinal cord injury (Himes et al., 1995; Eaton et al., 1996; Liu et al., 1999a). In general, reports on engineered immortalized neural stem-like cells focused on neuroprotection and complementary cellular or enzymatic deficiencies. Thus far, their potential on promoting CNS regeneration has received little study.

Figure 6 Photomicrographs of midbrain showing fluorogold (FG) retrograde tracing of Red Nucleus (RN) neurons (From Liu et al., 1999b). Neurons in both RNs were retrogradely traced by injection of FG into both sides of the spinal cord in normal animals (a,b) or in recipients of gelfoam (c,d), fibroblasts (e,f) and BDNF-producing fibroblasts (g,h) transplants. Survival after transplantation was one month In gelfoam recipients virtually no RN neurons are labeled by FG on the left (c), whereas labeling on the right is normal (d). In fibroblast transplant recipients, very few RN neurons are labeled in the left RN (e), whereas the right RN is normally labeled (f). In recipients of BDNF-producing transplants, numerous RN neurons are labeled in the left RN (g) and labeling is normal in the right RN (h). Scale bars: 100 mm. The FG-labeled RN neurons were counted and compared by one-way ANOVA, followed by Fisher post hoc, 1 or 2 months after transplantation. Significantly more RN neurons (175-200 neurons) were labeled contralateral to surgery in animals receiving BDNF-producing fibroblast transplants than those receiving fibroblats alone (30-40 neurons) or gelfoam (~10 neurons).

5. Neural stem cells

In the past several years, we have used neural stem cells for *ex vivo* gene transfer to promote CNS repair and regeneration (Chow et al., 1997 a, b, c, 1998). We have isolated precursor cells from embryonic rat spinal cord that showed several characteristics of neural stem cells. These cells remain proliferative in culture for more than 2 years and spontaneously differentiate into astrocytes, oligodendrocytes and neurons with a variety of phenotypes (e.g. cholinergic, GABAergic etc.). Interestingly, these cells can be guided toward neuronal differentiation with exogenous factors such as retinoic acid (Moul et al., 1998). We have genetically modified these cells with adenoviral vectors and grafted them into both intact and lesioned spinal cord of adult rats (Fig. 2). The neural stem cells survived well after transplantation and differentiated into both neuronal and glial phenotypes. Our preliminary studies also have shown that stem cells alone or mixed with BDNF-producing fibroblasts transplanted into a cervical partial hemisection cavity promoted recovery of function.

6. Other types of cells

Several other cells have also been modified and employed for *ex vivo* gene transfer into the CNS. A mouse neuroblastoma cell line was modified by a retroviral vector carrying the temperature-sensitive mutant of SV 40 large T antigen. Under non-permissive temperature, these cells differentiated into neurons that expressed bioactive NGF. When xenografted into a fimbria-fornix lesion of adult rats, they rescued about 50% of septal cholinergic neurons destined to undergo retrograde death (Whittermore et al., 1991).

Rat phenochromocytoma PC 12 cells engineered to produce mouse β-NGF were xenografted into mouse striatum to study their value for Parkinson's disease. Even though these cells expressed NGF *in vivo*, they lost tyrosine hydroxylase expression and showed only limited survival and neuronal differentiation following implantation. They were therefore not considered suitable for replacement of nigrostriatal dopamine neurons in the mouse model of Parkinson's disease (Cunningham et al., 1991b).

B. Application of *in vivo* Gene Therapy

In vivo gene therapy for CNS lesions has received less attention because of the lack of an appropriate vector system. During mid-80's to early-90's, HSV and retroviral vectors were the main gene delivery tools available. However, as discussed earlier, HSV vectors are problematic because of immunogenicity and cytotoxicity, whereas conventional retroviral vectors are not suitable for *in vivo* gene transfer. The breakthrough occurred in 1993, when several groups demonstrated the feasibility of *in vivo* gene transfer into the CNS using adenoviral vectors. The approach has become even more promising with the refinement of adenoviral vectors (see Section IIA3) and the development of AAV and lentivirus vectors (see Sections IIA4 and IIA5). Most *in vivo* gene therapy experiments have focused on neuroprotection for neurodegenerative diseases, with only a few studies aimed at promoting CNS regeneration. In the following section, we will briefly review studies on *in vivo* gene delivery into the CNS; the available studies on regeneration will be discussed in greater detail.

1. Herpes simplex virus vectors

Most experiments on HSV-mediated *in vivo* gene transfer into the CNS have been feasibility studies using reporter genes but several studies with HSV vectors encoding genes of NGF, BDNF, GAP-43 or bcl-2 have suggested their therapeutic potential in neuroprotection and neuroregeneration (Federoff et al., 1992; Geschwind et al., 1994, 1996; Verhaagen et al., 1994; Linnik et al., 1995; Lawrence et al., 1996). Other therapeutic genes that have been transferred into the CNS using HSV vectors include genes of β-glucuronidase (Wolfe et al., 1992), tyrosine hydroxylase (During et al., 1994) and glucose transporters (Ho et al., 1993; Lawrence et al., 1995; Dash et al., 1996), for specific disease. No direct evidence is yet available on whether this approach will promote CNS regeneration.

2. Adenoviral vectors

Adenovirus mediated *in vivo* gene transfer has attracted the most attention since the demonstration of efficient gene delivery into a variety of CNS regions [cerebral cortex (Doran et al., 1995), brain stem nuclei (Liu et al., 1997), striatum (Horellou et al., 1994; Lisovoski et al., 1995; Byrnes et al., 1995), hippocampus (Le Gal La Salle et al., 1993), olfactory neurons (Zhao et al., 1996), cerebellum (Hashimoto et al., 1996) and spinal cord (Lisovoski et al., 1995; Liu et al., 1997)], using adenoviral vectors encoding the lacZ or GFP reporter gene (Fig.7). Evidence remains scant on the efficacy of *in vivo* gene therapy with adenoviral vector to promote axon regeneration in mammalian CNS environment but several studies have provided promising results.

Following axotomy in adult rats, the central processes of DRG neurons normally fail to regenerate through the dorsal root entry zone into the spinal cord. Adenoviral vectors were used to deliver NT-3 or control lacZ genes into the ventral horn of lumbar cord. The transgenes were expressed at high levels in motor neurons and glial cells for at least 40 days. Dorsal root axon regeneration into the cord demonstrated that transgenic NT-3 expression in ventral horn significantly enhanced the number of DRG axons that had regenerated into the spinal cord.

The distance of axon growth within the cord was also greatly increased in animals receiving the NT-3 (Zhang et al., 1998). *In vivo* gene therapy with adenoviral vectors encoding a neurotrophin therefore promoted dorsal root axon regeneration into and through the CNS environment.

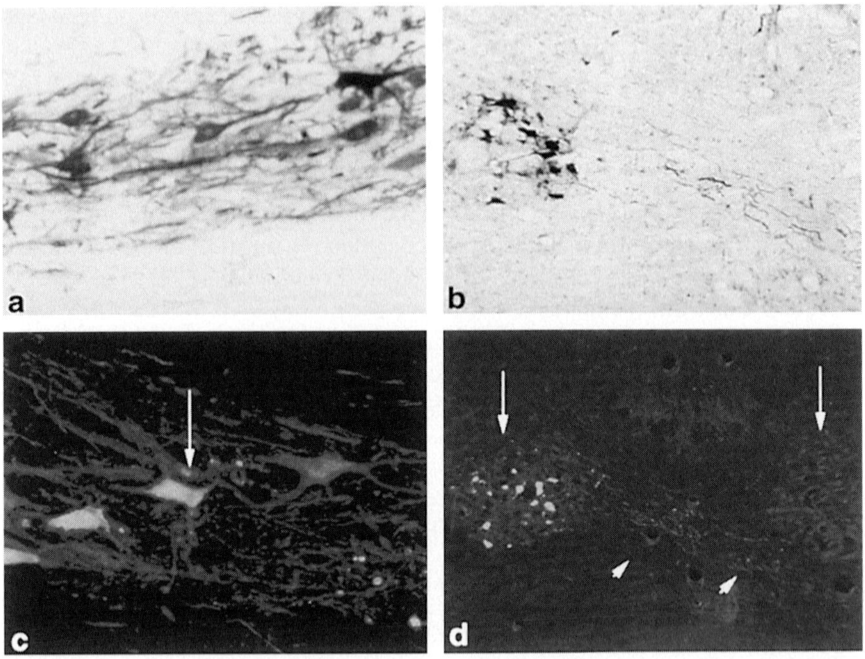

Figure 7 The recombinant adenovirus Ad.CMV.lacZ (a,b) or Ad.CMV.GFP (c,d) was injected into the right side of the spinal cord at the T7-8 level of adult rats (From Liu et al., 1997). The spinal cord was removed at 1 week and stained for b-galactosidase (a,b) or directly visualized using fluorescent microscopy (c,d). Transgene expression is readily detected at the injection site (a,c, 200X), where a variety of cells were infected. There was also expression of the transgene in neurons whose axons project to the injection site from rostral or caudal regions. Among labeled neurons were those of the contralateral left, but not right Red Nucleus (c and arrows in d, 25X). Note the staining of rubrospinal tract axons (b,arrowheads in d).

An adenoviral vector constructed to encode the B-50/GAP-43 gene was used to infect mouse olfactory neuroepithelium, which resulted in transduction of 20-50% mature olfactory neurons that normally do not express this gene. The transduced neurons exhibited spontaneous axon growth and morphological changes suggesting enhanced ability for axon regeneration (Holtmaat et al., 1997). The efficacy of this vector in promoting CNS axon regeneration has not yet been examined using a lesion paradigm.

Adenoviral vectors encoding cell-adhesion molecules, such as NgCAM and axonin-1, also have been engineered (Vogt et al., 1996, Giger et al., 1997). Even though *in vitro* studies with cultured neurons transduced by these vectors suggested enhanced growth cone formation, direct *in vivo* evidence on their role in neuroregeneration is not yet available.

More data are available on neuroprotection in animal models of neurodegenerative disease. *In vivo* gene therapy with adenoviral vectors was employed to introduce genes of tyrosine hydroxylase (TH), dopamine D2-receptor or neurotrophic/neurotropic factors into the striatum, basal forebrain cholinergic neurons and motor neurons in the facial and hypoglossal nuclei. These studies have provided encouraging results in experimental models of Parkinson's, Alzheimer's, Huntington's and motor neuron disease (Horellou et al., 1994; Ikari et al., 1995; Castel-Barthe et al., 1996; Baumgartner and Shine, 1997; Haase et al., 1997; Bilang-Bleuel et al., 1997)

3. AAV vectors

AAV vectors have drawn attention in recent years because of their potential in gene therapy (reviewed by Xiao et al., 1997). AAV mediated *in vivo* gene therapy with GDNF and TH was studied in a rat model of Parkinson's disease with promising neuroanatomical and behavioral results (Kaplitt et al., 1994; Mandel et al., 1997). In addition when NGF was delivered to the medial septum by recombinant AAV in a degenerative model of lesioned fimbria-fornix, there was a significant attenuation of cholinergic cell loss (Mandel et al., 1999). No data are available as yet on promoting regeneration with this vector.

4. Lentivirus vectors

HIV-based vectors (lentivirus vectors) have been developed only in the past few years (Naldini et al., 1996; Blomer et al., 1997; Miyoshi et al., 1997). Safety is the major challenge for their future application. Although initial studies using *in vivo* protocols with reporter genes demonstrated high gene transfer efficiency and stable transgene expression in neurons in several CNS regions, vectors encoding therapeutic genes remain to be constructed. Nothing is known therefore about their efficacy in CNS regeneration as yet.

5. Other vectors

We have explored the possibility of *in vivo* gene delivery with non-viral vectors. Plasmid constructs with either bcl-2 or lacZ gene were injected into the spinal cord of animals with a mid-thoracic hemisection. Transgene expressing was detected in Clarke's nucleus in the lumbar spinal cord and the red nucleus in the brain stem. Bcl-2 completely prevented axotomy-induced neuron loss and atrophy in the Clarke's nucleus ipsilateral to the lesion (Takahashi et al., 1999) and preliminary results indicate similar findings for the Red nucleus. This vector system has not been used to study regeneration, but studies with mice that overexpress Bcl-2 have shown that it can promote regeneration of axotomized retinal ganglion cells (Chen et al., 1997).

IV. FUTURE DIRECTIONS

As evident from this review there is no single ideal system for gene therapy, but rather a growing choice of vectors, cells and therapeutic genes that can be used to promote regeneration in CNS. The need for developing, trying and selecting the best combination for an efficient and safe treatment is particularly important in the "nongenetic illnesses" of brain trauma and spinal cord injury where the option of *ex vivo* gene therapy includes not only delivery of therapeutic genes, but also grafting of cells that can differentiate into specific phenotypes, integrate with host tissue and contribute to recovery of function.

The rapid advances in gene therapy promise continued and improved selection of vectors, cells and genes. New generations of vectors are designed to have higher titer, more cloning capacity, less immune response, and most importantly, better control of transgene expression. Recombinant vectors constructed with regulated genes will allow targeting into a specific population of cells, high level production of proteins and the ability to turn off transgene expression. One of the most important developments in CNS grafting is the improvement in methods for preparation and manipulation of neural stem cells. The continued use of stem cells for grafting will not only contribute to understanding the mechanism of cell differentiation in the CNS, but will also provide the means of cell replacement together with the delivery of therapeutic genes. The recent progress in promoting axon regeneration in CNS described in this chapter is an excellent example of how the emerging technology of gene therapy can be effectively applied to what has been learned from basic science on the intrinsic properties of neurons, the inhibitory influence of the CNS environment, and the role of neurotrophic factors, anti-apoptotic proteins and genes associated with axon growth and regeneration.

ACKNOWLEDGEMENTS

The work described and presented in this review was carried out in collaboration with Drs. Marion Murray, Alan Tessler, Evan Snyder, Tim Himes, Duckhyun Kim, Darwin Prockop, Stella Chow, Joanna Solowska-Bairs and Timothy Schallert. We wish to thank Dr. Laura Lillien for initiating our work with retroviruses and acknowledge the technical help of Theresa Connors, Maryla Obrocka and Kathy Bozek. Supported by NIH grants NS24707, NS10090, HD074677, the Research Service of the Veteran Administration, the Eastern Paralyzed Veterans Association, the International Spinal Cord Research Trust and the Center of Excellence grant of MCP Hahnemann University.

REFERENCES

Akli S, Caillaud C, Vigne E, Stratford-Perricaudet LD, Poenaru L, Perricaudet M, Kahn A, Peschanski, MR (1993) Transfer of a foreign gene into the brain using adenovirus vectors. Nature Genetics 3:224-228.

Almazan G, McKay, R (1992) An oligodendrocyte precursor cell line from rat optic nerve. Brain Res 579:234-245.

Andersen JK, Garber DA, Meaney CA, Breakefield X O (1992) Gene transfer into mammalian central nervous system using herpes virus vectors: extended expression of bacterial lacZ in neurons using the neuron-specific enolase promoter. Human Gene Therapy 3:487-99.

Anton R, Kordower JH, Maidment NT, Manaster JS, Kane DJ, Rabizadeh S, Schueller SB, Yang J, Rabizadeh S, Edwards RH, et al. (1994) Neural-targeted gene therapy for rodent and primate hemiparkinsonism. Exp Neurol 127:207-18.

Azizi SA, Stokes D, Augelli BJ, DiGirolamo C, Prockop, D (1998) Enraftment and migration of human bone marrow stromal cells implanted in the brains of albino rats - similarities to astrocyte grafts. Proc. Nat. Acad. Sci USA 95:3908-3913.

Bahr M, Bonhoeffer F (1994). Perspectives on axonal regeneration in the mammalian CNS. Trends in Neurosciences 17:473-479.

Bajocchi G, Feldman SH, Crystal RG, Mastrangeli A (1993) Direct *in vivo* gene transfer to ependymal cells in the central nervous system using recombinant adenovirus vectors. Nature Genetics 3: 229-34.

Barkats M, Nakao N, Grasbon-Frodl EM, Bilang-Bleuel A, Revah F, Mallet J, Brundin P (1997) Intrastriatal grafts of embryonic mesencephalic rat neurons genetically modified using an adenovirus encoding human Cu/Zn superoxide dismutase. Neurosci 78:703-13.

Baumgartner BJ, Shine HD (1997) Targeted transduction of CNS neurons with adenoviral vectors carrying neurotrophic factor genes confers neuroprotection that exceeds the transduced population. J Neurosci 17:6504-11.

Bilang-Bleuel A, Revah F, Colin P, Locquet I, Robert JJ, Mallet J, Horellou P (1997) Intrastriatal injection of an adenoviral vector expressing glial-cell-line-derived neurotrophic factor prevents dopaminergic neuron degeneration and behavioral impairment in a rat model of Parkinson disease. Proc Natl Acad Sci 94:8818-8823.

Blomer U, Naldini L, Verma IM, Trono D, Gage FH (1996) Applications of gene therapy to the CNS. Human Molecular Genetics, 1397-404.

Blomer U, Naldini L, Kafri T, Trono D, Verma IM, Gage FH (1997) Highly efficient and sustained gene transfer in adult neurons with a lentivirus vector. J Virol 71:6641-6649.

Boer GJ, van Esseveldt KE, Hermens WT, Liu R, Verhaagen J (1997) Long-term transgene expression in fetal rat suprachiasmatic nucleus neurografts following *ex vivo* adenoviral vector-mediated gene transfer. Exp Neurol 145:536-545.

Brook GA, Lawrence JM, Shah B, Raisman G (1994) Extrusion transplantation of Schwann cells into the adult rat thalamus induces directional host axon growth. Exp Neurol 126:31-43.

Byrnes A P, Rusby JE, Wood MJ, Charlton HM (1995) Adenovirus gene transfer causes inflammation in the brain. Neurosci 66:1015-1024.

Castel-Barthe MN, Jazat-Poindessous F, Barneoud P, Vigne E, Revah F, Mallet J, Lamour Y (1996) Direct intracerebral nerve growth factor gene transfer using a recombinant adenovirus: effect on basal forebrain cholinergic neurons during aging. Neurobiol Dis 3:76-86.

Cattaneo E, Magrassi, L, Butti G, Santi L, Giavazzi A, Pezzotta S (1994) A short term analysis of the behaviour of conditionally immortalized neuronal progenitors and primary neuroepithelial cells implanted into the fetal rat brain. Dev Brain Res 83:197-208.

Chen KS, Gage FH (1995) Somatic gene transfer of NGF to the aged brain: behavioral and morphological amelioration. J Neurosci 15:2819-2825.

Chen DF, Schneider GE, Martineu J-C, Tonegawa S (1997) Bcl-2 promotes regeneration of severed axons in mammalian CNS. Nature 385:434-439.

Chiocca EA, Choi BB, Cai W Z, DeLuca NA, Schaffer PA, DiFiglia M, Breakefield, XO, Martuza R L (1990) Transfer and expression of the lacZ gene in rat brain neurons mediated by herpes simplex virus mutants. New Biologist 2:739-46.

Chow SY, Liu, Y, Himes, BT, Moul J, Goold RG, Obrocka M, Tessler A, Fischer I (1997a). Survival and differentiation of stem cells from embryonic spinal cord grafted into adult spinal cord. J Neurochem 69:S26B.

Chow SY, Liu Y, Himes BT, Moul J, Obrocka M, Tessler A, Fischer I (1997b) Survival and differentiation of virally infected stem cells grafted into adult spinal cord. J NeuroVirology 3: 95.

Chow SY, Liu Y, Moul J, Himes BT, Obrocka M, Hao J, Tessler A, Fischer I. (1998) Isografts of neural stem cells into spinal cord of Fischer 344 rats. Soc Neurosci. Abstr 24: 68.

Chow SY, Moul J, Liu Y, Himes B T, Obrocka M, Tessler A, Fischer I. (1997c) Survival and differentiation of rat spinal cord stem cells grafted into normal and injured adult spinal cord. Soc Neuorsci Abstr 23, 905.

Crystal RG (1995) Transfer of genes to humans: early lessons and obstacles to success. Science 270:404-10.

Cunningham LA, Hansen JT, Short MP, Bohn, MC (1991a) The use of genetically altered astrocytes to provide nerve growth factor to adrenal chromaffin cells grafted into the striatum. Brain Res 561:192-202.

Cunningham LA, Short MP, Breakefield XO, Bohn MC (1994) Nerve growth factor released by transgenic astrocytes enhances the function of adrenal chromaffin cell grafts in a rat model of Parkinson's disease. Brain Res 658:219-31.

Cunningham LA, Short MP, Vielkind U, Breakefield XO, Bohn MC (1991b) Survival and differentiation within the adult mouse striatum of grafted rat pheochromocytoma cells (PC12) genetically modified to express recombinant beta-NGF. Exp Neurol 11:174-82.

Dash R, Lawrence M, Ho D, Sapolsky R (1996) A herpes simplex virus vector overexpressing the glucose transporter gene protects the rat dentate gyrus from an antimetabolite toxin. Exp Neurol 137:43-48.

Davidson BL, Allen ED, Kozarsky KF, Wilson JM, Roessler BJ (1993) A model system for *in vivo* gene transfer into the central nervous system using an adenoviral vector. Nature Genetics 3:219-223.

Davidson BL, Bohn MC (1997) Recombinant adenovirus: a gene transfer vector for study and treatment of CNS diseases. Exp Neurol 144:125-130.

Doering LC (1994) Nervous system modification by transplants and gene transfer. Bioessays 16:825-831.

Doran S E, Ren XD, Betz AL, Pagel MA, Neuwelt EA, Roessler BJ, Davidson BL (1995) Gene expression from recombinant viral vectors in the central nervous system after blood-brain barrier disruption. Neurosurgery 36: 965-970.

Eaton MJ, Santiago DI, Dancausse HA, Whittemore SR (1997) Lumbar transplants of immortalized serotonergic neurons alleviate chronic neuropathic pain. Pain 72:59-69.

Eaton MJ, Whittemore SR (1996) Autocrine BDNF secretion enhances the survival and serotonergic differentiation of raphe neuronal precursor cells grafted into the adult rat CNS. Exp Neurol 140:105-114.

Emerich DF, Lindner MD, Winn SR, Chen EY. Frydel BR, Kordower JH (1996) Implants of encapsulated human CNTF-producing fibroblasts prevent behavioral deficits and striatal degeneration in a rodent model of Huntington's disease. J Neurosci 16:5168-5181.

Engelhardt JF, Ye X, Doranz B, Wilson JM (1994) Ablation of E2A in recombinant adenoviruses improves transgene persistence and decreases inflammatory response in mouse liver. Proc Natl Acad Sci 91: 6196-6200.

Eves EM, Kwon J, Downen M, Tucker MS, Wainer BH, Rosner MR (1994) Conditional immortalization of neuronal cells from postmitotic cultures and adult CNS. Brain Res 656: 396-404.

Fawcett JW (1997) Astrocytic and neuronal factors affecting axon regeneration in the damaged central nervous system. Cell Tissue Res 290: 371-377.

Federoff HJ, Geschwind MD, Geller, AI, Kessler JA (1992) Expression of nerve growth factor *in vivo* from a defective herpes simplex virus 1 vector prevents effects of axotomy on sympathetic ganglia. Proc Natl Acad Sci USA 89:1636-1640.

Fisher LJ, Jinnah HA, Kale LC, Higgins GA, Gage FH (1991) Survival and function of intrastriatally grafted primary fibroblasts genetically modified to produce L-dopa. Neuron 6: 371-80.

Fisher LJ (1997) Neural precursor cells: Applications for the study and repair of the central nervous system. Neurobiology of Diseases 4:1-22.

Flotte TR, Afione SA, Conrad C, McGrath SA, Solow R, Oka H, Zeitlin PL, Guggino WB, Carter BJ (1993) Stable *in vivo* expression of the cystic fibrosis transmembrane conductance regulator with an adeno-associated virus vector. Proc Natl Acad Sci USA 90:10613-10617.

Friedlander DR, Brittis PA, Sakurai T, Shif B, Wirchansky W, Fishell G, Grumet M. (1998) Generation of radial-like glial cell line. J Neurobiol 37:291-304.

Gage FH, Ray J, Fisher LJ (1995) Isolation, characterization, and use of stem cells from the CNS. Ann Rev Neurosci 18:159-192.

Gage FH, Wolff J A, Rosenberg MB, Xu L, Yee JK, Shults C, Friedmann T (1987) Grafting genetically modified cells to the brain: possibilities for the future. Neurosci 23: 795-807.

Geschwind MD, Hartnick CJ, Liu W, Amat J, Van De Water TR, Federoff, HJ (1996) Defective HSV-1 vector expressing BDNF in auditory ganglia elicits neurite outgrowth: model for treatment of neuron loss following cochlear degeneration. Human Gene Therapy 7:173-182.

Geschwind MD, Kessler JA, Geller AI, Federoff HJ (1994) Transfer of the nerve growth factor gene into cell lines and cultured neurons using a defective herpes simplex virus vector. Transfer of the NGF gene into cells by a HSV-1 vector. Mol Brain Res 24:327-35.

Giger RJ, Ziegler U, Hermens WT, Kunz B, Kunz S, Sonderegger P. (1997) Adenovirus-mediated gene transfer in neurons: construction and characterization of a vector for heterologous expression of the axonal cell adhesion molecule axonin-1. J Neurosci Meth 71:99-111.

Giordano M, Takashima H, Herranz, A, Poltorak M., Geller, H.M., Marone, M. and Freed, W.J. (1993). Immortalized GABAergic cell lines derived from rat striatum using a temperature-sensitive allele of the SV40 large T antigen. Exp Neurol 124:395-400.

Goldman MJ, Litzky LA, Engelhardt JF, Wilson JM (1995) Transfer of the CFTR gene to the lung of nonhuman primates with E1-deleted, E2a-defective recombinant adenoviruses: a preclinical toxicology study. Human Gene Therapy 6: 839-51.

Grill R, Murai K, Blesch A, Gage FH., Tuszynski MH (1997) Cellular delivery of neurotrophin-3 promotes corticospinal axonal growth and partial functional recovery after spinal cord injury. J Neurosci 17:5560-72.

Guest JD, Hesse D, Schnell L, Schwab ME, Bunge MB, Bunge RP (1997) Influence of IN-1 antibody and acidic FGF-fibrin glue on the response of injured corticospinal tract axons to human Schwann cell grafts. J Neurosci Res 50:888-905.

Haase G, Kennel, P, Pettmann B, Vigne E, Akli S, Revah F, Schmalbruch H, Kahn A (1997) Gene therapy of murine motor neuron disease using adenoviral vectors for neurotrophic factors. Nature Medicine 3:429-36.

Hashimoto M, Aruga J, Hosoya Y, Kanegae Y, Saito I, Mikoshiba K (1996) A neural cell-type-specific expression system using recombinant adenovirus vectors. Human Gene Therapy 7:149-58.

Hermens WT Verhaagen J (1998) Viral vectors, tools for gene transfer in the nervous system. Prog Neurobiol 55:399-432.

Himes BT, Chow S, Jin H, Prockop D, Tessler A Fischer I (1999a) Grafting human bone marrow stromal cells into injured spinal cord of adult rats. Soc Neurosci Abst (in press).

Himes BT, Liu Y, Snyder EY, Fischer I, Tessler A,. (1999b) Transplants of cells genetically modified to express NT-3 keep alive axotomized Clarke's nucleus neurons after spinal cord hemisection in adult rats. (submitted).

Himes BT, Solowska-Baird J, Boyne L, Snyder EY, Tessler A, Fischer, I. (1995) Grafting of genetically modified cells that produce neurotrophins in order to rescue axotomized neurons in rat spinal cord. Soc Neurosci Abstr 21:537.

Ho DY, Mocarski ES, Sapolsky RM (1993) Altering central nervous system physiology with a defective herpes simplex virus vector expressing the glucose transporter gene. Proc Natl Acad Sci USA 90:3655-3659.

Holtmaat AJ, Hermens WT, Sonnemans MA, Giger RJ, Van Leeuwen FW, Kaplitt MG, Oestreicher AB, Gispen WH, Verhaagen J (1997) Adenoviral vector-mediated expression of B-50/GAP-43 induces alterations in the membrane organization of olfactory axon terminals *in vivo*. J Neurosci 17:6575-6586.

Honmou O, Felts PA, Waxman SG, Kocsis JD (1996) Restoration of normal conduction properties in demyelinated spinal cord axons in the adult rat by transplantation of exogenous Schwann cells. J Neurosci 16: 3199-3208.

Horellou P, Brundin P, Kalen P, Mallet J, Bjorklund A (1990) *In vivo* release of dopa and dopamine from genetically engineered cells grafted to the denervated rat striatum. Neuron 5:393-402.

Horellou P, Sabate O, Buc-Caron MH, Mallet, J (1997) Adenovirus-mediated gene transfer to the central nervous system for Parkinson's disease. Exp Neurol 144:131-138.

Horellou P, Vigne E, Castel MN, Barneoud P, Colin P, Perricaudet M, Delaere P, Mallet J (1994) Direct intracerebral gene transfer of an adenoviral vector expressing tyrosine hydroxylase in a rat model of Parkinson's disease. Neuroreport 6: 49-53.

Horwitz, M. S. (1994). Adenovirudae and their replication. In Virology, B. N. e. a. Fields, ed. (New York: Raven Press), pp. 1679-1721.

Ikari H, Zhang L, Chernak JM, Mastrangeli A, Kato S, Kuo H, Crystal RG, Ingram DK., Roth GS (1995) Adenovirus-mediated gene transfer of dopamine D2 receptor cDNA into rat striatum. Mol Brain Res 34:315-320.

Jiao S, Wolff JA (1992) Long-term survival of autologous muscle grafts in rat brain. Neurosci Lett 137:207-210.

Kaplitt M G, Leone P, Samulski RJ, Xiao X, Pfaff DW, O'Malley KL, During MJ (1994) Long-term gene expression and phenotypic correction using adeno-associated virus vectors in the mammalian brain. Nature Genetics 8:148-54.

Kaplitt MG, Pfaus JG, Kleopoulos SP, Hanlon BA, Rabkin SD, Pfaff DW (1991) Expression of a functional gene in adult mammalian brain following *in vivo* gene transfer via a herpes simplex virus type I defective viral vector. Mol. Cell Neurosci. 2:320-330.

Karpati G, Lochmuller H, Nalbantoglu J, Durham H (1996) The principles of gene therapy for the nervous sytem. Trends in Neuroscience 19:49-54.

Kawaja MD, Fagan AM, Firestein BL, Gage FH (1991) Intracerebral grafting of cultured autologous skin fibroblasts into the rat striatum: an assessment of graft size and ultrastructure. J Comp Neurol 307:695-706.

Kawaja MD, Rosenberg MB, Yoshida K, Gage FH (1992) Somatic gene transfer of nerve growth factor promotes the survival of axotomized septal neurons and the regeneration of their axons in adult rats. J Neurosci 12:2849-2864.

Kim DH, Gutin PH, Noble LJ, Nathan D, Yu JS, Nockels RP (1996) Treatment with genetically engineered fibroblasts producing NGF or BDNF can accelerate recovery from traumatic spinal cord injury in the adult rat. Neuroreport 7:2221-2225.

Kobayashi, S., Miura, M., Asou, H., Inoue, H. K., Ohye, C. and Uyemura, K. 1995. Grafts of genetically modified fibroblasts expressing neural cell adhesion molecule L1 into transected spinal cord of adult rats. Neurosc. Lett. 188, 191-4.

Kochanek S, Clemens PR, Mitani K, Chen H, Chan S, Caskey CT (1996) A new adenoviral vector: Replacement of all viral coding sequences with 28 kb of DNA independently expressing both full-length dystrophin and B-galactosidase. Proc Natl Acad Sci USA 93:5731-5736.

Lacorazza HD, Flax JD, Snyder EY, Jendoubi M (1996) Expression of human beta-hexosaminidase alpha-subunit gene (the gene defect of Tay-Sachs disease) in mouse brains upon engraftment of transduced progenitor cells. Nature Medicine 2:424-429.

La Gamma EF, Weisinger G, Lenn NJ, Strecker RE (1993) Genetically modified primary astrocytes as cellular vehicles for gene therapy in the brain. Cell Transplant 207-214.

Lawrence MS, Ho DY, Dash R, Sapolsky RM (1995) Herpes simplex virus vectors overexpressing the glucose transporter gene protect against seizure-induced neuron loss. Proc Natl Acad Sci USA 92:7247-7251.

Lawrence MS, Ho DY, Sun GH, Steinberg GK, Sapolsky, RM (1996) Overexpression of Bcl-2 with herpes simplex virus vectors protects CNS neurons against neurological insults *in vitro* and *in vivo*. J Neurosci 16:486-96.

Lee MG, Abina MA, Haddada H, Perricaudet M (1995) The constitutive expression of the immunomodulatory gp19k protein in E1-, E3- adenoviral vectors strongly reduces the host cytotoxic T cell response against the vector. Gene Therapy 2:256-262.

Le Gal La Salle G, Robert JJ, Berrard S, Ridoux V, Stratford-Perricaudet L D, Perricaudet M, Mallet J (1993) An adenovirus vector for gene transfer into neurons and glia in the brain. Science 259: 988-990.

Le Gros Clark WE (1942) The problem of neuronal regeneration in the central nervous system. I. The influence of spnal ganglia and nerve fragments grafted in the brain. J Anat 77:20-48.

Levi ADO, Guenard V, Aebischer P, Bunge RP (1994) The functional characteristics of Schwann cells cultured from human peripheral nerve after transplantation into a gap within the rat sciatic nerve. J Neurosci 14:1309-1319.

Levivier M, Przedborski S, Bencsics C, Kang UJ (1995) Intrastriatal implantation of fibroblasts genetically engineered to produce brain-derived neurotrophic factor prevents degeneration of dopaminergic neurons in a rat model of Parkinson's disease. J Neurosci 15:7810-7820.

Lieber A, He CY, Kirillova I, Kay MA (1996) Recombinant adenoviruses with large deletions generated by Cre-mediated excision exhibit different biological properties compared with first-generation vectors *in vitro* and *in vivo*. J Virol 70:8944-60.

Li Y, Raisman G (1994) Schann cells induce sprouting in motor and sensory axons in the adult rat spinal cord. J Neurosci 14:4050-4063.

Li Y, Field PM, Raisman G (1997) Repair of adult corticospinal tract by transplant of olfctory ensheating cells. Science 277:2000-2002.

Linnik, M. D., Zahos, P., Geschwind, M. D., and Federoff, H. J. (1995). Expression of bcl-2 from a defective herpes simplex virus-1 vector limits neuronal death in focal cerebral ischemia. Stroke *26*, 1670-4; discussion 1675.

Lisovoski F, Cadusseau J, Akli S, Caillaud C, Vigne E, Poenaru L, Stratford-Perricaudet L, Pericaudet M, Kahn A, Peschanski M (1994) *In vivo* transfer of a marker gene to study motoneuronal development. Neuroreport 5:1069-72.

Liu Y, Himes BT, Moul, J., Chow SY, Park KI, Tessler A, Murray M, Snyder EY, Fischer I (1999a) Intraspinal delivery of neurotrophin-3 (NT-3) using neural stem cells genetically modified by recombinant retrovirus. Exp Neurol. 158: 9-26.

Liu Y, Himes BT, Moul J, Huang WL, Chow SY, Tessler A, Fischer I (1997) Application of recombinant adenovirus for *in vivo* Gene Delivery to Spinal Cord. Brain Res 768:19-29.

Liu Y, Himes B.T., Murray M., Tessler, A. and Fischer, I. (1999c). Grafts of BDNF-producing fibroblasts that promote regeneration of axotomized rubrospinal neurons also rescue most neurons from retrograde death and prevent their atrophy. (submitted).

Liu Y, Himes BT, Tryon B, Moul J, Chow SY, Jin H, Murray M, Tessler A, Fischer I (1998) Intraspinal grafting of fibroblasts genetically modified by recombinant adenoviruses. NeuroReport 9:, 1075-1079.

Liu Y, Kim D, Himes BT, Chow SY, Schllart T, Murray M, Tessler A, Fischer I (1999b) Transplants of fibroblasts genetically modified to express BDNF promote regeneration of adult rat rubrospinal axons. J Neurosci 19: 4370-4387.

Lundberg C, Bjorklund A (1996) Host regulation of glial markers in intrastriatal grafts of conditionally immortalized neural stem cell lines. Neuroreport 7:847-52.

Lundberg C, Field PM, Ajayi YO, Raisman G, Bjorklund A (1996a) Conditionally immortalized neural progenitor cell lines integrate and differentiate after grafting to the adult rat striatum. A combined autoradiographic and electron microscopic study. Brain Res 737:295-300.

Lundberg C, Horellou P, Mallet J, Bjorklund A (1996b) Generation of DOPA-producing astrocytes by retroviral transduction of the human tyrosine hydroxylase gene: *in vitro* characterization and *in vivo* effects in the rat Parkinson model. Exp Neurol 139:39-53.

Lundberg C, Martinez-Serrano A, Cattaneo E, McKay RD, Bjorklund A (1997) Survival, integration, and differentiation of neural stem cell lines after transplantation to the adult rat striatum. Exp Neurol 145:342-360.

Luskin MB (1994) Neuronal cell lineage in the vertebrate central nervous system. FASEB Journal 8:722-730.

Mandel RJ, Gage F.H, Clevenger DG, Spratt SK, Snyder RO Leff SE (1999). Nerve growth factor expressed in the medial septum following *in vivo* gene delivery using a recombinant adeno-associated viral vector protects cholinergic neurons from fimbria-fornix lesion-induced degeneration. Exp. Neurol. 155:59-64.

Mandel RJ, Spratt SK, Snyder RO, Leff SE (1997) Midbrain injection of recombinant adeno-associated virus encoding rat glial cell line-derived neurotrophic factor protects nigral neurons in a progressive 6-hydroxydopamine-induced degeneration model of Parkinson's disease in rats. Proc Natl Acad Sci 94: 14083-14088.

Martinez-Serrano A, Bjorklund A (1996) Protection of the neostriatum against excitotoxic damage by neurotrophin-producing, genetically modified neural stem cells. J Neurosci 16:4604-16.

Martinez-Serrano A, Bjorklund A (1997) Immortalized neural progenitor cells for CNS gene transfer and repair. Trends in Neuroscience 20:530-538.

Martinez-Serrano A, Fischer W, Bjorklund A (1995b) Reversal of age-dependent cognitive impairments and cholinergic neuron atrophy by NGF-secreting neural progenitors grafted to the basal forebrain. Neuron 15:473-84.

Martinez-Serrano A, Fischer W, Soderstrom S, Ebendal T., Bjorklund A (1996a) Long-term functional recovery from age-induced spatial memory impairments by nerve growth factor gene transfer to the rat basal forebrain. Proc Natl Acad Sci 9: 6355-60.

Martinez-Serrano A, Hantzopoulos PA, Bjorklund, A (1996b) *Ex vivo* gene transfer of brain-derived neurotrophic factor to the intact rat forebrain: neurotrophic effects on cholinergic neurons. Eur J Neurosci 8:727-735.

Martinez-Serrano A, Lundberg C, Horellou P, Fischer W, Bentlage C, Campbell K, McKay RD, Mallet J, Bjorklund A (1995a) CNS-derived neural progenitor cells for gene transfer of nerve growth factor to the adult rat brain: complete rescue of axotomized cholinergic neurons after transplantation into the septum. J Neurosci 15:5668-80.

McCown TJ, Xiao X, Li J, Breese GR, Samulski RJ (1996) Differential and persistent expression patterns of CNS gene transfer by an adeno-associated virus (AAV) vector. Br Res 713:99-107.

McKay R (1997) Stem cells in the central nervous system. Science 276:66-71.

McTigue DM, Horner PJ, Stokes BT, Gage FH (1998) Neurotrophin-3 and brain-derived neurotrophic factor induce oligodendrocyte proliferation and myelination of regenerating axons in the contused adult rat spinal cord. J Neurosci 18:5354-65.

Mehler MF, Rozental R, Dougherty M, Spray DC, Kessler JA (1993) Cytokine regulation of neuronal differentiation of hippocampal progenitor cells. Nature 362: 62-65.

Menei P, Monteromenei C, Whittemore SR, Bunge RP, Bunge MB (1998) Schwann cells genetically modified to secrete human Bdnf promote enhanced axonal regrowth across transected adult rat spinal cord. Eur J Neurosci 10: 607-621.

Michael SI, Curie, DT (1994) Strategies to achieve targeted gene delivery via the receptor-mediated endocytosis pathway. Gene Therapy 1:223-232.

Miller AD (1992) Human gene therapy comes of age. Nature 357:455-60.

Miller N, Vile R (1995) Targeted vectors for gene therapy. FASEB J 9:190-199.

Miyoshi H, Blomer U, Takahashi M, Gage FH Verma IM (1998) Development of a self-inactivating lentivirus vector. J Virol *72*:8150-8157.

Miyoshi H, Takahashi M, Gage FH, Verma IM (1997) Stable and efficient gene transfer into the retina using an HIV-based lentiviral vector. Proc Natl Acad Sci 94:10319-23.

Moul J, Chow S, Obrocka M, Tessler A, Fischer I (1998) The influence of extrinsic factors on differentiation of embryonic spinal cord stem cells. Soc Neurosci Abstr 24, 1992.

Muir E, Du JS, Fok-Seang J, Smith-Thomas LC, Housden ES, Rogers J, Fawcett JW (1998) Increased axon growth through astrocyte cell lines transfected with urokinase. Glia 23:24-34.

Mulligan RC (1993) The basic science of gene therapy. Science 260:926-32.

Nakahara Y, Gage FH, Tuszynski MH (1996) Grafts of fibroblasts genetically modified to secrete NGF, BDNF, NT-3, or basic FGF elicit differential responses in the adult spinal cord. Cell Transplantation 5:191-204.

Naldini L, Blomer U, Gallay P, Ory D, Mulligan R, Gage FH, Verma IM, and Trono D (1996) *In vivo* gene delivery and stable transduction of nondividing cells by a lentiviral vector. Science 272: 263-267.

Neve RL (1993) Adenovirus vectors enter the brain. Trends in Neurosciences 16, 251-3.

Onifer SM, Whittemore SR, Holets VR (1993) Variable morphological differentiation of a raphe-derived neuronal cell line following transplantation into the adult rat CNS. Exp Neurol 122:130-42.

Paino CL, Bunge, MB (1991) Induction of axon growth into Schwann cell implants grafted into lesioned adult rat spinal cord. Exp Neurol 114:254-257.

Park KI, Jensen FE, Steig PE, Himes T, Fischer I Snyder EY (1997) Transplantation of neurotrophin-3 (NT-3) expressing stem-like cells into hypoxic-ischemic (HI) brain injury. Soc Neurosci Abstr 23:346.

Peel AL, Zolotukhin S, Schrimsher GW, Muzyczka N, Reier PJ (1997) Efficient transduction of green fluorescent protein in spinal cord neurons using adeno-associated virus vectors containing cell type-specific promoters. Gene Therapy 4:16-24.

Podsakoff G, Wong KK, Jr, Chatterjee S (1994) Efficient gene transfer into nondividing cells by adeno-associated virus-based vectors. J Virol 68:5656-66.

Radany EH, Brenner M, Besnard F, Bigornia V, Bishop JM Deschepper CF (1992) Directed establishment of rat brain cell lines with the phenotypic characteristics of type 1 astrocytes. Proc Natl Acad Sci USA 89:6467-6471.

Ramono-Cueto A, Planat GW, Avila J, Bunge MB (1998) Long-distance axonal regeneration in the transected adult rat spinal cord is promoted by olfactory ensheathing glia transplants. J Neurosci 18:3803-3815.

Raymon HK, Thode S, Gage FH (1997) Application of *ex vivo* gene therapy in the treatment of Parkinson's disease. Exp Neurol 144:82-91.

Reiser J, Harmison G, Kluepfel-Stahl S, Brady RO, Karlsson S, Schubert, M (1996) Transduction of nondividing cells using pseudotyped defective high-titer HIV type 1 particles. Proc Natl Acad Sci USA 93:15266-71.

Renfranz, P. J., Cunningham, M. G., and McKay, R. D. (1991). Region-specific differentiation of the hippocampal stem cell line HiB5 upon implantation into the developing mammalian brain. Cell 66:713-29.

Ridoux V, Robert JJ, Zhang X, Perricaudet M, Mallet J, Le Gal La Salle, G. (1994) The use of adenovirus vectors for intracerebral grafting of transfected nervous cells. Neuroreport 5:801-4.

Rosenberg MB, Friedmann T, Robertson RC, Tuszynski M, Wolff JA, Breakefield XO, Gage FH (1988) Grafting genetically modified cells to the damaged brain: restorative effects of NGF expression. Science 242:1575-8.

Russell DW, Miller AD, Alexander IE (1994) Adeno-associated virus vectors preferentially transduce cells in S phase. Proc Natl Acad Sci USA 91:8915-9.

Ryder EF, Snyder EY, Cepko CL (1990) Establishment and characterization of multipotent neural cell lines using retrovirus vector-mediated oncogene transfer. J Neurobiol 21:356-75.

Sabate O, Horellou P, Vigne E, Colin P, Perricaudet M, Buc-Caron MH, Mallet J (1995) Transplantation to the rat brain of human neural progenitors that were genetically modified using adenoviruses. Nature Genetics 9:256-60.

Scherman D, Bessodes M, Cameron B, Herscovici J, Hofland H, Pitard B, Soubrier F, Wils P, Crouzet J (1998) Application of lipids and plasmid design for gene delivery to mammalian cells. Curr Op Biotechnol 9:480-485.

Schinstine M, Fiore DM, Winn SR, Emerich DF (1995) Polymer-encapsulated schwannoma cells expressing human nerve growth factor promote the survival of cholinergic neurons after a fimbra-fornix transection. Cell Transplantation 4:93-102

Senut, M. C., Tuszynski, M. H., Raymon, H. K., Suhr, S. T., Liou, N. H., Jones, K. R., Reichardt, L. F., and Gage, F. H. (1995). Regional differences in responsiveness of adult CNS axons to grafts of cells expressing human neurotrophin 3. Exp Neurol 135:36-55.

Shihabuddin, L. S., Hertz, J. A., Holets, V. R, Whittemore, S. R. (1995). The adult CNS retains the potential to direct region-specific differentiation of a transplanted neuronal precursor cell line. J Neurosci 15: 6666-78.

Shihabuddin LS, Holets, VR, Whittemore SR (1996) Selective hippocampal lesions differentially affect the phenotypic fate of transplanted neuronal precursor cells. Exp Neurol 139:61-72.

Smith GM, Hale J, Pasnikowski, EM, Lindsay RM, Wong V, Rudge, JS (1996) Astrocytes infected with replication-defective adenovirus containing a secreted form of CNTF or NT3 show enhanced support of neuronal populations *in vitro*. Exp Neurol 139:156-66.

Snyder EY (1994) Grafting immortalized neurons to the CNS. Curr Op Neurobiol 4, 742-51.

Snyder, EY, Deitcher DL, Walsh C, Arnold-Aldea S, Hartwieg EA, Cepko CL (1992). Multipotent neural cell lines can engraft and participate in development of mouse cerebellum. Cell 68:33-51.

Snyder EY., Macklis, JD (1995) Multipotent neural progenitor or stem-like cells may be uniquely suited for therapy for some neurodegenerative conditions. Clin Neurosci 3:310-316.

Snyder EY, Park KI, Flax JD, Liu S, Rosario, CM, Yandava BD, Aurora S (1997). Potential of neural "stem-like" cells for gene therapy and repair of the degenerating central nervous system. Adv Neurol 72:121-32.

Snyder EY, Senut MC (1997) The use of nonneuronal cells for gene delivery. Neurobiology of Disease 4:69-102.

Snyder EY, Taylor RM, Wolfe JH (1995) Neural progenitor cell engraftment corrects lysosomal storage throughout the MPS VII mouse brain. Nature 374: 367-70.

Snyder EY, Wolfe JH (1996) Central nervous system cell transplantation: a novel therapy for storage diseases?. Curr Op Neurol 9:126-36.

Stemple DL, Mahanthappa NK (1997) Neural stem cells are blasting off. Neuron 18:1-4.

Stichel CC, Muller HW (1998) Experimental strategies to promote axonal regeneration after traumatic central nervous system injury. Prog Neurobiol 56: 119-148.

Takahashi K, Schwarz E, Ljubetic C, Murray M, Tessler A, Saavedra RA (1999) DNA plasmid that codes for human Bcl-2 gene preserves axotomized Clarke's nucleus neurons and reduces atrophy after spinal cord hemisection in adult rats. J Comp Neurol 404:159-71.

Tello F (1911) La influencia del neurotropismo en la regeneracion de las centro nerviosos. Trab Lab Invest Biol Univ Madrid 9:123-159.

Temin, H. M. (1990). Safety considerations in somatic gene therapy of human disease with retrovirus vectors. Human Gene Therapy 1:111-23.

Tessler A, Fischer I, Giszter S, Himes BT, Miya D, Mori F, Murray M (1997) Embryonic spinal cord transplants enhance locomoter performance in spinalized newborn rats, Volume 72, F. J. Seil, ed. (New York: Raven Press).

Tornatore, C., Baker-Cairns, B., Yadid, G., Hamilton, R., Meyers, K., Atwood, W., Cummins, A., Tanner, V., and Major, E. (1996) Expression of tyrosine hydroxylase in an immortalized human fetal astrocyte cell line, *in vitro* characterization and engraftment into the rodent striatum. Cell Transplantation. 5: 145-163.

Tuszynski, MH (1998) Gene therapy: applications to the neurosciences and to neurological disease. Neuroscientist 4:398-407.

Tuszynski MH, Gabriel K, Gage FH, Suhr S, Meyer S, Rosetti A (1996) Nerve growth factor delivery by gene transfer induces differential outgrowth of sensory, motor, and noradrenergic neurites after adult spinal cord injury. Exp Neurol 137:157-73.

Tuszynski, M. H., Peterson, D. A., Ray, J., Baird, A., Nakahara, Y., and Gage, F. H. (1994) Fibroblasts genetically modified to produce nerve growth factor induce robust neuritic ingrowth after grafting to the spinal cord. Exp Neurol 126:1-14.

van Esseveldt KE, Liu R, Hermens WT, Verhaagen J, Boer GJ (1997) Adenoviral vector-mediated gene transfer and neurotransplantation: possibilities and limitations in grafting of the fetal rat suprachiasmatic nucleus. J Neurosci Meth 71:113-23.

Verhaagen, J., Hermens, W. T., Oestreicher, A. B., Gispen, W. H., Rabkin, S. D., Pfaff, D. W., and Kaplitt, M. G. (1994). Expression of the growth-associated protein B-50/GAP43 via a defective herpes-simplex virus vector results in profound morphological changes in non-neuronal cells. Brain Research. Molecular Br Res 26:26-36.

Verma IM, Somia N (1997) Gene therapy -- promises, problems and prospects. Nature 389:239-42.

Vogt L, Giger RJ, Ziegler U, Kunz B, Buchstaller A, Hermens W, Kaplitt MG, Rosenfeld MR, Pfaff DW, Verhaagen J, Sonderegger P (1996) Continuous renewal of the axonal pathway sensor apparatus by insertion of new sensor molecules into the growth cone membrane. Curr Biol 6:1153-8.

Wang Q, Finer MH (1996). Second-generation adenovirus vectors. [Review]. Nature Medicine 2:714-6.

Weiss, S., Dunne, C., Hewson, J., Wohl, C., Wheatley, M., Peterson, A. C., and Reynolds, B. A. (1996). Multipotent CNS stem cells are present in the adult mammalian spinal cord and ventricular neuroaxis. Journal of Neuroscience 16:7599-609.

Weiss, S., Reynolds, B. A., Vescovi, A. L., Morshead, C., Craig, C. G., and van der Kooy, D. (1996). Is there a neural stem cell in the mammalian forebrain? Trends in Neurosciences 19:387-393.

White, L. A., Eaton, MJ, Castro MC, Klose, K. J., Globus, M. Y., Shaw, G., and Whittemore, S. R. (1994). Distinct regulatory pathways control neurofilament expression and neurotransmitter synthesis in immortalized serotonergic neurons. J Neurosci 14:6744-53.

Whittemore SR, Holet, VR, Keane RW, Levy DJ, McKay RD (1991) Transplantation of a temperature-sensitive, nerve growth factor-secreting, neuroblastoma cell line into adult rats with fimbria-fornix lesions rescues cholinergic septal neurons. J Neurosci Res 28:156-170.

Whittemore SR, Snyder EY (1996) Physiological relevance and functional potential of central nervous system-derived cell lines. Mol Neurobiol 12:13-38.

Whittemore, SR, and White, L. A. (1993). Target regulation of neuronal differentiation in a temperature-sensitive cell line derived from medullary raphe. Br Res 615:27-40.

Wolfe JH, Deshmane SL, Fraser NW (1992) Herpesvirus vector gene transfer and expression of beta-glucuronidase in the central nervous system of MPS VII mice. Nature Genetics 1:379-84.

Xiao X, Li J, McCown TJ, Samulski RJ (1997). Gene transfer by adeno-associated virus vectors into the central nervous system. Exp Neurol 144:113-124.

Xiao X, McCown TJ, Li J, Breese GR, Morrow AL, Samulski RJ (1997) Adeno-associated virus (AAV) vector antisense gene transfer *in vivo* decreases GABA(A) alpha1 containing receptors and increases inferior collicular seizure sensitivity. Brain Res 756:76-83.

Xu XM, Guenard V, Kleitman N, Aebischer P, Bunge, MB (1995b) A combination of BDNF and NT-3 promotes supraspinal axonal regeneration into Schwann cell grafts in adult rat thoracic spinal cord. Exp Neurol 134:261-72.

Xu XM, Guenard V, Kleitman N, Bunge MB (1995a) Axonal regeneration into Schwann cell-seeded guidance channels grafted into transected adult rat spinal cord. J Comp Neurol 351:145-60.

Yang Y, Nunes FA, Berencsi K, Furth EE, Gonczol E, Wilson JM (1994) Cellular immunity to viral antigens limits E1-deleted adenoviruses for gene therapy. Proc Natl Acad Sci USA 91:4407-4411.

Zhang Y, Dijkhuizen PA, Anderson PN, Lieberman AR, Verhaagen J (1998) NT-3 delivered by an adenoviral vector induces injured dorsal root axons to regenerate into the spinal cord of adult rats. J Neurosci Res 54:554-62

Zhang Y, Schneider RJ (1994) Adenovirus inhibition of cell translation facilitates release of virus particles and enhances degradation of the cytokeratin network. J Virol 68:2544-55.

Zhao H, Otaki JM, Firestein, S (1996) Adenovirus-mediated gene transfer in olfactory neurons *in vivo.* J Neurobiol 30:521-30.

23

Spinal Cord Injury and Fetal CNS Tissue Transplantation: An Initial "Bench-to-Bedside" Translational Research Experience

Paul J. Reier, Floyd J. Thompson, R. G. Fessler, Douglas K. Anderson, and E. D. Wirth, III

University of Florida College of Medicine and Brain Institute, and Malcolm Randall Veterans Administration Medical Center Gainesville, Florida

I. INTRODUCTION

As underscored by several contributing chapters to this volume, the last decade of central nervous system (CNS) injury research has introduced many new insights into the cellular dynamics that influence neuronal survival and axonal elongation after trauma. This especially applies to the growing body of information regarding cellular transplantation, neural stem cell biology and *in vivo* and *ex vivo* gene delivery. Coupled with dramatic progress in molecular biology, developmental neurobiology, immunology, and rehabilitation research, these technological and conceptual advances have stimulated unprecedented discussion about improved functional outcomes *via* interventions to enhance neuronal survival, regeneration, replacement, and plasticity at various post-injury milestones (e.g., Young, 1995; Gray, Dunnett, 1999). This new mindset constitutes a significant philosophical breakthrough in itself, given the long-standing pessimism that has clouded the prospect of any hope for those having sustained CNS trauma or other neurological disorders.

This heightened optimism about future cures for head and spinal cord injury also led to a greater public awareness and an increasingly proactive dialogue about the facilitated transfer of laboratory findings to the clinical arena (e.g., Fawcett,

1998). Understandably, a tremendous sense of urgency comes from those who have sustained CNS injury, their families, various private funding agencies and the political sector. As a result, there now exists more than ever before a stronger partnership between scientists and the general public at large.

While the impetus for converting scientific discoveries about CNS repair into clinical reality continues to build, the process clearly represents a formidable and costly task which embarks upon uncharted scientific and ethical territory. In view of the many biological problems and unknowns related to functional recovery (Tuszynski et al., 1999), a fundamental question is when is it the right time to initiate a clinical study (Reier et al., 1994a)? From another perspective, the predictably multifactorial nature of functional CNS repair (see Chapter 24) also poses immense challenges with respect to clinical designs and procedural implementation. Those considerations hardly take into account the myriad other issues ranging from tremendous functional/pathological diversity, even within a subset of individuals, to the expected risk-benefits. The ethical and appropriate development of control groups adds another layer of complexity and debate. The latter, for example, assumes greater significance in the case of surgically-based interventions. Placebo controls (Freeman et al., 1999; Macklin, 1999) and other experimental designs that can be easily carried out in the laboratory are more difficult, if not impossible, to employ clinically in a responsible and ethical manner.

The immediate issue thus becomes a matter of how and when to move judiciously forward with translational research focusing on regeneration after brain or spinal cord injury (SCI). It is unquestionably daunting to consider the many challenges of formulating rigorously designed clinical trials to test strategies for promoting functional regeneration. Still, many of the hurdles and their actual complexities are conjectural until directly encountered. It is equally difficult to dismiss the many valuable practical insights that could be gained from interfacing laboratory animal and human biology. A clinical study undeniably represents an integral part of a research continuum if appropriately meshed with a core of applied or fundamental basic science. As such, a well-conceived initial clinical study can actually be vitally instructive in shaping future bench science so that it comes in closer register with the human condition while at the same time offering some promise of patient benefit.

In this chapter, we review the inception and early results of an on-going, small-scale clinical "experience" in which we are testing the safety and feasibility of intraspinal transplantation of human fetal spinal cord (FSC) tissue in a population of SCI subjects with progressive posttraumatic syringomyelia (PPTS). This condition also has served as the basis for a similar clinical study being carried out concurrently in Sweden (Falci et al., 1997). In our decision to move forward with this study, we were concerned about the highly criticized precedent set by past surgical procedures that were performed in an effort to promote regeneration in the injured human spinal cord (e.g., see De La Torre, 1999). Therefore, it was our immediate intent to ensure scientific credibility by acquainting the research community with what we were planning to do and eliciting constructive feedback. We, therefore, outlined the rationale, goals, preclinical foundation, and study design at two major scientific meetings[1] in advance of the first transplantation procedure being done by our team of basic scientists and clinicians.

This chapter represents our first published documentation of the substance of those presentations and a description of early findings. We start by discussing issues related to the basic histopathology of SCI which helps to establish the underlying rationale for the emphasis on intraspinal transplantation and selection of the type of donor tissue used. Since this incorporates many considerations already discussed in this volume and elsewhere (Beattie et al., 1988; Reier et al., 1992a; Bunge, 1994; Reier et al., 1994a; Reier et al., 1994b; Young, 1995; Zompa et al., 1997; Bregman et al., 1997; Bregman, 1998; Fawcett, 1998; Vrbová et al., 1994), our intent is only to provide a selective overview largely for the purpose of general orientation. The chapter then progresses to a discussion of the clinical study matrix itself, followed by a summary of this project's current status. More detailed accounts of results are being prepared for peer-reviewed publications (Wirth et al., in preparation; Thompson et al., in preparation).

II. A CELLULAR-BASED STRATEGY SEEMS NECESSARY FOR SPINAL CORD REPAIR

A. The Stereotypic Lesion Setting

Human SCI can present a range of histopathological profiles extending from a solid cord injury with disrupted white matter and no concomitant necrosis of central gray matter (Quencer et al., 1992), to massive laceration/maceration injuries causing obliteration of recognizable anatomical features with formation of a dense fibrotic scar at the lesion epicenter (Bunge et al., 1993; Bunge, 1994). The most frequently cited type of injury, however, involves a contusive insult, rather than a direct physical transection (Kakulas, 1985; Hayes, Kakulas, 1997), which usually triggers a series of pathophysiological (recently reviewed in Velardo et al., 1999) and catastrophic neuropathological events resulting in the demise of both gray and white matter (Balentine, 1988; Wrathall, 1995). The extent of the primary and secondary tissue damage and degree of functional disability are dependent upon the spinal level and severity of the injury. In the worst case scenario, a very massive insult can lead to progressive, complete tissue destruction at the lesion epicenter analogous to a total transection. Injuries of lesser magnitude, however, typically display end-stage features characterized by central hemorrhagic necrosis of gray matter and the formation of fluid-filled cysts, with sparing of varying

---

[1] Neurotrauma Society Annual Meeting (PJR) November, 1996; Paralyzed Veterans of America Spinal Cord Research Foundation's 20th Anniversary Symposium, December, 1996 (PJR, EW).

amounts of surrounding white matter (Fig. 1) (Kakulas, 1999; Wrathall, 1995). In addition to the primary and secondary loss of neurons and white matter tracts, apoptosis of oligodendrocytes (Springer et al., 1999; Yong et al., 1998; Crowe et al., 1997; Liu et al., 1997; Shuman et al., 1997; Li et al., 1996) also occurs which can contribute to primary demyelination of spared axons (Blight 1983). As this cursory overview of the histopathology of SCI illustrates, a cellular-based intervention will more than likely constitute one component of a combined therapeutic strategy to promote functional recovery in the chronically injured spinal cord. This represents the operational bias of the clinical study described later.

B. The Theoretical Background for Intraspinal Repair Experimentally and Clinically Involves Many Donor Cell Choices and Interventional Options

A partial list of candidate donor cells includes: (i) Schwann cells (Chapter 21), (ii) primary fetal CNS tissue (reviewed in Chapter 24), (iii) olfactory ensheathing cells (Chapter 21), (iv) genetically-modified non-neural or neural tissue (Chapter 23);

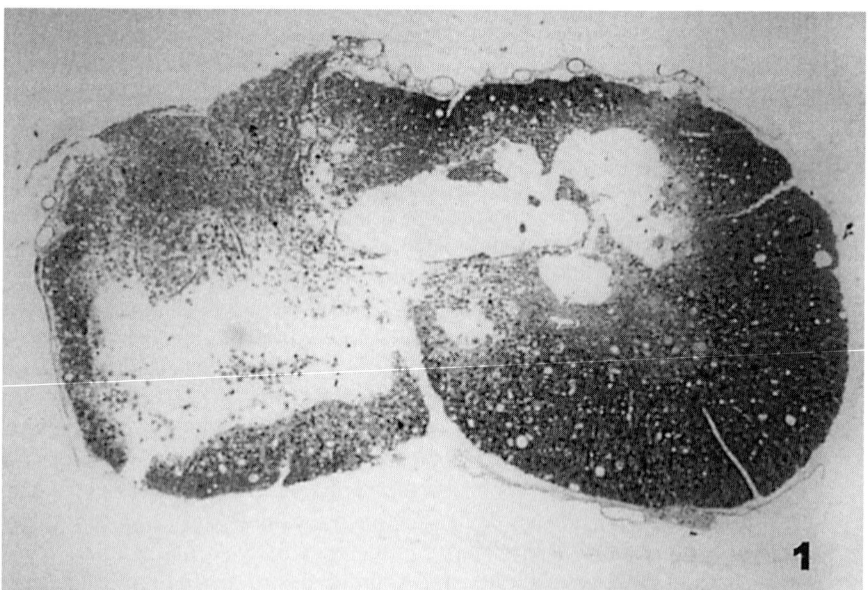

Figure 1 An intentionally prepared lateralized contusion injury is shown in this 2μm plastic transverse section of an adult rat spinal cord at the lesion epicenter as seen 3 months after injury. Only a small rim of ventral and lateral white matter is seen on the more severely damaged side, whereas some gray matter is present contralaterally along with substantial white matter preservation. This type of histopathology closely resembles lesion morphologies seen in some MR images of injured human spinal cords (e.g., Fig. 2b, Fig. 11c).

(v) various transgenic cell lines, (vi) pluripotent neural elements, and (vii) non-neural stem cells (also refer to Chapter 24). Some of these cell or tissue types have more appeal than others from biological, clinical, and logistical perspectives. However, it is still unknown which donor cell type will be most beneficial and these options are not mutually exclusive. A co-grafting approach may ultimately be required in order to encourage certain improvements over others in some SCI individuals. A "designer" cell therapy would require the neuropathological and neurophysiological underpinnings of specific functional deficits – many of which have yet to be conclusively defined. More immediate and direct targets for a cell-based intervention in SCI involve remyelination, axonal regeneration, and neuronal replacement. These considerations not only help to formulate useful therapeutic approaches, but also focus on some less-than-heroic realities of spinal cord repair, as well as inherent risk factors that are often overlooked.

1. White Matter Repair Will Require Remyelination of Spared Axons and Regrowth of Injured Fibers, But How Many Axons Will Be Required?

SCI is traditionally viewed as being a "white matter" (i.e., long-tract) problem involving both long descending supraspinal and ascending second-order axonal projections. One experimental emphasis pertaining to cellular grafting and SCI centers on enhancing remyelination of spared, but dysfunctional, axons with myelin-producing glia (Blakemore et al., 1987; Blakemore, Franklin, 1991; Rosenbluth et al., 1997; Utzschneider et al., 1994; Imaizumi et al., 1998). For example, recent neurophysiological studies of human SCI suggest that focal deficits in impulse conduction at the lesion epicenter may be primarily responsible for a protracted latency in transcranial magnetic stimulation-evoked muscle responses below the injury (Becerra et al., 1995; Calancie et al., 1999). Thus, even a geographically-restricted remyelination of denuded axons could be beneficial. While this has been seen at the electrophysiological level, specific experiments demonstrating behavioral improvements via remyelination in a clinically relevant SCI animal model remain to be performed.

A complementary and well-established goal relevant to white matter repair is to establish a terrain capable of stimulating axonal regeneration through the wound site (i.e., tissue "bridges") and, ideally to more distant caudal and rostral levels. As discussed in Chapter 24, this approach has been energized by some of the latest advances in spinal cord regeneration. Recent studies of bridging techniques have been especially instrumental in crystallizing the concept of combination strategies (Blesch, Tuszynski, 1997; Chen et al., 1996; Grill et al., 1997; Guest et al., 1997; Xu et al., 1995; Xu et al., 1999; Bregman et al., 1997; Bregman, McAtee, 1995)– a view that has been expressed many times (e.g., (Reier et al., 1994b)) but is only now gaining acceptance. In addition, these recent findings have been valuable in showing a capacity for stimulating axonal regrowth from neurons whose cell bodies are far from the site of injury and cell grafting. Many of these investigations in the acute hemitransection spinal injury setting will undoubtedly be extended to chronic lesion models including the use of spinal contusion injury. Some grafting experiments already have shown that certain axotomized supraspinal neuronal populations can be induced to regenerate in response to a peripheral nerve graft and specific neurotrophic factors in the chronically injured spinal cord (Ye, Houle, 1997).

An obvious and long-standing question related to axonal remyelination and regeneration is the magnitude of long-tract system repair needed to subserve meaningful degrees of functional improvement? The answer presently available is one that generates optimism, but at the same time makes an assumption that requires periodic reevaluation. Studies have indicated that the preservation of a small fraction of the original descending fiber projections can mediate spontaneous locomotor rebound after SCI and permanent paralysis (Fehlings, Tator, 1995; Noble, Wrathall, 1989; Blight, Decrescito, 1986). This principle also seems to apply to SCI in humans provided that a threshold number of functioning axons is present in a specific tract rather than being distributed randomly (Kakulas, 1999). It is worthy of note, that Kakulas' data also suggest that more axonal sparing may be required for the preservation of some sensory modalities below the injury than appears to be required for the expression of any residual motor function. Nevertheless, the number of fibers critical to whether an individual is functionally incomplete versus complete seems to range between 8-25% based on available data and consideration of various technical caveats.

An understandable extrapolation of the principle that a few axons may be required to subserve spontaneous locomotor recovery after SCI is that the remyelination and/or regrowth of a relatively modest contingent of fibers should stimulate functional recovery. One proof of principle has been derived from studies of lamprey spinal cord regeneration showing that a small number of regenerated descending fibers can activate locomotor networks below the injury (McClellan, 1998). It remains to be shown conclusively in higher species that the minimum requirement for promoting behavioral improvements *via* regeneration is equivalent to that needed for spontaneous functional improvement after SCI. The injured spinal cord is likely to be undergoing continuous remodeling in terms of cellular pathology and neuronal interactions over time, and this could place a different demand on axonal regrowth. The success that should continue to manifest itself in continuing studies of spinal cord regeneration and combined therapies will undoubtedly offer numerous opportunities to garner more definitive data.

2. *Neuronal Replacement Is A More Complex Theoretical and Practical Issue*

While the introduction of surrogate neuronal populations is frequently cited as another therapeutic objective for chronic SCI, the specific objectives and associated rationales are rarely articulated in much detail. From one perspective, the value of this approach seems self-evident in view of the extensive intraspinal, neuronal apoptosis and necrosis (Yong et al., 1998; Liu et al., 1997) after SCI and resultant loss of gray matter after spinal injuries at either cervical or lumbar levels. Most emphasis, however, is directed at motoneuron and autonomic cell replacement, which raises a host of biological issues in both the spinal cord and periphery.

Other intraspinal neurons at risk, and thereby potential candidates for replacement, include: (i) long ascending and descending propriospinal neurons; (ii) supraspinally-targeted, long ascending projection neurons (e.g., spinocerebellar neurons), and (iii) short inter- and intrasegmental cells. In principle, the former two neuronal population types are actually more related to the problem of white matter sparing and repair than gray matter reconstitution *per se*.

From another viewpoint, relatively little functional significance is usually attached to gray matter necrosis and secondary damage, especially in terms of thoracic injuries. Some literature suggests that even very extensive gray matter loss in humans may be of little motoric consequence (Goldstein et al., 1998). This agrees with experiments in which complete lateral hemisections were made on opposite sides of the spinal cord with a separation of 1-3 spinal segments between them. Despite the presence of a continous propriospinal circuit between the lesions, hindlimb function was permanently compromised (Stelzner, Cullen, 1991).

The modest behavioral contribution of gray matter is rather paradoxical since quantitative studies in the cat have indicated that in a surgically isolated S_2 spinal segment, as much as 60% of the fibers are of propriospinal origin (Chung, Coggeshall, 1988). The seemingly modest importance of gray matter also is difficult to reconcile when considering certain propriospinal short distance cells mediating descending input onto motoneurons. A notable example are the C_3-C_4 propriospinal neurons that project monosynaptically onto motoneurons and Ia inhibitory interneurons at the forelimb segments of C_6-T_1(Alstermark et al., 1987; Alstermark, Sasaki, 1986a; Alstermark, Sasaki, 1986b; Alstermark, Kummel, 1986; Yezierski, 1996). Cortico-, rubro-, tecto-, and reticulospinal projections converge on these cells which mediate the command for visually guided target-reaching movements and conjoint control of axial muscles to stabilize the trunk during target reaching (Tantisira et al., 1996).

Part of the difficulty in assigning a clinically useful rationale for gray matter repair, in the shadow of the more obvious and compelling long-tract problem, is that what is known about gray matter and function is still very incomplete. Some evidence shows, however, that central gray destruction alone can lead to enhanced tonic and driven discharges of spinal neurons bordering a central gray lesion (Yezierski, Park, 1993). Other recent findings suggest that small lesions of spinal gray matter can effect segmental and sensory sensitivity for thermal input over segments remote from the lesions (Acosta-Rua, Vierck, 1999). Other on-going experiments (Vierck, C.J., unpublished observations) are suggesting that focal lesions restricted only to spinal gray matter can result in hyperactivity among cells in the diffusely connected system of short propriospinals leading to spasticity. Along similar lines, Yezierski (1996) has noted that local circuit changes in GABA could account for allodynia after SCI due to decreased inhibitory tone in the injured cord contributing to an increased excitability of spinal neurons. These early findings point to the possibility that a cascade of short- and intermediate-range intersegmental coupling, analogous to what has been more extensively investigated in lower vertebrates (e.g., lampreys, (McClellan, Hagevik, 1999; Mellen et al., 1995)), could contribute to the manifestation of some functional consequences of SCI. In that sense, restoration of the continuity of spinal gray matter may have more significance than previously considered.

3. *Neuronal Substitution for Damaged Bulbospinal Projections*

A third option for a transplantation-based intervention, which has been considered for many years (Björklund et al., 1983), entails the introduction of catecholaminergic neurons below the level of injury (Privat et al., 1988). It is now well established that both serotonergic and noradrenergic pharmacological agents can exert an effect on hindlimb locomotion in spinalized animals (Rossignol et al., 1998). Furthermore, pharmacological protocols, based on these findings and combined with locomotor training or functional electrical stimulation, seem to have promise for improving locomotor recovery in the human SCI patient (Barbeau, Rossignol, 1994). In the case of serotonergic projections, those boutons terminate mostly on proximal dendrites of motoneurons (Alvarez et al., 1998)and exert considerable influence over motoneuron excitability (Hounsgaard et al., 1988; Kiehn, Eken, 1998). Previous experiments have shown that transplants of fetal raphé neurons can compensate for the reduction of such inputs after SCI. In fact, such transplants show a remarkable fidelity in their reinnervation of appropriate regions of spinal gray matter even after chronic denervation (reviewed in Reier et al. (Reier et al., 1994b). Other recent data suggest that graft-mediated restoration of catecholaminergic innervation of lumbar motoneuron pools can influence hindlimb motor patterns (Yakovleff et al., 1995) and neurophysiology based on electrophysiological and kinematic analyses (Gimenez y Ribotta et al., 1998a; Gimenez y Ribotta et al., 1998b; Feraboli-Lohnherr et al., 1997).

C. The Cardinal Rule of Medicine Is "Do No Harm"

In certain respects, the task of functional spinal cord repair may not represent as much of a heroic effort as it would seem when considering the various degrees of substantive improvement that can be sought (Bunge, 1994; Young, 1995). Functional repair over a distance as little as one cervical spinal segment could represent a profound difference in a person's level of independence and quality of life. With that in mind, the evidence and theories just discussed can effectively shape a compelling rationale for clinically applied SCI research using intraspinal transplantation as a model interventional modality. Of the three approaches outlined, each has its own unique merits. However, to launch a clinical study of this nature under the most ideal conditions, three fundamental questions need to be addressed. Is there adequate information to indicate which donor cell type would be the most suitable graft prototype? Is there sufficient evidence of therapeutic efficacy available from laboratory experiments involving a clinically-relevant lesion model to warrant a focused clinical endeavor? In the context of SCI, where it now seems that a combined strategy will be required, how well has each component intervention been tested in terms of safety and feasibility? Clearly, the issue of safety is of paramount importance especially since there is growing recognition of the existence of intrinsic repair processes (Brook et al., 1998; Beattie et al., 1997; Guth et al., 1985) that could someday translate into detectable subacute or chronic functional recoveries. For an initial clinical study, safety would encompass minimizing any life-threatening risk or potential of additional functional deterioration. Safeguards also would have to be considered to avoid compromising the opportunity to benefit from other therapies as they evolve.

III. PROGRESSIVE POSTTRAUMATIC SYRINGOMYELIA (PPTS) OFFERS A VIABLE PATIENT PROFILE FOR AN INITIAL CLINICAL EXPERIENCE

When our human study was initiated, grafting into SCI subjects with stable lesions and neurological status, transplantation at mid- to high cervical levels, or the introduction of cells into intact spinal parenchyma above or below the site of injury would be difficult to reconcile in terms of a risk-to-benefit ratio. We thus reasoned in developing the following study that the ideal patient profile for the purpose of evaluating safety and feasibility would be one in which a clear medical need existed for intraspinal surgery due to incipient neurological deterioration. Furthermore, a well-established preclinical technology and base of experimental information should already be at hand that could be readily superimposed onto the standard of medical care with little risk of negating the efficacy of that treatment. Finally, the approach should be able to offer some potential of therapeutic benefit.

PPTS is documented as being a very rare event affecting approximately 0.3-3.4% of chronic SCI individuals (Piatt, Jr., 1996; Biyani, el Masry, 1994; Umbach, Heilporn, 1991). The condition is characterized by a progressive myelomalacia (i.e., liquification of the cord) with ascending cyst expansion that can become life-threatening if brainstem involvement occurs. Presenting signs and symptoms typically include intractable pain and an onset of deteriorating upper extremity motor and sensory function. Progressive cystic necrosis also can have a descending component; however, the pathology is usually masked by the original deficits.

Figure 2 presents one example of a male PPTS patient who subsequently had an intraspinal fetal graft procedure performed on him. In brief, this individual had an injury at T_{12} nearly 30 years ago which resulted in severe lower extremity weakness and partial paralysis. This individual was, nonetheless, able to regain significant ambulatory capacity with the assistance of bracing and a single-point cane or walker (i.e., a community ambulator status). This person began experiencing upper extremity weakness and some additional signs suggestive of a progressive, ascending myelomalacia. However, neither allodynia nor deterioration of upper extremity function was noted either in terms of overall mobility or grip strength. Routine pulmonary function testing also revealed performance within normal limits. Quite surprisingly, subsequent MRI revealed extensive and continuous cavitation of the spinal cord from the original level of injury at T_{12} to C_1-

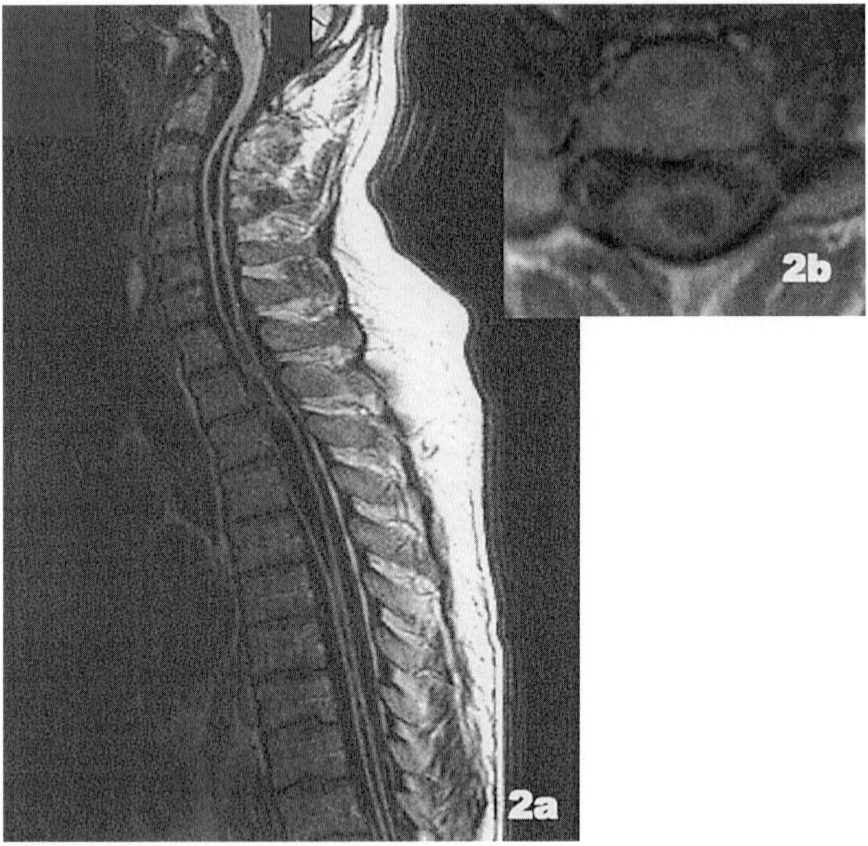

Figure 2 In panel "a," a sagittal FLAIR-weighted MRI of patient PPTS-6 shows the status of his spinal cord 30 years after sustaining an injury at T_{12}. A continuous, large syrinx extends from the original injury site up to C_2. Essentially the entire cyst was paracentrally located (panel "b," T1-weighted image) except from T_6 up to T_3 where the cyst widened considerably and encompassed all but a thin rim of spared tissue. As a matter of general interest, the configuration of the lesion in 2b closely resembles a lateralized contusion that can be produced experimentally as shown in Fig. 1.

C_2 (Fig. 2). At cervical levels, a single, large eccentrically positioned cyst was observed which was partially bordered by a peripheral rim of tissue on the most involved side of the cord and by more substantial spinal parenchyma contralaterally which exhibited a very mottled pattern of grayscale intensity (Fig. 11b).

This particular individual not only serves as a dramatic example of PPTS but also as a reminder of several fundamental considerations related to PPTS specifically and SCI in a more general sense. As this patient's history indicates, PPTS is essentially a silent condition that has both a chronic and acute/subacute component. For that reason, PPTS may have a higher undetected incidence than the recorded frequency of diagnosed cases indicates. What is particularly intriguing is the overall neurological status of this individual relative to the devasting nature of his cord pathology. An analogous patient profile has been recently described by Goldstein et al. (1998). This type of picture argues very strongly in favor of the functional significance of even a limited amount of spared tissue. Even moreso, these data could reflect a much greater degree of spinal cord neuroplasticity potential (Goldstein et al., 1998) than is usually acknowledged. From an interventional perspective, more gain of function may be attainable by amplifying inherent repair mechanisms.

The remarkable degree of plasticity suggested in this individual also draws attention to another issue related to safety. Namely, as much consideration as possible should be given to ensuring that intrinsic repair mechanisms are not at risk in designing new therapies and clinical trials. As discussed below (Section IV.B.5), experimental paradigms are available that could provide useful indices of safety in that regard while also providing an opportunity to assess whether compensatory neuroplasticity mechanisms can be enhanced.

Treatment of PPTS entails stabilization of the syrinx requiring various draining or shunting procedures (Biyani, el Masry, 1994; Van Calenbergh, Van den Bergh, 1993), as well as other approaches to curtail refilling of the cysts (Williams, 1990). While such procedures can be successful in reducing clinical symptoms in most, if not all, patients for the first year after surgery, some reports cite data showing that half the cases will require follow-up surgery due to occlusion of shunts or reestablishment of tissue filling conditions (Sgouros, Williams, 1995; Aschoff, Kunze, 1993). Lytic destruction of arachnoid scars also is performed as an adjunct to shunting but these adhesions generally reemerge unless other surgical measures are taken (Lee et al., 1997).

Since most of the laboratory procedures used for intraspinal fetal cell transplantation are very analogous to the surgical treatment of PPTS, it seemed reasonable that an initial safety-feasibility study could be conducted on a small group of these individuals without invoking additional risk or substantial modification of the accepted method of treatment. The current absence of documented long-term cyst stabilization with any of the existing surgical procedures also presents the possibility of offering patient benefit should successful grafting either slow or completely suppress the refilling of cysts, particularly in individuals with a history of failed shunts.

IV. FETAL CNS TISSUE PROVIDES A WINDOW OF OPPORTUNITY AND IMPORTANT TEMPLATE FOR OTHER CELL-BASED STRATEGIES

The decision to focus on fetal CNS transplants in the clinical study detailed below, took into consideration a wealth of experience derived from numerous independ-

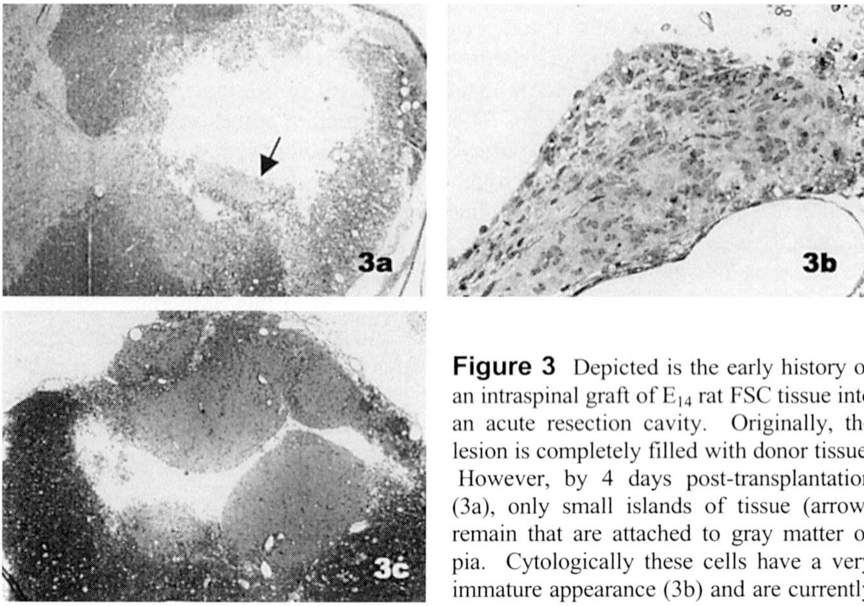

Figure 3 Depicted is the early history of an intraspinal graft of E_{14} rat FSC tissue into an acute resection cavity. Originally, the lesion is completely filled with donor tissue. However, by 4 days post-transplantation (3a), only small islands of tissue (arrow) remain that are attached to gray matter or pia. Cytologically these cells have a very immature appearance (3b) and are currently being characterized to determine the extent of their differentiation. Nevertheless, by 2 weeks post-transplantation, these islands of tissue give rise to large masses of maturing graft tissue (3c) that ultimately fill the entire lesion defect in most cases.

ently conducted experiments over the last 15-20 years involving intracerebral and intraspinal fetal cell transplantation. That collective scientific enterprise has not only shown neurotransplantation to be a valuable experimental tool but also drew rapid attention to the clinical implications of this technique as most notably exemplified in the case of Parkinson's disease (Freed et al., 1992; Freeman et al., 1995; Kordower et al., 1995; Lindvall et al., 1994; Palmeri et al., 1999; Houlé et al., 1999; Yakovleff et al., 1995). Fetal CNS grafts in both animal and human recipients are capable of long-term survival and function (Kiehn, Eken, 1998; Kim et al., 1999a; Kiehn, Kjaerulff, 1996). Such transplants also exhibit comparable cytological and cytoarchitectonic features (Kordower et al., 1998) in recipients ranging from mice to humans. The availability of protocols for fetal CNS grafts into human subjects provides a level of assurance related to the safe use of such donor material for which there is virtually no other precedent as thoroughly documented.

Taken collectively, existing information strongly argues in favor of fetal neural grafts as a model for the future clinical use of other evolving cellular strategies about which much less is currently known. A small-scale study of fetal CNS allografts in human subjects could provide a fundamental proof of principle independently of the usual ethical and practical objections that are expressed. In that regard, a close parallel with neural stem cell biology represents one of the more striking facets of fetal cell grafts that illustrates their importance as a template for other evolving approaches.

It is a well known, though rarely acknowledged, fact that soon after transplantation, fetal CNS tissue shows a very substantial, initial cellular attrition under many experimental conditions. This is most often noted in relation to specific cellular populations, such as tyrosine hydroxylase-producing cells in fetal ventral mesencephalic transplants (Zawada et al., 1998; Boonman, Isacson, 1999; Bjorklund et al., 1997; Dunnett, 1991; Brundin et al., 1985). The extent of early graft cell loss, however, is more widespread, as illustrated by the initial fate of rat fetal (E_{14}) spinal cord (FSC) grafts into acute hemilesions of the adult rat spinal cord. Although the prepared cavities are initially filled completely with donor tissue, by 4 days post-transplantation (Fig. 3a), small islands (Fig. 3b) of very immature-appearing cells are the only vestiges of the original FSC grafts (Theele, Reier, 1996). Within the next 7-10 days, however, these transplants exhibit a striking rebound (Fig. 3c) such that by one month post-transplantation, the lesion cavities are typically filled by matured donor neural tissue. This early life history of an embryonic CNS graft serves to illustrate that such transplants probably represent neural progenitor/precursor implants more than previously considered. In that regard, primary fetal CNS grafts continue to be a valuable experimental tool through which one can garner a better understanding of the cellular requirements for successful functional repair. They also provide a gold-standard against which one can compare outcomes with other alternative sources of fetal-like donor tissue, particularly neural precursor cell populations. Our choice of primary human fetal tissue for the clinical investigation described below thus extends, in principle, well beyond fetal tissue *per se*.

A. Fetal Spinal Cord (FSC) Tissue Can Compensate For Gray And White Matter Tissue Loss

Experiments addressing the use of fetal CNS grafts in models of neurodegenerative disease and trauma have suggested a variety of potential mechanisms whereby functional improvements may be obtained: (i) reconstruction of synaptic circuitries, (ii) replaced afferent inputs to denervated regions, (iii) neuropharmacological restoration, (iv) bridges for axonal elongation, (v) sources of trophic support, (vi) contribution of myelin-forming glia, and (vii) recruitment of endogenous repair mechanisms. With regard to SCI, the theoretical framework for intraspinal fetal cell transplantation has largely centered on the potential to serve as bridges or functional relays (Reier et al., 1986; Tessler, 1991; Bregman et al., 1993) between separated regions of the spinal cord. Either or both mechanisms could effectively help circumvent gray and white matter destruction after SCI. To date, various lines of anterograde/retrograde (Jakeman, Reier, 1991)and transsynaptic (Schrimscher et al., 1998) neuroanatomical evidence support the concept of fetal grafts being able to establish short, propriospinal-like relays. Such novel circuits would be theoretically more fitting to the reconstruction of polysynaptic descending projection systems, rather than those involving direct projections to motoneurons, although the latter cannot be arbitrarily dismissed. However, a compelling demonstration of the functionality of such novel circuits still awaits neurophysiological analyses of reconstructed pathways involving appropriate neurotransmitter-receptor matching between host-graft, afferent, and graft-host, efferent, projections.

In neonatal recipients, intraspinal grafts of FSC tissue also can serve as bridges for the elongation of host axons through the site of injury (Bernstein Goral, Bregman, 1993; Bregman, Bernstein Goral, 1991). In contrast, while host axons can enter these transplants in adult animals, they typically form extensively ramified branches and establish synaptic interactions after crossing the host-graft interface. Their elongation within the graft domain is thus very limited. However, as discussed elsewhere in this volume (Chapters 8,15,16,18), the addition of neurotrophic factors or blocking of myelin inhibitory proteins can effectively promote the extension of host axons through intraspinal fetal grafts (Bregman et al., 1997). A frequently cited shortcoming of fetal grafts has been the limited degree of axonal growth that these tissues appear to support (Bunge, 1994). The effects of exogenous growth factors challenges this perspective and raises the possibility of achieving even more substantial host-graft interactions that could contribute to enhanced functional outcomes (Bregman, 1998). Even without growth factors, however, the seemingly limited host and graft axonal growth does not rule out a possible functional impact of fetal grafts when placed into cervical or lumbar lesions or sites of injury in close proximity to specific motoneuron pools.

B. Experimental Fetal Cell Transplantation Experiments Have Established a Pre-Clinical Foundation

Aside from the above theoretical framework that postures a potential graft benefit from different points of view, more direct lines of preclinical evidence also are available that set the stage for an initial safety and feasibility clinical study of intraspinal fetal CNS transplantation.

1. Fetal CNS Grafts Can Obliterate Chronic Lesion Cavities in the Rat and Cat Spinal Cord

Relative to our focus on PPTS, the most dramatic base of information relates to the simple fact that grafts of FSC tissue can, in the majority of cases, completely fill lesions of the adult rat spinal cord. This is a commonly reproducible finding that has been independently reported by this and many other laboratories. We have thus observed high rates of graft success in acute and chronic resection lesions, as well as in both acute/subacute and chronic contusion injuries (Horner et al., 1991; Stokes, Reier, 1992; Reier et al., 1994b; Horner et al., 1995) of the adult rat spinal cord. For example, over 95% of the grafts made into chronic (i.e., 1-3 month post-injury delays) contusions survived for extended posttransplantation intervals of up to at least one year with complete filling of the epicenters. These transplants also were in close approximation to host and graft tissue at the rostral and caudal margins of the contusion cavities. These transplants thus completely filled what would have been regions of extensive cystic cavitation. At the epicenter, fetal tissue blended with spared subpial axons by infiltrating expansive extracellular spaces in the wake of neuronal and fiber degeneration. While considerable radial expansion of the donor tissue had occurred, no obvious compression of persisting host fibers has ever been indicated. A more comprehensive description of the cytological and neuroanatomical features of these grafts is presented elsewhere (Reier et al., 1994b).

It should be noted parenthetically that while we have had high levels of FSC graft survival in 1-3 month-old, chronic contusion lesions of the adult rat spinal cord, the success rate plummets precipitously to approximately 15 percent with graft delays extending beyond 3 months (Reier, Schrimsher, and Thompson unpublished observations). The successful grafts in those cases are, however, as robust in terms of their growth and differentiation as those obtained with shorter pregraft delay intervals (e.g., Fig. 4). Therefore, a long-term lesion may not be absolutely inhospitable to fetal cell grafting; however, the overall biology of those established injuries may require different methods of donor tissue placement in order to optimize graft survival. In that light, it is serendipitous that the PPTS condition involves both a chronic, as well as acute/subacute, component which should be a favorable setting in which to test the feasibility of intraspinal transplantation in the human.

The results obtained in rats subsequently led to experiments in which the feasibility of intraspinal transplantation was determined in another species where the logistics of this approach would be more complicated due to differences in lesion volume, graft-host histocompatibility, and the availability of appropriately timed fetal tissue. We chose the cat as an animal model because considerable work on neurophysiology, neuroanatomy, behavior, and neuroprotection had already been done in relation to the normal and injured spinal cord in this species. Our results showed that either solid grafts or suspensions of dissociated cells could survive, undergo cytoarchitectonic differentiation, and integrate with the host CNS in both acute and chronic lesions of the adult cat spinal cord (Anderson et al., 1989; Anderson et al., 1991; Howland et al., 1995; Anderson et al., 1995; Anderson et al., 1996; Reier et al., 1992b). The extent of cavity filling by fetal tissue varied based on lesion size, amount of available tissue and initial cell survivability, and mode of graft tissue preparation. Thus, in some cases entire regions of cavitation were replaced by donor tissue, whereas in others (Fig. 4), only partial occlusion of the cysts was achieved. This was not limited to homotopic grafts alone since similar results were obtained with tissue obtained from several regions of the embryonic neuraxis. From a functional perspective, it still remains to be explored whether the degree of recovery obtained is related to the volume of tissue or types and percentages of cells present in the graft.

Many studies have demonstrated a close parallel in the cytological differentiation of human-to-rat and rat-to-rat, intrastriatal xeno-and allografts respectively.

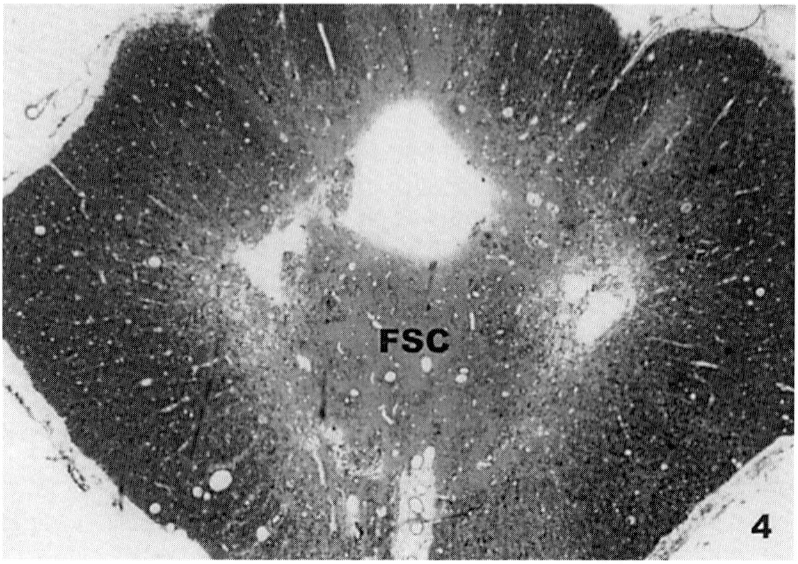

Figure 4 A 2μm plastic, toludine blue stained section of an adult cat spinal cord that had sustained a static-load compression thoracic injury and subsequently grafted with fetal cat (E_{26}) spinal cord tissue (FSC). In this particular example, the cavity is not completely filled though otherwise viable donor tissue is evident. This specimen is illustrated because it depicts a graft outcome that may be very similar to what has been indicated thus far in our study of PPTS patients (e.g., Figs. 10f, 11d). A companion MRI related to this histological sample is shown in Wirth et al., 1992.

The same principle appears to apply to xenografts of human FSC tissue into lesions of the rat spinal cord (Akesson et al., 1998; Gilerovich et al., 1996; Giovanini et al., 1997; Giovanini et al., 1997) where this tissue can survive, grow, and integrate with surrounding host spinal cord tissue. As with rat or cat FSC grafts, analogous human embryonic tissue has the capacity to fill large cavities produced by aspiration or resection, as well as extensive cysts resulting from contusion injury in the rat spinal cord. The pattern of differentiation and degree of host-graft integration, however, appear to be dependent upon lesion conditions and grafting techniques (Giovanini et al., 1997). One report indicates that in contrast to rat FSC tissue, neurons in human FSC xenografts can extend axons over longer distances (Wictorin, Bjorklund, 1992).

2. Excellent Diagnostic Value of Graft Survival by MRI

Early work on MR imaging of fetal tissue transplants in the injured spinal cords of live cats showed that these grafts could be clearly visualized and readily distinguished from areas of cystic degeneration (Wirth et al., 1992). Subsequently, quantitative approaches to assessing conventional T1 and T2 images, confirmed the predictive value of T2 images for assessing graft survival in hemisection cavities (Wirth et al., 1995). Although signals on T1 images were not predictive of graft viability, these images were still a helpful adjunct to the T2 images for evaluation of the graft site morphology. While these early data provided convincing evidence of the ability of MR imaging to demonstrate the gross morphology of the transplant site *in vivo*, it was also clear that the MR images could not reveal some features that were readily appreciated in post-mortem histological sections, such as the degree of interdigitation between the donor tissue and host parenchyma. Despite these limitations in spatial resolution, MRI still proved to be an essential tool for monitoring graft status, primarily because of its noninvasive nature, which allowed for repeated scans over time. This temporal information is critical for assessing potential correlations between changes in the graft site and variations in other experimental parameters, such as immunosuppression and locomotor function. Since MRI is the only diagnostic tool with sufficient spatial resolution and tissue contrast to study the spinal cord in intact living subjects, these animal data were a vital component of the preclinical foundation for this pilot clinical study.

3. Immunological Rejection of Fetal Grafts Does Not Exacerbate Histopathology or Compromise Spared Host Neurological Function

The issue of graft rejection and its effects on spinal cord anatomy and function after injury have been addressed using both allograft and xenograft models. These preliminary experiments were carried out to determine whether the rejection of transplanted tissue could lead to adjacent host pathology and/or an additional loss of neurological function. Also, since the adverse side-effects of long-term immunosuppression would far outweigh any benefit of a transplantation therapy for SCI, it was important to determine from a safety perspective whether the possibility of ensuing graft rejection would represent a significant risk factor in the design of a clinical study.

The susceptibility of intraspinal fetal CNS grafts to immunological rejection has been observed both in rats (Theele, Reier, 1996) and cats (Anderson et al., 1991). In one set of experiments (Theele et al., 1996), we grafted fetal tissue from ACI rats (RT1.A/B^{a}) into spinal lesion made in Wistar-Furth (RT1.A/B^{u}) recipients. These strains were selected since they represent high-responder allograft mismatch pairs having a high probability of donor tissue rejection. In the absence of immunosuppression, all ACI grafts were rejected routinely over the course of 10-45 days post-transplantation. By comparison, grafts of Sprague-Dawley (SD) FSC tissue to Wistar recipients showed 38% survival rates (Theele, Reier, 1996). Under all circumstances studied to date, the pathology associated with tissue rejection was restricted to donor cells with no obvious involvement of host white or gray matter. In addition, the neurological status of animals with actively rejecting, young grafts showed no overt deterioration in function.

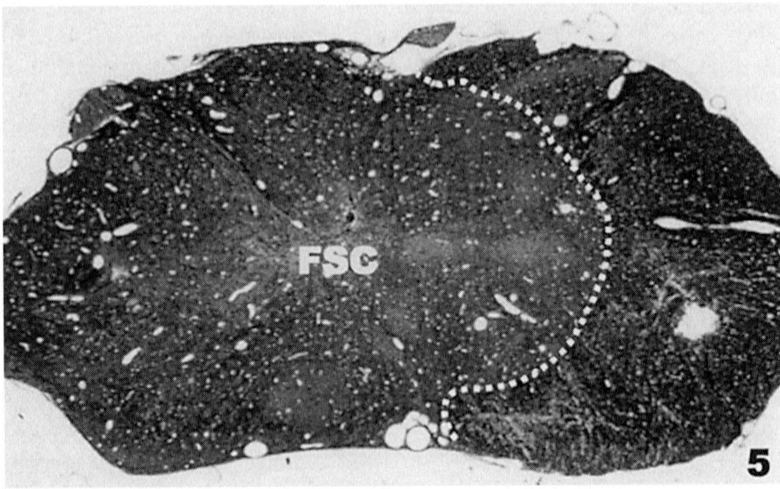

Figure 5 An example of long-term graft survival following temporary immunosuppression (see text) with CsA of a Wistar-Furth recipient of E_{14} FSC tissue from an ACI maternal donor. The graft was placed into an acute hemisection cavity made at $C_{4\text{-}5}$ 28 weeks prior to post-mortem study. As seen in this 2μm plastic, toludine blue stained section, a healthy, highly vascularized transplant (FSC) is present. The dotted line indicates the host-graft interface which extends well across the midline in this preparation.

Even under the circumstances of a xenograft rejection, no adverse neurological changes were observed. Four cats received a "mild" compression injury of their thoracic spinal cord which resulted in minimal hindlimb involvement leaving bowel and bladder function intact. Twelve to fourteen weeks post-injury, suspensions of E_{14} rat FSC and brainstem tissue were injected into the chronic compression lesions of these non-immunosuppressed cats. Hindlimb motor function was evaluated for approximately 14 months. The lesion site was assessed using MRI immediately prior to grafting, at approximately 6 months post-grafting, and at the time of sacrifice. The spinal cords were then removed for routine histological analysis. During the entire 14 month period of evaluation, hindlimb movement in all four cats was unchanged from pre-graft levels. In addition, there was no measurable change in the size or configuration of the lesion at either 6 or 14 months post-grafting as assessed by MRI. At 6 months, there was no evidence of surviving graft tissue in the lesion cavity in the MR images which was confirmed by histological analysis at 14 months.

4. Temporary Immunosuppression May Be Sufficient for Long-term Graft Survival

It is presently unknown whether chronic immunosuppression will be required for long-term viability of fetal allografts in the human spinal cord. Evidence from the

Parkinson's disease trials suggests that intracerebral transplants of fetal mesencephalic tissue can survive at least 18 months following withdrawal of cyclosporine A (CsA) (Kordower et al., 1995). We also have found that only temporary immunomodulation of the host might be required with intraspinal grafts. A single dose of antilymphocyte serum was sufficient enough to enhance FSC graft survival in SD-to-Wistar grafting experiments from 38% to 75% over a period of at least 60 days post-transplantation (Theele, Reier, 1996).

Experiments were subsequently extended to a study of allograft survival following cessation of temporary CsA immunosuppression. Using the ACI-to-Wistar-Furth model described above, recipients were maintained on a daily regimen of 10mg/kg CsA starting one day prior to grafting and continued for two months post-transplantation. CsA administration was then stopped, and the host animals survived for an additional 5-28 weeks. Healthy transplants were found in 75% of the recipients (n=16). At the latest post-graft intervals, the grafts showed no overt signs of ongoing or incipient rejection (Fig. 5). Commonly, however, a cadre of small, darkly stained mononuclear cells infiltrated the graft site. These cells were often distributed near the host-graft interface, and this low-level inflammatory response did not appear to be associated with any obvious pathology. Such profiles were virtually absent from adjacent host tissue.

The issue of fetal neural cell transplantation immunology is a complex problem that is still very poorly understood. The studies described above, thus represent only one perspective and were largely designed to obtain a basic index of safety. To the extent that one can extrapolate from the rat to human in this regard, our findings provide an indication of short-term immunosuppression efficacy.

5. *Intraspinal Fetal Grafts Do Not Restrict Expression of Intrinsic Plasticity Following SCI*

In view of some of the compensatory functions and partial recovery that have been reported in victims of SCI, consideration also should be given to impact of a therapy on inherent repair dynamics. This is of importance from both the viewpoint of treatment safety, as well as efficacy. As noted earlier (e.g., Fig. 2 and related discussion), this issue has come into greater focus for us because of the striking discrepancy we have noted between neurological status and the extent of spinal tissue destruction in some patients in our study.

Therefore, in parallel with our clinical investigation, we have begun experiments to test the effects of intraspinal fetal cell transplantation in the phrenic motor system (Schrimscher et al., 1998; Reier et al., 1998), which shows a significant degree of neuroplasticity in the form of what is referred to as the "crossed phrenic phenomenon" (CPP) (Nantwi, Goshgarian, 1998). While the CPP has been viewed primarily as the activation of a latent pathway under rigorously controlled, terminal neurophysiological conditions, we have recently obtained evidence suggesting that it is spontaneously expressed in adult rats under normal eupnic condit-

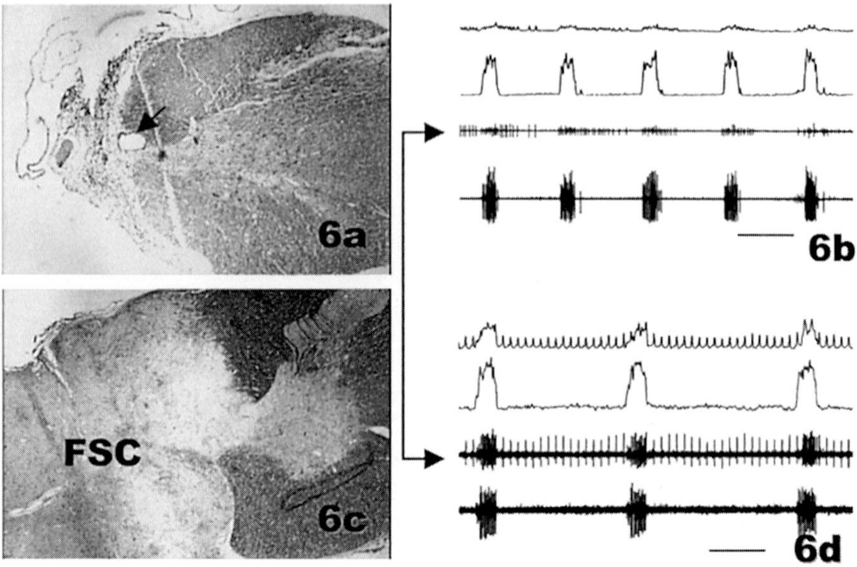

Figure 6 The absence of a deleterious effect of transplants on the expression of spontaneously recovered phrenic activity is illustrated. In panel 6a a transverse section is shown at the level of C_2 4 months after a hemiresection cavity was made. The arrow points to an intact, but enlarged, central canal. The traces shown in 6b are recordings of phrenic nerve activity under rigorously controlled terminal electrophysiological conditions thus reflecting bulbospinal drive to the phrenic motor nucleus at $C_{3\text{-}5}$. Despite complete interruption of descending pathways, some spontaneous bursting activity is ultimately recovered (arrow in 6b), albeit considerably below normal levels (lowest unrectified traces in 6b and 6d). In an animal from the same series of experiments which had received a transplant of FSC tissue (6c), phrenic activity (6d) ipsilateral to the lesion at C_2 is substantially greater (arrow in 6d).

ions (Nantwi et al., 2000). Following hemisection at C_2, the ipsilateral diaphragm is paralyzed; however, by 6-10 weeks postinjury phrenic neurograms and diaphragm EMGs show an appearance of functional recovery, though the level of improvement is well-below normal (Fig. 6a, b). In an initial series of studies, transplants of E_{14} FSC tissue were made into acute lesion cavities at C_2. Interestingly, these grafts which filled the entire lesion cavity did not interfere with the expression of intrinsic recovery (Fig. 6c, d). In fact, at 4 mos. post-injury the level of phrenic activity actually appeared greater than seen in lesion-only animals.

These early results thus provide some indication of three levels of safety in a functionally critical level of the spinal cord. First, the grafts do not appear to compromise the expression of at least one intrinsic repair mechanism. Second, the transplants do not appear to affect phrenic motoneuron function on the contralateral intact side. Lastly, these early results suggest safety related to transplantation into an enlargement region of the spinal cord.

6. Neurophysiological and Behavioral Evidence of Functional Improvement in Animal Models

It also is intriguing that the FSC transplants may be enhancing plasticity in the phrenic motor system (e.g., Fig. 6b vs. 6d). This would be consistent with the fact that several other investigations over the years have independently demonstrated that intraspinal fetal grafts alone can promote changes in locomotor performance in both neonatal and adult rats (Bregman et al., 1993; Kunkel-Bagden, Bregman, 1990; Kunkel-Bagden et al., 1991; Stokes, Reier, 1990; Kim et al., 1999b; Diener, Bregman, 1998; Miya et al., 1997; Tessler et al., 1997) and cats (Anderson et al., 1991; Howland et al., 1995; Howland et al., 1995).

While these observations alone would not justify a clinical investigation of transplant efficacy in SCI at the present time, the reported effects, for example, on altered motoneuron excitability after contusion injury (Thompson et al., 1992; Thompson et al., 1993; Thompson et al., 1998b) does imply the possibility of another element of patient benefit that in PPTS subjects could be coupled with a more permanent obliteration of the cysts and prevention of refilling. Work in animal models has show that the neurophysiological regulation of reflex excitability during repetitive peripheral nerve stimulation is significantly altered following midthoracic contusion injury (Thompson et al., 1992) in the rat. Some evidence also indicates that this may be linked to the expression of hindlimb spasticity in this model. Fetal tissue transplantation at a variety of post-injury time times, ranging from 1-90 days promotes significant normalization of motoneuron excitability under those physiological test conditions (Reier et al., 1992a; Thompson et al., 1993; Thompson et al., 1998a). These protocols also have been extended to human spinal cord injury as an assay of the integrity of reflex modulation (Calancie et al., 1993; Nielsen et al., 1993). Therefore, neurophysiological paradigms that have been used to study intraspinal transplants also represent an important template for human studies since much of the technology and approaches used can be translated from bench-to-bedside and vice versa.

V. CLINICAL TRANSLATION

A. The Primary Goals Are To Test Safety and Feasibility

Intraspinal fetal tissue transplantation has been performed on humans in Russia (Blagodatskii et al., 1994; Katunian, Pogos reported in Reier et al., 1994a), but few documented details are available. In one case (Blagodatskii et al., 1994), the grafts were tested as a treatment of syringomyelia in 5 subjects. From information that is available, no adverse effects of the grafting procedure were observed in these two investigations. More recently, this application of intraspinal fetal cell transplantation has been explored by Falci et al. (1997) in Sweden who described initial evidence for graft survival at 7 months post-transplantation with no complications. In that case study, transplantation was performed within 9-10 hours of the elective termination procedure. Federal guidelines in the United States, however, require that the elective termination be decided completely independent of any knowledge about the option of donating tissue from the aborted fetus for medical research. Consent on both levels is typically not obtained until immediately before the termination procedure is performed. For that reason, donor fetal tissue must be stored for a minimum of two days to allow for virological and bacteriological screening.

In the clinical study described below, the first transplantation procedure was performed on July 11,1997. From the earliest inception of this endeavor, prompted by discussions at a workshop that was held at the University of Florida three years earlier (Reier et al., 1994a), the focus has been exclusively on the issues of safety and feasibility. In contrast to the stated goals of the studies by Blagodatskii *et al.* and Falci *et al.*, noted above, the primary mission of our clinical study has never been to develop another generation of treatment for PPTS. Instead, we envisioned that anything gained as far as the surgical management and treatment of this condition to represent an added element of patient benefit. Essentially the same point can be made with regard to therapeutic efficacy insofar as each recipient's post-transplantation neurological status was concerned. As described below, we perform a comprehensive battery of functional evaluations pre- and post-operatively on each person enrolled in the study. The emphasis, however, is on determining the safety of the procedure. Beyond that, this investigation is not designed to be a direct test of any form of graft-mediated functional improvement *per se*. A more looming early concern was the question of how to differentiate on one hand between possible graft-associated functional deterioration relative to that caused by the ongoing pathology itself versus improvements in neurological status resulting from untethering and cyst drainage as part of the primary surgical procedure.

B. Study Design and Technical Approaches

The following section highlights some of the major considerations related to operational infrastructure of the trial. A more detailed discussion will be presented in a forthcoming manuscript (Wirth, et al., in preparation). The following reflects protocols that have been employed on all individuals who have participated in this study thus far.

1. Candidate Selection and Initial Testing

This study represents a non-randomized, open label pilot investigation. Aside from a history of PPTS or clear radiological and neurological evidence of PPTS, potential participants had to exhibit ASIA (American Spinal Cord Injury Association) scoring at Grade A-C or Grade D with significant loss of function. Candidates for the study were initially examined by the team neurosurgeon and, based on his clinical judgment, individuals considered to be good subjects were then told of the fetal cell transplantation study. After being given due opportunity to weigh the risk-benefits of the procedure and to gain a better appreciation of the underlying scientific principles, the neurosurgeon then obtained informed consent. Thereafter, each subject underwent an intensive and comprehensive initial evaluation which included: ASIA neurological exam, functional independence measure (FIM) for disability, comprehensive pain assessment, and psychosocial assessment. In addition, MRI scans were performed using a 1.5 Tesla (T) system (Vision, Siemens) and standard protocols for syringomyelia along with sagittal FLAIR (fluid attenuation by inversion recovery)-weighted imaging. Each patient also was given extensive neurophysiological testing, including measurements of spasticity, H-reflexes, spinal- and somatosensory-evoked potentials. One month later, each subject returned for a repeat testing session. The two preoperative evaluations were thus used to compute average baseline scores against which postoperative analyses would be compared. Within approximately one month after the second visit, the patients were admitted for syrinx drainage and implantation of fetal neural tissue. Follow-up clinical, neurophysiological and MRI evaluations were performed before discharge and at 1.5, 3, 6, 9, 12, and 18 months after discharge. All evaluations were done in blinded fashion. Thus, no one other than the radiologist and neurosurgical team was fully aware of the patient's MRI profiles before or after surgery.

1. Transplantation Considerations

One week prior to surgery, CsA immunosuppression was started and continued until 6 months post-transplantation. Blood chemistry and urinalysis were performed routinely in order to monitor for toxicity.

Human FSC donor tissue was procured after elective abortions in strict accordance with federal and state laws, as well as the guidelines developed by the NIH Advisory Committee for Human Fetal Tissue Transplantation Research. Only FSC tissue obtained at 6-9 weeks post-conception was used. Subsequent treatment of the donor tissue closely mirrored published protocols (Kawamoto, Barrett, 1986; Freeman, Kordower, 1991). This involved a series of washes and subsequent microdissection, and cold storage of tissue (Freeman, Kordower, 1991) for 2-3 days prior to surgery. Cultures for bacterial, viral, and fungal agents were performed.

The final preparation of donor tissue was fashioned according to the lesion setting identified in each person's MRI. For example, the cyst in the first patient consisted of numerous, small compartments in the inferior portion of his syrinx. For that procedure, minced pieces of donor tissue were made for multiple 100μl injections of tissue. By comparison, the second graft recipient had a large continuous cavity extending from C_6-T_5 and a smaller cyst at the T_7-T_8 interface. Experience with animal models with analogous cyst morphology argued against the use of an injection approach. Accordingly, ~10 mm long strands of tissue were prepared for grafting into the upper cyst, whereas shorter pieces were prepared for the lower cavity.

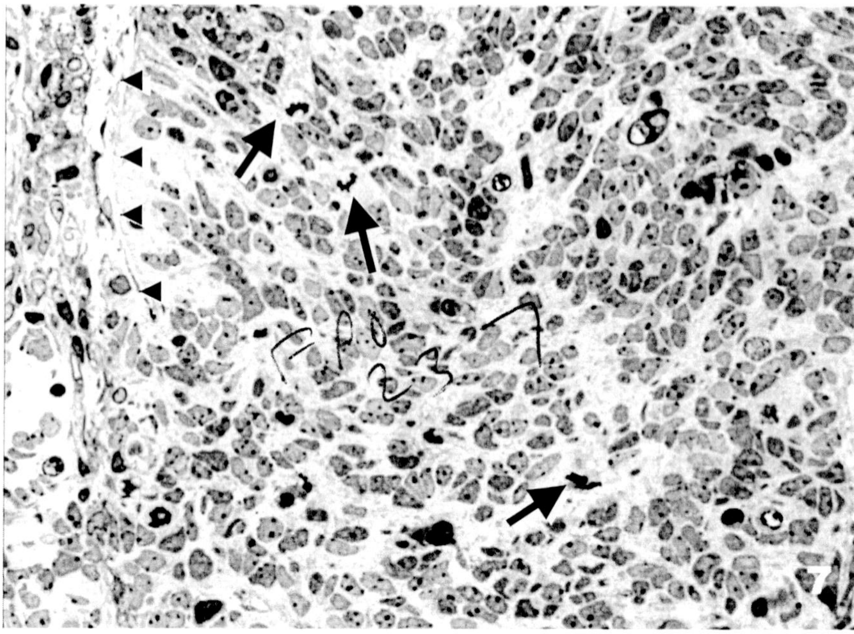

Figure 7 As mentioned in the text, one measure of the human fetal tissue used for transplantation in PPTS subjects is a xenografting analysis involving tissue obtained at either the end of the final dissection phase immediately prior to transplantation or following the surgical procedure itself. This figure shows an example of viable xenograft tissue grafted to the adult rat spinal cord. Note the very germinal appearance of this tissue and frequent mitotic figures (arrows) in this 2μm plastic, toludine blue stained section. Arrowheads point to the establishment of an external glial limiting membrane adjacent to mesodermal infiltration.

For viability determination, a segment of dissected FSC tissue was removed for assays using a dye-exclusion technique. Half of this sample was used to check viability immediately after the initial dissection and viability of the remaining half was recorded 1-2 hours prior to transplantation. No tissue was used if the viability fell below 50%. In addition, some residual tissue obtained either during the final tissue dissection step or immediately following surgery was implanted into acute resection lesions of the rat spinal cord (Fig. 7).

Screening and testing of maternal donor and fetal tissue were performed in accordance with Florida law and the FDA Guidelines regarding tissue intended for human transplantation and donors of reproductive tissue. Both maternal and candidate recipient serological screenings were performed. Furthermore, donor tissue was screened for infectious agents that may be present in the reproductive tract.

VI. INITIAL FINDINGS INDICATE PROCEDURAL SAFETY AND FEASIBILITY

The following is a summary of the status of this investigation as of November, 1999. The original plan was to enroll a total of 10 patients over the course of two years. As of this writing, we have performed intraspinal FSC allografts on seven subjects. For the purposes of this chapter, a more general review is provided with reference to specific case vignettes. The reader is advised that any commentary regarding functional outcome is purely to emphasize procedural safety and in no way is intended to convey specific conclusions or implications related to therapeutic efficacy in terms of direct graft-mediated recoveries.

A. Review of Patient Histories and Specific Surgical Procedures

As outlined in Table 1, six males and one female, ranging between 45-66 years of age, have been entered into this trial. All sustained a spinal injury at thoracic levels between 12-31 years prior to their first pre-transplant clinical visit. The first diagnosed onset of PPTS ranged from 2-17 years which is consistent with published accounts of this condition. Presenting symptoms were variable and most typically involved manifestation of pain, upper and/or lower extremity weakness, as well as spasms. The first four subjects had histories of 1-5 previous shunting procedures, whereas the other three were being considered for their first post-injury spinal surgery. In cases where shunting had been previously performed, relief of presenting symptomology ranged from no change to symptom reduction for up to 3 years before another surgery was required or considered. Determination of pre-operative syrinx sizes by MRI revealed cavitations of 1-20 cm in length.

In each case, cyst decompression was performed by either needle aspiration or myelotomy along with detethering of all intradural adhesions as necessary. Apart from the introduction of donor tissue, no other procedure was carried out in 5 cases. Shunting was required in two cases and these were threaded rostrally similar to the procedure described by Falci *et al.* (Falci et al., 1997). Localized grafts were made at various levels ranging from C_6 to L_1 (Table 1). In several instances, graft placement was verified by ultrasound. As depicted by Figure 7, donor tissue viability was confirmed by xenografting experiments involving random preoperative samples of donor tissue.

B. MRI Findings in Three Recipients With Extensive Pre-Graft Intraspinal Cavities Suggest Partial Cavity Filling by Donor Tissue

Demonstration of feasibility in this clinical study is clearly dependent upon MRI interpretation. To provide a conservative cross-section of observations thus far, MRI findings from the first, second, and sixth patient (herein referred to as PPTS-1, PPTS-2, and PPTS-6) have been selected for this review.

As illustrated by comparison of pre- and post-operative MRIs of these three graft recipients, significant changes were routinely observed in the sizes of cysts

Table 1. Summary of PPTS subjects enrolled in a study of the feasibility and safety of intraspinal fetal spinal allografts. Italics denote individuals whose preoperative and postoperative MRI and neurological status are discussed in the text.

Sex/Age	*M/45*	*M/53*	M/66	M/56	*F/52*	*M/53*	M/50
Cause of Injury/ Level	*Resection mass/T6*	*Motorcycle accid./ T6*	Fall /T9-10	MVA/ ischemic injury/ T4-5	*MVA/T5 +cervical involve-ment*	*Hit by falling pipe/T12*	Fall/T5
Yr. of Injury	*1979*	*1977*	1983	1987	*1968*	*1969*	1985
Cyst Diagnosis	*1991*	*1994*	1992	1989	*1986*	*1991*	1987
Preop MRI Levels of Cyst	*T2-L1*	*C6-T8*	C4/5-T11	C6-T8	*T5-6*	*C2-T10*	T8-T10
# Previous Shunts	*3 Shunts*	*1 (1995)/ CT guided drain-age in 1997*	1 (1992)	5 + C6-7 myelot-omy	*0*	*0*	0
Length of Relief post-shunt	*Minor reduction of Sx with 1st revision, then constant progression of Sx*	*Relief of Sx for ~ 7mos.; no relief after CT drain.*	No relief of pain after 1st shunt	Minor change after each revision			
Radiologic Evidence of Refilling	*1yr/3mos./1yr*	*7 months*	Thoracic cyst reex-panded	<1yr/3y/3 y/3y/2y			
Transplant Date	*7/11/97*	*10/10/97*	6/26/98	7/24/98	*2/5/99*	*3/26/99*	5/21/99
Levels Transplanted/ Other Rx	*T11-L1/detethering*	*Injected just caudal to T6/strands placed into myelotomy @ T4;detethering @ T5-T6*	Myelot. @T10; myelot. @ T12-L1/deteth ering @ C6	Injections @ C7-T2	*T5-6– injected pieces*	*Shunt T5-C7; graft T5-6*	Shunt T9; graft T10

and their overall morphology following transplantation. Prior to surgery, very well defined cavities could be observed with both T1- and T2-weighted images, whereas following transplantation, the diameter of the spinal cord in affected regions was significantly reduced and approximated normal limits. At spinal levels where tissue was introduced, the cavities appeared either completely or partially filled. Even after 2 years in PPTS-1 and -2, the cavities were only partially obliterated. Accordingly, there was no evidence of tissue overgrowth. In addition, there was no indication of cyst refilling either above or at levels of graft placement. Thus far, only the second patient has shown progressive cyst re-enlargement that will require another surgery. The region of expansion, however, is below the transplantation site. Some re-expansion of the cyst also has been seen in the first patient after the first year, but to date (> 2 years) this has not warranted any consideration of additional surgical intervention. As in the second patient, refilling of the cyst is in a region where no graft tissue was introduced.

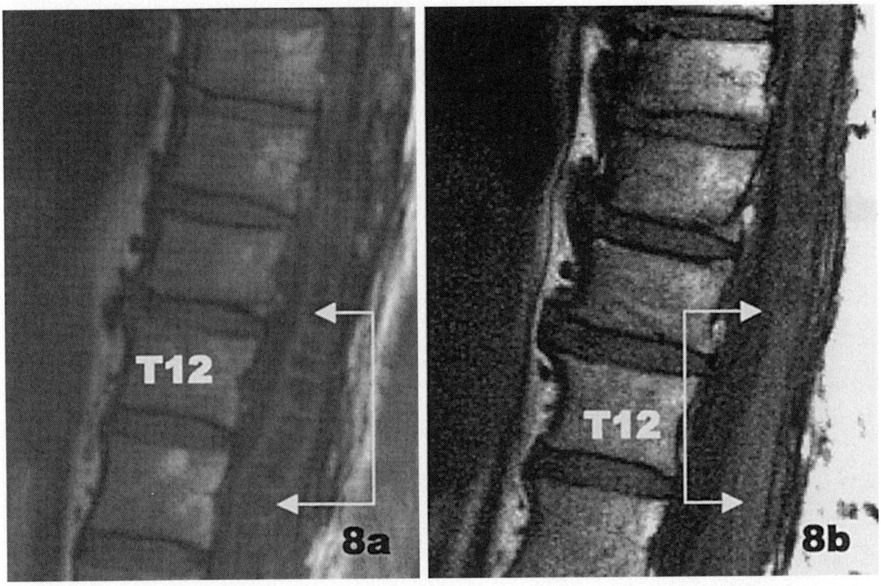

Figure 8 Sagittal pre- (8a, T1-weighted) and post-operative (3 mos., 8b, FLAIR) MRIs of the lower thoracic spinal cord of the first transplant recipient (PPTS-1) in this study are shown where donor tissue was introduced (double arrows). Prior to surgery this individual's spinal cord was distended and exhibited highly locular cystic profiles including at the level of the lumbar enlargement as panel 8a depicts. Following surgery, the cyst was collapsed at the level of graft placement, whereas immediately rostral to that region, little change was evident. Axial images (not shown) indicate an absence of cavitation at $T_{11\text{-}12}$.

Preoperative sagittal MRIs of the first patient's spinal cord revealed highly partitioned cysts from T_2- L_1 that were most prevalent caudally beginning at approximately vertebral T_8 (Fig. 8a). Minced pieces of donor FSC tissue from two fetuses were injected into the syrinx at the T_{11} vertebral level overlying an extensively cavitated lumbar enlargement. Tissue also was introduced at vertebral T_{12}-L_1 and T_{10-11}. Postoperative MR sagital and transverse images revealed a general reduction in syrinx size. At graft levels, the previously cavitated spinal cord appeared as a solid mass of tissue (Fig. 8b). This has remained a static picture through 18 months after transplant surgery.

In the case of PPTS-2, the MR images present a more challenging picture to interpret. Pre-grafting sagittal MR images (Fig. 9a) revealed a syrinx extending from vertebral levels C_6-T_8. The transplantation procedure was carried out as a two-staged process. In the first phase, minced tissue from four donor cords was injected into the syrinx caudal to the original site of injury (i.e., at T_7). For the other phase of this grafting procedure, a myelotomy was performed immediately

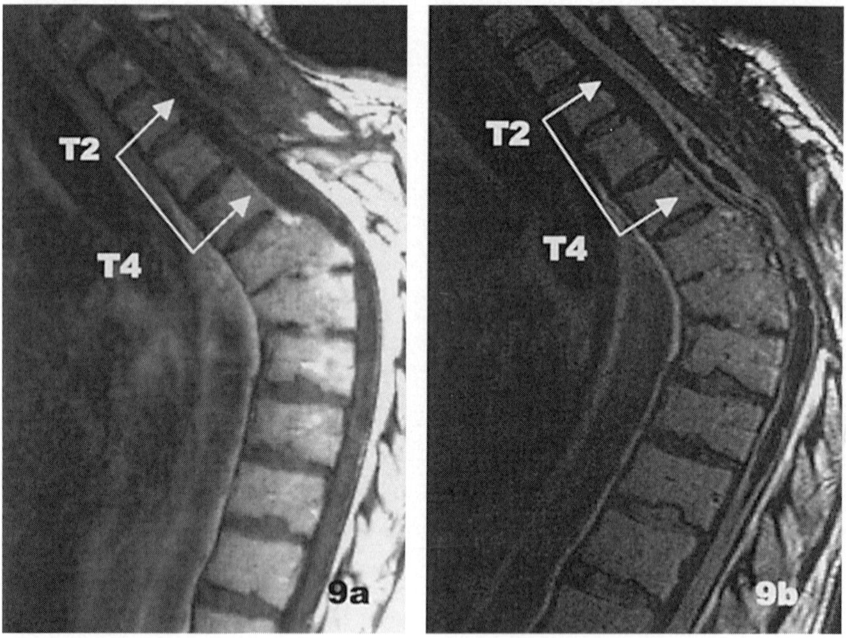

Figure 9 Sagittal, T1-weighted pre- (9a) and FLAIR (9b) postoperative MRIs are shown of the graft site in the second participant in the clinical study (PPTS-2). Before surgery very expanded cavitation is seen between $T_{2\text{-}4}$. At 3 mos. post-transplantation and maintained thereafter, the cord is reduced in size immediately rostral to the graft site which is immediately above a kyphosis. At T_4, some cavitation was present, but the walls of the cavity appeared thickened relative to the preoperative images. This was the region at which strands of donor tissue had been placed adjacent to spared host tissue.

above the level of spinal cord injury in an area where the cyst wall was very thin (T_2-T_4). Visual inspection of the myelotomy site revealed spared tissue with prominent microvasculature. Long strands of FSC from four fetuses were placed directly into the cavity, and the myelotomy was then closed.

Postoperatively, the cyst was reduced at T_2-T_4 in PPTS-2, whereas at T_7 there was little difference from the preoperative MRI. At T_2-T_3, the original cyst seemed nearly obliterated (Fig. 9b). A prominent cyst lumen was still present at T_4, but it appeared reduced relative to the preoperative images. FLAIR imaging (Fig. 9b) also revealed that the walls of the cyst at that level had an undulated contour. Regions of intracystic hyperintensity suggestive of linearly positioned tissue strands also could be viewed extending to T_4, but there wasn't enough intensity demarcation between host and graft tissue to render an unequivocal interpretation.

A preoperative sagittal MRI of the sixth patient's spinal cord is shown in Fig. 2. A shunt and donor fetal tissue were both introduced through a single myel-

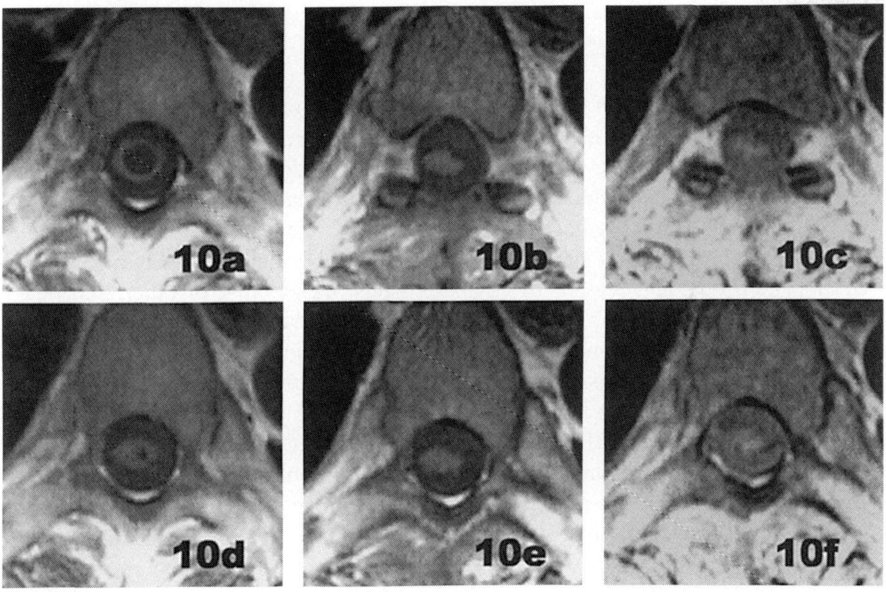

Figure 10 T1-weighted axial images of patient PPTS-6 (see Fig. 2 for preoperative sagittal MRI) obtained at 3 months post-transplantation. The top row represents images taken at the upper region to T_5; the second row shows images obtained at the more rostral aspect of T_6. Figures 10a and d represent preoperative T1-weighted MRIs; Figures 10 b and e and 10c and f are postoperative T1-weighted and proton density images, respectively. At both levels, comparisons of pre- and postoperative images indicate reduction of the cyst and replacement by what appears to be a solid mass of tissue. This appears even more apparent with proton density imaging, and the image in Fig. 10f has features depicted in Fig. 4 of a cat spinal cord with a partially filled cyst.

otomy made at the widest portion of the cyst at T_5, thereby minimizing surgical damage to the cord. First a 1.5 mm endoscope was introduced into the opening and the syrinx cavity was visualized. Multiple septations were noted, but none appeared to be complete, and most appeared to be based on bridging blood vessels. The endoscope was then removed. The syrinx to pleural shunt was then inserted and threaded cephalad for approximately 15 cm. Next, long strands of tissue from a total of eight donor spinal cords were injected through the myelotomy immediately caudal to the shunt. The strands ranged from 3-27 mm length (mean approx. 15 mm), and were introduced using a 500μl Hamilton syringe. Three injections of 325, 400, and 420 μl were made for a total of 1145 μl.

On the postoperative MR images the cervical and upper thoracic portions of the cyst appeared to be almost completely collapsed. The shunt was visible from T_5-T_2 and at T_6-T_7 the cord appeared as a solid mass of tissue. As with the previous images in this chapter, it was not possible to distinguish any donor-host boundaries with certainty on sagittal images, and a small residual cyst was visible in the lower thoracic cord. Axial MR imaging, however, demonstrated extensive filling of a cyst that was pronounced in the preoperative MRI at the same spinal level (Figs. 10a-f).

The most compelling indication from these MR observations of the presence of a graft is the absence of pronounced cavitation (seen preoperatively) in many regions where fetal tissue had been introduced. In addition, some graft sites exhibited small regions of moderately hypertense signal suggestive of tissue masses. Very similar observations have been described by Falci et al. (1997). In our animal experiments (both rat and cat), failed or rejected grafts tend not to be replaced by fibrotic tissue, and regions of cavitation show no collapse or other significant alteration even after decompression related to transplantation. If those findings translate to the human spinal cord under these pathological conditions, then by default one would have to assume that the MR images are indicative of donor tissue survival.

The capacity of MRI to demonstrate viable fetal CNS grafts in cats served as a major basis of our advance to a clinical trial. In contrast to those experimental results, however, MR has not provided an unequivocal definition of the host-graft interface either in terms of different signal intensities or general morphology in our human recipients. This is likely to be due to significant differences in the MR imaging requirements for animal models of SCI versus human subjects with post-traumatic syringomyelia cysts. In addition, there are important differences in the capabilities of animal and human MR scanners. Regarding the former, cats typically receive a controlled injury in which the majority of cystic degeneration is confined to ~1-2 cm of the spinal cord, whereas post-traumatic cysts in human subjects can extend over 30 cm. Since the entire spinal cord must be visualized for adequate surgical planning and follow-up, the radiofrequency (rf) coils used to image human subjects have to be relatively large (50 cm length), whereas much smaller coils (6 cm length) can be used in the animal studies. In general, smaller rf coils perform much better than larger ones and can thus be used to acquire images with much better spatial resolution. For example, for our previous cat studies (Wirth, III et al., 1992; Wirth, III et al., 1995), we produced images with a 2 mm slice thickness and an in-plane resolution of 0.23 x 0.23 mm, which results in image elements ("voxels") with volumes of 0.11 mm^3. Corresponding images in our human subjects have a 4 mm slice thickness and in-plane resolution of 0.7 x 0.7 mm, which results in 1.96 mm^3 voxels. Thus, the spatial resolution is nearly 20-fold worse on the MR images of the human subjects. While this is certainly adequate for visualizing cysts that are up to 100-fold larger than those in the cats, it is less optimal for detecting small islands of grafted fetal tissue that are of similar size to those observed in cats (e.g., Fig. 4). We anticipate that our recent acquisition of a 3T human scanner should improve our imaging capabilities significantly, along with other protocols such as diffusion-weighted and proton (Figs. 10 c, f) imaging.

C. Neurological and Neurophysiological Evaluations Do Not Indicate Adverse Procedural Effects

To date, our composite neurological and neurophysiological evaluations show that none of the patients have exhibited any adverse signs or symptoms following the transplantation procedure. The most conservative interpretation of the results of this investigation in progress is that neither the introduction of fetal tissue from multiple donors, irrespective of the ultimate survival or demise of the grafts, nor associated protocols (e.g., short-term immunosuppression) impose additional undo risk to the subject beyond those normally involved with the detethering/decompression procedure itself. Furthermore, there is no indication that the placement of these grafts interferes with the benefits of the standard of medical care for PPTS patients. A general trend, which is still being analyzed, is that after surgery there are immediate neurological improvements. This is subsequently followed by a period during which the subjects consistently relate perceptions of worsening function. However, thereafter, there appears to be a progressive improvement indicated in various measures over time.

Detailed description and discussion of the first two patients will be forthcoming (Wirth et al., in preparation; Thompson et al., in preparation). As one example of these findings, the first patient's (Fig. 8) neurological status has remained stable during the first 12 months postoperative. By the first month after transplant surgery, he reported a slight return of strength in his left leg and was experiencing tingling dysesthesias in both lower extremities. He also indicated partial sensation of bowel and bladder fullness and had not experienced either a bowel or bladder accident in several weeks. Prior to the grafting procedure, he was having daily accidents. He also perceived increased spasticity in both lower extremities. His bowel and bladder function, tingling dysesthesias, and sensation of lower extremity spasms remained essentially unchanged from 6-weeks through 18-months postoperative.

Neurophysiological evaluations were also performed of lower extremity spasticity, segmental reflexes, and conduction in long white matter tracts. In addition, these assessments included ankle torque testing for spasticity, measurement of H-reflexes, and recording of spinal- and somatosensory-evoked potentials (Thompson et al, in preparation). Interestingly, despite the first patient's greater perception of spasticity various electrophysiological measures of reflex function tended to progressively approximate normal after surgery. For example, recordings of right soleus H-reflexes prior to transplantation revealed low amplitude waveforms at the control frequency of 0.1 Hz, and marked potentiations at 5 and 10 Hz stimulation frequencies. The largest potentiation, a mean of 854.5% of the 0.1Hz control, was produced at 5 Hz. At 1.5 months, the 5 Hz low frequency potentiation of this person's waveforms had decreased to 203% of the 0.1 Hz control, and was observed to decrease even moreso at subsequent quarterly recording intervals. At 18 months, the potentiation was 128% of the 0.1 Hz control. The pre-grafting H-reflex control amplitudes were approximately 0.1 mV, and progressively increased to approximately 1.0 mV by the 18 month recording interval.

As an example of the neurological observations in one of the more recent graft recipients (PPTS-6, Figs. 2, 10), this individual reported feeling generally weaker for the the first several weeks after surgery, but then reported a slow and steady improvement that has continued through 3 and 6 months postoperative. Anecdotally, the patient also noted at his 3 month visit that his foot drop on the right, present since his original injury in 1969, had improved considerably. As noted earlier in reference to Fig. 2, this individual has remained ambulatory since his accident, and this status has not changed since the transplantation surgery.

VII. OBLITERATION OF SMALL CYSTS WITH FSC GRAFTS APPEARS FEASIBLE

As seen in the patient vignettes provided above, there are indications of feasibility and graft survival; however, as anticipated, extensive filling of these cavities has not occurred. In once sense, this underscores a commonly stated limitation of fetal CNS transplantation – namely, the insufficient amount of tissue required to promote, at the very least, anatomical repair. For extensive cavitations this is certainly a reasonable perspective, although there is no evidence presently available demonstrating that entire lesions need to be filled in order to promote functional improvement.

On the other hand, for lesions of more limited size, this impression may require some qualifiers. An illustration of this point is the fifth patient in the study, who presents a striking contrast with other graft recipients in that her preoperative cyst was only 1 cm long (Fig. 11a). Axial images showed that the syrinx was eccentrically positioned (Fig. 11c) with fairly substantial tissue still present. That lesion thus approximated a type of stable, chronic injury which would be especially amenable to a transplantation approach by virtue of its anatomical configur-

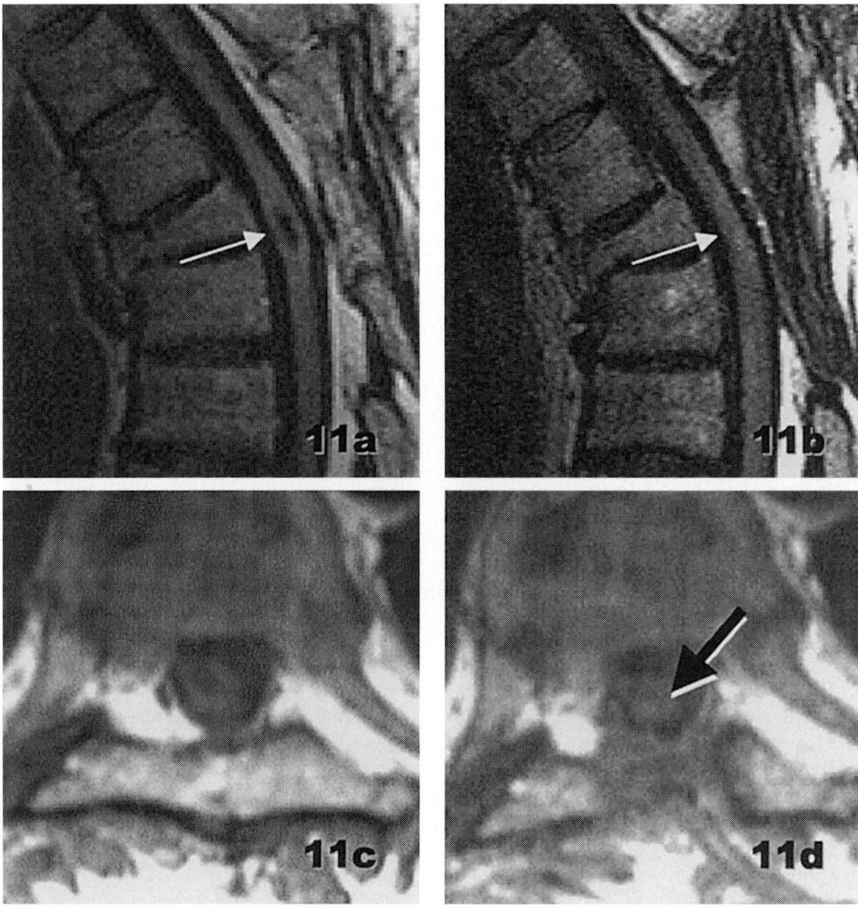

Figure 11 By comparison with the other subjects enrolled in this study, the fifth person to be included exhibited only a small cyst preoperatively (11a) that was eccentrically positioned as seen on inspection of axial images (11c). At 3 months after transplantation, the cyst was no longer evident on sagittal images (11b), and suggestion of graft tissue was indicated in axial T1-weighted images (arrow).

ation and size. Furthermore, the dimensions of this lesion paralleled what we have encountered in our previous studies in the cat. As summarized in Table 1, this individual sustained a T_5 plus lower cervical injury over 30 years ago with an initial intraspinal cyst diagnosis obtained 18 years after her injury. She remained ambulatory after her accident, but then began to experience progressive lower extremity weakness and gait instability resulting in more wheelchair dependence. Longitudinal MRI analysis indicated an expanding syrinx. However, in view of the acutely progressive nature of her condition and the extensive amount of residual spinal cord tissue still involved, we did not consider this person as a viable candidate for the transplantation procedure. A major concern was that it would be virtually impossible to dissociate continued pathology and functional decline from any possible adverse effects of the graft and vice versa. This individual, however, was independently well informed. She was thus fully aware of all the risks involved and determined to have the grafting procedure performed.

Solid pieces of FSC tissue from two donor fetuses were introduced into the cavity *via* a cannula attached to a Hamilton syringe. For this particular case, enough donor fetal tissue remained after the procedure to have been used for at least one other patient with a comparable preoperative profile. T1-weighted sagittal MRI at 3 months post-operatively showed filling of the original cyst (Fig. 12b). Partial filling of the cyst was seen in axial MR images with some remaining cavitation seen primarily in the more inferior aspect of the cord (Fig. 12d). Otherwise, much of the original cavity seemed to be reduced in size. Neurologically, this individual showed no deterioration in function after surgery and, to date, has made steady progress in becoming more independently ambulatory on a daily basis.

VIII. INITIAL CLINICAL FINDINGS: SUMMARY AND CURRENT INTERPRETATIONS

While it is premature to raise many interpretations from the MRI results at this early stage of investigation, it is worth noting that there is a trend suggesting stabilization of the cavitation process in all but one of the graft recipients. In the case of PPTS-1, for example, who had three shunts done at yearly intervals prior to the grafting surgery, there has been no indication of refilling to the degree requiring another procedure (currently at 2.5 years post-transplantation). What cyst expansion has been seen in this individual is in regions distant from the graft site. On the other hand, Patient PPTS-2, who is also beyond two years, does require a second procedure; however, as in the first subject, the refilling is occurring below and distant to the level of graft placement. Should this trend be sustained, it would be indicative of the potential patient benefit that we hoped to see beyond the primary emphasis on safety and feasibility. Given the limited growth of the grafts, as far as our MRI findings suggest, we have to conclude at this point that at least FSC tissue may be limited in its capacity to obliterate cysts in PPTS patients. While filling of small cysts is a possibility, the capacity to populate the extensive cysts seen in several of these individuals (with at least FSC tissue) is unlikely. Whether such extensive filling will actually be necessary, however, is an open consideration.

Regarding neurological outcomes, any speculation concerning a potentially direct graft-mediated effect would be highly premature. Instead, the fact that none of the graft recipients to date have experienced any further functional compromise or debilitating sensory effects points toward procedural safety. It is interesting also that even grafts into an enlargement region (i.e., patient PPTS-1) has not adversely affected residual lower extremity function. The fact that this and a few other patients have shown some modest, but progressive, qualitative and quantitative signs of improvement also speaks to the issue of safety. Presently, we favor the view that the improvements seen 3 months and longer after grafting reflect intrinsic plasticity that is being expressed as a result of stabilization of spinal cord pathology.

VIII. FINAL REMARKS

In this chapter, we have provided a detailed overview of the collective practical and theoretical foundation of basic science experience that has led to a proverbial "bench-to-bedside" translational endeavor in one realm of SCI research. While the emphasis of this scientific/clinical pursuit is on primary fetal CNS tissue transplantation *per se*, a re-examination of the early life-history of these grafts under specific lesion conditions suggests that these transplants may be more representative of the next generation of donor tissue – namely, precursor/progenitor cells – that many laboratories are actively investigating in an effort to circumvent the use of human donor material. The multidimensional characteristics of fetal tissue thereby underscores its importance as an experimental tool, a gold-standard to which other analogous approaches can be compared, as well as a window to the future in terms of other evolving therapeutic approaches.

The impetus for extending basic research on intraspinal transplantation to the clinical setting takes into account many considerations including over 15 years of experience and independent research confirmations world-wide. Additionally, it seems reasonable that some form of cellular transplantation will be a key component in one or more combinatorial strategies for promoting functional repair of the injured spinal cord. Therefore, it is of considerable interest to learn how amenable approaches are to human application that have had some measure of success in rodents and other species. Reciprocally, even a limited clinical experience can be instrumental in shaping laboratory investigations to be in closer register with the human condition. As in many other areas of biomedical research, neuroscience is in an era where basic and clinical investigatons are more likely to run in parallel to a much greater degree than in the past. It thus becomes very essential to begin dealing with the establishment of translational research templates that can facilitate this process.

Our emphasis on PPTS as a clinical "model" in which to begin addressing the very basic issues of safety and feasibility represents both a conservative, as well as biologically challenging, test condition. Because this is an on-going study, the results presented here have to be viewed as very preliminary. Therefore, a concerted effort has been made to present these findings and related speculations as conservatively as possible. In terms of our primary objectives, the MRI observations provide strong suggestions of graft survival, though limitations have been openly considered. While the ultimate test of feasibility will require more definitive imaging approaches, it does appear at this time that many of the basic approaches used for fetal CNS grafts in animal experiments can be effectively translated to the clinical arena in nearly a point-to-point fashion. The final word on safety also requires unequivocal demonstration of surviving graft tissue. However, from the existing results, it seems reasonable to conclude that from a procedural perspective, the introduction of fetal CNS tissue and related protocols neither contribute to an acceleration of the existing pathology nor represent an impediment to the principle surgical management of PPTS.

Functional observations, which have been presented in a more anectodal framework here, also indicate a clear margin of safety in that we have not seen any adverse change relative to preoperative status. In fact, the relatively modest improvements that have been noted so far may be foreshadowing the signature outcome of this clinical endeavor beyond the issue of intraspinal transplantation itself. As seen in one of these patients prior to surgery, an individual's neurological status can be substantially better than would be predicted from her/his MRI. This is probably a more common finding than the clinical literature reflects. One interpretation is that such a mismatch is a compelling suggestion of intrinsic compensatory repair mechanisms in the injured spinal cord. These are being constantly expressed where there is a slow progression of pathology. By stabilizing cysts in the subjects enrolled in our study, the improvements that have been seen could very well be the result of a re-emergence of these repair mechanisms that might be further amplified by other treatments and/or locomotor training approaches (Edgerton et al., 1997; Barbeau et al., 1998; Harkema et al., 1997; Ladouceur et al., 1997; Rossignol et al., 1996; Freeman et al., 1999; Wernig et al., 1995). In light of the debate related to intraspinal sprouting and spinal neuroplasticity (Goldberger, Murray, 1988), it is ironic that one of the more controversial issues in SCI research at one time could represent the greatest ally to functional recovery in the injured spinal cord. In view of the existence of experimental models of SCI plasticity, it is intriguing to consider parallel animal and clinical studies to test this notion more directly.

IX. ACKNOWLEDGMENTS

The authors wish to acknowledge their appreciation to Thomas Freeman, M.D. who has been extremely instrumental in our development of the clinical study based upon his extensive experience with fetal cell transplantation in neurodegenerative disease clinical trials. We also are very grateful to Dr. M. Jo Velardo for her input to this chapter and Dr. Dena Howland for the useful discussions. Funding of the preclinical laboratory experiments cited in this chapter derived from NIH (1PO1NS35702), the State of Florida Brain and Spinal Cord Injury Research Trust Fund, the Department of Veterans Affairs, and the Mark F. Overstreet and C.M. and K.E. Overstreet Chairs for Spinal Cord Injury Research. The clinical study was funded solely through non-federal sources *via* the University of Florida Brain Institute and College of Medicine.

X. REFERENCES

Acosta-Rua AJ, Vierck CJ (1999) Effects of excitatory amino acid (EAA) lesions of thoracic spinal gray matter on escape and withdrawal/licking responses of rats to thermal stimulation. Soc.Neurosci.Abst. 25:1680.

Akesson E, Kjaeldgaard A, Seiger A 1998. Human embryonic spinal cord grafts in adult rat spinal cord cavities: survival, growth, and interactions with the host. Exp Neurol 149:262-276.

Alstermark B, Kummel H 1986. Transneuronal labelling of neurones projecting to forelimb motoneurones in cats performing different movements. Brain Res. 376:387-391.

Alstermark B, Kummel H, Pinter MJ, Tantisira B 1987. Branching and termination of C3-C4 propriospinal neurones in the cervical spinal cord of the cat. Neurosci.Lett. 74:291-296.

Alstermark B, Sasaki S 1986b. Integration in descending motor pathways controlling the forelimb in the cat. 14. Differential projection to fast and slow motoneurones from excitatory C3-C4 propriospinal neurones. Exp.Brain Res. 63:530-542.

Alstermark B, Sasaki S 1986a. Integration in descending motor pathways controlling the forelimb in the cat. 15. Comparison of the projection from excitatory C3-C4 propriospinal neurones to different species of forelimb motoneurones. Exp.Brain Res. 63:543-556.

Alvarez FJ, Pearson JC, Harrington D, Dewey D, Torbeck L, Fyffe RE 1998. Distribution of 5-hydroxytryptamine-immunoreactive boutons on alpha- motoneurons in the lumbar spinal cord of adult cats. J Comp.Neurol. 393:69-83.

Anderson DK, Howland DR, Reier PJ 1995. Fetal neural grafts and repair of the injured spinal cord. Brain Pathol. 5:451-457.

Anderson DK, Howland DR, Reier PJ (1996) Characteristics of intraspinal grafts and locomotor function after spinal cord injury. In: Proceedings of the Third Altshul Symposium (Juurlink BHJ, Doucette R eds), pp 249-266. New York: Plenum Press.

Anderson DK, Reier PJ, Theele DP, Munson JB, Ritz LA , Brown SA, Zeller BE 1989. Development of fetal cat neural grafts in acute and chronic lesions of the adult cat spinal cord. Soc.Neurosci.Abst. 15:1242-1242.

Anderson DK, Reier PJ, Wirth III ED, Theele DP, Brown SA 1991. Transplants of fetal CNS grafts in chronic compression lesions of the adult cat spinal cord. Restorative Neurol. Neurosci 2:309-325.

Aschoff A, Kunze S 1993. 100 Years syrinx-surgery--a review. Acta Neurochir (Wien) 123:157-159.

Balentine JD (1988) Impact injuries of the spine and spinal cord. In: Forensic Neuropathology (Leestma JE, Kirkpatrick JB eds), pp 254-275. New York: Raven Press.

Barbeau H, Norman K, Fung J, Visintin M, Ladouceur M 1998. Does neurorehabilitation play a role in the recovery of walking in neurological populations? Ann.N.Y.Acad.Sci. 860:377-392.

Barbeau H, Rossignol S 1994. Enhancement of locomotor recovery following spinal cord injury. Curr.Opin.Neurol. 7:517-524.

Beattie MS, Bresnahan JC, Komon J, Tovar CA, Van-Meter M, Anderson DK, Faden AI, Hsu CY, Noble LJ, Salzman S, Young W 1997. Endogenous repair after spinal cord contusion injuries in the rat. Exp.Neurol. 148:453-463.

Beattie MS, Stokes BT, Bresnahan JC (1988) Experimental spinal cord injury -- strategies for acute and chronic intervention based on anatomic, physiological, and behavioral studies. In: Pharmacological Approaches to the Treatment of Brain and Spinal Cord Injury (Stein DG, Sabel BA eds), pp 43-74. New York: Plenum Pub. Corp.

Becerra JL, Puckett WR, Hiester ED, Quencer RM, Marcillo AE, Post MJ, Bunge RP 1995. MR-pathologic comparisons of wallerian degeneration in spinal cord injury. AJNR.Am.J Neuroradiol. 16:125-133.

Bernstein Goral H, Bregman BS 1993. Spinal cord transplants support the regeneration of axotomized neurons after spinal cord lesions at birth: a quantitative double- labeling study. Exp.Neurol. 123:118-132.

Biyani A, el Masry WS 1994. Post-traumatic syringomyelia: a review of the literature. Paraplegia 32:723-731.

Bjorklund L, Spenger C, Stromberg I 1997. Tirilazad mesylate increases dopaminergic neuronal survival in the *in oculo* grafting model. Exp Neurol 148:324-333.

Björklund A, Stenevi U, Dunnett SB (1983) Transplantation of brainstem monoaminergic "command" systems: models for functional reactivation of damaged CNS circuitries. In: Spinal Cord Reconstruction (Kao CC, Bunge RP, Reier PJ eds), pp 397-413. New York: Raven Press.

Blagodatskii MD, Sufianov AA, Larionov SN, Kibort RV, Seminskii IZ, Manokhin PA 1994. [The transplantation of embryonic nerve tissue in syringomyelia: initial clinical experience]. Zh Vopr Neirokhir Im N N Burdenko 27-29.

Blakemore WF, Crang AJ, Patterson RC 1987. Schwann cell remyelination of CNS axons following injection of cultures of CNS cells into areas of persistent demyelination. Neurosci.Lett. 77:20-24.

Blakemore WF, Franklin RJM 1991. Transplantation of glial cells into the CNS. Trends Neurosci. 14:323-327.

Blesch A, Tuszynski MH 1997. Robust growth of chronically injured spinal cord axons induced by grafts of genetically modified NGF-secreting cells. Exp.Neurol. 148:444-452.

Blight AR, Decrescito V 1986. Morphometric analysis of experimental spinal cord injury in the cat: the relation of injury intensity to survival of myelinated axons. Neurosci. 19:321-341.

Boonman Z, Isacson O 1999. Apoptosis in neuronal development and transplantation: role of caspases and trophic factors. Exp Neurol 156:1-15.

Bregman BS 1998. Regeneration in the spinal cord. Curr. Opin.Neurobiol. 8 :800-807.

Bregman BS, Bernstein Goral H 1991. Both regenerating and late-developing pathways contribute to transplant-induced anatomical plasticity after spinal cord lesions at birth. Exp.Neurol. 112:49-63.

Bregman BS, Diener PS, McAtee M, Dai HN, James C 1997. Intervention strategies to enhance anatomical plasticity and recovery of function after spinal cord injury. Adv.Neurol. 72:257-275.

Bregman BS, Kunkel Bagden E, Reier PJ, Dai HN, McAtee M, Gao D 1993. Recovery of function after spinal cord injury: mechanisms underlying transplant-mediated recovery of function differ after spinal cord injury in newborn and adult rats. Exp.Neurol. 123:3-16.

Bregman BS, McAtee M (1995) Neurotrophic factors increase axonal growth after spinal cord lesions and transplants in adult rats. Soc.Neurosci.Abst. 21:1056(Abstract)

Bregman BS, McAtee M, Dai HN, Kuhn PL 1997. Neurotrophic factors increase axonal growth after spinal cord injury and transplantation in the adult rat. Exp.Neurol. 148 :475-494.

Brook GA, Plate D, Franzen R, Martin D, Moonen G, Schoenen J, Schmitt AB, Noth J, Nacimiento W 1998. Spontaneous longitudinally orientated axonal regeneration is associated with the Schwann cell framework within the lesion site following spinal cord compression injury of the rat. J Neurosci.Res. 53:51-65.

Brundin P, Nilsson OG, Gage FH, Bjorklund A 1985. Cyclosporin A increases survival of cross-species intrastriatal grafts of embryonic dopamine-containing neurons. Exp Brain Res 60:204-208.

Bunge RP (1994) Clinical implications of recent advances in neurotrauma research. In: The Neurobiology of Central Nervous System Trauma (Salzman SK, Faden AI eds), pp 329-339. New York: Oxford Univ. Press.

Bunge RP, Puckett WR, Becerra JL, Marcillo A, Quencer RM 1993. Observations on the pathology of human SCI - a review and classification of 22 new cases with details from a case of chronic cord compression with extensive focal demyelination. Adv.Neurol. 59:75-90.

Calancie B, Alexeeva N, Broton JG, Suys S, Hall A, Klose KJ 1999. Distribution and latency of muscle responses to transcranial magnetic stimulation of motor cortex after spinal cord injury in humans. J Neurotrauma 16:49-67.

Calancie B, Broton JG, Klose KJ, Traad M, Difini J, Ayyar DR 1993. Evidence that alterations in presynaptic inhibition contribute to segmental hypo- and hyperexcitability after spinal cord injury in man. Electroencephalogr Clin Neurophysiol . 89:177-186.

Chen A, Xu XM, Kleitman N, Bunge MB 1996. Methylprednisolone administration improves axonal regeneration into Schwann cell grafts in transected adult rat thoracic spinal cord. Exp.Neurol. 138:261-276.

Chung K, Coggeshall RE 1988. Propriospinal fibers in the white matter of the cat sacral spinal cord. J Comp.Neurol. 269:612-617.

Crowe MJ, Bresnahan JC, Shuman SL, Masters JN, Beattie MS 1997. Apoptosis and delayed degeneration after spinal cord injury in rats and monkeys [published erratum appears in Nat Med 1997 Feb;3(2):240]. Nat. Med. 3:73-76.

De La Torre JC 1999. Collagen-omentum reconstructive approach. J.Neurotrauma 16:747

Diener PS, Bregman BS 1998. Fetal spinal cord transplants support the development of target reaching and coordinated postural adjustments after neonatal cervical spinal cord injury. J Neurosci 18:763-778.

Dunnett SB 1991. Transplantation of embryonic dopamine neurons: what we know from rats [editorial]. J Neurol 238:65-74.

Edgerton VR, De-Leon RD, Tillakaratne N, Recktenwald MR, Hodgson JA, Roy RR 1997. Use-dependent plasticity in spinal stepping and standing. Adv.Neurol. 72:233-247.

Falci S, Holtz A, Akesson E, Azizi M, Ertzgaard P, Hultling C, Kjaeldgaard A, Levi R, Ringden O, Westgren M, Lammertse D, Seiger A 1997. Obliteration of a posttraumatic spinal cord cyst with solid human embryonic spinal cord grafts: first clinical attempt. J Neurotrauma 14:875-884.

Fawcett JW 1998. Spinal cord repair: from experimental models to human application. Spinal.Cord. 36:811-817.

Fehlings MG, Tator CH 1995. The relationship among severity of spinal cord injury, residual neurological function, axon counts, and counts of retrogradely labeled neurons after experimental spinal cord injury. Exp.Neurol. 132:220-228.

Feraboli-Lohnherr D, Orsal D, Yakovleff A, Gimenez, Privat A 1997. Recovery of locomotor activity in the adult chronic spinal rat after sublesional transplantation of embryonic nervous cells: specific role of serotonergic neurons. Exp.Brain Res. 113:443-454.

Freed CR, Breeze RE, Rosenberg NL, Schneck SA, Kriek E, Qi JX, Lone T, Zhang YB, Snyder JA, Wells TH, et al 1992. Survival of implanted fetal dopamine cells and neurologic improvement 12 to 46 months after transplantation for Parkinson's disease [see comments]. N.Engl.J.Med. 327:1549-1555.

Freeman TB, Kordower JH (1991) Human cadaver embryonic substantia nigra grafts: effects of ontogeny, preoperative graft preparation, and tissue storage. In: Intracerebral transplantation in movement disorders (Lindvall O, Bjorklund A, Widner H eds), pp 163-170. Amsterdam: Elsevier.

Freeman TB, Olanow CW, Hauser RA, Nauert GM, Smith DA, Borlongan CV, Sanberg PR, Holt DA, Kordower JH, Vingerhoets FJ, et al 1995. Bilateral fetal nigral transplantation into the postcommissural putamen in Parkinson's disease. Ann.Neurol. 38:379-388.

Freeman TB, Vawter DE, Leaverton PE, Godbold JH, Hauser RA, Goetz CG, Olanow CW 1999. The use of placebo surgery in controlled trials of a cellular-based therapy for Parkinson's Disease. N.Engl.J.Med. 341:988-992.

Gilerovich EG, Fedorova EA, Otellin VA 1996. [The development of human embryonic spinal cord transplants in the spinal cord of adult rats]. Morfologiia 110:43-46.

Gimenez y Ribotta M, Orsal D, Feraboli-Lohnherr D, Privat A, Provencher J, Rossignol S 1998a. Kinematic analysis of recovered locomotor movements of the hindlimbs in paraplegic rats transplanted with monoaminergic embryonic neurons. Ann.N.Y.Acad.Sci. 860:521-3:521-523.

Gimenez y Ribotta M, Orsal D, Feraboli-Lohnherr D, Privat A 1998b. Recovery of locomotion following transplantation of monoaminergic neurons in the spinal cord of paraplegic rats. Ann.N.Y.Acad.Sci. 860:393-411:393-411.

Giovanini MA, Reier PJ, Eskin TA, Anderson DK 1997. MAP2 expression in the developing human fetal spinal cord and following xenotransplantation. Cell Transplant. 6:339-346.

Giovanini MA, Reier PJ, Eskin TA, Wirth E, Anderson DK 1997. Characteristics of human fetal spinal cord grafts in the adult rat spinal cord: influences of lesion and grafting conditions. Exp.Neurol. 148:523-543.

Goldberger ME, Murray M (1988) Patterns of sprouting and implications for recovery of function. In: Functional Recovery in Neurological Disease. In: *Advances in Neurology*, Vol. 47 (Waxman SG ed), pp 361-386. New York: Raven Press.

Goldstein B, Hammond MC, Stiens SA, Little JW 1998. Posttraumatic syringomyelia: profound neuronal loss, yet preserved function. Arch.Phys.Med.Rehabil. 79:107-112.

Gray J, Dunnett SB (1999) Neural transplantation in neurodegenerative disease. Symposium No. 231, in press.

Grill R, Murai K, Blesch A, Gage FH, Tuszynski MH 1997. Cellular delivery of neurotrophin-3 promotes corticospinal axonal growth and partial functional recovery after spinal cord injury. J Neurosci. 17:5560-5572.

Guest JD, Hesse D, Schnell L, Schwab ME, Bunge MB, Bunge RP 1997. Influence of IN-1 antibody and acidic FGF-fibrin glue on the response of injured corticospinal tract axons to human Schwann cell grafts. J Neurosci.Res. 50:888-905.

Guth L, Barrett CP, Donati EJ, Anderson FD, Smith MV , Lifson M 1985. Essentiality of a specific cellular terrain for growth of axons into a spinal cord lesion. Exp Neurol 88:1-12.

Harkema SJ, Hurley SL, Patel UK, Requejo PS, Dobkin BH, Edgerton VR 1997. Human lumbosacral spinal cord interprets loading during stepping. J Neurophysiol. 77:797-811.

Hayes KC, Kakulas BA 1997. Neuropathology of human spinal cord injury sustained in sports-related activities. J Neurotrauma 14 :235-248.

Horner PJ, Reier PJ, Stokes BT 1995. Quantitative analysis of vascularization and cytochrome oxidase following fetal transplantation in the contused rat spinal cord. J.Comp.Neurol. 363:1-14.

Horner PJ, Stokes BT, Reier PJ, Sharp FR 1991. Increased vascularity and cytochrome oxidase levels in fetal suspension grafts of the adult rat spinal cord. Soc.Neurosci.Abst. 17:

Houle JD, Morris K, Skinner RD, Garcia-Rill E, Peterson CA 1999. Effects of fetal spinal cord tissue transplants and cycling exercise on the soleus muscle in spinalized rats. Muscle Nerve 22:846-856.

Hounsgaard J, Hultborn H, Jespersen B, Kiehn O 1988. Bistability of α-motoneurones in the decerebrate cat and in the acute spinal cat after intravenous 5-hydroxytryptophan. J.Physiol. 345-367.

Howland DR, Bregman BS, Tessler A, Goldberger ME 1995. Transplants enhance locomotion in neonatal kittens whose spinal cords are transected: a behavioral and anatomical study. Exp.Neurol. 135:123-145.

Howland DR, Reier PJ, Anderson DK 1995. Intraspinal transplantation of fetal tissue: Therapeutic potential for spinal cord repair. In: Neurotrauma: A Comprehensive Textbook on Head and Spinal Injury (Narayan RK, Wilberger JE, Povlishock JT eds), pp 1507-1520. New York: McGraw-Hill, Inc.

Imaizumi T, Lankford KL, Waxman SG, Greer CA, Kocsis JD 1998. Transplanted olfactory ensheathing cells remyelinate and enhance axonal conduction in the demyelinated dorsal columns of the rat spinal cord. J Neurosci. 18:6176-6185.

Jakeman, LB, Reier, PJ. 1991. Axonal projections between fetal spinal cord transplants and the adult rat spinal cord: a neuroanatomical tracing study of local interactions. J.Comp.Neurol. 307: 311-334.

Kakulas BA 1985. Pathology of spinal injuries. Cent.Nerv.Syst.Trauma 1:117-129.

Kakulas BA 1999. A review of the neuropathology of human spinal cord injury with emphasis on special features. J.Spinal Cord Med. 22:119-124.

Kawamoto JC, Barrett JN 1986. Cryopreservation of primary neurons for tissue culture. Brain Res 384:84-93.

Kiehn O, Eken T 1998. Functional role of plateau potentials in vertebrate motor neurons. Curr.Opin.Neurobiol. 8:746-752.

Kiehn O, Kjaerulff O 1996. Spatiotemporal characteristics of 5-HT and dopamine-induced rhythmic hindlimb activity in the in vitro neonatal rat. J Neurophysiol. 75:1472-1482.

Kim D, Adipudi V, Shibayama M, Giszter S, Tessler A, Murray M, Simansky KJ 1999a. Direct agonists for serotonin receptors enhance locomotor function in rats that received neural transplants after neonatal spinal transection . J Neurosci. 19:6213-6224.

Kim D, Adipudi V, Shibayama M, Giszter S, Tessler A, Murray M, Simansky KJ 1999b. Direct agonists for serotonin receptors enhance locomotor function in rats that received neural transplants after neonatal spinal transection . J Neurosci 19:6213-6224.

Kordower JH, Freeman TB, Olanow CW 1998. Neuropathology of fetal nigral grafts in patients with Parkinson's disease. Mov.Disord. 13 Suppl 1:88-95:88-95.

Kordower JH, Freeman TB, Snow BJ, Vingerhoets FJ, Mufson EJ, Sanberg PR, Hauser RA, Smith DA, Nauert GM, Perl DP, et al 1995. Neuropathological evidence of graft survival and striatal reinnervation after the transplantation of fetal mesencephalic tissue in a patient with Parkinson's disease [see comments]. N.Engl.J.Med. 332:1118-1124.

Kunkel-Bagden E, Bregman BS 1990. Spinal cord transplants enhance the recovery of locomotor function after spinal cord injury at birth. Exp.Brain Res. 81:25-34.

Kunkel-Bagden E, Reier PJ, Dai H-N, Bregman BS 1991. Influence of fetal spinal cord transplants on recovery of motor function after spinal cord injury. Soc.Neurosci.Abst. 17:236

Ladouceur M, Pepin A, Norman KE, Barbeau H 1997. Recovery of walking after spinal cord injury. Adv.Neurol. 72:249-255.

Lee TT, Arias JM, Andrus HL, Quencer RM, Falcone SF, Green BA 1997. Progressive posttraumatic myelomalacic myelopathy: treatment with untethering and expansive duraplasty. J Neurosurg 86:624-628.

Li GL, Brodin G, Farooque M, Funa K, Holtz A, Wang WL, Olsson Y 1996. Apoptosis and expression of Bcl-2 after compression trauma to rat spinal cord. J Neuropathol.Exp.Neurol. 55 :280-289.

Lindvall O, Sawle G, Widner H, Rothwell JC, Bjorklund A, Brooks D, Brundin P, Frackowiak R, Marsden CD, Odin P, et al 1994. Evidence for long-term survival and function of dopaminergic grafts in progressive Parkinson's disease. Ann.Neurol. 35:172-180.

Liu XZ, Xu XM, Hu R, Du C, Zhang SX, McDonald JW, Dong HX, Wu YJ , Fan GS, Jacquin MF, Hsu CY, Choi DW 1997. Neuronal and glial apoptosis after traumatic spinal cord injury. J Neurosci. 17:5395-5406.

Macklin R 1999. The ethical problems with sham surgery in clinical research. N.Engl.J Med. 341:992-996.

McClellan AD 1998. Spinal cord injury: lessons from locomotor recovery and axonal regeneration in lower vertebrates. The Neuroscientist 4:250-263.

McClellan AD, Hagevik A 1999. Coordination of spinal locomotor activity in the lamprey: long-distance coupling of spinal oscillators. Exp.Brain Res. 126:93-108.

Mellen N, Kiemel T, Cohen AH 1995. Correlational analysis of fictive swimming in the lamprey reveals strong functional intersegmental coupling. J Neurophysiol. 73:1020-1030.

Miya D, Giszter S, Mori F, Adipudi V, Tessler A, Murray M 1997. Fetal transplants alter the development of function after spinal cord transection in newborn rats. J Neurosci 17:4856-4872.

Nantwi KD, El-Bohy A, Schrimscher GW, Reier PJ, Goshgarian HG 2000. Spontaneous functional recovery in a paralyzed hemidiaphragm following upper cervical spinal cord injury in adult rats. Neurorehab.Neural Repair In Press:

Nantwi KD, Goshgarian HG 1998. Theophylline-induced recovery in a hemidiaphragm paralyzed by hemisection in rats: contribution of adenosine receptors. Neuropharmacology 37:113-121.

Nielsen J, Petersen N, Ballegaard M, Biering-Sorensen F, Kiehn O 1993. H-reflexes are less depressed following muscle stretch in spastic spinal cord injured patients than in healthy subjects. Exp Brain Res 97:173-176.

Noble LJ, Wrathall J 1989. Correlative analyses of lesion development and functional status after graded contusive injuries in the rat. Exp.Neurol. 103:34-40.

Palmeri A, Sapienza S, Giuffrida R, Bellomo M, Rampello L, Vecchio I, Raffaele R 1999. Modulatory action of noradrenergic system on spinal motoneurons in humans. Neuroreport. 10:1225-1229.

Piatt JH, Jr. (1996) Post-traumatic syringomyelia. In: Neurosurgery (Wilkins RH, Rengachary SS eds), pp 3063-3066. New York: McGraw-Hill.

Privat A, Mansour H, Geffard M (1988) Transplantation of fetal serotonin neurons into the transected spinal cord of adult rats: morphological development and functional influence. In: Transplantation into the Mammalian CNS (Gash DM, Sladek JR, Jr. eds), pp 155-166. Amsterdam: Elsevier.

Quencer RM, Bunge RP, Egnor M, Green BA, Puckett W, Post MJD 1992. MR/Pathological correlations in acute traumatic central cervical spinal cord syndrome. Neuroradiol. 34:85-94.

Reier PJ, Anderson DK, Schrimsher GW, Bao J, Friedman RM, Ritz LA, Stokes B (1994b) Neural cell grafting: anatomical and functional repair of the spinal cord. In: The Neurobiology of Central Nervous System Trauma (Salzman SK, Faden AI eds), pp 288-311. New York: Oxford University Press.

Reier PJ, Anderson DK, Stokes BT 1992a. Neural tissue transplantation and CNS trauma: anatomical and functional repair of the injured spinal cord. In: Central Nervous System Status Report (Jane JA, Anderson DK, Torner JC, and Young W eds.). J.Neurotrauma 9(Supp 1):S223-S248

Reier PJ, Anderson DK, Young W, Michel ME, Fessler R 1994a. Workshop on intraspinal transplantation and clinical application. J.Neurotrauma 11:369-377.

Reier PJ, Bregman BS, Wujek JR (1986) Intraspinal transplantation of fetal spinal cord tissue: an approach toward functional repair of the injured spinal cord. In: Proceedings of the International Symposium on Plasticity and Development of the Mammalian Spinal Cord (M.Goldberger, A.Gorio, M.Murray eds), pp 251-269. Padova: Liviana Press.

Reier PJ, Schrimsher GW, El-Bohy A, Goshgarian HG (1998) Residual phrenic motoneuron function following fetal spinal cord (FSC) tissue grafting to the cervical spinal cord in rats. *Soc. for Neurosci.* , 24: 70. Soc.Neurosci.Abst. 24:70(Abstract)

Reier PJ, Stokes BT, Thompson FJ, Anderson DK 1992b. Fetal cell grafts into resection and contusion/compression injuries of the rat and cat spinal cord. Exp.Neurol. 115:177-188.

Rosenbluth J, Schiff R, Liang WL, Menna G, Young W 1997. Xenotransplantation of transgenic oligodendrocyte-lineage cells into spinal cord-injured adult rats. Exp.Neurol. 147:172-182.

Rossignol S, Chau C, Brustein E, Belanger M, Barbeau H, Drew T 1996. Locomotor capacities after complete and partial lesions of the spinal cord. Acta Neurobiol.Exp.Warsz. 56:449-463.

Rossignol S, Chau C, Brustein E, Giroux N, Bouyer L, Barbeau H, Reader TA 1998. Pharmacological activation and modulation of the central pattern generator for locomotion in the cat. Ann.N.Y.Acad.Sci. 860:346-59:346-359.

Schrimscher GW, Hubscher CH, Johnson RD, Reier PJ (1998) Neuroanatomical evidence for intraspinal fetal grafts establishing relay connectivity in the phrenic motor system of adult rats. Soc.Neurosci.Abst. 24:70.

Sgouros S, Williams B 1995. A critical appraisal of drainage in syringomyelia. J Neurosurg 82:1-10.

Shuman SL, Bresnahan JC, Beattie MS 1997. Apoptosis of microglia and oligodendrocytes after spinal cord contusion in rats. J Neurosci.Res. 50:798-808.

Springer JE, Asbill RD, Knapp PE 1999. Activation of the caspase-3 apoptotic cascade in traumatic spinal cord injury. Nat.Med. 5:943-946.

Stelzner DJ, Cullen JM 1991. Do propriospinal projections contribute to hindlimb recovery when all long tracts are cut in neonatal or weanling rats? Exp.Neurol. 114:193-205.

Stokes BT, Reier PJ (1990) Fetal grafts alter chronic behavioral outcome after contusion damage to the adult rat spinal cord. Soc.Neurosci.Abst. 16:37(Abstract)

Stokes BT, Reier PJ 1992. Fetal grafts alter chronic behavioral outcome after contusion damage to the adult rat spinal cord. Exp.Neurol. 116:1-12.

Tantisira B, Alstermark B, Isa T, Kummel H, Pinter M 1996. Motoneuronal projection pattern of single C3-C4 propriospinal neurones. Can.J Physiol.Pharmacol. 74:518-530.

Tessler A 1991. Intraspinal transplants. Ann.Neurol. 29:115-123.

Tessler A, Fischer I, Giszter S, Himes BT, Miya D, Mori F, Murray M 1997. Embryonic spinal cord transplants enhance locomotor performance in spinalized newborn rats. Adv Neurol 72:291-303.

Theele DP, Reier PJ 1996. Immunomodulation with intrathymic grafts or anti-lymphocyte serum promotes long-term intraspinal allograft survival. Cell Transplant. 5:243-255.

Theele DP, Schrimsher GW, Reier PJ 1996. Comparison of the growth and fate of fetal spinal iso- and allografts in the adult rat injured spinal cord. Exp.Neurol. 142:128-143.

Thompson FJ, Parmer R, Reier PJ 1998b. Alteration in rate modulation of reflexes to lumbar motoneurons after midthoracic spinal cord injury in the rat. I. Contusion injury. J Neurotrauma 15:495-508.

Thompson FJ, Reier PJ, Lucas CC, Parmer R 1992. Altered patterns of reflex excitability subsequent to contusion injury of the rat spinal cord. J.Neurophysiol. 68:1473-1486.

Thompson FJ, Reier PJ, Parmer R, Lucas CC (1993) Inhibitory control of reflex excitability following contusion injury and neural tissue transplantation. In: Advances in Neurology, Vol. 59 (Seil FJ ed), pp 175-184. New York: Raven Press.

Thompson FJ, Uthman B, Mott S, Remson EJ, Wirth III ED, Fessler RG, Reier PJ, Behrman A, Trimble M, Anderson DK (1998a) Neurophysiological assesment of neural tissue transplantation in syringomyelia patients. Soc.Neurosci.Abstr. 24:70.

Tuszynski M, Edgerton R, Dobkin B 1999. Recovery of locomotion after experimental spinal cord injury: axonal regeneration or modulation of intrinsic spinal cord walking? A course synopsis. J.Spinal Cord Med. 22:143

Umbach I, Heilporn A 1991. Review article: post-spinal cord injury syringomyelia. Paraplegia 29:219-221.

Utzschneider DA, Archer DR, Kocsis JD, Waxman SG, Duncan ID 1994. Transplantation of glial cells enhances action potential conduction of amyelinated spinal cord axons in the myelin- deficient rat. Proc.Natl.Acad.Sci.USA 91:53-57.

Van Calenbergh F, Van den Bergh R 1993. Syringo-peritoneal shunting: results and problems in a consecutive series. Acta Neurochir (Wien) 123:203-205.

Velardo MJ, Reier PJ, Anderson DK (1999) Acute Spinal Cord Injury. In: Neurosurgery: The Scientific Basis of Clinical Practice (Crockard A, Hayward R, Hoff J eds), pp In PressOxford: Blackwell Science Ltd.

Vrbová G, Clowry G, Nógrádi A, Sieradzan K (1994) Transplantation of Neural Tissue into the Spinal Cord. Austin: R. G. Landes Co.

Wernig A, Muller S, Nanassy A, Cagol E 1995. Laufband therapy based on rules of spinal locomotion is effective in spinal cord injured persons. Eur.J Neurosci. 7:823-829.

Wictorin K, Bjorklund A 1992. Axon outgrowth from grafts of human embryonic spinal cord in the lesioned adult rat spinal cord. NeuroReport 3:1045-1048.

Williams B 1990. Post-traumatic syringomyelia, an update. Paraplegia 28:296-313.
Wirth ED, III, Theele DP, Mareci TH, Anderson DK, Brown SA, Reier PJ 1992. *In vivo* magnetic resonance imaging of fetal cat neural tissue transplants in the adult cat spinal cord. J.Neurosurg. 76:261-274.
Wirth ED, III, Theele DP, Mareci TH, Anderson DK, Reier PJ 1995. Dynamic assessment of intraspinal neural graft survival using magnetic resonance imaging. Exp.Neurol. 136:64-72.
Wrathall JR (1995) Weight-drop models of experimental spinal cord injury. In: Neurotrauma (Narayan RJ, Wilberger JE, Povlishock JT eds), pp 1381-1394. New York: McGraw-Hill.
Xu XM, Guénard V, Kleitman N, Aebischer P, Bunge MB 1995. A combination of BDNF and NT-3 promotes supraspinal axonal regeneration into Schwann cell grafts in adult rat thoracic spinal cord. Exp.Neurol. 134:261-272.
Xu XM, Zhang SX, Li H, Aebischer P, Bunge MB 1999. Regrowth of axons into the distal spinal cord through a Schwann-cell-seeded mini-channel implanted into hemisected adult rat spinal cord. Eur.J Neurosci. 11:1723-1740.
Yakovleff A, Cabelguen JM, Orsal D, Gimenez, Rajaofetra N, Drian MJ, Bussel B, Privat A 1995. Fictive motor activities in adult chronic spinal rats transplanted with embryonic brainstem neurons. Exp.Brain Res. 106:69-78.
Ye JH, Houle JD 1997. Treatment of the chronically injured spinal cord with neurotrophic factors can promote axonal regeneration from supraspinal neurons. Exp.Neurol. 143:70-81.
Yezierski RP 1996. Pain following spinal cord injury: the clinical problem and experimental studies [see comments]. Pain 68:185-194.
Yezierski RP, Park SH 1993. The mechanosensitivity of spinal sensory neurons following intraspinal injections of quisqualic acid in the rat. Neurosci.Lett. 157:115-119.
Yong C, Arnold PM, Zoubine MN, Citron BA, Watanabe I , Berman NE, Festoff BW 1998. Apoptosis in cellular compartments of rat spinal cord after severe contusion injury. J Neurotrauma 15:459-472.
Young W (1995) Spinal cord injury pathophysiology and therapy. In: Neurotrauma (Narayan RJ, Wilberger JE, Povlishock JT eds), pp 1075-1093. New York: McGraw-Hill.
Zawada WM, Zastrow DJ, Clarkson ED, Adams FS, Bell KP, Freed CR 1998. Growth factors improve immediate survival of embryonic dopamine neurons after transplantation into rats. Brain Res 786:96-103.
Zompa EA, Cain LD, Everhart AW, Moyer MP, Hulsebosch CE 1997. Transplant therapy: recovery of function after spinal cord injury. J Neurotrauma 14:479-506.

24

Therapies to Promote CNS Repair

Marion Murray
MCP Hahnemann University, Philadelphia, Pennsylvania

I. INTRODUCTION

The dramatic advances in research into regeneration have encouraged us in the hope that a treatment for CNS injuries that can restore function will soon be available. Studies of the biological basis for the robust and successful regeneration that occurs naturally in the brains of lower vertebrates and in the peripheral nervous system of all vertebrates have provided directions for developing experimental strategies that will encourage similar regeneration in the adult mammalian CNS. The studies of Aguayo and his colleagues have convincingly demonstrated that adult mammalian CNS neurons can regenerate their axons. Progress in understanding the requirements for regeneration in the CNS has reinforced the idea that the failure of regeneration that normally occurs is due to a conspiracy of intraneuronal and extraneuronal elements that converge to impede outgrowth. The encouraging corollaries are that none of these impediments individually prevents regeneration and that what is necessary is to modify the intrinsic properties of neurons and to improve the environment. A combination of treatments, however, is likely to be necessary to achieve functional regeneration in the adult CNS. Specific and separate treatments may be required to deal with the vulnerability of injured neurons to apoptosis, the intrinsically poor ability of the adult central neuron to mount a successful regenerative campaign, the development of an astrocytic barrier at the site of the lesion, the cytotoxic consequences of the immune response to injury, the inhospitality of the environment in the adult CNS, and the difficulties posed to the regenerating axon of identifying an appropriate target. The solutions to some of these problems are closer than others but none seem insurmountable. We now know that axotomized neurons can be rescued (this volume, chapter by Himes and

Tessler), gene therapy can be used to modify neuronal responses to injury (this volume, chapter by Fischer and Liu), astrocytic barriers can be overcome (this volume, chapters by Hirsch and Bähr, Raisman, Plant et al.,), inhibitory factors can be neutralized (this volume, chapter by Schwab), the immune response can be modulated (this volume, chapter by Ravich and Kreutzberg) and regenerating axons can sometimes find their targets (this volume, chapter by So and Yip). Development of an effective combined treatment, given the many contributors to regenerative failure, remains daunting. This is particularly important when considering the requirements of governmental regulatory agencies for application of experimental findings to the treatment of patients. It is difficult to gain approval for combined treatments since each component must be examined individually in patient populations before multiple interventions can be considered for use therapeutically. The prospect of expensive and complex clinical trials contributes to the lack of involvement of industry and the need to rely on governmental and private agencies for support. The challenge for animal research in the next phase of the search for a treatment for CNS injury is to identify convincingly which interventions will be most useful in encouraging functional regeneration in acutely and chronically injured patients.

In this chapter I will review the requirements for repair that suggest useful components of a combinatorial treatment. We need to continue to develop strategies to provide the factors that will rescue injured neurons, stimulate neurite outgrowth, replace lost cells and neutralize intrinsic inhibitory factors. The optic nerve and the spinal cord have provided particularly favorable models to study injury, regeneration and functional recovery because their anatomical organization facilitates analysis, and most of the work reviewed here reflects that experimental bias. Nevertheless, the lessons from these systems should apply to most other parts of the CNS.

II. INTRINSIC NEURONAL INCOMPETENCY: HOW TO MAKE INJURED CNS NEURONS SURVIVE AND REGENERATE

The adult mammalian CNS neuron is intrinsically a poor regenerator, in contrast to, for example, the goldfish retinal ganglion cell. Mammalian CNS neurons may die following axotomy and even under conditions that allow survival, they may become atrophic and they do not regenerate unaided. The ability of mammalian neurons to respond to interventions that promote regeneration varies among regions, types of neurons and age of the neurons (this volume, chapter by Fernandes and Tetzlaff). A great deal of effort has been directed at developing strategies that will promote both neuronal survival and axonal regeneration in adult CNS neurons.

A. Injured neurons are vulnerable but can be rescued

Axotomized neurons may die (retrograde degeneration). Neonatal neurons are in general more vulnerable to axotomy than are mature neurons, but careful studies in adults have shown that most mammalian retinal ganglion cells (this volume, chapter by Benowitz et al.,), 50% of subcortically axotomized corticospinal neurons (this volume, chapter by Fernandes and Tetzlaff), 30 to 40% of Clarke's and Red Nucleus neurons (this volume, chapter by Himes and Tessler), and some ascending spinal neurons (Bradbury et al., 1998) will die following axotomy. Others that survive do so in an atrophic state. It is clearly important for successful repair to rescue neurons that would otherwise die in order to maximize the number of neurons available for regeneration. Indeed those that are rescued may be the neurons most likely to regenerate (Liu et al., 1999b). Since the retrograde death is apoptotic (e.g. Berkelaar et al., 1994; Rabacchi et al., 1994; Shibayama et al., 1998c, this volume, chapter by Chaudhary and Sharma), and may result from loss of target derived factors, early efforts at rescuing these neurons used direct administration of trophic factors or transplantation of tissues or cells that provide these factors. Thus, grafting fetal tissue that expressed specific trophic factors, exogenous administration of trophic factors and implanting cells genetically modified to secrete trophic factors have been reported to rescue axotomized neurons. In most of these experiments the intervention was made at the site of the lesion; in others, rescue could be demonstrated after injection of trophic factors near the soma of axotomized neurons (Giehl, Tetzlaff 1996). Some populations of neurons are rescued by supplying a single neurotrophic factor (e.g. NT3 for Clarke's Nucleus, Shibayama et al., 1998a); others are rescued by more than one trophic factor (as many as 7 different peptides can promote retinal ganglion cell survival *in vitro* (Meyer–Franke et al., 1995). It remains difficult, however, to distinguish whether the rescue of axotomized neurons by neurotrophic factors indicates that their survival normally depends on these factors or whether axotomy renders them vulnerable to withdrawal of neurotrophic support.

In most studies of neuronal rescue, the intervention was carried out at the time of the injury, a condition unlikely to be obtained in a clinical situation. Shibayama et al., (1998b), however, also transplanted fetal tissue into hemisection sites at different post-transplantation delays in rats. Their results showed that delay of the graft for as much as a week had little effect on survival but if the graft was delayed for two weeks, all of the protective effects were lost (Fig 1). This important observation suggests that there is a critical and limited period during which treatments to rescue injured neurons should be initiated. It will be important to learn the effective and safe interval for humans. Interestingly, Houle has shown that surviving neurons can regenerate even several months post-injury (Ye and Houle, 1997), further increasing the pool of neurons that survive should increase the efficiency of regeneration.

While supplying trophic factors can prevent most or all of the retrograde cell death, these treatments usually do not prevent the atrophy of the survivors. This of

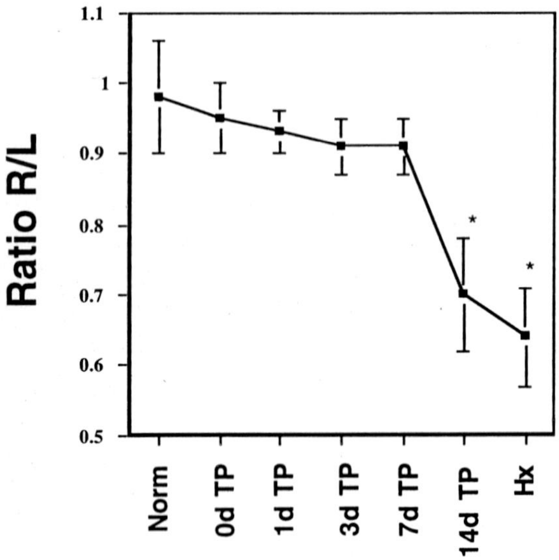

Figure 1 Survival of axotomized Clarke's neurons following hemisection and transplantation. The ratio of the number of R (axotomized) to L (uninjured) Clarke's neurons after transplantation of fetal tissue at delays of 0 days to 2 weeks post hemisection. Transplantation rescues virtually all of the axotomized neurons if performed within 1 week but fails to rescue neurons if delayed by 2 weeks. (Shibayama et al. 1998a).

course raised the question, still unanswered, as to how functional are the rescued neurons. Physiological experiments that compare function in atrophic neurons with function in neurons that have been rescued with retention of normal morphology will be needed to answer this question. Furthermore since different neuronal populations are sensitive to different trophic factors, the administration of a cocktail of trophic factors will be needed for efficient rescue of a mixed population of axotomized neurons. We still do not know how many factors need to be provided or indeed if all of the factors needed for survival of CNS neurons have been identified. We also do not know how to control the effective concentrations of the factor *in vivo*.

Other neuroprotective strategies have aimed at blocking the apoptotic pathway at the level of the signal transduction cascade. Our group has provided the antiapoptotic molecule Bcl2 by injection of a plasmid encoding this gene into the spinal cord adjacent to lesions that severed the dorsal spinocerebellar tract (Takahashi et al. 1999) or rubrospinal tract (Saavedra, preliminary data). The plasmid is taken up by axons in the vicinity of the injury and retrogradely transported to the cell body. Since Bcl2 acts downstream of trophic factors in the apoptotic cascade, providing this protein may have a broader range of efficacy in preventing apoptosis than supplying individual neurotrophins. Bcl2 administration successfully rescued most of the Clarke's neurons and the Red nucleus neurons, which are dependent on NT3 and BDNF respectively, and moreover, largely prevented their atrophy. We do not know whether the effect of the Bcl2 administration on survival of supraspinal neurons reflects a direct effect on those neurons or is secondary to neuroprotective effects at the lesion site, which diminishes the toxic environment locally. We also do not know if administration of genes by plasmid injection is the most efficient strategy or whether administration by other methods, such as recombinant adenovirus, would be preferable. Finally, a number of other antiapoptotic proteins have been discovered which may also be neuroprotective and the effects of administering these will need to be explored (this volume, chapters by Chaudhary and Sharma; Himes and Tessler). In addition, there is evidence that Bcl2 has some regeneration supporting activity (Chen et al., 1997; Holm and Isacson, 1999). There is, therefore, the possibility that the requirements for survival and for regeneration may overlap; not only is survival necessary for regeneration, but those interventions that promote survival may also promote regeneration.

There are therefore methods available for preventing retrograde cell death, at least one of which, Bcl2 injection, also preserves the morphology of the neurons (Fig. 2). The post injury period during which these neurons can be rescued appears to be limited. Transplanting cells or grafting tissue might not be feasible for treatment of patients during the acute post-injury period. The injection of a plasmid encoding Bcl2 or other antiapoptotic genes may be a more suitable acute treatment for CNS injury than the more invasive grafting procedures.

B. Adult central neurons are not good regenerators

Adult mammalian CNS neurons are intrinsically limited in their ability to regenerate compared to goldfish and tadpoles. Goldfish retinal ganglion cells robustly regenerate their severed axons and reinnervate their targets in a retinotopic fashion that enables recovery of visual function. Adult rat retinal ganglion cells die after axotomy; if they are rescued, they may regenerate, e.g. through peripheral nerve grafts (this volume, chapter by So and Yip), but even when some degree of reinnervation is achieved, it is spatially restricted. While regenerating rat optic axons may mediate some functions (Thanos 1997) the reinnervation is not sufficient for recovery of patterned vision (this volume, Part I and chapters by So and Yip; Fischer and Liu). Some of the limited capability of adult mammalian neurons is due to maturation - embryonic mammalian neurons may regenerate under circumstances in which adult neurons will not (Fawcett 1992; Chen et al. 1995; Li et al.1995; Bates et al.1999). Some of these limitations in mammalian central neuron regeneration are at the level of gene expression. Since we now have methods by which genes may be introduced into damaged neurons (this volume, chapter by Fischer and Liu), the identification of those genes whose products participate in regeneration is possible.

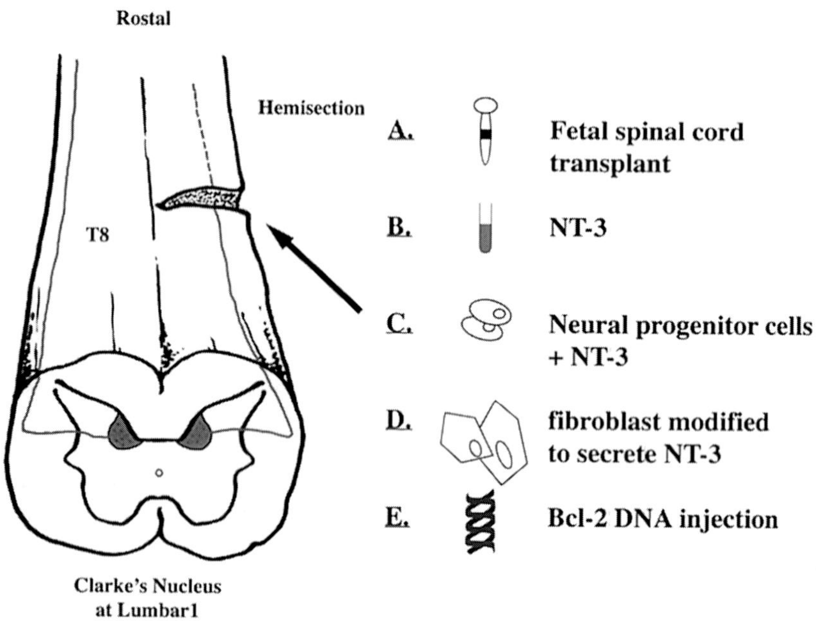

Figure 2 Clarke's nucleus is a model to study neuronal survival after axotomy. Midthoracic hemisection results in 30 to 40% neuron loss in ipsilateral Clarke's nucleus at L1. A) Fetal transplants into the lesion rescue all of the neurons, but rescued neurons are atrophic (Himes et al 1994); B) Application of NT-3 by minipump or in gelfoam implants rescues about 50% of neurons destined to die but rescued neurons are atrophic (Shibayama et al 1998a); C. Implantation of C-17 progenitor cells and gelfoam implants with NT-3 rescues all neurons but the rescued neurons are atrophic (Himes et al 1999a); D. Fibroblasts modified to secrete NT-3 rescue all neurons but the rescued neurons are atrophic (Himes); E. Injection of a plasmid encoding BCl-2 gene into the spinal cord rostral to the lesion rescues all of the neurons destined to die, and also preserves the morphology (Takahashi et al. 1999).

1. Which genes to express?

Studies of genes whose expression is modified after axotomy have produced an enormous catalogue of candidates but the genetic program that is required for regeneration is still unknown. Studies of systems in which axonal outgrowth occurs (PNS regeneration: this volume, chapters by Fernandes and Tetzlaff; Gillen; goldfish optic system regeneration, this volume, chapters by Benowitz et al., Beasley; development: this volume, Part II) suggest that expression of some genes (Regeneration Associated Genes, RAGs) is closely associated with axonal growth. The evidence is circumstantial but, as is the case of the fish found in the pail of milk, not to be ignored. At the least, these observations suggest that the expression of some genes is necessary, even if not sufficient, for regeneration.

a. Cytoskeletal proteins. The reconstitution of the axon in the PNS requires that certain cytoskeletal components, e.g. tubulins, be synthesized at a high level by the injured neuron and transported to the regenerating axon (Mikucki, Oblinger 1991), and that others, e.g. neurofilaments, be downregulated (Tetzlaff et al., 1996). Injured CNS neurons show only modest or transient changes in expression of these genes. When provided with a regeneration permissive environment (a peripheral nerve graft) the expression of some of these genes increases (Fournier and McKerracher 1997) indicating a relationship between expression of these genes, induced by factors extrinsic to the neuron, and axonal growth.

b. GAP-43. GAP-43 expression is high in all instances where regeneration occurs (this volume, chapter by Benowitz et al.,) as befits a constituent of the regenerating growth cone (Skene, 1989). Thus GAP-43 is thought to be an intrinsic determinant of neurite outgrowth (Aigner et al., 1995). Cells that are the poorest regenerators, e.g. Purkinje cells, do not express GAP-43 after injury or when presented with an environment favorable to regeneration (Zagrebelsky et al., 1998). GAP-43 expression by itself is not sufficient for regeneration since Purkinje cells modified to overexpress GAP43 still do not regenerate (Buffo et al., 1997). Expression of GAP-43 may be accompanied by high levels of other molecules [(GAP-43 and CNTF (Jo et al., 1999); GAP-43 and L1 (Becker et al., 1998, Meiri et al., 1998; GAP-43 and NCAM (Meiri et al., 1998); GAP43 and CAP-23 (Caroni et al., 1997)]. Combined expression of several genes is therefore likely to be required for successful regeneration.

c. Cell adhesion molecules. The families of cell adhesion molecules (CAMs) are also important in axonal growth through their interactions with other proteins, including GAP-43 (Meiri et al., 1998). They regulate fasciculation of growing axons by creating a balance of permissive and non-permissive conditions that modulate the environment through which axons grow. L1 is one CAM that has been shown to be expressed at high levels by neurons that regenerate. This transmembrane protein is a constituent of the growth cone in addition to mediating cell adhesion. The importance of molecules that modify cell-cell interactions is supported by the observation that cultured rodent retinal ganglion cells lose the ability to regenerate in fascicles at the same time that they lose the ability to express the adhesion molecules L1 and n-cadherin (Bates et al., 1999). L1 (and GAP-43) expression is induced in rat neurons that regenerate into a peripheral nerve graft but not if the same neurons are axotomized without being offered a graft (Zhang et al., 1995; Jung et al., 1997). Thus environments that induce regeneration also induce expression of regeneration associated genes.

d. Transcription factors. Studies of expression of individual genes are of utmost importance since they identify candidates for gene transfer. If regeneration of axons, like development of axons, requires an orchestrated pattern of expression of different genes, supplying individual genes or gene products may not be adequate for efficient regeneration. Stimulating expression of specific transcription factors that can regulate coordinated expression of regeneration associated genes may be a more efficient strategy. Certain transcription factors, notably the proto-oncogene c-jun, are upregulated after axotomy in regenerating systems but not in those that do not regenerate, e.g. Purkinje cells (Herdegen, Leah 1998; Vaudano et al., 1998; Zagrebelsky et al., 1998). c-jun appears to be particularly important in regulating transcription of mRNAs for regeneration associated genes (Herdegen, Leah 1998). Its expression is greater in rat retinal ganglion cells that are induced to regenerate into peripheral nerve grafts than in those that are only axotomized (Robinson, 1995) and it is upregulated in axotomized brainstem-spinal neurons but only in the presence of fetal tissue grafts or trophic factor administration (Broude et al., 1999). These results may reflect the fact that expression of transcription genes is enhanced by supplying trophic factors via the grafts that promote regeneration (Haas et al., 1998; Houle et al., 1998). There is also evidence that expression of c-jun is associated with degeneration and cell death (Estus et al., 1994; Herdegen et al., 1997), a reminder that many of the interventions that we consider to be beneficial to regeneration may also have detrimental effects.

We are beginning to understand the pattern of gene expression by which regeneration is stimulated. The genes implicated in goldfish retinal ganglion cell and peripheral nerve regeneration appear to be similar to those required for rat retinal ganglion cell regeneration (this volume, Chapters by Benowitz et al.; Fernandes and Tetzlaff; Gillen). However complicated regeneration of CNS axons may be, the process is surely less complex than brain development. There is likely to be some redundancy in the mechanisms that contribute to regeneration and therefore the possibility that adequate regeneration may be achieved with enhanced expression of a limited number of genes for a limited time.

III. EXTRINSIC FACTORS CONTRIBUTE TO FAILURE: CNS AXONS WILL ELONGATE IN AN APPROPRIATE ENVIRONMENT

During development, CNS neurons grow axons that reach their proper targets. This ability is lost during postnatal development in mammals, in part because of the appearance of growth inhibitors and loss of growth promotors in the environment. Aguayo and his colleagues have shown that most adult mammalian CNS axons will regenerate readily if the environment is modified (this volume, Chapter by So and Yip). The modifications include those that stimulate expression of the genes necessary to support axon outgrowth, neutralize inhibitory signals and provide growth promoting molecules. This growth may be impressive, for example in the distance through which CNS axons may extend in a peripheral nerve graft, but limited, for example, in the extent of growth into the denervated neuropil and, therefore, the extent of reinnervation that is possible. Identifying the components of an appropriate environment is essential to developing methods for promoting regeneration. Molecular dissection of the regeneration promoting properties of Schwann cells that largely provide the permissive environment of peripheral nerve grafts has identified a mix of trophic factors, adhesion molecules and extracellular matrix molecules that contribute to a favorable environment. Similarly, identifying the inhibitory components has allowed development of strategies to neutralize their effects (this volume, Chapters by Schwab; David and McKerracher).

A. Trophic factors need to be supplied

Endogenous levels of trophic factors in the adult CNS are inadequate to rescue vulnerable axotomized neurons; they are also inadequate to support regeneration. Fetal grafts (Jakeman, Reier 1991) or unmodified fibroblasts (Liu et al., 1999, Grill et al., 1997) placed into the adult CNS also do not elicit regeneration beyond the graft-host interface. Trophic factors stimulate CNS axonal regeneration *in vivo* when combined with other interventions, e.g. providing a permissive terrain through grafts of peripheral nerves (Xu et al., 1995), fetal tissue (Bregman et al., 1997), or fibroblasts (Grill et al., 1997; Liu et al., 1999) or in conjunction with blockade of inhibitors (Von Meyerberg et al., 1998). Virtually all classes of brain-stem-spinal axons have been stimulated to regenerate when provided with grafts supplemented by trophic or other factors (Table 1). Different populations of CNS neurons have different requirements for some of these factors. Purkinje neurons, for example, will not regenerate into peripheral nerve grafts even after supplementation with additional growth factors. In contrast bulbospinal neurons will regenerate their axons robustly into peripheral nerve grafts if specific growth factors are added (Ye, Houle, 1997; Xu et al., 1995) and the administration of two (or more) trophic factors increases the number of axons that regenerate into the graft. Retinal ganglion cells respond to the neurotrophin BDNF and to the cytokine CNTF, and the response is greater when both are provided (Jo et al., 1999). Identifying the trophic factor requirements of specific neuronal populations may soon enable us to customize cocktails of trophic factors. There is further encouraging information suggesting that trophic factor administration in combination with peripheral grafts can induce even chronically injured axons to regenerate (Ye, Houle 1997).

Trophic factors can be supplied by exogenous sources, e.g. minipumps, or by grafting genetically engineered cells. Exogenous administration may be more difficult to control but engineered cells may downregulate their production with time. Prolonged release of trophic factors may also lead to downregulation of their receptors and decreased efficacy. We do not yet know the time during which the trophic factors need to be supplied, although it is reasonable to suppose that trophic factors need be available for only the length of time necessary to activate a regenerative program. Prolonged supply may be unnecessary and perhaps undesirable. We also need to know whether introduction of trophic factors into an injury site will have untoward effects. Some growth factors (IGF-1 and PDGF) decrease the number of axons regenerating into a Schwann cell channel (Oudega et al., 1997). It is also possible that high levels of trophic factor introduced into the spinal cord could increase sprouting by dorsal root axons and therefore contribute to the development of central pain syndromes.

Table 1 Trophic Factors Stimulate Regeneration of Spinal Pathways in the Adult Rat in Permissive Environments

Pathway	Trophic Factor	Additional Intervention	Lesion	Regeneration	Ref
Cortico-spinal	BDNF	fetal graft	cervical over-Hx	into graft	1
	NT3	fetal graft	cervical over-HX	into graft	1
	NT3	modified fibroblast graft	dorsal HX	adjacent to graft	4
	NT3	IN-1	dorsal HX	around lesion	8
	aFGF	PNG	transection	into graft and caudal to lesion	2
Rubro-Spinal	BDNF	fetal graft	cervical over-HX	into graft	1
	BDNF	modified fibroblast graft	cervical HX	into, through around, 10 segments caudal	6
	BDNF	PNG	cervical HX	into graft	5
	BDNF	PNG	cervical HX	into graft	10
	NT3	PNG	cervical HX	into graft	9
Coerulo-spinal	BDNF	fetal TP	cervical over-HX	into graft	1
	NT3	fetal TP	cervical over-HX	into graft	1
	NGF	modified fibroblast graft	dorsal HX	near graft	4
Raphé spinal	BDNF	fetal TP	cervical over-HX	into graft	1
	BDNF	PNG	cervical HX	into graft	10
	NT3	fetal TP	cervical over-HX	into graft	2
Vestibulo-spinal	BDNF	Schwann cell bridge + NT3	transection	into graft	9
	BDNF	PNG	cervical HX	into graft	10

Table 1 (cont'd) Trophic Factors Stimulate Regeneration of Spinal Pathways in the Adult Rat in Permissive Environments

Pathway	Trophic Factor	Additional Intervention	Lesion	Regeneration	Ref
	NT3	Schwann cell bridge + BDNF	transection	into graft	9
Retriculo-Spinal	NT3	PNG	cervical HX	into graft	10
Proprio-spinal	NT3	Schwann cell graft +BDNF	transection	into graft	9
	BDNF +NT-3	Schwann cell graft	transection	into graft	9
Dorsal root	NGF	modified fibroblast	dorsal HX	near graft	3
	NGF	PNG	dorsal column	into graft, dorsal column	7
	NT-3	Schwann cell bridge + BDNF	transection	into graft	10
	NT-3	PNG	dorsal column	into graft, dorsal column	7
	BDNF	PNG	dorsal column	into graft dorsal column	7

Abbreviations: HX- hemisection; PNG –peripheral nerve graft; TP - transplant
Refs: 1 Bregman et al. 1997; 2 Cheng et al 1995.; 3. Grill et al., 1997a.; 4. Grill et al.1997b.; 5. Kobayashi et al. 1997' 6..Liu et al.1999; 7. Oudega,,Hagg 1999. 8. von Meyenberg et al.1998; 9. Xu et al. 1995; 10. Ye, Houle 1997

B. Bridges are important

Transplanted dorsal root ganglion neurons will regenerate axons unaided through a microlesion site in which a scar does not form (Davies et al., 1997). In most cases, however, injury to spinal cord or brain results in formation of a cyst or a scar that blocks outgrowth of axons. A large lesion will therefore need to be repaired by providing a bridge that is permissive to regenerating axons.

Fetal tissue readily survives and integrates with adult host tissue, often with minimal cyst formation. Unless supplemented by additional treatments, e.g. growth factors or antibodies that block inhibitors, grafts of fetal tissue do not encourage extensive regeneration by host axons. Grafting of genetically modified cell lines can provide a permissive bridge that encourages regeneration; this strategy also obviates the political, logistical and ethical problems associated with the use of fetal tissue. Neural stem cell grafts are attractive candidates for bridges because they can differentiate into neurons and glial cells and thus have the potential to replace lost neurons and glial cells (Weiss et al. 1996; Whittemore, Snyder 1996; McKay 1997). Their utility in CNS repair is only just beginning to be appreciated (Fisher et al., 1997). Grafts of fibroblasts can also provide a suitable substrate in immunosuppressed rats, and, if the fibroblasts are modified to secrete BDNF, the grafts will stimulate regeneration of rubrospinal axons into, through, and around the graft (Liu et al., 1999). Fibroblasts modified to produce NT3 have also served as grafts that induce regeneration of corticospinal and other axons in adult rats (Grill et al., 1997). Marrow stromal cells, used clinically for gene therapy, also survive, integrate and provide a permissive environment for axonal regeneration (Azizi et al., 1998; Himes et al., 1999b). The advantage of stromal cells or fibroblasts is that they can be harvested from the patient, modified as necessary, and implanted in injured CNS without eliciting an immune response. These cells, however, will not replace neural cells and will not provide a target for synaptogenesis by regenerating axons. Finally, development of artificial substrates that will provide a bridge or matrix that is both permissive and directive is another attractive strategy for promoting regeneration (this volume, Chapter by Plant et al.,).

C. Barriers exist

Once the regenerative program is launched, the neurites are faced with the unwelcoming environment of the adult CNS neuropil. This has proved to be a formidable problem. In most cases, regeneration stimulated by trophic factors has resulted in only very minimal invasion of the denervated territory. The inhospitality of the adult CNS is largely a result of the failure of the glial cells to support regeneration. The favorable molecular environment that is present during development and which can be provided by Schwann cells and olfactory ensheathing cells includes extracellular matrix and adhesion molecules such as laminin, L1, and NCAM but these molecules are absent or present at low levels in the adult mammalian CNS. Proteins associated with oligodendrocytes and myelin inhibit outgrowth (this volume, Chapters by Steeves, Schwab, David and McKerracher). In addition, high levels of other putative inhibitory molecules, e.g. proteoglycans, are present particularly near the lesion site. There are, therefore, molecular obstacles to axonal growth (Fitch, Silver 1999; this volume, Chapter by Grumet).

The astrocytes form another barrier, the glial scar that acts to seal the injury site, but also poses a mechanical obstacle to regenerating axons. The scar contains components inhibitory to growth which thus contribute to the molecular barrier (Fitch, Silver 1999). Astrocytes activated in response to injury also secrete substances that support growth, e.g. NCAM, trophic factors, etc. (Eddelston , Mucke 1993; Fitch, Silver 1999, this volume, Chapter by Hirsch and Bähr). Indeed, axons stimulated to regenerate in the CNS elongate *in vivo* on astrocytes (Lavie et al. 1990; Kawaja and Gage 1991; Dezawa et al. 1999).

D. Barriers can be overcome

Progress is being made in countering the hostile environment of the CNS. When the inhibitory proteins associated with the myelin sheath are neutralized by an antibody, transected corticospinal axons can grow around the site of injury and extend some distance caudal to the injury (Bregman et al. 1995; Raineteau et al. 1999). Dyer et al., (1998) using a different protocol, imunnological disruption, to eliminate myelin inhibitors showed regeneration of axotomized rubrospinal axons in adult rats. Even in the absence of inhibitors of the myelin proteins, regeneration can occur if the lesion itself is small and scarring does not develop (Davies et al., 1997; Davies et al., 1999). Growth cones from DRG cells that overexpress GAP43 are also more resistant to myelin inhibitors (Aigner and Caroni 1995) and trophic factor administration may also override the inhibitors (Cai et al., 1999). Finally, regenerating axons may in some cases progress through degenerating myelin suggesting that disrupted myelin may be permissive or at least no longer inhibitory (Stichel et al. 1995; Davies et al., 1997; Davies et al., 1999; Liu et al., 1999; Raineteau et al., 1999).

Countering other inhibitory molecules, e.g. proteoglycans, has proven to be more difficult although *in vitro* methods using proteases, e.g. urokinases or metalloproteases, diminished their inhibitory effects (La Fleur et al., 1996, Zuo et al., 1998, Muir et al., 1998). Even without these interventions, the presence of these inhibitory molecules does not prevent dorsal root axons from regenerating into a permissive environment (Sugawara et al., 1999) perhaps because of their content of metalloproteinases (Zuo et al., 1998). Preventing the development of the glial scar by inhibiting collagen synthesis *in vivo* has led to successful regeneration by fimbria-fornix axons through the injury site and along their normal pathway to their target (Stichel et al., 1999). X-irradiation has also been reported to disrupt the formation of a glial scar and to allow regeneration of corticospinal axons (Kalderon, Fuks 1996). The rapid development of gene therapy techniques may make it easier to provide some of the molecules that facilitate outgrowth, e.g. L1,

NCAM and laminin, and thus to provide another strategy to counterbalance the inhibitory effects of myelin and other proteins (David et al., 1995).

Finally, the extraordinary properties of olfactory ensheathing cells (this volume, Chapter by Plant et al.,) in promoting regeneration of axons are just beginning to be appreciated. Long distance regeneration of brainstem-spinal axons into and through a Schwann cell channel has been shown following injection of olfactory ensheathing cells into transected spinal cord (Ramon-Cueto et al., 1998). Transplants of olfactory ensheathing cells at the lesion site have also promoted regeneration of corticospinal axons (Li et al., 1997). In addition to providing trophic factors and permissive adhesion and matrix molecules, these cells when implanted in a lesion site will accompany the growing neurites, providing them with a permissive environment as the neurites enter the neuropil.

Thus, blocking the inhibitory influence of myelin and providing stimulatory molecules and a permissive substrate are interventions that can enhance the regenerative response. There are therefore several strategies available to override one or more of the barriers that are present in the normal adult CNS neuropil or that develop after injury.

E. Where is the target?

Another barrier to successful functional regeneration may be the absence of adequate guidance cues. Developmental neurobiology is rapidly expanding our understanding of guidance molecules, e.g. ephrins, semaphorins, netrins, etc. Developing axons elongate toward or are repulsed by concentrations of specific guidance molecules along their pathway, best described for the Zebrafish embryo (this volume, Chapter by Stuermer and Leppert). While there is some evidence from *in vitro* studies that guidance cues are reexpressed in the injured retinotectal pathway in adults (Weitzenmann et al., 1997), we do not yet know whether guidance molecules are expressed at all in the adult mammalian CNS or whether they are upregulated after injury. The fear has been that, in the absence of specific guidance cues, regenerating CNS axons would be undirected and fail to find targets that could contribute to functional repair. There is evidence to support this fear; axons that have been induced to regenerate often grow only in gray matter (e.g. Cheng et al., 1997; Raineteau et al., 1999) and in regions which do not appear to be their normal pathway. Under other circumstances, however, axons have been shown to grow substantial distances in the white matter and to enter the gray matter, apparently terminating in appropriate targets (Li et al., 1997; Liu et al., 1999; Stichel et al., 1999) (Fig 3). It is possible that these regenerating CNS axons are tracking along degenerating pathways and thus, as is the case with regenerating PNS axons, are led to the region of their appropriate target. Another strategy is to provide the pathway. Menei et al., created a trail of Schwann cells genetically modified to secrete BDNF that led regenerating axons into the spinal cord distal to the lesion site (Menei et al., 1998), opening the possibility of selectively guiding specific axonal populations to appropriate targets.

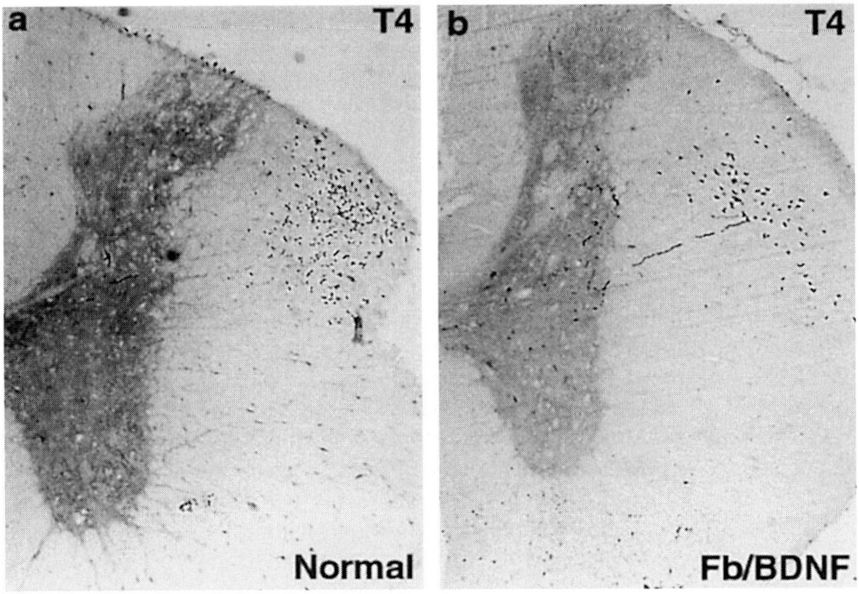

Figure 3 Long distance regeneration into white matter. A. Normal rubrospinal axons labeled by BDA injection in the contralateral Red nucleus are localized in the dorsolateral quadrant of the lateral funiculus at the T4 segment. B. Rubrospinal axons, labeled by BDA, that have regenerated from a lesion site at C3-4 to T4 occupy a position similar to that of control rubrospinal axons. (Liu et al., 1999a).

IV. THE IMMUNE RESPONSE- WHEN IS IT HELPFUL, WHEN IS IT HARMFUL AND CAN IT BE MODIFIED?

A CNS lesion breaches the blood brain barrier, engages the immune system and thus adds another dimension to the complexity of the response to injury. The function of the immune response is to protect the organism by contributing to the formation of a scar that isolates the lesion site and to remove debris or foreign matter. As a side effect of this protective response, a toxic environment is created at the site of injury. In the brain and spinal cord, the initial injury is often followed by an expansion of the lesion site resulting from the toxic environment created by resident and invading macrophages and by injured and dying cells. This expansion produces cysts and eliminates cellular pathways permissive to regeneration.

In the peripheral nervous system (this volume, Chapter by Ravich and Kreutzberg) and in lower vertebrates that successfully regenerate their CNS axons (Murray 1982, Battisti et al., 1995), the immune cells, including microglia, together with astrocytes, contribute to repair by supplying factors that support regeneration, by removing sources of inhibition, and by efficient removal of degenerative debris. After CNS injury in mammals, the response includes rapid activation of the resident immune cells, the microglia, and recruitment of peripheral macrophages which act with activated astrocytes to establish a post-injury environment that inhibits regeneration, and a very slow removal of degenerated axons. The activated microglia release both pro- and anti-inflammatory cytokines with a complex and poorly understood temporal pattern. Both activated microglia (Banati et al., 1993; Kreutzberg, 1996) and activated astrocytes (Fitch, Silver 1997) secrete molecules that are neurotoxic or block regeneration but they also secrete trophic factors and other molecules (microglia: Elkabes et al., 1996, Mallat et al., 1989; Kreutzberg 1996; Rabshevsky and Streit 1997; astrocytes: Eddelston, Mucke 1993) that may be permissive to regeneration. In order to develop effective targeted therapies against the immune response we will have to distinguish those responses that are deleterious and those that are helpful to regeneration.

Two kinds of interventions have been used to counter the immune response: immune suppression and transplantation of activated macrophages. Immune suppression is in fact the only therapy approved in the U.S. for treatment of spinal cord injury. Administration of methylprednisolone within 8 hours of injury has been shown to improve modestly the functional outcome (Bracken et al., 1992). It is thought that the efficacy is largely a consequence of its anti-inflammatory properties that reduce secondary injury. However, it is also possible that this rather broadly acting agent may have additional features that contribute to its effectiveness. Methylprednisolone administration improves axonal regeneration into peripheral nerve grafts in rats (Chen et al., 1996) which may be due to decreased secondary or bystander injury (Bartoldi, Schwab 1995) or direct enhancement of axonal outgrowth. Administration of another immunosuppressant drug, Tacrolimus, increased GAP43 expression and improved functional outcome following spinal injury in rats (Madsen et al., 1998) and administration of Cyclosporin A has been shown to decrease axonal injury following traumatic brain injury (Okonkwo et al., 1999). Continued investigation of other steroids and reagents that neutralize free radicals is likely to identify more targeted drugs that when administered soon after the injury can reduce the secondary damage.

A second approach has been to implant cultured microglia (Rabchevsky, Streit 1997) or peripheral macrophages activated by exposure to damaged peripheral nerves (Rapalino et al., 1998; Schwartz et al., 1999) into injured spinal cord. Both strategies take advantage of the growth promoting effects of brain or peripheral macrophages. Implantation of cultured microglia elicited ingrowth of neurites into the grafted cells (Rabchevsky, Steit 1997). Since activated peripheral macrophages which contribute to peripheral regeneration may be better able to promote central regeneration than microglia, Rapalino et al., (1998) incubated peripheral macrophages with sciatic nerve segments for 24 hours and then implanted the macrophages into a midthoracic transection site in adult rats. The rats showed behavioral, physiological and anatomical signs of improvement compared to rats with spinal transections but no transplants, suggesting that these stimulated peripheral macrophages created a growth-permissive environment. As we learn more about the permissive elements provided by these macrophages, more targeted strategies can be developed.

V. INTERACTIVE TRAINING - CAN ACTIVITY DEPENDENT MECHANISMS ENHANCE TARGETING OR CENTRAL LEARNING?

We know that axons induced to regenerate by peripheral nerve (Vidal-Sanz et al., 1989; Keirstead et al., 1989) or fetal (e.g. Itoh et al., 1993; Itoh et al., 1996) grafts can make functional synaptic contact with neurons in host or graft tissue. The density of innervation that has been achieved is limited and novel connections may sometimes be formed, but functional recovery may be achieved by these novel connections. Hindlimb motor function is largely organized by the central pattern generators for locomotion (CPG), a system of interneuronal networks that extends through the lumbar spinal cord (Kjaerulff, Kiehn 1996). The CPG remains functional after complete transection and even limited regeneration and formation of synaptic contacts with neurons within the CPG may be sufficient to gain supraspinal access to the networks that produce patterned locomotor activity.

In recent years considerable interest has been directed to interactive training methods to improve function. The hypothesis is that activity dependent plasticity can be used to strengthen pathways required for specific activities (de Leon et al., 1998), to shape reorganization following injury (Nudo et al., 1996), to increase the likelihood of survival (Meyer-Franke et al., 1995) or perhaps, in the case of transplants, to stabilize novel connections. The mechanisms responsible may include LTP (Dobkin et al., 1998; Walpow, Carp 1990), exercise stimulated production of trophic factors (Neeper et al., 1995; Oliff et al., 1998) and the morphologically demonstrated changes in synapses (Feng-Chen and Walpow, 1996) or dendrites (Jones and Schallert 1994). One example of this approach, providing partial weight support during treadmill locomotion training, has been shown to be remarkably effective in improving performance in humans with incomplete spinal injury (Barbeau et al., 1993; Wernig et al., 1995). Excessive activity may, however, be deleterious since intensive training during the first postoperative week was shown to enlarge the lesion, presumably through excitotoxic mechanisms (Humm, Schallert 1998). In any combination therapy to be developed, appropriate types and levels of activity should play an important part in achieving the most successful functional outcome.

VI. FUTURE DIRECTIONS

Our hope is that the combination of factors that prevent regeneration can be overcome by targeted treatments (Fig. 4). These therapies will need to be administered in stages. Immediately after the injury inflammatory and toxic effects need to be modified using relatively non-invasive approaches. A second stage should include

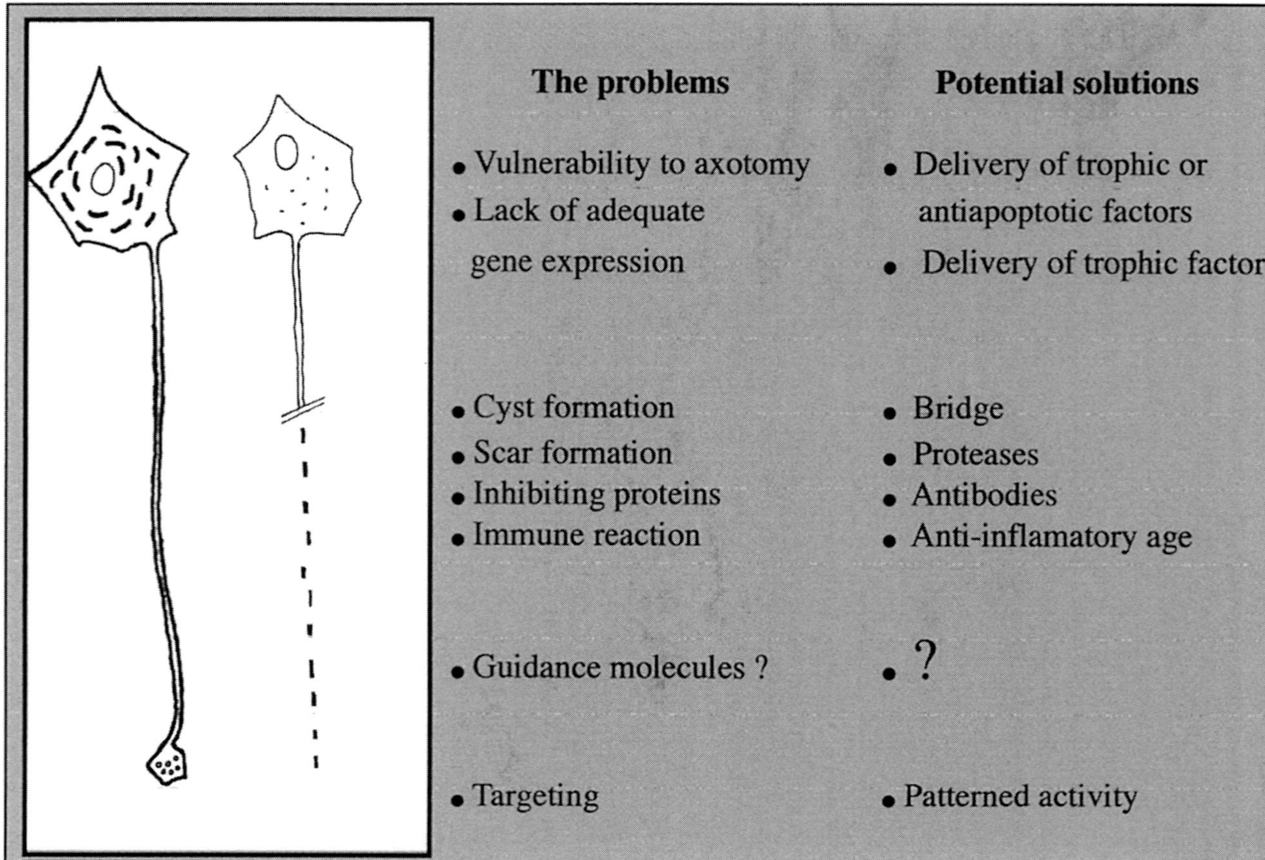

Figure 4 Summary of some of the impediments to regenation of adult CNS neurons and how these impediments might be overcome.

treatments designed to promote regeneration, e.g. transplants, administration of trophic factors and blocking inhibitors. The final stage may include targeting with guidance molecules and an appropriate program of patterned training. The redundancy of neural systems may work in favor of some degree of recovery of function even if complete repair is not achieved. Recovery of useful motor function after injury is frequently considered to require only a fraction of the normal pathways (Mitz, Humphrey 1986; Blight, de Cresito 1997; Bregman et al., 1997; Liu et al., 1999). As we enter the next stage of investigations into CNS injury we can expect that the extraordinary achievements of basic science in developing an understanding of the problems in and potential treatments for CNS repair will be translated into clinical practice and that the outcome for persons with CNS injury will be much brighter.

ACKNOWLEDGMENTS

The continued support by NS 24707, the Eastern Paralyzed Veterans Association, the Spinal Cord Research Foundation, the International Spinal cord Research Trust, the American Paralysis Association, the International foundation for Research into Paraplegia and grants from the Medical College of Pennsylvania to the Center of Excellence for Spinal Cord Research is gratefully acknowledged. I would also like to thank my colleagues at MCP for their helpful comments in the preparation of this chapter.

REFERENCES

Aigner L, Caroni P 1995. Absence of persistent spreading, branching and adhesion in GAP-43 depleted growth cones. J. Cell Biol.128:647-660.

Aigner L, Arber S, Kapfhammer JP, Laux T, Schneider C, Botteri F, Brenner H-R, Caroni P. 1995. Overexpression of the neural growth-associated protein GAP43 induces nerve sprouting in the adult nervous system of transgenic mice. Cell 83:269-278.

Azizi SA, Stokes D, Augelli BJ, DiGarolamo C, Prockop DJ. 1998. Engraftment and migration of human bone marrow stromal cells implanted in brains of albino rats. Proc. Natl. Acad.Sci. 95:3508-3513

Banati RB, Gehrmann J, Schubert P, Kreutzberg GW. 1993. Cytotoxicity of microglia Glia 7:111-118

Barbeau H, Danakas M, Arsenault B 1993. The effects of locomotor training in spinal cord injured subjects. Restor. Neurol Neurosc. 5:81-84.

Bartholdi D, Schwab ME 1995. Methylprednisolone inhibits early inflammatory processes but not ischemic cell death after experimental spinal cord lesion in the rat. Brain Res. 672:177-186.

Bates CA, Becker CG, Miotke JA, Meyer RL 1999 Expression of polysialylated NCAM but not L1 or N-Cadherin by regenerating adult mouse optic fibers in vitro. Exp. Neurol.155:128-139.

Battisti,WP, Wang J, Bozek K, Murray, M. 1995. Macrophages, microglia and astrocytes are rapidly activated after crush injury of the goldfish optic nerve. J. Comp. Neurol. 354:306-320.

Becker T, Bernhardt RR, Reinhard E, Wullimann MF, Tongiorgi E, Schachner M 1998. Readiness of zebrafish brain neurons to regenerate a spinal axon correlates with differential expression of specific cell recognition molecules. J. Neurosc. 18:5789-803.

Berkelaar M, Clarke DB, Wang YC, Bray GM, Aguayo AJ 1994. Axotomy results in delayed death and apoptosis of retinal ganglion cells in adult rats. J. Neurosc. 14:4368-4374.

Blight A, De Cresito V. 1987. Morphometric analysis of experimental spinal cord injury in the cat. Neurosc. 19:321-341.

Bracken MB, Shepard MJ, Collins WF, Jr., Holford TR, Baskin DS, Eisenberg HM, Flamm E, Leo-Summers L, Maroon JC, Marshall LF, Perot PL, Piepmeier J, Sonntag VKH, Wagner FC, Wilberger JL, Winn HR, Young W. 1992. Methylprednisolone or naloxone treatment after acute spinal cord injury: 1-year follow-up data: Results of the second National Acute Spinal Cord Injury Study. J. Neurosurg. 76:23-31.

Bradbury EJ, King, VR, Simmons, LJ, Priestley JV, McMahon SB 1998. NT-3, but not BDNF, prevents atrophy and death of axotomized spinal cord projection neurons. Eur. J. Neurosc. 10:3058-3068.

Bregman BS, Kunkel-Bagden E, Schnell L, Dai HN, Gao D and Schwab ME 1995. Recovery from spinal cord injury mediated by antibodies to neurite growth inhibitors. Nature 378:498-501.

Bregman BS, McAtee M, Dai HN, Kuhn PI. 1997. Neurotrophic factors increase axonal growth after spinal cord injury and transplantation in the adult rat. Exper. Neurol. 148:475-94.

Broude E, McAtee M, Kellely MS, Bregman BS 1999. Fetal spinal cord transplants and exogenous neurotrophic support enhance c-jun expression in mature axotomized neurons after spinal cord injury. Exper. Neurol. 155:65-78.

Buffo A, Holtmaat AJ, Savio T, Verbeek JS, Oberdick J, Oestreicher AB, Gispen WH, Verhaagen J, Rossi F, Strata P 1997. Targeted overexpression of the neurite growth associated protein B-50/GAP-43 in cerebellar Purkinje cells induces sprouting after axotomy but not axon regeneration into growth permissive transplants. J. Neurosc.17:8778-8791.

Cai DM, Shen YJ, De Bellard M, Tang S, Filbin MT 1999. Prior exposure to neurotrophins blocks inhibition of axonal regeneration by MAG and myelin via a cAMP-dependent mechanism. Neuron 22:89-101.

Caroni P 1997. Intrinsic neuronal determinants that promote axonal sprouting and elongation. Bioessays 19:767-75.

Chen A, Xu SM, Kleitman N, Bunge MB. 1996. Methylprednisolone administration improves axonal regeneration into Schwann cell grafts in transected adult rat thoracic spinal cord. Exp. Neurol. 138:261-276.

Chen DF, Jhaveri S, Schneider GE 1995. Intrinsic changes in developing retinal neurons results in regenerative failure of their axons. Proc.Natl. Acad. Sci.92:7287-7291.

Chen DF, Schneider GE, Martinou JC, Tonegawa S 1997. Bcl2 promotes regeneration of seevered axons in mammalian CNS. nature 385:434-439.

Cheng H, Cao Y, Olson L. 1996. Spinal cord repair in adult paraplegic rats. Science 273:510-513.

David S, Braun PE, Jackson DL, Kottis V, McKerracher L 1995. Laminin overrides the inhibitory effects of peripheral nervous system and central nervous system inhibitors of neurite growth. J. neurosc. Res. 42:594-602.

Davies SJA, Fitch MT, Memberg SP, Hall AK, Raisman G, Silver J. 1997. Regeneration of adult axons in white matter tracts of the central nervous system. Nature 390:680-683.

Davies SJA, Goucher DR, Doller C, Silver J 1999.Robust regeneration of adult sensory axons in degenerating white matter of the adult rat spinal cord. J. Neurosc. 19:5810-5822.

De Leon, RD, Hodgson JA, Roy RR, Edgerton VR 1998. Locomotor capacity attributable to step training versus spontaneous recovery after spinalization in adult cats. J. Neurophysiol 79:1329-1340.

Dezawa M, Kawana K, Negishi H, Adachi-Usami E. 1999. Glial cells in degenerating and regenerating optic nerve of the adult rat. Brain Res.Bull. 48:573-9

Dobkin BH 1998 Activity dependent learning contributes to motor recovery. Ann. Neurol. 44:158-160,

Dyer J, Bourque JA, Steeves JD. 1998. Regeneration of brainstem-spinal axons after lesion and immunological disruption of myelin in adult rat. Exp.Neurol. 154:12-22.

Eddelston M , Mucke L 1993 Molecular profile of reactive astrocytes - implications for their role in neurologic disease. Neurosc. 54:15 -36.

Elkabes S, DiCicco Bloom EM, Black IB 1996. Brain microglia/macrophages express neurotrophins that selectively regulate microglial proliferation and function. J. Neurosc. 16:2508-2521.

Estus S, Zaks WJ, Freeman RS, Gruda M, Bravo R, Johnson EM, Jr. 1994. Altered gene expression in neurons during programmed cell death: identification of c-jun as necessary for neuronal apoptosis. J. Cell Biol. 127:1717-27.

Fawcett J 1992. Intrinsic neuronal determinants of regeneration. Trends in Neurosci.15:5-8.

Feng-Chen KC, Wolpaw JR 1996. Operant conditioning of H-reflex changes synaptic terminals on primate motorneurons. Proc. Nat. Acad. Sci. 93:9206-9211.

Fisher LJ 1997 Neural precursor cells: Applications for the study and repair of the central nervous system. Neurobiology of Disease 4:1-22

Fitch MT, Silver J 1997. Activated macrophages and the blood brain barrier: inflammation after CNS injury leads to increases in putative inhibitory molecules. Exp. Neurol 148:587-603.

Fitch MT, Silver J 1999. Beyond the glial scar. In CNS Regeneration. MJH Tuszinski, JH Kordower (eds). Academic Press.

Fournier AE, McKerracher L. 1997. Expression of specific tubulin isotypes increases during regeneration of injured CNS neurons, but not after application of brain-derived neurotrophic factor (BDNF). J.Neurosc.17:4623-4632.

Giehl KM, Tetzlaff W 1996 BDNF and NT-3, but not NGF, prevent axotomy-induced death of rat corticospinal neurons in vivo. Eur. J. Neurosc.8:1167-1175.

Grill R, Blesch A, Tuszinski MH 1997a. Robust growth of chronically injured spinal cord axons induced by grafts of genetically modified NGF secreting cells. Exp. Neurol. 148:444-452.

Grill R, Murai K, Blesch A, Gage FH, Tuszinski M. 1997b. Cellular delivery of NT-3 promotes corticospinal axonal growth and partial functional recovery after spinal cord injury. J.Neurosc.17:5560-5572.

Haas, CA, Bach A, Heimrich B, Linke R, Otten U, Frotscher M. 1998. Axotomy induced c-jun expression in young medial septal neurons is regulated by nerve growth factor. Neurosc.87:831-844.

Herdegen T, Skene P, Bahr M 1997 The c-Jun transcription factor- bipotential mediator of neuronal death, survival and regeneration. Trends in Neurosc. 20:227-31.

Herdegen T, Leah JD 1998. Inducible and constitutive transcription factors in the mammalian nervous system: control of gene expression by Jun, Fos and Krox, and CREB/ATF proteins. Brain Res. Reviews 28:370-490.

Himes BT, Goldberger ME, Tessler A 1994. Grafts of fetal CNS tissue rescue axotomized Clarke's nucleus neurons in adult and neonatal operates. J. Comp. Neurol. 239:117-31.

Himes BT, Liu Y, Solowska JM, Snyder EY, Fischer I, Tessler A. 1999. Transplants of cells genetically modified to express NT-3 rescue axotomized Clarke's nucleus neurons after spinal cord hemisection in adult rats. Submitted.

Holm K, Isacson O. 1999. Factors intrinsic to the neuron can induce and maintain its ability to promote axonal outgrowth: a role for BCL2? Trends in Neurosciences 22:269-272.

Houle JD, Schramm P, Herdegen T. 1998. Trophic factor modulation of c-Jun expression in supraspinal neurons after chronic spinal cord injury. Exp. Neurol.154:602-611.

Humm JL, Kozlowski DA, James DC, Gotts JE , Schallert T 1998. Use dependent exacerbation of brain damage occurs during an early post-lesion vulnerable period. Brain Res. 783:269-292.

Itoh Y, Sugawara T, Kowada M , Tessler A 1993. Time course of dorsal root axon regeneration into transplants of fetal spinal cord: an electron microscopic study Exp. Neurol 123:133-146.

Itoh Y, Waldeck RF, Tessler A, Pinter MJ 1996. Regenerated dorsal root fibers form functional synapses in embryonic spinal cord transplants. J. Neurophysiol. 76:1236-1245.

Jakeman LB, Reier PJ 1991 Axonal projections between fetal spinal cord transplants and the adult rat spinal cord. J. Comp. Neurol 307:311-334.

Jo SA, Wang E, Benowitz LI 1999. Ciliary neurotrophic factor is an axogenesis factor for retinal ganglion cells. Neurosc. 89:579-591.

Jones TA, Schallert T 1994. Use dependent growth of pyramidal neurons after neocortical damage. J.Neuroscience 14:2140-52.

Jung M, Petrausch B, Stuermer CAO. 1997. Axon-regenerating retinal ganglion cells in adult rats synthesize the cell adhesion molecule L1 but not TAG-1 or SC-1. Molec. Cell. Neurosc. 9:116-131.

Kalderon N, Fuks Z 1996. Structural recovery in lesioned adult mammalian spinal cord by x-irradiation of the lesion site. Proc. Natl. Acad.Sc.93:11179-11184.

Kawaja MD, Gage FH 1991. Reactive astrocytes are substrates for the growth of CNS in the presence of elevated levels of nerve growth factor. Neuron 7:1019-1030.

Keirstead SA, Rasminsky M, Fukuda Y, Carter DA, Aguayo AJ, Vidal-Sanz M. 1989. Electrophysiologic responses in hamster superior colliculus evoked by regenerating retinal axons. Science 246:255-257.

Kjaerulff O, Kiehn O 1996. Distribution of networks generating and coordinating locomotor activity in the neonatal rat spinal cord *in vitro*. J. Neurosc. 15:5777-5794.

Kreutzberg GW. 1996. Microglia: a sensor for pathological events in the CNS. TINS 19:312-318.

La Fleur M, Underwood JL, Rappolee DA, Werb Z. 1996. Basement membrane and repair of injury to peripheral nerve: defining a potential role for macrophages, matrix metalloproteinases, and tissue inhibitor of metalloproteinases-1. J. Exp. Med. 184:2311-2326.

Lavie V, Murray M, Solomon A, Schwartz M. 1990. Growth of injured rabbit optic axons in the degenerating optic nerve. J. Comp. Neurol. 298:293-314.

Li D, Field P, Raisman G. 1995. Failure of axon regeneration in postnatal rat entorhino-hippocampal slice coculture is due to maturation of the axon not that of the pathway or target. Eur. J. Neurosc. 7:1164-1171.

Li Y, Field PM, Raisman G. 1997. Repair of adult corticospinal tract by transplant of olfactory ensheathing cells. Science 277:2000-2002.

Liu Y, Himes BT, Murray M, Tessler A, Fischer I 1999. Grafts of BDNF-producing fibroblasts that promote regeneration of axotomized rubrospinal neurons also rescue most neurons from retrograde death and prevent their atrophy. Submitted.

Liu Y, Kim, D, Himes BT, Chow SY, Schallert T, Murray M, Tessler A, Fischer I. 1999a Transplants of fibroblasts genetically modified to express BDNF promote regeneration of adult rat rubrospinal axons. J. Neurosc.19:4370-87.

Madsen JR, MacDonald P, Irwin N, Goldberg DE, Yao GL, Meiri, KF, Rimm IJ, Stieg, PE, Benowitz LI. 1998. Tacrolimus (FK506) increases neuronal expression of GAP-43 and improves functional recovery after spinal cord injury in rats. Exp. Neurol.154:673-683.

Mallat M, Houlgatte R, Brachet P, Prochiantz A. 1989 Lipopolysaccharide stimulated rat brain macrophages release NGF in vitro. Dev. Biol. 122:309-311.

McKay R 1997 Stem cells in the central nervous system. Science 276:66-71.

Menei P, Montero-Menei C, Whittemore SR, Bunge RP, Bunge MB. 1998. Schwann cells genetically modified to secrete human BDNF promote enhanced axonal regrowth across transected adult spinal cord. Eur. J. Neurosc.10:607-621.

Merei KF, Saffell JL, Walsh FS, Doherty P 1998. Neurite outgrowth stimulated by neural cell adhesion molecules requires growth associated protein -43 (GAP43) function and is associated with GAP-43 phosphorylation in growth cones. J. Neurosc. 18:10429-37.

Meyer-Franke A, Kaplan MK, Pfrieger FW, Barres BA 1995. Characterization of the signaling interactions that promote the survival and growth of developing retinal ganglion cells in culture. Neuron 15:805-819.

Mikucki SA, Oblinger MM 1991. Corticospinal neurons exhibit a novel pattern of cytoskeletal gene expression after injury. J. Neurosc. Res. 30:213-225.

Mitz AR, Humphrey DR 1986. Intracortical stimulation in pyramidotomized monkeys. Neurosc. Lett. 64:59-64.

Mori F, Himes BT, Kowada M , Murray M and Tessler A 1997. Fetal spinal cord transplants rescue some axotomized rubrospinal neurons from retrograde cell death in adult rats. Exp. Neurol.143:45-60.

Muir E, Du J-S, Fok-Seang J, Smith -Thomas LC, Rogers JH, Fawcett JW 1998. Increased axon growth through astrocyte cell lines transfected with urokinase. Glia 23:24-34.

Murray M. 1982. A quantitative study of regenerative sprouting by optic axons in goldfish. J. Comp. Neurol. 209:352-362.

Neeper SA, Gomez-Pinilla F, Choi JK, Cotman C. 1995. Exercise and brain neurotrophins. Nature 373:109-110.

Nudo, RJ, Wise BM, SiFuentes F, Milliken GW 1996. Neural substrates for the effects of rehabilitative training on motor recovery after ischemic infarct. Science 272:1791-94.

Okonkwo DO, Buki A, Siman R, Povlishock JT. 1999. Cyclosporin A limits calcium-induced axonal damage following traumatic brain injury. NeuroReport 10:353-358.

Oliff HS, Berchtold NC, Isackson P, Cotman CW. 1998. Exercise-induced regulation of brain-derived neurotrophic factor (BDNF) transcripts in the rat hippocampus. Molec. Br. Res. 61:147-153

Oudega M, Hagg T 1999 Neurotrophins promote regeneration of sensory axons into the adult rat spinal cord. Br. Res. 818:431-438.

Oudega M, Xu XM, Guenard V, Kleitman N, Bunge MB 1997 A combination of insulin like growth factor-1 and platelet derived growth factor enhances myelination but diminishes axonal regeneration into Schwann cell grafts in the adult rat spinal cord. Glia 19:247-258.

Rabacchi SA, Bonfanti L, Liu XH, Maffei 1994. Apoptotic cell death induced by optic nerve lesion in the neonatal rat. J. Neurosc.14:5292-5301.

Rabchevsky AG, Streit WJ 1997 Grafting of cultured microglial cells into the lesioned spinal cord of adult rats enhances neurite outgrowth. J. Neurosc. Res. 47:344-48.

Raineteau O, Z'Graggen WJ, Thallmair M, Schwab ME. 1995. Sprouting and regeneration after pyramidotomy and blockade of the myelin-associated neurite growth inhibitors NI 35/250 in adult rats. Eur. J. Neurosc.11:1486-90/

Ramon-Cueto A, Plant GW, Avila J, Bunge MB 1998. Long distance axonal regeneration in the transected adult rat spinal cord is promoted by olfactory ensheathing cells. J. Neurosc. 18:3803-5.

Rapaolino O, Lazarov-Spiegler O, Agranov E, Velan GJ, Yoles E, Fraidakis, M, Solomon A, Gepstein R, Katz A, Belkin M, Hadani M, Schwartz M 1998 Implantation of stimulated homologous macrophages results in partial recovery of paraplegic rats. Nature Medicine 4:814-821.

Robinson GA 1995 Axotomy-induced regulation of c-jun expression in regenerating rat retinal ganglion cells. Mol. Brain Res. 30:61-69.

Schwartz M, Moalem G, Leibowitz-Amit R, Cohen IR 1999. Innate and adaptive immune responses can be beneficial for CNS repair. Trends in Neurosc.22:295-9.

Shibayama M, Hattori S, Himes BT, Murray M, Tessler A 1998a. Neurotrophin-3 (NT-3) prevents death of axotomized Clarke's Nucleus neurons in the adult rat. J. Comp. Neurol. 390:102-11.

Shibayama M., Matsui N, Himes BT, Murray M, Tessler A. 1998b. Critical interval for rescue of axotomized neurons by transplants. NeuroReport 9:11-14.

Shibayama M, Nothias JM, Battisti W, Tessler A, Murray M. 1998c Axotomized Clarke's neurons die by apoptosis. Soc. for Neurosc.24:1302.

Skene, JHP 1989. Axonal growth-associated proteins. Ann. Rev. Neurosc. 12:127-158.

Stichel CC, Hermanns S, Luhmann HJ, Lausberg F, Niermann H, D'Urso D, Servos G, Hartwig H-G, Muller HW. 1999. Inhibition of collagen IV deposition promotes regeneration of injured CNS axons. Eur J. Neurosc. 11:632-647.

Stichel CC,Wunderlich G, Schwab ME, Muller HW 1995. Clearance of myelin constituents and axonal sprouting in the transected postcommissural fornix of the adult rat. Eur. J. Neurosc. 7:401-11.

Sugawara T, Himes BT, Kowada M, Muray M, Tessler A, Battisti WP. 1999. Relationship between putative inhibitory extracellular matrix molecules and dorsal root regeneration into fetal spinal cord transplants. In press.

Takahashi K, Schwarz E, Ljubetic C, Murray M, Tessler A, Saavedra R. 1999. A DNA plasmid that codes for the human BCl2 gene preserves axotomized Clarke's nucleus neurons and reduces atrophy after spinal cord hemisection in adult rats. J.Comp.Neurol..404:159-171.

Tetzlaff W, Alexander SW, Miller FD, Bisby MA 1991.Responses of facial and rubrospinal neurons to axotomy. J. Neurosc. 11:2528-2544

Tetzlaff W, Leonard C, Krekoski GA, Parhod M, Bisby MA 1996. Reduction in motoneuronal filament synthesis by successive axotomies. Exp. Neurol 139:95-106

Thanos S, Naskar R, Heiduschka P. 1997. Regenerating ganglion cell axons in the adult rat establish retinofugal topography and restore visual function. Exp. Br. Res. 114:483-91.

Vaudano E, Campbell G, Hunt SP, Lieberman AR.1998. Axonal injury and peripheral nerve grafting in the thalamus and cerebellum of the adult rat: upregulation of c-jun and correlation with regenerative potential. Eur. J. Neurosc. 10:2644-2656.

Vidal-Sanz M, Bray GM, Aguayo AJ 1991. Regenerated synapses persist in the superior colliculus after regrowth of retinal ganglion cell axons. J. Neurocyt. 20:940-952.

Von Meyenburg J, Brosamle C, Metz GA, Schwab ME. 1998. Regeneration and sprouting of chronically injured corticospinal tract fibers in adult rats promoted by NT-3 and the mAB IN-1 which neutralizes myelin associated neurite growth inhibitors. Exp. Neurol. 154:583-594.

Walpow JR, Carp JS 1990 Memory traces in the spinal cord. Trends Neurosc. 13:137-142.

Weiss S, Dunne C, Hewson J, Wohl C, Wheatley M, Peterson, AC, Reynolds BA 1996. Multipotent CNS stem cells are present in the adult mammalian spinal cord and ventricular neuroaxis. J. Neurosc. 16:7599-7609.

Wernig A, Muller S, Nanassy A, Cagol E. 1995. Laufband therapy based on rules of spinal locomotion is effective in spinal cord injured persons. Eur. J. Neurosc. 7:823-9.

Whittemore SR, Snyder EY 1996. Physiological relevance and functional potential of central nervous system-derived cell lines. Mol. Neurobiol. 12:13-38.

Wizenmann A, Thies E, Klostermann S, Bonhoeffer F, Bahr M. 1993. Appearance of target specific guidance information for regenerating axons after CNS lesions. neuron 11:975-983.

Xu XM, Guenard V, Kleitman N, Aebischer P, Bunge MB 1995 A combination of BDNF and NT-3 promotes supraspinal axonal regeneration into Schwann cell grafts in adult rat thoracic spinal cord. Exp. Neurol 134:261-272.

Ye, J-H, Houle JD. 1997. Treatment of the chronically injured spinal cord with neurotrophic factors can promote axonal regeneration from supraspinal neurons. Exp. Neurol. 143:70-81.

Zagrebelsky M, Buffo A, Skerra A, Schwab ME, Strata P, Rossi F. 1998. Retrograde regulation of growth-associated gene expression in adult rat Purkinje cells by myelin associated neurite growth inhibitory proteins. J. Neurosc. 18:7912-7929.

Zhang Y, Campbell G, Anderson PN, Martini R, Schachner M, Lieberman AR 1995 Molecular basis of interactions between regenerating adult rat thalamic axons and Schwann cells in peripheral nerve grafts. I. Neural cell adhesion moleculues. J. Comp. Neurol. 361:193-209. .

Zuo J, Ferguson TA, Hernandez YJ, Stetler-Stevenson WG, Muir D. 1998. Neuronal matrix mettalo proteinase -2 degraded and inactivated a neurite inhibiting chondroitin sulfate proteoglycan. J. Neurosc. 18:5203-5211.

25

Treatment of Degenerative Disorders of the Nervous System: From Helpless Descriptive Categorization to Rational Therapeutic Approaches

Hans Thoenen
Max-Planck-Institute of Neurobiology, Martinsried, Germany

I. INTRODUCTION

The understanding of the basic mechanisms of the functions of the nervous system is advancing at a breathtaking rate, opening up possibilities to envisage the treatment of degenerative disorders—including the consequences of traumatic and vascular lesions—on a rational basis. For a long time, clinical neurology was a field of refined, descriptive diagnostics, accommodating countless syndromes that were preferentially labeled with the names of those who first described them. Beyond palliative measures, however, there were no rational perspectives for therapy. This is also reflected by the complementary descriptive histopathological documentation, which did not permit any understanding of the underlying mechanisms. In spite of visionary views of possible molecular concepts (DeFelipe and Jones, 1991), such visions could not be brought to life, since the basic knowledge and the necessary experimental technology were insufficiently advanced to permit the identification of possible underlying cellular and molecular mechanisms. This situation changed at an ever-increasing rate, with the identification of the conventional neurotransmitter substances and a still-growing number of neuropeptides,*

* No references given; see neurobiological textbooks.

the identification and molecular characterization of the corresponding receptors (Green et al., 1998), the detection of molecules that determine the site, period, and extent of neuron production, the elucidation of the regionally differential regulation of neuronal survival (Barde, 1989; Davies, 1994; Edlund and Jessel, 1999), and the characterization of the correct formation and activity-dependent refinement of neuronal circuits (Katz and Shatz, 1996). Last but not least, a rapidly increasing number of (mono-) genetically determined diseases of the nervous system have been characterized at the molecular level (Green et al., 1998). This has also yielded valuable information on similar, sporadic disorders for which possible epigenetic causes and polygenetic dispositions are not yet known.

In the following, I will briefly delineate how rational approaches for the treatment of degenerative diseases developed, thereby outlining the present situation and possible perspectives for the future. In order to do so, I have chosen representative examples, their selection being unavoidably arbitrary and the cited references incomplete. As far as possible, I have quoted recent reviews; groundbreaking, original papers could only be quoted in rare cases. Since this chapter had to be written in parallel with the others in this volume, it was not possible to take account of overlaps or possible discrepancies.

II. REPLACEMENT OF NEUROTRANSMITTERS AND ENHANCEMENT OF THEIR FUNCTION

Following the identification of dopamine as a potential neurotransmitter in the central nervous system, Hornykiewicz (1966) made the seminal observation that levels of dopamine in the nigrostriatal system were drastically reduced in autoptic material of Parkinson patients. This observation led to the L-Dopa therapy, the basis of which is an increased availability of dopamine for the residual, still-functioning dopaminergic neurons of the substantia nigra, thus enhancing their residual function (Hornykiewicz, 1988; Agid, 1998). However, treatment with the dopamine precursor L-Dopa does not interfere with the further degeneration of dopaminergic neurons (Fischer and Gage, 1995). It has even been debated whether prolonged L-Dopa treatment can lead to neurotoxic effects, as demonstrated for the oxidation products of dopamine *in vitro*, although to a much lesser extent than is the case with 6-hydroxydopamine (Agid, 1998). Accordingly, the beneficial effects of L-Dopa treatment are of limited duration, with subsequent "L-Dopa resistance" and an increased incidence of side effects. Since up to 80% of dopaminergic neurons of the substantia nigra have to degenerate before the first clinical manifestations become apparent (Agid, 1998), it will be essential to develop procedures for early diagnosis and interference with the progression of the degeneration of dopaminergic neurons, and/or to replace these neurons by transplantation. These aspects will be discussed below.

The situation for Parkinson's disease was mirrored by the first rational efforts to treat Alzheimer's disease. After combined clinical and neuropathological investigations provided compelling evidence that the basal forebrain cholinergic neurons are consistently affected at a relatively early stage of Alzheimer's disease, and that the malfunction of these neurons is largely responsible for the characteristic cognitive deficits (Hefti and Weiner, 1986), it was a logical consequence to attempt to enhance the function of the residual, still-functioning cholinergic neurons of the basal forebrain. The cholinergic neurotransmitter acetylcholine is predominantly inactivated enzymatically by acetylcholinesterase. Hence, therapeutic efforts were directed towards the development of drugs that either interfere with the degradation of acetylcholine by acetylcholinesterase, or exhibit cholinomimetic actions that are preferentially restricted to the central nervous system (Farlow and Evans, 1998; Imbimbo et al., 1998; Winkler et al., 1998). Again, however, these therapies do not interfere with the progression of the degenerative processes.

In spite of very significant advances in the understanding of the pathophysiological mechanisms that result in Alzheimer's disease (Selkoe, 1996; Beyreuther and Masters, 1997; Hardy, 1997; Masters and Beyreuther, 1998; Spillantini and Goedert, 1998; Van Leewen et al., 1998), the elucidation of the neuropathological mechanisms has not (yet) led to direct, practicable therapeutic consequences. Although a causal therapy is the ultimate goal for the treatment of degenerative disorders, alternative (symptomatic) therapies must be envisaged, in view of the uncertainty as to whether a causal therapy will at all be possible.

III. POSSIBILITIES AND LIMITATIONS FOR THE USE OF NEUROTROPHIC MOLECULES IN THE TREATMENT OF DEGENERATIVE DISORDERS

The use of neurotrophic molecules, together with the knowledge evolving from their biological actions, represents one of the most promising approaches yet developed to interfere with the progression of degenerative disorders. Neurotrophic molecules of different gene families have been shown to inhibit or delay degenerative processes in neurons in a great variety of experimental systems (reviewed by Hefti 1997). It must be emphasized, however, that the treatment of degenerative disorders with neurotrophic factors is not a causal therapy since, to date, no human degenerative disorder has been identified as being caused by the absence or defective production of a neurotrophic molecule. The reduced Brain-Derived Neurotrophic Factor (BDNF) mRNA levels reported for autoptic material of Alzheimer patients (Phillips et al., 1991) are more likely a reflection of the consequences of the degenerative processes rather than being their cause. Moreover, the inactivation of the human Ciliary Neurotrophic Factor (CNTF) gene, resulting from a point mutation, is not directly correlated with an increased incidence of degenerative diseases, in particular Amyotrophic Lateral Sclerosis (ALS) (Takahashi et al., 1994; Orrell et al., 1995; Giess et al., 1998). However, in this relatively frequent human mutation (the frequency of homozygous CNTF null mutants in both Asian and Caucasian populations is about one in forty), there was a particularly early onset of ALS in patients homozygous for CNTF gene inactivation. This might suggest that the CNTF null mutation leads to an augmented disposition to ALS, together with other cryptic genetic defects or epigenetic damaging influences. This is reminiscent of the observations made in CNTF and Leukemia Inhibitory Factor (LIF) knockout mice (Sendtner et al., 1996), which demonstrated that inactivation of the LIF gene alone did not elicit degenerative processes in motoneurons. However, the gradual motoneuron degeneration in adult CNTF knockout animals began much earlier, and was much more severe when the LIF gene was also inactivated.

Although there is no evidence to suggest that a defective production of neurotrophic factors is a direct cause of neurodegenerative diseases, the exploitation of the biological actions of neurotrophic molecules nevertheless represents an attractive possibility for their treatment. Molecules of different gene families, in particular neurotrophins (the name coined for the NGF gene family), Insulin-like Growth Factor 1 (IGF-1), members of the Glial-Derived Neurotrophic Factor (GDNF), Transforming Growth Factor (TGFß), and Fibroblast Growth Factor (FGF) gene families, as well as cytokines acting via the gp130/LIFß receptor signal transduction unit (CNTF, LIF, oncostatin-M, cardiotrophin), have shown impressive neuroprotective effects in a great variety of experimental systems, both *in vitro* and *in vivo* (see Hefti, 1997). The evolving high therapeutic expectations, together with the possibility of commercial exploitation, initially blurred the view for the biological reality. Accordingly, the first clinical trials, which were based on insufficient pre-clinical investigations, led to failures (Verral, 1994; ALS CNTF Treatment Study Group, 1996; Miller et al., 1996; Sendtner, 1997). There is now the danger of neurotrophic molecules being discredited as indiscriminately as they had initially been welcomed as "miracle drugs" with unrealistic expectations, a case of "throwing out the baby with the bath-water." However, it is essential to recognize that the concept of the use of neurotrophic molecules for the treatment of degenerative disorders was not wrong, but rather the manner in which the initial therapeutic procedures had been designed. I would like to exemplify this by the unsuccessful treatment of ALS patients by the subcutaneous administration of CNTF and BDNF: long before the advent of cloning and the availability of recombinant CNTF and BDNF, it had been demonstrated that intravenously injected NGF is efficiently accumulated in sympathetic and NGF-responsive sensory neurons, predominantly by retrograde axonal transport (Stoeckel et al., 1976). This might have led to the wrong conclusion that this is also the case for systemically administered CNTF and BDNF. Although the motoneurons of the spinal cord and the brain stem project to the periphery, no experimental evidence has been provided to indicate an accumulation of CNTF or BDNF in motoneurons after the systemic injection (either intravenous or subcutaneous) of these molecules. We approached the question of the uptake and retrograde axonal transport of CNTF in motoneurons in my own laboratory. We demonstrated that, after intravenous injection of labeled CNTF, there was no accumulation in either motoneurons or sympathetic neurons, which also respond to CNTF (Dittrich et al., 1994). However, there was a very high accumulation in the liver. This seems to reflect the high level of soluble CNTFα receptors in the serum (the CNTF receptor complex consists of the signal-transducing units gp130 and LIFβ receptor and the GPI-link CNTFα receptor) (Stahl and Yancopoulos, 1994). Accordingly, the labeled CNTF—injected intravenously—was trapped by soluble CNTFα receptors, and the ligand-receptor complex docked into the abundant LIF receptors in the liver, activating them via the gp130 and LIFβ signal-transduction subunits. In this way, the injected CNTF activated the LIF receptors and initiated the production of acute phase proteins, resulting in general inflammatory reactions (Dittrich et al., 1994; Hirano et al., 1997).

The evidence for the retrograde transport of BDNF to motoneurons was based on experiments in which labeled BDNF had been injected directly into the sciatic nerve or administered to lesioned axons, although there was no such evidence after systemic or even direct injection into the skeletal muscle (DiStefano et al., 1992; Lindsay et al., 1994). It is conceivable that systemically administered NGF penetrates much better to the "naked" nerve terminals of sympathetic or NGF-responsive sensory neurons than does BDNF to the nerve terminals of motoneurons, which are localized in the highly specialized structures of the motor endplate, well shielded by Schwann cells.

I would like to emphasize that the demonstration of retrograde axonal transport of CNTF or BDNF in motoneurons after systemic administration would not have been a guarantee for the successful treatment of ALS, since the motor axons are "dying back" (Rowland, 1991; Chou, 1992). However, when not even evidence can be provided that—in animals under physiological conditions—subcutaneously injected BDNF or CNTF reaches the therapeutic target, i.e., the motoneurons, the chances for a successful clinical treatment are very poor, unless it were to be assumed that the pathogenetic process of ALS facilitates the penetration of CNTF and/or BDNF to the motor axons in an unknown manner.

A rational approach for the appropriate administration of neurotrophic factors has been demonstrated by Sendtner and collaborators (Dittrich et al., 1996), in careful pre-clinical experiments to provide a rational basis for the use of BDNF to treat ALS patients. They first established a procedure for the continuous intrathecal administration (by battery-driven pumps) of BDNF in sheep, monitoring the evolving concentrations of BDNF in the cerebrospinal fluid in relation to the site of infusion. Using immunohistochemistry, they also demonstrated the accumulation of BDNF in the motoneurons of the sheep spinal cord (Dittrich et al., 1996). Based on these careful, focussed, pre-clinical experiments, a small number of ALS patients have been treated, and the initial results appear promising (Ochs et al., 1998), although final conclusions cannot yet be drawn from this small group of patients. However, even such carefully designed experiments are not yet a guarantee for real clinical success, and I would like to mention a few possible pitfalls that have to be borne in mind in designing future therapeutic procedures. When using BDNF, an optimal dosage schedule is crucial, since the administration of large quantities of BDNF leads to "desensitization" and, in turn, to a limitation of the supportive action of BDNF on lesioned motoneurons (Eriksson, 1994: Vejsada et al., 1994; 1995). This limitation of the duration of the BDNF action most likely results from a downregulation of the signal-transducing Trk-B receptors (Knusel et al., 1997). Therefore, it is necessary to determine the optimal therapeutic dosage that permits the maintenance of the BDNF effect. That this is indeed possible can be deduced from the observation that the continuous BDNF supply by adenoviral gene transfer into the proximal stump of the facial nerve resulted in a prolonged supportive effect on lesioned motoneurons (Gravel et al., 1997), with no evidence of desensitization, as observed after the local administration of very high quantities of BDNF (Eriksson, 1994; Vejsada et al., 1994). In this context, the recent observations of Meyer-Franke et al. (1998) might be of importance. These authors found that depolarization and an increase in cyclic AMP levels, at least in culture, resulted in an enhanced insertion of Trk-B receptors into the plasma membrane of motoneurons, opening up the possibility to counteract the downregulation of Trk receptors by the administration of Trk-B receptor ligands. Moreover, the use of a combination of several neurotrophic factors seems to be advisable, since their actions might be additive or even superadditive (Thoenen et al., 1993; Sendtner et al., 1994; Sendtner 1997; Wong et al., 1997). In this way, the necessary dosage for the individual neurotrophic factors could be reduced and potential side effects minimized. Additionally, the effects of the different neurotrophic factors may complement one another, for instance by predominantly interfering with apoptosis, or by predominantly supporting the maintenance of specific neuronal functions. Such complementary functions have been reported for the combined administration of CNTF and BDNF, GDNF and NT-3, and NT-3 and CNTF (Haase et al., 1997; Sagot et al., 1998), respectively. Another important aspect to be considered is that a sufficient supply of neurotrophic factors to support the survival and function of the neuronal cell bodies does not result *eo ipso* in the regrowth of the corresponding axons to the periphery over longer distances. The opposite may in fact be the case. Even a supramaximal supply of neurotrophic molecules to the neuronal cell body could lead to a situation—as observed in transgenic mice—in which NGF was specifically overexpressed in sympathetic neurons by a dopamine β-hydroxylase promoter construct (Hoyle et al., 1993). In these neurons, there was not only no increase in the density of sympathetic innervation in the peripheral projection areas, but also even a decrease in the density of sympathetic innervation, despite a marked increase in the size of the sympathetic ganglia and the individual, sympathetic neuronal cell bodies (Hoyle et al., 1993). This indicates that a supramaximal neurotrophic supply to the cell bodies may have paradoxical consequences. The cell bodies become "self-sufficient" and no longer "recognize" any necessity to probe the projection field from where they are normally supplied by limited quantities of neurotrophic molecules under physiological conditions (Barde, 1989). This interpretation is further supported by the recent experiments of Ringstedt (1998), in which the overexpression of BDNF and NT-3 in transgenic mice by a nestin promoter construct (nestin is expressed in neuronal progenitor cells) resulted not only in a markedly increased survival of sensory neurons, but also in an insufficient peripheral target innervation by these neurons. Astonishingly, the phenotypes of these transgenic mice, which overexpress BDNF and NT-3, resemble the phenotypes of NT-3 and BDNF-knockout mice respectively (Snider, 1994; Lewin and Barde, 1996). I am aware that these possible pitfalls are not in every respect pertinent to the therapeutic situation for ALS. However, they serve to illustrate that the survival and even the hypertrophy of individual neuronal cell bodies do not imply a normal function, as reflected by an appropriate innervation of the peripheral target tissues.

In order to accomplish a restoration of the original innervation by motoneurons, a sufficiently high concentration of neurotrophic molecules has to become available all along the pathway to the peripheral target sites: in the case of ALS, the skeletal muscle. Although there exist conceptual possibilities to achieve this goal, there is in any case a long way to go before they will attain clinical practicability. In this context, I am thinking of the delivery of neurotrophic molecules by viral vectors (Gravel et al., 1997; Haase et al., 1997; Barkats et al., 1998), or by the systemic injection of activated, targeted T-cells that are engineered to overexpress neurotrophic molecules (Kramer et al., 1995; Flügel et al., 1999). Another possibility might also evolve from the observation that, after mechanical nerve lesion resulting in the degeneration of the peripheral axons, the production of BDNF, LIF, and GDNF is markedly upregulated in the distal part of the lesioned nerve (Meyer et al., 1992; Curtis et al., 1994; Henderson et al., 1994). A molecular analysis of the mechanisms underlying the upregulation of these neurotrophic molecules may open up possibilities to enhance their synthesis by pharmacological procedures, particularly in view of the fact that, in ALS, Schwann cells are deserted by motoneuron axons that are dying back (Rowland, 1991; Chou, 1992), creating similar conditions to those after mechanical lesion of the whole nerve.

For the design of therapeutic procedures for the treatment of degenerative disorders in which those populations of neurons of the central nervous system are affected that do not project to the periphery and that cannot be reached by peripheral systemic administration owing to the blood-brain barrier, a first straightforward approach was the delivery of these molecules directly into the brain (Hefti, 1986). Such approaches have been encouraged by the observation that not only could neuroprotective effects be demonstrated after mechanical or selective neurotoxic lesions (reviewed by Hefti, 1997), but also cognitive deficits in aged rats could be improved by the intraventricular infusion of NGF (Fisher et al., 1987). The cognitive performance of these rats was evaluated in the Morris Water Maze, and the deficits correlated with degenerative/atrophic processes of the cholinergic neurons of the basal forebrain. The improved performance in the Morris Water Maze resulting from NGF infusion was accompanied by a restoration of the structure and function of the cholinergic neurons towards normality, including a substantial increase in the levels of choline acetyltransferase (Fisher et al., 1987). Based on these observations, a small number of Alzheimer's patients in Sweden have been treated by intraventricular NGF infusion. After an initial, rather promising report (Olson et al., 1992), a very recent, more extensive study has shown that side effects, in particular pain, dominated over possible beneficial effects (Jonhagen et al., 1998). These side effects have their counterpart in animal experiments in which a broad spectrum of acute reactions has been observed, depending on the site of injection of NGF and other neurotrophins. These range from epileptic activity, through increased motor activity, to the initiation of theta rhythms and sedation (Thoenen, 1995; Berninger and Poo, 1996; Kobayashi et al., 1997a,b). Moreover, prolonged intraventricular infusion of large quantities of NGF resulted in Schwann cell hyperplasia and extensive sprouting of sensory and sympathetic nerve fibers in the subpial region of the brain stem (Winkler et al., 1997). All these observations demonstrate the limitations of intraventricular or intracerebral infusion, as well as the (uncontrolled) abundant production of neurotrophic molecules by transplanted, engineered cells. In this context, it should also be remembered that neurotrophins (in particular BDNF and NGF) are involved in the modulation of activity-dependent neuronal plasticity (Thoenen, 1995; Bonhoeffer, 1996; Cellerino and Maffei, 1996). The prolonged local infusion of BDNF or NGF, and also of corresponding blocking agents (blocking antibodies or corresponding Trk-receptor bodies*) to the visual cortex results in a dramatic disturbance of the activity-dependent development of ocular dominance in several species (Cellerino and Maffei, 1996; Cabelli et al., 1995, 1997). All these experiments demonstrate impressively that, in developing strategies for the treatment of degenerative disorders of the central nervous system with neurotrophic factors, it is not sufficient to supply the affected neurons with (uncontrolled) large quantities of neurotrophic molecules. The expected therapeutic effects have to be weighed up against the potentially occurring side effects. These side effects may be particularly severe if the therapeutic targets are neurons that are involved in highly specialized neuronal circuits. For neurons with larger projection areas, and whose function is mainly a modulatory one (for instance, noradrenergic neurons of the locus coeruleus, serotoninergic neurons of the raphe nucleus, or dopaminergic neurons of the substantia nigra), the expected side effects may not be as pronounced, provided that the neurotrophic molecules used do not also affect other populations of neurons involved in more refined functions.

I will refrain from discussing in detail the additional difficulties encountered when the goal is the treatment of lesions that require the regeneration of central neurons over long distances, as is the case, for instance, after traumatic lesions of the spinal cord. There, in the central nervous system (in contrast to the periphery, where the major problem is the supply of the appropriate neurotrophic molecules, not only to the cell bodies, but also all along the regeneration pathway), the blocking actions of inhibitory molecules have additionally to be overcome. These aspects are specifically addressed in this volume by Bregman, David, Raisman, and Schwab.

---

*Trk receptor bodies are IgG antibodies in which the variable domain is replaced by the specific binding domain of Trk receptors.

IV. REPLACEMENT OF DEGENERATED NEURONS BY TRANSPLANTATION

The replacement of degenerated neurons by transplantation is a complementary procedure to that of the administration of neurotrophic molecules to interfere with the degeneration of specific populations of neurons. To date, such efforts have mainly been focussed on the treatment of Parkinson's disease, in which the dopaminergic neurons of the substantia nigra, at least initially, are predominantly affected (Hornykiewicz, 1988; Agid, 1998). After extensive animal experimentation (Fisher and Gage, 1995; Gage, 1998a,b), the first clinical trials were performed in which dopaminergic neurons isolated from human fetuses were transplanted into the striatum, the main projection area of dopaminergic neurons of the substantia nigra. Moreover, autologous transplantations of adrenal medullary cells were performed (Lindvall et al., 1994; Kordower et al., 1997; Wenning et al., 1997). The long-term success of such transplantations was variable, the major problem being the generally poor and inconsistent survival of the transplanted cells, which came from both fetuses and the patient's own adrenal medullary cells. Additionally, the transplantation of human fetal dopaminergic neurons—for one transplantation, the dopaminergic neurons of several fetuses are necessary—required that the recipient patient be treated with immunosuppressants in order to prevent rejection of the transplants. The survival of the transplanted neurons was improved by the administration of neurotrophic factors that support them (Olson et al., 1991; Takayama et al., 1995).

Currently, a very active direction of research concerns the isolation of neuronal stem cells—from various brain areas of fetal and adult animals—that have the potential to be expanded *in vitro* and then to differentiate into either neurons or glial cells when transplanted into fetal and adult recipients (Brüstle et al., 1997, 1998; Flax et al., 1998; Gage, 1998a,b). Moreover, these neuronal stem cells can be manipulated to differentiate predominantly into either neurons or glial cells. Very recently, it became apparent that corresponding stem cells are also present in adult humans (Eriksson et al., 1998), opening up promising perspectives for future transplantation experiments. These aspects will be discussed below.

V. PERSPECTIVES FOR THE FUTURE

The primary goal for future therapeutic concepts is to interfere, as directly as possible, with the pathogenetic mechanisms, be they genetic or epigenetic. However, even the most detailed knowledge of the underlying molecular mechanisms does not, in general, lead to a straightforward causal therapy. I would like to document this by the following examples. A genetically determined familial form of ALS caused by a mutation in the gene coding for the copper zinc superoxide dismutase (Rosen et al., 1993; Deng et al., 1993) does not lead to a loss of function of this enzyme, but rather to a gain of (wrong) function (Borchelt et al., 1995; Pasinelli et al., 1998). Accordingly, it is not possible to supply the affected neurons with the normal, non-mutated enzyme.

In Huntington's disease, the expansion of a repetitive CAG sequence (CAG coding for glutamine) in a molecule of virtually ubiquitous expression in the brain leads to changes in the physico-chemical properties of huntingtin. These changes initiate degenerative processes only in selective populations of neurons of the central nervous system (Green et al., 1998; Gusella and Macdonald, 1998; Kim and Tanzi, 1998). The longer the CAG repetitive sequence, the more severe are the degenerative manifestations, and the earlier they begin. A direct correction of the underlying mechanism is not possible without the development of procedures that would enable the genetic defect in post-mitotic somatic cells to be corrected, in particular in neurons. Although such procedures are currently under intense investigation (Ye et al., 1998), the results obtained to date are as yet far from being clinically applicable. However, in animal models of Huntington's disease (Emerich et al., 1997) or in neurons transduced with a mutated (CAG extension) huntingtin gene leading to functional manifestations of Huntington's disease (Saudou et al., 1998), the administration of neutrotrophic molecules such as CNTF and GNDF impressively protected the affected neurons from degeneration (Emerich et al., 1997; Saudou et al., 1998). This observation is of particular importance, since the individuals who will potentially be affected (according to their family history) can be identified by genetic analysis before the outbreak of the disease (Green et al., 1998; Gusella and Macdonald, 1998), and a timely prophylactic treatment initiated.

The symptomatic, non-causal treatment of degenerative disorders will most likely remain of importance in the near future. However, this should by no means discourage efforts towards the most complete understanding of the normal molecular function of the nervous system and corresponding pathological deviations. Such investigations should be performed in the absence of excessive pressure to attain practicable therapeutic goals as directly and as quickly as possible. It cannot be overemphasized that important therapeutic concepts may evolve from investigations that are exclusively directed towards the basic understanding of physiological and pathophysiological mechanisms.

In the final stages of neuronal degeneration, apoptotic mechanisms come into play that show very similar features to those of physiologically regulated cell death. The detailed understanding of the signal transduction pathways that regulate apoptosis/antiapoptosis is advancing at a rapid rate (Jacobson et al., 1997; Susin et al., 1997; Chao and Korsmeyer, 1998). The pharmacological modification of these signal transduction pathways is the focus of the experimental efforts of many pharmaceutical/biotechnology firms. However, it has to be borne in mind that a general, ubiquitous interference with apoptotic mechanisms cannot be the solution for the treatment of degenerative disorders of the nervous system. The continuous turnover of cells in many biological systems is of crucial importance for normal physiological functions. Interference with such general mechanisms may lead to an uncontrolled production of cells, leading in turn to the formation of tumors. For instance, under pathophysiological conditions in the immune system, disregulated antiapoptopic molecules act as oncogens (Chao and Korsmeyer, 1998). Hence, cell-specific strategies need to be designed to achieve the therapeutic goal. However, even if this goal should be attained, an interference with neuronal cell death does not mean that the normal physiological function of a neuron is preserved. This already became apparent in the very first experiments reported by Garcia et al. (1992), in which the degeneration of sympathetic neurons deprived of NGF was prevented by the overexpression of the antiapoptotic molecule Bcl-2. Although the overexpression of Bcl-2 prevented the death of sympathetic neurons, they nevertheless did not show normal morphological characteristics as they did in the presence of NGF. In particular, the neuronal processes appeared very atrophic, and it must be assumed that these neurons did not regain their full physiological function. In this context, it would be illuminating if the inactivation of the NGF gene in transgenic mice were to be combined with the overexpression of Bcl-2 under the control of the dopamine β-hydroxylase promoter. This would make it possible to evaluate to what extent the normal function of the sympathetic neurons is preserved. That the prevention of neuronal cell death by the overexpression of antiapoptotic molecules does not correspond to a normal neuronal function is supported by the observation of Sagot et al. (1995). These authors found that the neuronal overexpression of Bcl-2 markedly reduces motoneuron cell body losses in the pmn mouse mutant (a model for ALS), but that this overexpression did not interfere with axonal degeneration, nor did it influence the survival time of this mouse mutant. Hence, the neuron-specific interference with apoptotic mechanisms may be complementary to the treatment with neurotrophic molecules (or the activation of the corresponding receptors) that preferentially regulate neuron-specific functions.

The importance of the site of administration of neurotrophic molecules has been discussed in detail above. In principle, an augmented supply could best be accomplished by enhancing the physiological regulatory mechanisms for the synthesis of neurotrophic factors (Thoenen et al., 1994; Skaper and Walsh, 1998). For BDNF and NGF, the mechanism of the regulation of their synthesis is relatively well understood (Lindholm et al., 1994; Shieh et al., 1998; Tao et al., 1998). However, since this regulation is mediated via glutamate (NMDA and non-NMDA), muscarinic, and also $GABA_A$ receptors (see Lindholm et al., 1994; Thoenen et al., 1994), which are also involved in a great variety of other physiological functions of the nervous system, any pharmacological regulation will most likely be hampered by disturbing side effects. Since all these receptors show a regionally differential expression, including many combinations of isoforms of the receptor subunits (Wisden et al., 1992; Seeburg, 1993; Hollmann and Heinemann, 1994; Green et al., 1998), there is the possibility to accomplish some selectivity. Again, a balance between the therapeutic goal and most likely unavoidable side effects will be a challenging task for the future. In addition to the enhancement of the synthesis of neurotrophic factors on the basis of the knowledge of their physiological regulatory mechanisms, a great variety of compounds have been identified that *in vitro*—and partially also *in vivo*—augment the production of neurotrophic factors, in particular NGF. Hefti (1997) has reviewed the present state of knowledge. It seems that the majority of these compounds evolved from classical screening procedures, in which the screening parameter was the evaluation of the changing levels of neurotrophic factors *in vitro*. It is to be expected that these compounds will be further investigated according to classical procedures for drug development.

To date, the local delivery of neurotrophic molecules by the transplantation of engineered cells has been based on strong (constitutive) promoters that resulted in stable, but unregulated gene expression (Rosenberg et al., 1988; Tuszynski et al., 1996). However, the unregulated, high expression of neurotrophic molecules may have serious consequences, since potentially occurring side effects cannot be controlled. Hence, for clinical applications, it will be necessary to regulate the expression of the transduced genes and to regulate individually the optimal expression of the neurotrophic molecule, avoiding side effects from too high an expression. In principle, such systems are already available, but they have not yet been developed to a level that would permit their immediate clinical application. The goal of these systems is a low baseline expression and then a regulation by a small molecule, preferentially acting by oral administration. These regulated expression systems are based on heterologous transcription factors and corresponding promoters, activated by molecules that ideally exhibit no physiological actions in mammalian systems. So far, these include derivatives of tetracycline (an antibiotic), ecdysone (a steroid of crucial importance in insect development), synthetic steroids, and also derivatives of immunosuppressants such as cyclosporin or FK-506. The derivatives used activate the heterologous transcription factors without interfering with the activity of calcineurin, a calcium-regulated phosphatase, and accordingly these derivatives do not exhibit immunosuppressive properties. The development of such expression systems is currently the focus of intense research (Freundlieb et al., 1997; Saez et al., 1997; Rossi and Blau, 1999; Baron et al., 1999; Ye et al., 1999).

Although a general activation of the receptors of neurotrophic molecules involves the same risks and limitations as the administration of their ligands, it is important to recognize that the activation of the same receptor with different ligands may lead to differences in the activation of the signal transduction pathway. I would like to exemplify this by the activation of the Trk-B receptor with BDNF as compared to NT-4/5. The differences between BDNF and NT-4/5 activation of the Trk-B receptor have become impressively apparent in recent experiments in which, in the Trk-B receptor, the Shc signal transduction pathway (important for neuronal differentiation and also, in part, survival) was inactivated by a point mutation, resulting in the substitution of a tyrosine residue by a phenylalanine (Minichiello et al., 1998). This substituted tyrosine residue in the Trk-B receptor is responsible for the binding and activation of the Shc adapter molecule. The consequences of this mutation of the Trk-B receptor for the activation by BDNF as compared to NT-4/5 were quite different, i.e., the isolated mutation at the Shc binding site almost exclusively affected the survival of NT-4/5 dependent neurons (Minichiello et al., 1998). This observation indicates that the activation of a receptor does not necessarily lead to the activation of a qualitatively and quantitatively identical signal transduction. This could, however, provide an opportunity to design new ligands, unrelated to the physiological ones—for instance by combinatorial phage display technology (Wilson and Finlay, 1998)—producing a great variety of peptides that can be screened for Trk receptor binding and activation. These newly developed peptides may lead to an activation spectrum that is different to that of the physiological ligands. Moreover, on the basis of these new identified peptides, non-peptide ligands may be derived (Tian et al., 1998) with better stability and also improved bioavailability. Similar procedures can be used for the selective modification of specific steps of the signal transduction pathways of neurotrophin receptors. The detailed elucidation of these pathways is advancing very rapidly (Green and Kaplan, 1995; Segal and Greenberg, 1996; Kaplan and Miller, 1997; Cattaneo and Pelicci, 1998; Qian et al., 1998), including not only the identification of the molecules involved, but also the characterization of the manner in which they interact with one another. This even extends to the precise identification of the molecular domains involved, and, in certain cases, their three-dimensional structure (Scheffzek et al., 1998). The more detailed the knowledge of these pathways, the better will be the possibilities to influence them in a specific manner.

For the local, non-invasive administration of neurotrophic factors, the development of T-cell lines appears to be very promising. However, in order to develop these towards clinical applicability, their endogenous inflammatory properties need to be reduced as much as possible. Moreover, a focussed targeting based on the recognition of cell-specific epitopes (both of the peripheral and central nervous system) could be of great importance, not only for the local delivery of neurotrophic factors, but also for immunosuppressive and anti-inflammatory molecules (see Kramer et al., 1995; Flügel et al., 1999). Such an approach, if successful, would be superior to the transfer of neurotrophic molecules across the blood-brain barrier (Friden et al., 1993: Wu and Pardridge, 1999), exploiting physiological transfer systems such as the transferin receptor. The use of such a transfer system results in an indiscriminate delivery of neurotrophic factors to the entire brain with the potential for all the side effects described above. Moreover, only a very small proportion of intravenously injected coupling products of transferin receptor antibodies reaches the brain (Friden et al., 1993; Wu and Pardridge, 1999) and, depending on the necessary concentrations and the nature of the neurotrophic molecule injected, substantial side effects may also be expected in the periphery (Hefti, 1997). My personal reservations concerning this method have not been eliminated by a recent report that a coupling product between derivatized, recombinant BDNF and an anti-transferin receptor antibody protected a particularly sensitive subpopulation of hippocampal neurons against systemic ischemia (Wu and Pardridge, 1999). Perhaps such an approach could be useful for the acute, relatively short-term administration of neurotrophic molecules, as for the treatment of strokes, where short-term, adverse side effects would be taken into account.

The very recent developments in the isolation and expansion of neuronal stem cells, even from adult brains (Brüstle et al., 1998; Flax et al., 1998; Gage 1998a,b; Björklund and Svendsen, 1999; Johansson et al., 1999), and also the possibility to expand them *in vitro* and to engineer them for the regulated expression of specific molecules, open up interesting and promising perspectives for future transplantation procedures. They could become important tools, not only for the treatment of Parkinson's disease, but also for a much broader spectrum of degenerative disorders. Very recently, a successful treatment of experimental Huntington's disease in monkeys by the transplantation of autologous, striatal stem cells has been reported (Palfi et al., 1998). The main challenge will be to develop cells that are fully integrated into the adult nervous system, to the extent that they assume the function of the degenerated neurons that they replace. So far, it has only been possible to accomplish a completely satisfactory integration with the transplantation of stem cells into the developing brains of embryos and early postnatal stages (Brüstle et al., 1998; Flax et al., 1998; Gage, 1998a,b). The recent report on the development of human embryonic stem cells (Shamblott et al., 1998; Thomson et al., 1998; reviewed by Solter and Gearhart, 1999) opens up an additional possibility to develop a great variety of tissues from these human cells, such as cardiac muscle, hematopoietic cells, but also neurons, as has been shown to be possible by the choice of appropriate culture conditions in mouse embryonic stem cells (Li et al., 1998). The use of human embryonic stem cells is an issue that is laden with ethical concerns, but to my mind these possibilities should be thoroughly and carefully evaluated (Solter and Gearhart, 1999) before premature, emotionally driven decisions are made. We must acknowledge that the transplantation issue now also includes parts of the brain, the organ that is the very seat of our personality and consciousness. This is a more delicate and sensitive matter than the mere replacement of a pump or filtration organ. However, we must remember that we also had to become acquainted with the idea of the possibility to transplant kidneys, and particularly hearts. I assume that at the turn of the century it would have been unthinkable that a French heart should beat in a German chest or vice versa, the heart being the seat of pride and patriotism.

ACKNOWLEDGMENTS

I would like to thank Martin Korte for his critical reading of the manuscript and constructive suggestions, Rainer Kramer for his helpful comments, and also Michael Ashdown for his linguistic revision.

REFERENCES

Agid, Y. (1998) Levodopa: is toxicity a myth? [Review] Neurology, 50: 858-863.ALS CNTF Treatment Study Group (1996) A double-blind placebo-controlled clinical trial of subcutaneous recombinant human ciliary neurotrophic factor (rHCNTF) in amyotrophic lateral sclerosis. Neurology, 46: 1244-1249.

Andrus, P.K., Fleck, T.J., Gurney, M.E., and Hall, E.D. (1998) Protein oxidative damage in a transgenic mouse model of familial amyotrophic lateral sclerosis. J. Neurochem., 71: 2041-2048.

Barde, Y.-A. (1989) Trophic factors and neuronal survival. Neuron, 2: 1525-1534.

Barkats, M., Bilang-Bleuel, A., Buc-Caron, M.H., Castel-Barthe, M.N., Corti, O., Finiels, F., Horellou, P., Revah, F., Sabate, O., and Mallet, J. (1998) Adenovirus in the brain: recent advances of gene therapy for neurodegenerative diseases. [Review] Prog. Neurobiol., 55: 333-341.

Baron, U., Schnappinger, D., Helbl, V., Gossen, M., Hillen, W., and Bujard, H. (1999) Generation of conditional mutants in higher eukaryotes by switching between the expression of two genes. Proc. Natl. Acad. Sci. USA, 96: 1013-1018.

Berninger, B., and Poo, M.-M. (1996) Fast actions of neurotrophic factors. Curr. Opin. Neurobiol., 6: 324-330.

Beyreuther, K., and Masters, C.L. (1997) Alzheimer's disease: the ins and outs of amyloid-β. Nature, 389: 677-678.

Björklund, A., and Svendsen, C. (1999) Breaking the blood-brain barrier. Nature, 397: 569-570.

Blau, H.M., and Rossi, F.M.V. (1999) Tet B or not tet B: advances in tetracycline-inducible gene expression. [Commentary] Proc. Natl. Acad. Sci. USA, 96: 797-799.

Bonhoeffer, T. (1996) Neurotrophins and activity-dependent development. Curr. Opin. Neurobiol., 6: 119-126.

Borchelt, D.R., Guarnieri, M., Wong, P.C., Lee, M.K., Slunt, H.S., Xu, Z.S., Sisodia, S.S., Price, D.L., and Cleveland, D.W. (1995) Superoxide dismutase 1 subunits with mutations linked to familial amyotrophic lateral sclerosis do not affect wild-type subunit function. J. Biol. Chem., 270: 3234-3238.

Broide, R.S., Grifman, M., Shapira, M., Ginzberg, D., and Soreq, H. (1997) Genetic manipulations of cholinergic communication reveal trans-acting control mechanisms over acetylcholine receptors. [Review] J. Recept. Signal Tr. R., 17: 279-291.

Brüstle, O., Choudhary, K., Karram, K., Hüttner, A., Murray, K., Dubois-Dalcq, M., and Mckay, R.D.G. (1998) Chimeric brains generated by intraventricular transplantation of fetal human brain cells into embryonic rats. Nat. Biotechnol., 16: 1040-1044.

Brüstle, O., Spiro, A.C., Karram, K., Choudhary, K., Okabe, S., and McKay, R.D.G. (1997) *In vitro*-generated neural precursors participate in mammalian brain development. Proc. Natl. Acad. Sci. USA., 94: 14809-14814.

Cabelli, R.J., Hohn, A., and Shatz, C.J. (1995) Inhibition of ocular dominance column formation by infusion of NT-4/5 or BDNF. Science, 267: 1662-1666.

Cabelli, R.J., Shelton, D.L., Segal, R.A., and Shatz, C.J. (1997) Blockade of endogenous ligands of trkB inhibits formation of ocular dominance columns. Neuron, 19: 63-76.

Campbell, K., Olsson, M., and Björklund, A. (1995) Regional incorporation and site-specific differentiation of striatal precursors transplanted to the embryonic forebrain ventricle. Neuron, 15: 1259-1273.

Cattaneo, E., and Pelicci, P.G. (1998) Emerging roles for SH2/PTB-containing Shc adaptor proteins in the developing mammalian brain. [Review] Trends Neurosci. 21: 476-481.
Cellerino, A., and Maffei, L. (1996) The action of neurotrophins in the development and plasticity of the visual cortex. Prog. Neurobiol., 49: 53-71.
Chao, D.T., and Korsmeyer, S.J. (1998) BCL-2 family: regulators of cell death. [Review] Annu. Rev. Immunol., 16: 395-419.
Chou, S.M. (1992) Pathology-light microscopy of amyotrophic lateral sclerosis. In: Handbook of amyotrophic lateral sclerosis (Smith, R.A., ed.), pp. 133-182. New York: Marcel Dekker, Inc.
Curtis, R., Scherer, S.S., Somogyi, R., Adryan, K.M., Ip, N.Y., Zhu, Y., Lindsay, R.M., and DiStefano, P.S. (1994) Retrograde axonal transport of LIF is increased by peripheral nerve injury: correlation with increased LIF expression in distal nerve. Neuron, 12: 191-204.
Davies, A.M. (1994) The role of neurotrophins in the developing nervous system. J. Neurobiol., 25: 1334-1348.
DeFelipe, J., and Jones, E.G., eds. (1991) Cajal's degeneration and regeneration of the nervous system. (Translated by Raoul M. May.) New York, Oxford: Oxford University Press, 768p.
Deng, H.X., Hentati, A., Tainer, J.A., Iqbal, Z., Cayabyab, A., Hung, W.Y., Getzoff, E.D., Hu, P., Herzfeldt, B., et al. (1993) Amyotrophic lateral sclerosis and structural defects in copper zinc superoxide dismutase. Science, 261: 1047-1051.
DiStefano, P.S., Friedman, B., Radziejewski, C., Alexander, C., Boland, P., Schick, C.M., Lindsay, R.M., and Wiegand, S.J. (1992) The neurotrophins BDNF, NT-3, and NGF display distinct patterns of retrograde axonal transport in peripheral and central neurons. Neuron, 8: 983-993.
Dittrich, F., Ochs, G., Grosse-Wilde, A., Berweiler, U., Yan, Q., Miller, J.A., Toyka, K.V., and Sendtner, M. (1996) Pharmacokinetics of intrathecally applied BDNF and effects on spinal motoneurons. Exp. Neurol., 141: 225-239.
Dittrich, F., Sendtner, M., and Thoenen, H. (1994) Ciliary neurotrophic factors: pharmocokinetics and acute phase response. Ann. Neurol., 35: 151-163.
Edlund, T., and Jessell, T.M. (1999) Progression from extrinsic to intrinsic signaling in cell fate specification: a view from the nervous system. Cell, 96: 211-224.
Emerich, D.F., Winn, S.R., Hantraye, P.M., Peschanski, M., Chen, E.Y., Chu, Y.P., Mcdermott, P., Baetge, E.E., and Kordower, J.H. (1997) Protective effect of encapsulated cells producing neurotrophic factor CNTF in a monkey model of Huntington's disease. Nature, 386: 395-399.
Eriksson, N.P., Lindsay, R.M., and Aldskogius, H. (1994) BDNF and NT-3 rescue sensory but not motoneurones following axotomy in the neonate. NeuroReport, 5: 1445-1448.
Eriksson, P.S., Perfilieva, E., Bjorkeriksson, T., Alborn, A.M., Nordborg, C., Peterson, D.A., and Gage, F.H. (1998) Neurogenesis in the adult human hippocampus. Nat. Med., 4: 1313-1317.
Farlow, M.R., and Evans, R.M. (1998) Pharmacologic treatment of cognition in Alzheimers dementia. [Review] Neurology, 51 (Suppl 1): 36-44.
Fisher, L.J., and Gage, F.H. (1995) Novel therapeutic directions for Parkinson's disease. [Review] Mol. Med. Today, 1: 181-187.
Fisher, W., Wictorin, K., Björkland, A., Williams, L.R., Varon, S., and Gage, F.H. (1987) Amelioration of cholinergic neuron atrophy and spatial memory impairment in aged rats by nerve growth factor. Nature, 329: 65-68.

Flax, J.D., Aurora, S., Yang, C.H., Simonin, C., Wills, A.M., Billinghurst, L.L., Jendoubi, M., Sidman, R.L., Wolfe, J.H., Kim, S.U., and Snyder, E.Y. (1998) Engraftable human neural stem cells respond to developmental cues, replace neurons, and express foreign genes. Nat. Biotechnol., 16: 1033-1039.

Flügel, A., Willem, M., Berkowicz, T., and Wekerle, H. (1999) Gene transfer into CD^{4+} T lymphocytes: green fluorescent protein-engineered, encephalitogenic T cells illuminate brain and autoimmune responses. Nat. Med., 5: 843-847.

Freundlieb, S., Baron, U., Bonin, A.L., Gossen, M., and Bujard, H. (1997) Use of tetracycline-controlled gene expression systems to study mammalian cell cycle. Method. Enzymol., 283: 159-173.

Friden, P.M., Walus, L.R., Watson, P., Doctrow, S.R., Kozarich, J.W., Backman, C., Bergman, H., Hoffer, B., Bloom, F., and Granholm, A.C. (1993) Blood-brain barrier penetration and in-vivo activity of an NGF conjugate. Science, 259: 373-377.

Gage, F.H. (1998a) Cell therapy. Nature, 392 (Suppl.): 18-24, 1998.

Gage, F.H. (1998b) Discussion point: stem cells of the central nervous system. Curr. Opin. Neurobiol., 8: 671-676.

Garcia, I., Martinou, I., Tsujimoto, Y., and Martinou, J.-C. (1992) Prevention of programmed cell death of sympathetic neurons by the *bcl-2* proto-oncogene. Science, 25: 302-304.

Giess, R., Goetz, R., Schrank, B., Ochs, G., Sendtner, M., and Toyka, K. (1998) Potential implications of a ciliary neurotrophic factor gene mutation in a German population of patients with motor neuron disease. Muscle Nerve, 21: 236-238.

Gravel, C., Gotz, R., Lorrain, A., and Sendtner, M. (1997) Adenoviral gene transfer of ciliary neurotrophic factor and brain-derived neurotrophic factor leads to long-term survival of axotomized motor neurons. Nature Medicine, 3: 765-770.

Green, T., Heinemann, S.F., and Gusella, J.F. (1998) Molecular neurobiology and genetics: investigation of neural function and dysfunction. [Review] Neuron, 20: 427-444.

Greene, L.A., and Kaplan, D.R. (1995) Early events in neurotrophin signaling via Trk and p75. Curr. Opin. Neurobiol., 5: 579-587.

Gusella, J.F., and Macdonald, M.E. (1998) Huntingtin: a single bait hooks many species. Curr. Opin. Neurobiol., 8: 425-430.

Haase, G., Kennel, P., Pettmann, B., Vigne, E., Akli, S., Revah, F., Schmalbruch, H., and Kahn A. (1997) Gene therapy of murine motor neuron disease using adenoviral vectors for neurotrophic factors. Nat. Med., 3: 429-436.

Hardy, J. (1997) Amyloid, the presenelins and Alzheimer's disease. Trends Neurosci., 20: 154-159.

Hefti, F. (1986) Nerve growth factor promotes survival of septal cholinergic neurons after fimbrial transections. J. Neurosci., 6: 2155-2162.

Hefti, F. (1997) Pharmacology of neurotrophic factors. [Review] Annu. Rev. Pharmacol., 37: 239-267.

Hefti, F., and Weiner, W.J. (1986) Nerve growth factor and Alzheimer's disease. Ann. Neurol., 20: 275-281.

Henderson, C.E., Phillips, H.S., Pollock, R.A., Davies, A.M., Lemeulle, C., Armanini, M., Simpson, L.C., Moffet, B., Vandlen, R.A., Koliatsos, V.E., and Rosenthal, A. (1994) GDNF: a potent survival factor for motoneurons present in peripheral nerve and muscle. Science, 266: 1062-1064.

Hirano T., Nakajima K., and Hibi M. (1997) Signaling mechanisms through gp130: a model of the cytokine system. [Review] Cytokine & Growth Factor Review, 8: 241-252.

Hollmann, M., and Heinemann, S. (1994) Cloned glutamate receptors. In: Annu. Rev. Neurosci., 17 (Cowan, W. M., ed.), ix+623p. Palo Alto: Annual Reviews Inc., pp. 31-108.
Hornykiewicz, O. (1966) Metabolism of brain dopamine in human parkinsonism: neurochemical and clinical aspects. In: Biochemistry and Pharmacology of the Basal Ganglia. (Costa, E., Côté, L.J., and Yahr, M.D., eds.) New York: Raven Press, pp. 171-185.
Hornykiewicz, O. (1988) Neurochemical pathology and the etiology of Parkinson's disease: basic facts and hypothetical possibilities. Mt. Sinai J. Med., 55: 11-20.
Hoyle, G.W., Mercer, E.H., Palmiter, R.D., and Brinster, R.L. (1993) Expression of NGF in sympathetic neurons leads to excessive axon outgrowth from ganglia but decreased terminal innervation within tissues. Neuron, 10: 1019-1034.
Imbimbo, B.P., Lucca, U., Lucchelli, F., Alberoni, M., and Thal, L.J. (1998) A 25-week placebo-controlled study of eptastigmine in patients with Alzheimer's disease. [In Process Citation] Alz. Dis. Assoc. Dis., 12: 313-322.
Jacobson, M.D., Weil, M., and Raff, M.C. (1997) Programmed cell death in animal development. Cell, 88: 347-354.
Johansson, C.B., Momma, S., Clarke, D.L., Risling, M., Lendahl, U., and Frisén J. (1999) Identification of a neural stem cell in the adult mammalian central nervous system. Cell, 96: 25-34.
Jonhagen, M.E., Nordberg, A., Amberla, K., Backman, L., Ebendal, T., Meyerson, B., Olson, L., Seiger, A., Shigeta, M., Theodorsson, E., Viitanen, M., Winblad, B., and Wahlund, L.O. (1998) Intracerebroventricular infusion of nerve growth factor in three patients with Alzheimers-disease. Dement. Geriat. Cogn., 9: 246-257.
Kaplan, D.R., and Miller, F.D. (1997) Signal transduction by the neurotrophin receptors. Curr. Opin. Cell Biol., 9: 213-221.
Katz, L.C., and Shatz, C.J. (1996) Synaptic activity and the construction of cortical circuits. Science, 274: 1133-1138.
Kempermann G., and Gage, F.H. (1998) Closer to neurogenesis in adult humans. Nat. Med., 4: 555-557.
Kim, T.-W. and Tanzi, R.E. (1998) Neuronal intranuclear inclusions in polyglutamine diseases: nuclear weapons or nuclear fallout? Neuron, 21: 657-659.
Kirschenbaum, B., Nedergaard, M., Preuss, A., Barami, K., Fraser, R.A.R., and Goldman, S. A. (1994) In vitro neuronal production and differentiation by precursor cells derived from the adult human forebrain. Cereb. Cortex, 4: 576-589.
Knusel, B., Gao, H., Okazaki, T., Yoshida, T., Mori, N., Hefti, F., and Kaplan, D.R. (1997) Ligand-induced down-regulation of trk messenger RNA, protein and tyrosine phosphorylation in rat cortical neurons. Neuroscience, 78: 851-862.
Kobayashi, S., Ogren, S.O., Ebendal, T., and Olson, L. (1997a) Dopamine receptor antagonists block nerve growth factor-induced hyperactivity. Eur. J. Pharmacol., 326: 1-5.
Kobayashi, S., Ogren, S.O., Ebendal, T., and Olson, L. (1997b) Intraventricular injection of NGF, but not BDNF, induces rapid motor activation that is inhibited by nicotinic receptor antagonists. Exp. Brain Res., 116: 315-325.
Kordower, J.J., et al. (1997) Neuropathological evidence of graft survival and striatal reinnervations after the transplantation of fetal mesencephalic tissue in a patient with Parkinson's disease. N. Engl. J. Med., 2717: 1118-1124.
Kramer, R., Zhang, Y.P., Gehrmann, J., Gold, R., Thoenen, H., and Wekerle, H. (1995) Gene transfer through the blood-nerve barrier: NGF-engineered neuritogenic T lymphocytes attenuate experimental autoimmune neuritis. Nat. Med., 1: 1162-1166.

Lewin, G.R., and Barde, Y.-A. (1996) Physiology of the neurotrophins. Annu. Rev. Neurosci., 19: 289-317.

Li, M., Pevny, L., Lovell-Badge, R., and Smith A. (1998) Generation of purified neural precursors from embryonic stem cells by lineage selection. Curr. Biol., 8: 971-974.

Lindholm, D., Castrèn, E., Berzaghi, M., Blöchl, A., and Thoenen, H. (1994) Activity-dependent and hormonal regulation of neurotrophin mRNA levels in the brain: implications on neuronal plasticity. J. Neurobiol., 25: 1362-1373.

Lindsay, R.M., Wiegand, S.J., Altar, C.A., and DiStefano, P.S. (1994) Neurotrophic factors: from molecule to man. Trends Neurosci., 17: 182-190.

Lindvall, O., Sawle, G., Widner, H., Rothwell, J.C., Björklund, A., Brooks, D., Brundin, P., Frackowiak, R., Marsden, C.D., Odin, P., et al. (1994) Evidence for long-term survival and function of dopaminergic grafts in progressive Parkinson's disease. Ann. Neurol., 35: 172-80.

Masters, C.L., and Beyreuther, K. (1998) Science, medicine, and the future: Alzheimers-disease. [Review] Brit. Med. J., 316: 446-448.

Meyer, M., Matsuoka, I., Wetmore, C., Olson, L., and Thoenen, H. (1992) Enhanced synthesis of brain-derived neurotrophic factor in the lesioned peripheral nerve: different mechanisms are responsible for the regulation of BDNF and NGF mRNA. J. Cell. Biol., 119: 45-54.

Meyer-Franke, A., Wilkinson, G.A., Kruttgen, A., Hu, M., Munro, E., Hanson, M.G., Reichardt, L.F., and Barres, B.A. (1998) Depolarization and cAMP elevation rapidly recruit TrkB to the plasma membrane of CNS neurons. Neuron, 21: 681-693.

Miller, R.G., Petajan, J.H., Bryan, W.W., Armon, C., Barohn, R.J., Goodpasture, J.C., Hoagland, R.J., Parry, G.J., Ross, M.A., Stromatt, S.C., Belsh, J.M., Buchman, A.S., Donofrio, P.D., Eisen, A.A., Gan, R.A., Gutmann, L., Horowitz, S.H., Jackson, W.S., Johnston, W.S., Kelly, J.J., Malta, E., Mandler, R.N., Massey, J.M., Mcguire, D., Newman, D.S., et al. (1996) A placebo-controlled trial of recombinant human ciliary neurotrophic (rhCNTF) factor in amyotrophic lateral sclerosis. Ann. Neurol., 39: 256-260.

Minichiello, L., Casagranda, F., Tatche, R.S., Stucky, C.L., Postigo, A., Lewin, G.R., Davies, A.M., and Klein R. (1998) Point mutation in trkB causes loss of NT4-dependent neurons without major effects on diverse BDNF responses. Neuron, 21: 335-345.

Ochs, G., Penn, R.D., Giess, R., Schrank, B., Sendtner, M., and Toyka, K.V. (1998) A trial of recombinant methionyl human Brain-Derived Neurotrophic Factor (BDNF) given by intrathecal (IT) infusion to patients with Amyotrophic Lateral Sclerosis (ALS). Neurology, 50: A246.

Olson, L., Backlund, E.-O., Ebendal, T., Freedman, R., Hamberger, B., Hansson, P., Hoffer, B., Lindblom, U., Meyerson, B., Strömberg, I., Sydow, O., and Seiger, A. (1991) Intraputaminal infusion of nerve growth factor to support adrenal medullary autografts in Parkinson's disease: one-year follow-up of first clinical trial. Arch. Neurol.-Chicago, 48: 373-381.

Olson, L., Nordberg, A., von Holst, H., Bäckman, L., Ebendal, T., Alafuzoff, I., Amberla, K., Hartvig, P., Herlitz, A., Lilja, A., Lundqvist, H., Långström, B., Meyerson, B., Persson, A., Viitanen, M., Winblad, B., and Seiger, A. (1992) Nerve growth factor affects ^{11}C-nicotine binding, blood flow, EEG, and verbal episodic memory in an Alzheimer patient (Case Report). J. Neural Transm.-Park., 4: 79-95.

Orrell, R.W., King, A.W., Lane, R.J., and de Belleroche, J.S. (1995) Investigation of a null mutation of the CNTF gene in familial amyotrophic lateral sclerosis. J. Neurol. Sci., 132: 126-128.

Palfi, S., Condé, F., Riche, D., Brouillet, E., Dautry, C., Mittoux, V., Chibois, A., Peschanski, M., and Hantraye, P. (1998) Fetal striatal allografts reverse cognitive deficits in a primate model of Huntington disease. Nat. Med., 4: 963-966.

Pasinelli, P., Borchelt, D.R., Houseweart, M.K., Cleveland, D.W., and Brown, R.H. (1998) Caspase-1 is activated in neural cells and tissue with amyotrophic lateral sclerosis-associated mutations in copper-zinc superoxide dismutase. Proc. Natl. Acad. Sci. USA, 95: 15763-15768.

Phillips, H.S., Hains, J.M., Armanini, M., Laramee, G.R., Johnson, S.A., and Winslow, J.W. (1991) BDNF mRNA is decreased in hippocampus of individuals with Alzheimer's disease. Neuron, 7: 695-702.

Qian, X., Riccio, A., Zhang ,Y., and Ginty, D.D. (1998) Identification and characterization of novel substrates of TrK receptors in developing neurons. Neuron, 21: 1017-1029.

Ringstedt, T. (1998) Neurotrophins during development: overexpression in neural stem cells. Thesis, Division of Molecular Neurobiology, Department of Neuroscience, Karolinska Institute, Stockholm.

Rosen, D.R., Siddique, T., Patterson, D., Figlewicz, D.A., Sapp, P., Hentati, A., Donaldson D., Goto, J., Oregan J .P., et al. (1993) Mutations in copper-zinc superoxide dismutase gene are associated with familial amyotrophic lateral sclerosis. Nature, 362: 59-62.

Rosenberg, M.B., Friedmann, T., Robertson, R.C., Tuszynski, M., Wolff, J.A., Breakefield, X.O., and Gage, F.H. (1988) Grafting genetically modified cells to the damaged brain: restorative effects of NGF expression. Science, 242: 1575-1578.

Rossi, F.M.V., and Blau, H.M. (1998) Recent advances in inducible gene expression systems. [Review] Curr. Opin. Biotechnol., 9: 451-456.

Rowland, L.P. (1991) Amyotrophic lateral sclerosis and other motor neuron diseases. Adv. Neurol., vol. 56, Raven Press, New York.

Saez, E., No, D., West, A., and Evans, R.M. (1997) Inducible gene expression in mammalian cells and transgenic mice. [Review] Curr. Opin. Biotech., 8: 608-616.

Sagot, Y., Dubois-Dauphin, M., Tan, S.A., De Bilbao, F., Aebischer, P., Martinou, J.C., and Kato, A.C. (1995) Bcl-2 overexpression prevents motoneuron cell body loss but not axonal degeneration in a mouse model of a neurodegenerative disease. J. Neurosci., 15: 7727-7733.

Sagot, Y., Rossé, T., Vejsada, R., Perrelet, D., and Kato, A.C. (1998) Differential effects of neurotrophic factors on motoneuron retrograde labeling in a murine model of motoneuron disease. J. Neurosci., 18: 1132-1141.

Sagot, Y., Tan, S.A., Hammang, J.P., Aebischer, P., and Kato, A.C. (1996) GDNF slows loss of motoneurons but not axonal degeneration or premature death of pmn/pmn mice. J. Neurosci., 16: 335-341.

Saudou, F., Finkbeiner, S., Devys, D., and Greenberg, M.E. (1998) Huntingtin acts in the nucleus to induce apoptosis but death does not correlate with the formation of intranuclear inclusions. Cell, 95: 55-66.

Scheffzek, K., Ahmadian, M.R., and Wittinghofer A. (1998) GTPase-activating proteins: helping hands to complement an active site. [Review] Trends Biochem. Sci., 23: 257-262.

Seeburg, P.H. (1993) The TINS/TiPS lecture. The molecular biology of mammalian glutamate receptors. Trends Neurosci., 16: 359-365.

Segal, R.A., and Greenberg, M.E. (1996) Intracellular signaling pathways activated by neurotrophic factors. [Review] Annu. Rev. Neurosci., 19: 463-489.

Selkoe, D.J. (1996) Cell biology of the beta-amyloid precursor protein and the genetics of Alzheimers-disease. Cold Spring Harb. Sym., 61: 587-596.

Sendtner, M. (1997) Gene therapy for motor neuron disease. Nat. Med., 3: 380-381.

Sendtner, M., Dittrich, F., Hughes, R.A., and Thoenen, H. (1994) Actions of CNTF and neurotrophins on degenerating motoneurons: preclinical studies and clinical implications. J. Neurol. Sci., 124 (Suppl.): 77-83.

Sendtner, M., Götz, R., Holtmann, B., Escary, J.L., Masu, Y., Carroll, P., Wolf, E., Brem, G., Brulet, P., and Thoenen, H. (1996) Cryptic physiological trophic support of motoneurons by LIF revealed by double gene targeting of CNTF and LIF. Curr. Biol., 6: 686-694.

Shamblott, M.J., Axelman, J., Wang, S.P., Bugg, E.M., Littlefield, J.W., Donovan, P.J., Blumenthal, P.D., Huggins, G.R., and Gearhart, J.D. (1998) Derivation of pluripotent stem cells from cultured human primordial germ cells. Proc. Natl. Acad. Sci. USA, 95: 13726-13731.

Shieh, P.B., Hu, S.C., Bobb, K., Timmusk, T., and Ghosh A. (1998) Identification of a signaling pathway involved in calcium regulation of BDNF expression. Neuron, 20: 727-740.

Skaper, S.D., and Walsh, F.S. (1998) Neurotrophic molecules: strategies for designing effective therapeutic molecules in neurodegeneration. [Review] Mol. Cell. Neurosci., 12: 179-193.

Snider, W.D. (1994) Functions of the neurotrophins during nervous system development: what the knockouts are teaching us. Cell, 77: 627-638.

Solter, D., and Gearhart, J. (1999) Putting stem cells to work. Science, 283: 1468-1470.

Spillantini, M.G., and Goedert, M. (1998) Tau protein pathology in neurogenerative diseases. [Review] Trends Neurosci., 21: 428-433.

Stahl, N., and Yancopoulos, G.D. (1994) The tripartite CNTF receptor complex: activation and signaling involves components shared with other cytokines. [Review] J. Neurobiol., 25: 1454-1466.

Stoeckel K., Guroff G., Schwab M., and Thoenen H. (1976) The significance of retrograde axonal transport for the accumulation of systemically administered nerve growth factor (NGF) in the rat superior cervical ganglion. Brain Res., 109: 271-284.

Susin, S.A., Zamzami, N., Castedo, M., Daugas, E., Wang, H.-G., Geley, S., Fassy, F., Reed, J.C., and Kroemer G. (1997) The central executioner of apoptosis: multiple connections between protease activation and mitochondria in Fas/AOP-1/CD95- and ceramide-induced apoptosis. J. Exp. Med., 186: 25-37.

Takahashi, R., Yokoji, H., Misawa, H., Hayashi, M., Hu, J., and Deguchi, T.A. (1994) A null mutation in the human CNTF gene is not causally related to neurological diseases. Nat. Genet., 7: 79-84.

Takayama, H., Ray, J., Raymon, H.K., Baird, A., Hogg, J., Fisher, L.J., and Gage, F.H. (1995) Basic fibroblast growth factor increases dopaminergic graft survival and function in a rat model of Parkinson's disease. Nat. Med., 1: 53-58.

Tao, X., Finkbeiner, S., Arnold, D.B., Shaywitz, A.J., and Greenberg, M.E. (1998) Ca^{2+} influx regulates BDNF transcription by a CREB family transcription factor-dependent mechanism. Neuron, 20: 709-726.

Thoenen, H. (1995) Neurotrophins and neuronal plasticity. [Review] Science, 270: 593-598.

Thoenen, H., Castrén, E., Berzaghi, M., Blöchl, A., and Lindholm, D. (1994) Neurotrophic factors: possibilities and limitations in the treatment of neurodegenerative disorders. In: International Academy for Biomedical and Drug Research, vol. 7. Recent advances in the treatment of neurodegenerative disorders and cognitive dysfunction; Collegium Internationale Neuro-Psychopharmacologicum President's Workshop, Capri, Italy, May 1-3, 1993. (Racagni, G., N. Brunello, and Langer, S.Z., eds.) vii+264p. Basle, New York: S. Karger AG.

Thoenen, H., Hughes, R.A., and Sendtner, M. (1993) Trophic support of motoneurons: physiological, pathophysiological, and therapeutic implications. Exp. Neurol., 124: 47-55.

Thomson, J.A., Itskovitzeldor, J., Shapiro, S.S., Waknitz, M.A., Swiergiel, J. J., Marshall, V. S., and Jones, J.M. (1998) Embryonic stem cell lines derived from human blastocysts. Science, 282: 1145-1147.

Tian, S.-S., Lamb, P., King, A.G., Miller, S.G., Kessler, L., Luengo, J.I., Averill, L., Johnson, R.K., Gleason, J.G., Pelus, L.M., Dillon, S.B., and Rosen J. (1998) A small, nonpeptidyl mimic of granulocyte-colony-stimulating factor. Science, 281: 257-259.

Tuszynski, M.H., and Gage, F.H. (1996) Somatic gene therapy for nervous system disease. In: Growth factors as drugs for neurological and sensory disorders. Ciba F. Symp., 196: 85-87.

Tuszynski, M.H., Roberts, J., Senut, M.C., U, H.S., and Gage, F.H. (1996) Gene therapy in the adult primate brain: Intraparenchymal grafts of cells genetically modified to produce nerve growth factor prevent cholinergic neuronal degeneration. Gene Ther., 3: 305-314.

Van Leewen, F.W., Burbach, J.P.H., and Hol, E.M. (1998) Mutations in RNA: a first example of molecular misreading in Alzheimer's Disease. Trends Neurosci., 21: 331-335.

Vejsada, R., Sagot, Y., and Kato, A.C. (1994) BDNF-mediated rescue of axotomized motor neurones decreases with increasing dose. Neuroreport, 5: 1889-1892.

Vejsada, R., Sagot, Y., and Kato, A.C. (1995) Quantitative comparison of the transient rescue effects of neurotrophic factors on axotomized motoneurons in vivo. Eur. J. Neurosci., 7: 108-115.

Verrall, M. (1994) Lay-offs follow suspension of clinical trials of protein. Nature, 370: 6.

Wakayama, T., Perry, A.C.F., Zuccotti, M., Johnson, K.R., and Yanagimachi, R. (1998) Full-term development of mice from enucleated oocytes injected with cumulus cell nuclei. Nature, 394: 369-374.

Wenning, G.K., Odin, P., Morrish, P., Rehncrona, S., Widner, H., Brundin, P., Rothwell, J.C., Brown, R., Gustavii, B., Hagell, P., Jahanshahi, M., Sawle, G., Björklund, A., Brooks, D.J., Marsden, C.D., Quinn, N.P., and Lindvall, O. (1997) Short- and long-term survival and function of unilateral intrastriatal dopaminergic grafts in Parkinson's disease. Ann. Neurol., 42: 95-107.

Wilson D.R., and Finlay, B.B. (1998) Phage display: applications, innovations, and issues in phage and host biology. [Review] Can. J. Microbiol., 44: 313-329.

Winkler, J., Ramirez, G.A., Kuhn, H.G., Peterson, D.A., Day-Lollini, P.A., Stewart, G.R., Tuszynski, M.H., Gage, F.H., and Thal, L.J. (1997) Reversible Schwann cell hyperplasia and sprouting of sensory and sympathetic neurites after intraventricular administration of Nerve Growth Factor. Ann. Neurol., 41: 82-93.

Winkler, J., Thal, L.J., Gage, F.H., and Fisher, L.J. (1998) Cholinergic strategies for Alzheimer's disease. [Review] J. Mol. Med., 76: 555-567.

Wisden, W., Laurie, D.J., Monyer, H., and Seeburg, P.H. (1992) The distribution of 13 $GABA_A$ receptor subunit mRNAs in the rat brain. I. Telencephalon, diencephalon, mesencephalon. J. Neurosci., 12: 1040-1062.

Wong, V.V., Glass, D.J., Arriaga, R., Yancopoulos, G.D., Lindsay, R.M., and Conn, G. (1997) Hepatocyte growth factor promotes motor neuron survival and synergizes with ciliary neurotrophic factor. J. Biol. Chem., 272: 5187-5191.

Wu, D., and Pardridge, W.M. (1999) Neuroprotection with noninvasive neurotrophin delivery to the brain. Proc. Natl. Acad. Sci. USA, 96: 254-259.

Ye, S.Z., Cole-Strauss, A., Frank, B., and Kmiec, E.B. (1998) Targeted gene correction: a new strategy for molecular medicine. [Review] Mol. Med. Today, 4: 431-437.

Ye, X., Rivera, V.M., Zoltick, P., Cerasoli Jr., F., Schnell, M.A., Guang-ping, G., Hughes, J.V., Gilman, M., and Wilson, J.M. (1999) Regulated delivery of therapeutic proteins after in vivo somatic cell gene transfer. Science, 283: 88-91.

Index

about the editors...

NICHOLAS A. INGOGLIA is Professor of Pharmacology, Physiology, and Neuroscience, New Jersey Medical School–UMDNJ, Newark. The author or coauthor of numerous scientific articles in the areas of axon regeneration and cellular neurobiology, he is a member of the Society for Neuroscience, Society for Neurochemistry, and New York Academy of Sciences. He received the Ph.D. degree (1969) from New York University, New York.

MARION MURRAY is Professor of Neurobiology and Anatomy, MCP Hahnemann University, Philadelphia. The author or coauthor of numerous scientific articles dealing with regeneration, neuroprotection, and recovery and function, she is an editorial board member of the *Journal of Comparative Neurology*, *Experimental Neurology*, and *Neurorehabilitation and Neural Repair*, and a member of the Scientific Advisory Board of the Paralyzed Veterans of America. She received the Ph.D. degree (1964) in physiology from the University of Wisconsin, Madison.